Khonsari's

CARDIAC SURGERY

Safeguards and Pitfalls in Operative Technique

Khonsari's

CARDIAC SURGERY

Safeguards and Pitfalls in Operative Technique

FIFTH EDITION

Abbas Ardehali, MD
Professor of Surgery and Medicine
Division of Cardiothoracic Surgery
William E. Connor Endowed Chair in Cardiothoracic Transplantation
Director, UCLA Heart, Lung, and Heart-Lung Transplant Programs
David Geffen School of Medicine at UCLA
Los Angeles, California

Jonathan M. Chen, MD
Professor of Surgery
Sam and Althea Stroum Endowed Chair in Pediatric Cardiovascular Surgery
Chief of Congenital Cardiac Surgery
Seattle Children's Hospital
University of Washington School of Medicine
Seattle, Washington

ILLUSTRATORS

Timothy C. Hengst, CMI, FAMI
BodyScientific International, LLC

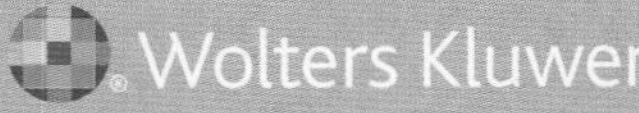

Philadelphia • Baltimore • New York • London
Buenos Aires • Hong Kong • Sydney • Tokyo

Acquisitions Editor: Keith Donnellan
Product Development Editor: Brendan Huffman
Production Project Manager: Priscilla Crater
Design Coordinator: Elaine Kasmer
Senior Manufacturing Coordinator: Beth Welsh
Marketing Manager: Dan Dressler
Prepress Vendor: S4Carlisle Publishing Services

Fifth Edition

9 8 7 6 5 4 3 2 1

Printed in China

Library of Congress Cataloging-in-Publication Data

Names: Ardehali, Abbas, author. | Chen, Jonathan M., author. | Preceded by (work): Khonsari, Siavosh. Cardiac surgery.
Title: Khonsari's cardiac surgery: safeguards and pitfalls in operative technique / Abbas Ardehali, Jonathan Chen.
Other titles: Cardiac surgery
Description: Fifth edition. | Philadelphia: Wolters Kluwer Heath, [2017] | Includes index. | Preceded by: Cardiac surgery / Siavosh Khonsari, Colleen Flint Sintek, in collaboration with Abbas Ardehali. 4th ed. c2008.
Identifiers: LCCN 2016025071 | ISBN 9781451183689
Subjects: | MESH: Cardiac Surgical Procedures—methods | Cardiovascular Diseases—surgery
Classification: LCC RD598 | NLM WG 169 | DDC 617.4/12—dc23 LC record available at https://lccn.loc.gov/2016025071

LWW.com

RRS1607

To our families:
Mitra, Leila, and Sara Ardehali
and
Abbie, Maddie, and Atlas Chen

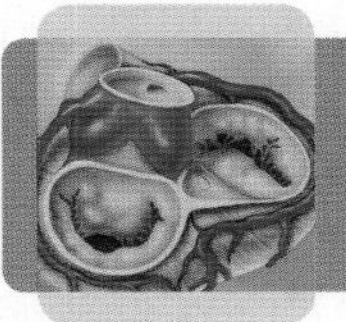

Foreword

The concept of *Cardiac Surgery: Safeguards and Pitfalls in Cardiac Surgery* came to me over 35 years ago. I wanted to provide a tool to help surgical residents master the techniques of cardiac surgery while avoiding the pitfalls that often result in suboptimal or even fatal outcomes. After five years of preparation, the work was completed and published in late 1987. Many prominent cardiac surgeons from Europe and the United States reviewed each chapter and made useful suggestions, thus benefitting the work with their vast experiences.

The book would not have been completed without the support and invaluable encouragement of the late Professor Gerry Brom of Leiden. The superb "telling" illustrations by Joanie Livermore and Timothy Hengst have been the hallmark of the work. The success of the book is reflected in the present (fifth) edition and the fact that it has been translated into Portuguese, Japanese, and Chinese. It has been gratifying to visit operating rooms in many countries and see a copy of the book or photocopies of its various chapters there. My partner and colleague of close to 30 years, Dr. Colleen Sintek, was my coauthor on the second, third, and fourth editions, and I am very much indebted to her and grateful for her support.

My good fortune does not end here. For this fifth edition, I have been blessed to have Dr. Abbas Ardehali, professor of surgery, David Geffen School of Medicine at University of California, Los Angeles, an esteemed friend and colleague, accept the baton of responsibility to ensure the continued success of the book. Dr. Jonathan Chen, professor of surgery and chief of pediatric cardiovascular surgery at University of Washington, Seattle, has been gracious to edit and update the Congenital section. I am very impressed with their contributions and am grateful for their efforts in bringing the fifth edition of *Cardiac Surgery: Safeguards and Pitfalls in Cardiac Surgery* to fruition.

Siavosh Khonsari, MB, FRCS, FACS, FACC
Clinical Professor of Surgery
University of California
Los Angeles, California

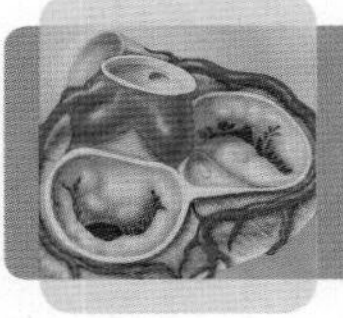

Preface

Khonsari's Cardiac Surgery: Safeguards and Pitfalls in Operative Technique is a unique book in the field of cardiac surgery. It details the important technical aspects of cardiac surgery in a concise, readable, and illustrative format. It also highlights technical misadventures and offers preventive and corrective measures. It serves as a great resource for the novice and/or trainee as well as the seasoned surgeon.

The popularity of this book since the first edition has been due to Dr. Khonsari's unmatched surgical intuition, wisdom, judgment, and attention to details, as is evident throughout this book. Illustrative and detailed figures have been and continue to be an important feature that emphasizes salient points. Dr. Sintek's collaboration on the previous two editions has only enhanced these qualities of this popular book. We, the present editors, have tried very hard to maintain the character of this book: emphasizing technical aspects of cardiac surgery, highlighting pitfalls, striving for brevity, and using clear illustrations to convey the message to the readers.

Organizationally, the first two sections remain dedicated to adult cardiac surgery, while the third section covers pediatric cardiac surgery. All chapters have been updated, new illustrations have been added, and some of the illustrations have been colorized for greater clarity. Additionally, new topics have been added to reflect the advances in the field: endovascular procedures, transcatheter aortic valve replacement, new approaches to the Norwood reconstruction, repair of Ebstein anomaly, and alternative anatomic repairs of congenitally corrected transposition.

The format of this book follows the previous editions: the technical pitfalls are denoted by a hazard sign ⊘. The mechanism of technical errors and the techniques to prevent and correct these errors are emphasized. Important points are highlighted by special Nota Bene NB notations.

Khonsari's Cardiac Surgery: Safeguards and Pitfalls in Operative Technique has long been considered a great reference text in technical aspects of cardiac surgery. We have worked hard to maintain the core strengths of this book: a concise, illustrative, and focused description of techniques in cardiac surgery. We believe that with the many improvements implemented in this fifth edition, it will continue to be a valuable resource for cardiac surgery trainees and senior surgeons alike.

Abbas Ardehali, MD
Los Angeles, California
June 2016

Jonathan Chen, MD
Seattle, Washington
June 2016

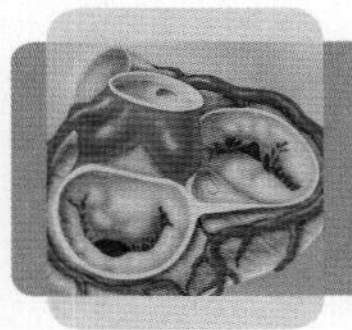

Acknowledgments

First and foremost, Dr. Chen and I would like to thank Dr. Khonsari and Dr. Sintek for their many contributions to the field of cardiac surgery and the legacy they have left with this book. I am privileged to have been trained by them, and I remain grateful for the imparted wisdom, support, and importantly their friendship. I would also like to thank Dr. Peyman Benharash of the Division of Cardiac Surgery at UCLA for his contributions to endovascular procedure topics and many helpful suggestions in other chapters.

Finally, we would like to thank the editorial staff at Wolters Kluwer, particularly Brendan Huffman and Keith Donnellan, for their assistance and dedication. We also would like to thank Lik Kwong and Carolina Hrejsa from BodyScientific for their tireless work to create and update the artwork in this new edition. We believe that the fifth edition carries on the tradition of its predecessors while delivering the most current and concise reference book on techniques and pitfalls in the field of cardiac surgery.

Abbas Ardehali

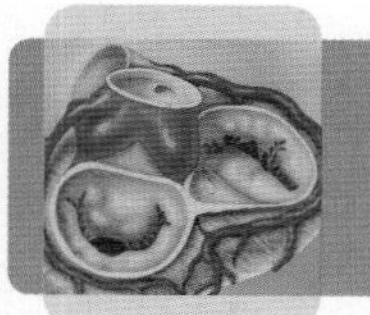

Contents

SECTION

I

General Considerations

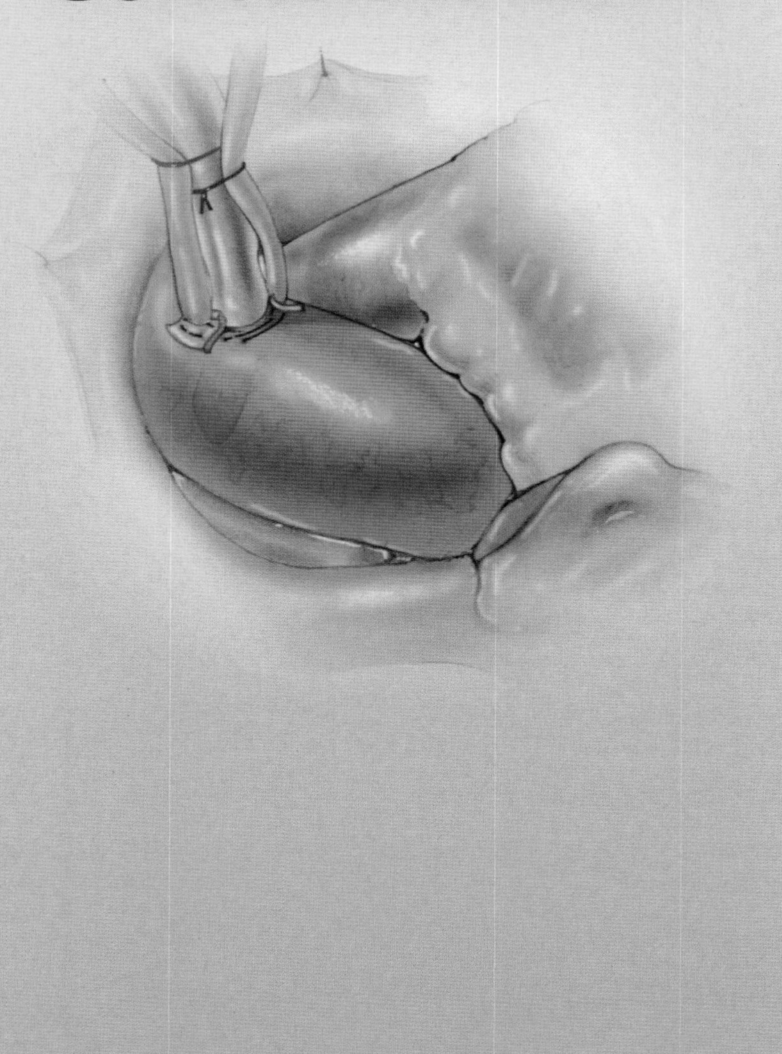

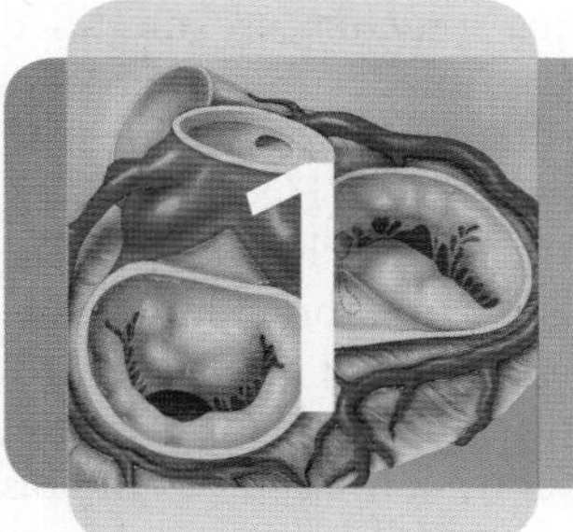

1 Surgical Approaches to the Heart and Great Vessels

PRIMARY MEDIAN STERNOTOMY

Median sternotomy remains the most widely used incision in cardiac surgery because it provides excellent exposure for most surgeries involving the heart and great vessels.

Technique

The skin incision normally extends from just below the suprasternal notch to the tip of the xiphoid process. A saw with a vertical blade is most commonly used to divide the sternum. In young infants, the sternum is divided with heavy scissors. An oscillating saw is used for repeat sternotomies and some primary surgeries through limited skin incisions. Its use requires that the surgeon develop a "feel" for when the blade has penetrated the posterior table of the sternum (see Repeat Sternotomy section).

⊘ Bleeding

A small vein is usually evident running transversely in the suprasternal notch. At times, however, it may be large and engorged, particularly in patients with elevated right heart pressure. Excessive bleeding may occur if this vein is inadvertently injured. It is important to be aware of its presence and to coagulate it (if tiny) or to occlude it with a metal clip. If the vein has been cut and its ends have retracted, thereby making hemostasis difficult, control of bleeding can be gained by packing the suprasternal notch area and proceeding with the sternotomy. After the two sides of the sternum have been spread apart, the sites of bleeding can be easily identified and controlled. ⊘

⊘ Sternal Infection

Not only is dissection of the suprasternal notch unnecessary, but it can also open up tissue planes in the neck. Tracheostomy is now rarely necessary but always remains a possibility. Whenever tracheostomy is performed, a separate incision is kept as high in the neck as possible so that a superficial tracheostomy wound infection does not spread into the suprasternal notch and eventually into the mediastinum, leading to wound complications and mediastinitis. ⊘

⊘ Entry into the Peritoneal Cavity

During the division of the linea alba or the lower part of the pericardium, the peritoneal cavity may be entered. The opening should be closed immediately to prevent any spillage of blood or cold saline used for topical cooling into the peritoneal cavity, which may promote postoperative ileus. ⊘

⊘ Asymmetric Division of the Sternum

The sternotomy should be in the midline of the sternum. By dipping the thumb and index finger into the incision and spreading them against the lateral margins of the sternum into the intercostal spaces, the proper site for sternal splitting can be located and marked by an electrocautery on the periosteum. Unequal division may leave one side of the sternum too narrow and allow the closure wires to cut through the narrower segments of the bone, leading to an increased incidence of sternal dehiscence. Similarly, the costochondral junction may be damaged (Fig. 1.1). ⊘

⊘ Pneumothorax and Hemothorax

The anesthesiologist is always asked to deflate the lungs while the surgeon is using the sternal saw so that the pleural cavities can be kept intact. This is particularly important in patients with chronic obstructive pulmonary disease and hyperinflated lungs. Occasionally, however, the pleural cavities are opened by the sternal saw or during dissection of the thymus and pericardium. If the opening is small and no fluid has entered the pleural cavity, at the close of the procedure, the tip of the mediastinal chest tube may be introduced for 2 to 3 cm into the pleural defect. The pleura may be opened fully, particularly in patients undergoing harvesting of internal thoracic arteries. In these cases, a separate chest tube is inserted subcostally over the lateral aspect of the diaphragm for drainage of fluid and blood and evacuation of air. ⊘

⊘ Use of Bone Wax

Excessive use of bone wax to control bleeding from the sternal marrow should be avoided. It can be associated with increased rates of wound infection, impaired wound

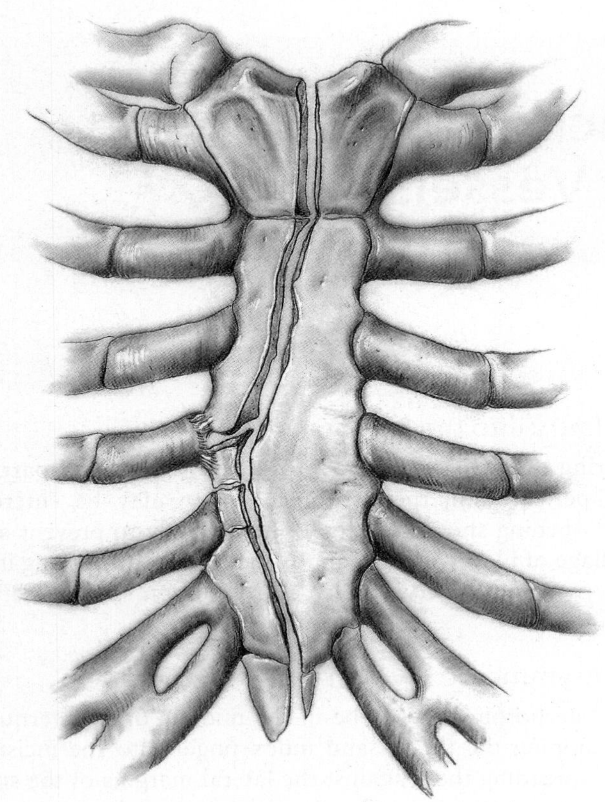

⊘ FIG. 1.1 Fracture resulting from improper division of the sternum.

healing, and, most serious of all, wax embolization to the lungs. However, the use of small amounts of bone wax is an effective tool to control bleeding from sternal edges. We have found that vancomycin paste (mixing of vancomycin powder with 2.5 ml of saline) is an effective agent for sternal bone marrow oozing, with possible antimicrobial properties. ⊘

⊘ Brachial Plexus Injury

Brachial plexus injury has been associated with median sternotomy. Stretching of the plexus by hyperabduction of the arm and compression of the nerve trunks between the clavicle and first rib during sternal retraction has been implicated as a cause of injury. Introduction of a Swan–Ganz catheter through the internal jugular vein can injure the brachial plexus, either directly by the introducer itself or indirectly by the formation of a hematoma in the vicinity. The most serious cause of brachial plexus injury is fracture of the first rib (Fig. 1.2). The sternal retractor should be placed with its crossbar superiorly so that the blades spread apart the lower third of the sternal edges. It is then opened gradually in a stepwise manner (one to two turns at a time) to prevent fractures of the first rib or sternum (Fig. 1.3A). If for some reason the crossbar of the retractor is to be placed inferiorly, it is important for the blades to be in the lower part of the incision. Many surgeons use modified sternal retractors with two or three blades on either side, placing the crossbar inferiorly. These retractors are opened just enough to provide adequate exposure (Fig 1.3B). ⊘

Retractors (e.g., Favaloro) used in harvesting the internal thoracic artery can also cause brachial plexus injury. Therefore, sudden excessive upward pull on the retractor should be avoided. The surgeon should ensure good exposure by manipulating the operating room table and his or her headlight to minimize traction of the upper sternum. Moreover, when the proximal internal thoracic artery is freed, the degree of upper sternal retraction is reduced. These simple measures can often eliminate or reduce the incidence of brachial plexus injury.

⊘ Innominate Vein Injury

The innominate vein may be injured during dissection and division or resection of the thymus or its remnant, particularly when scarring is present from a previous surgery. The scar tissue on each side of the injured vein is dissected free. Brisk bleeding can then be controlled by simple suturing. In rare instances of severe damage to the vein, it is divided and its right end is suture ligated. The other end of the vein is left open for drainage of venous return from left internal jugular tributaries until the patient is ready to come off cardiopulmonary bypass when it is similarly suture ligated. ⊘

The innominate vein is a useful channel for an additional intravenous line, which can be used to monitor central venous pressure, particularly in infants and patients with poor peripheral veins. The catheter is introduced percutaneously into the center of a 7-0 Prolene purse-string suture buttressed with fine pericardial pledgets on the innominate vein. The purse-string suture must be tied snugly to prevent any bleeding after removal of the venous line. Sometimes, a large thymic vein can be used for the same purpose.

REPEAT STERNOTOMY

An increasing number of patients require surgical intervention a second, third, or even fourth and fifth time for replacement of prosthetic valves, definitive correction or revision of congenital heart defects, or repeat myocardial revascularization. Because it is anticipated that this trend will continue, all cardiac surgeons must acquire expertise in preoperative procedures. When making the skin incision, it is not always necessary to excise the previous scar unless it is gross and thick. The subcutaneous tissue is incised in the customary manner, and using electrocoagulation, the sternum is marked along the midline.

Technique

Previous wires or heavy nonabsorbable sutures are divided anteriorly but are not removed. They provide some resistance posteriorly to the oscillating saw, which helps

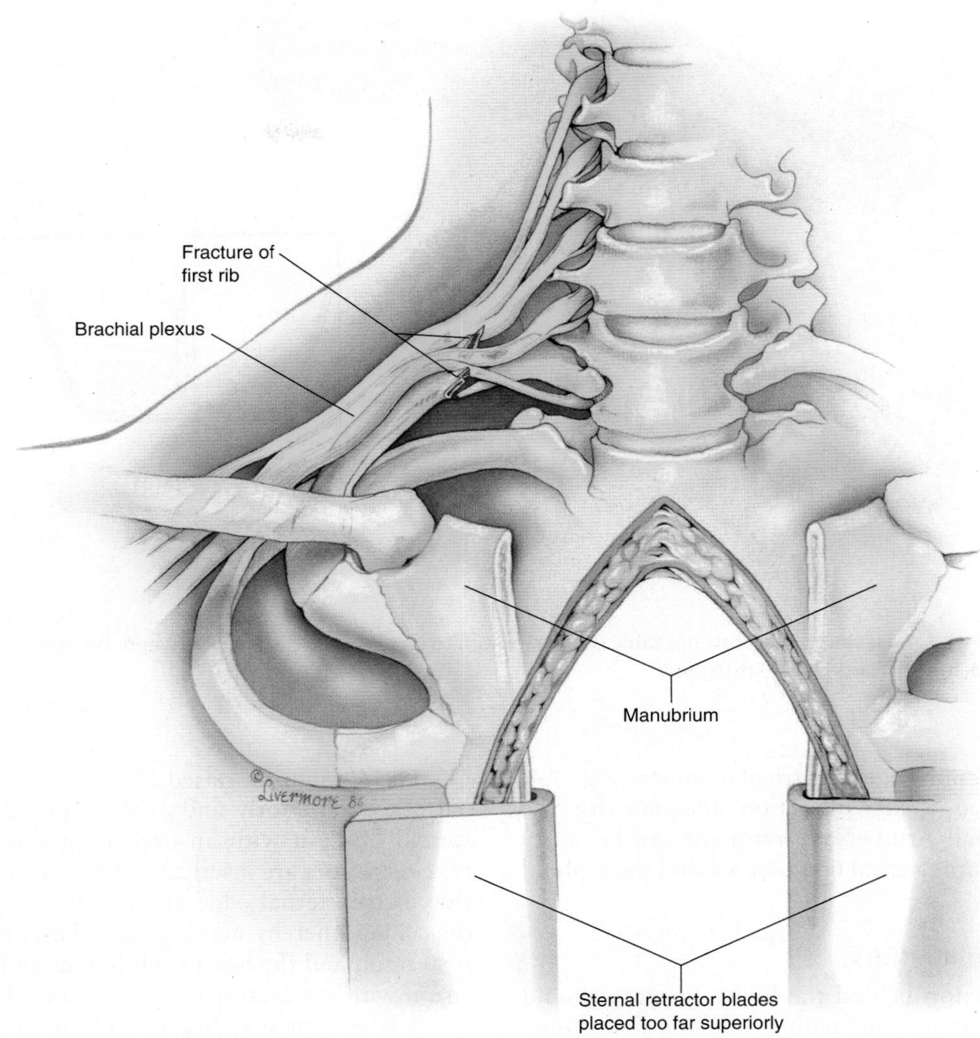

⊘ **FIG. 1.2** Mechanism of a brachial plexus injury.

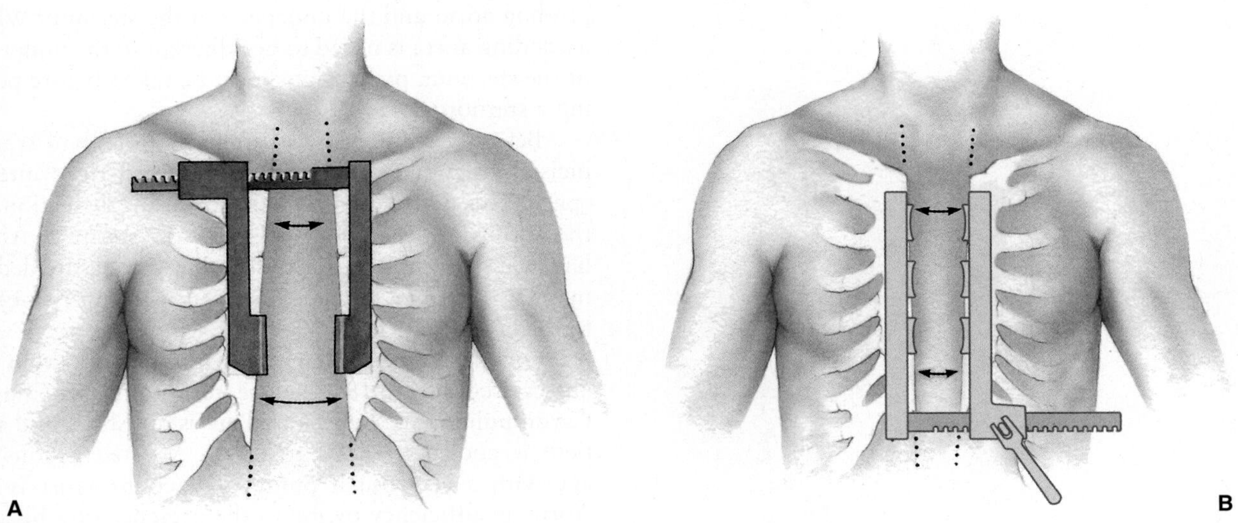

FIG. 1.3 **A** and **B:** Techniques for sternal retractor placement.

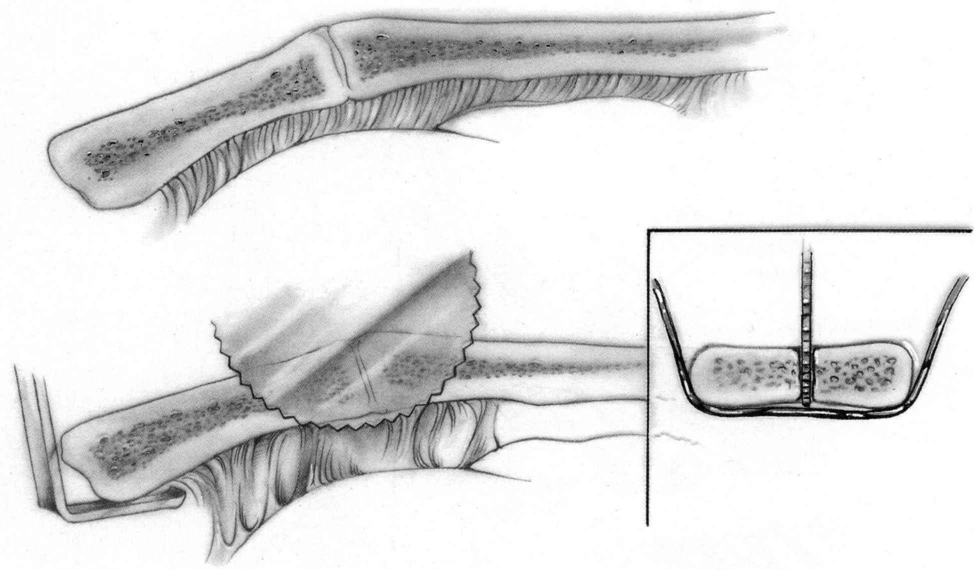

FIG. 1.4 Elevating the posterior table of the sternum to increase the distance between the saw blade and underlying structures.

to prevent any possible right ventricular injury (Fig. 1.4, inset). Only limited, sharp dissection adequate for the placement of a small Army–Navy retractor can be safely carried out in the suprasternal notch or around the xiphoid process.

⊘ Right Ventricular Injury

Blunt digital dissection behind the lower sternum should rarely be practiced in patients with a previous sternotomy because of possible injury to the friable right ventricular wall (Fig. 1.5). ⊘

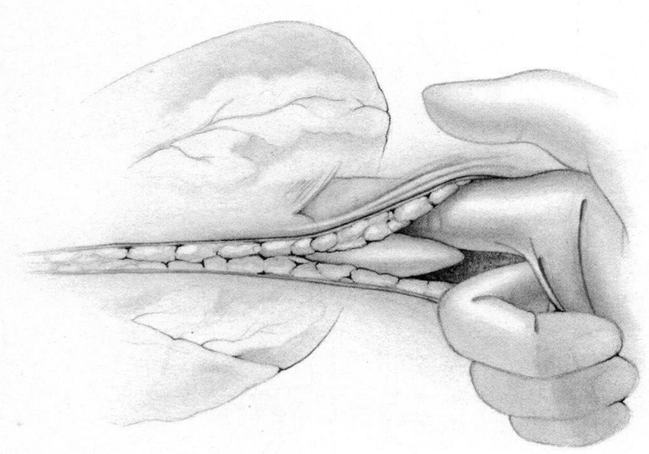

⊘ FIG. 1.5 Right ventricular injury caused by blunt digital dissection.

The sternum is raised by retractors at the suprasternal notch superiorly and at the xiphoid inferiorly during sternal division with an oscillating saw (Fig. 1.4). Small rake retractors are inserted into the marrow cavity on each side of the sternal edge and gently lifted upward toward the ceiling, thereby making the adhesions between the retrosternum and the heart slightly taut and accessible for division with the cautery or scissors (Fig. 1.6).

A lateral chest radiograph often reveals the proximity of the right ventricle and ascending aorta to the undersurface of the sternum. However, a computed tomography scan will accurately identify the relation between the ascending aorta and the underside of the sternum. When the ascending aorta is noted to be adherent to the undersurface of the sternum, precautions must be taken before performing a sternotomy.

Before a sternotomy is attempted, a small transverse incision is made in the second or third right intercostal space. This allows a lateral approach for dissection to free the aorta from the undersurface of the sternum. After this has been accomplished, the sternum can be divided in the manner described for repeat surgery without risk of injury to the aorta (Fig. 1.7).

Our preference is femoral artery–femoral vein bypass and core cooling to 18°C before sternotomy (see Chapter 2). Cardiopulmonary bypass is then established, and the patient is cooled to 18°C to 20°C. Assisted venous drainage with a centrifugal pump or vacuum assist is useful. Aortic insufficiency owing to the presence of a bileaflet or a single-disc mechanical prosthesis or a disrupted aortic

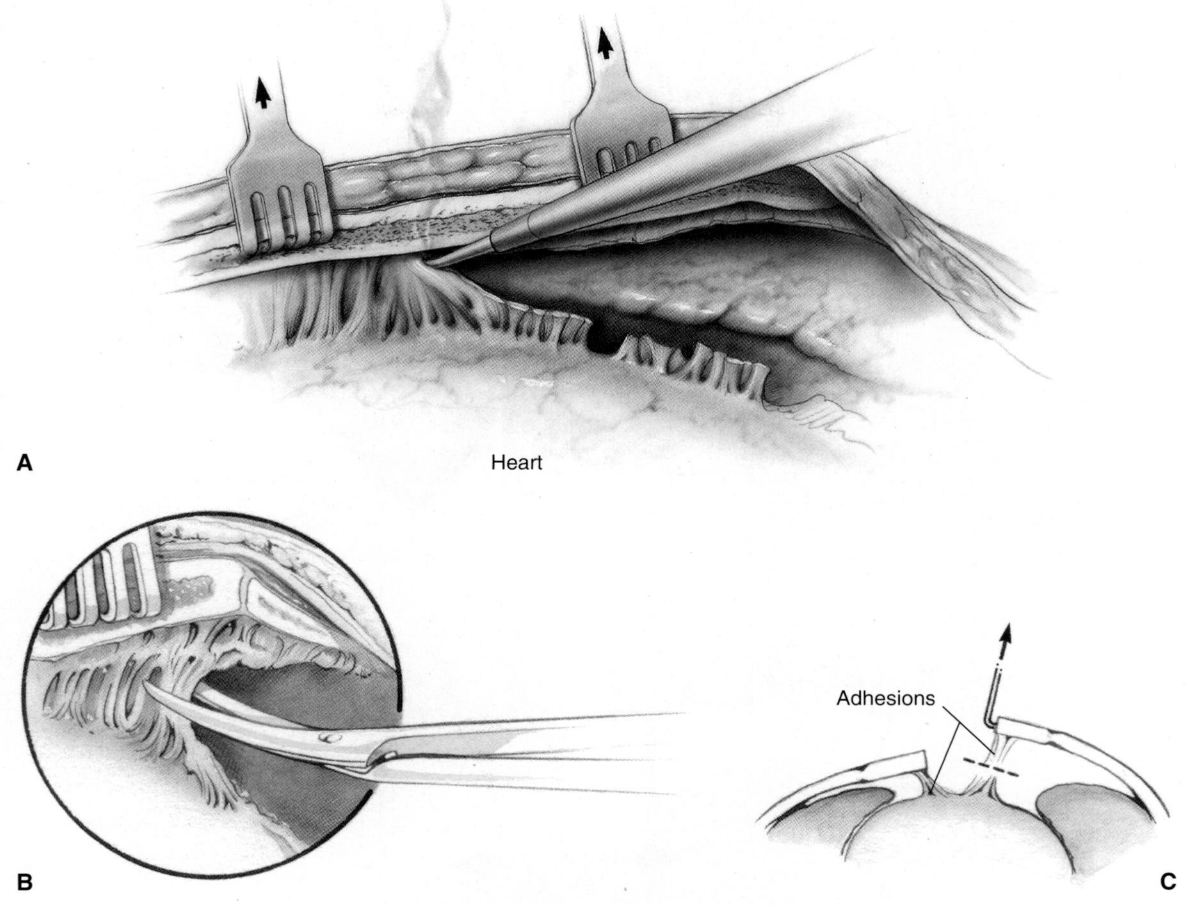

FIG. 1.6 **A–C:** Stepwise division of fibrous adhesions from the undersurface of the sternum.

bioprosthesis may result in left ventricular distension. An appropriately sized vent is placed into the apex of the left ventricle through a small left anterior thoracotomy as cardiopulmonary bypass is being initiated to protect the heart from overdistension (see Left Ventricular Apical Venting section in Chapter 4). Transesophageal echocardiography is always used to monitor left ventricular volume. If left ventricular distension occurs either at the initiation of bypass or when the heart begins to fibrillate, a vent is placed immediately.

If the sternotomy is uneventful, the patient is gradually rewarmed and the surgery is completed in the usual manner. Conversely, if the aorta is torn or disrupted, hypothermic arrest is instituted and the ascending aorta is repaired or replaced. The intended surgery is then resumed to its completion.

NB This precaution may appear to be a very major undertaking with its own possible serious complications. However, it is the only way to prevent catastrophic hemorrhage with a frequently fatal outcome. NB

NB Unanticipated Aortic Entry

When the possibility of aortic injury is not anticipated and the aorta is entered during sternotomy, towel clamps are used to reapproximate the sternal edges in an effort to tamponade the bleeding site. Direct pressure should be applied by an assistant surgeon while cardiopulmonary bypass is established expeditiously through the femoral artery and vein, as noted in the preceding text. NB

NB Division of the Posterior Table

The division of the posterior table of the sternum may be accomplished with heavy scissors under direct vision. This is facilitated by elevating the sternum slightly with a rake retractor. Such a maneuver is particularly important at the manubriosternal junction, where the manubrium takes a posterosuperior course (Fig. 1.4). NB

Fibrous adhesions to the undersurface of the sternum are mainly along the previous sternotomy. After dividing these fibrous adhesions with an electrocautery or scissors, the sternum is relatively free (Fig. 1.6). An adequate

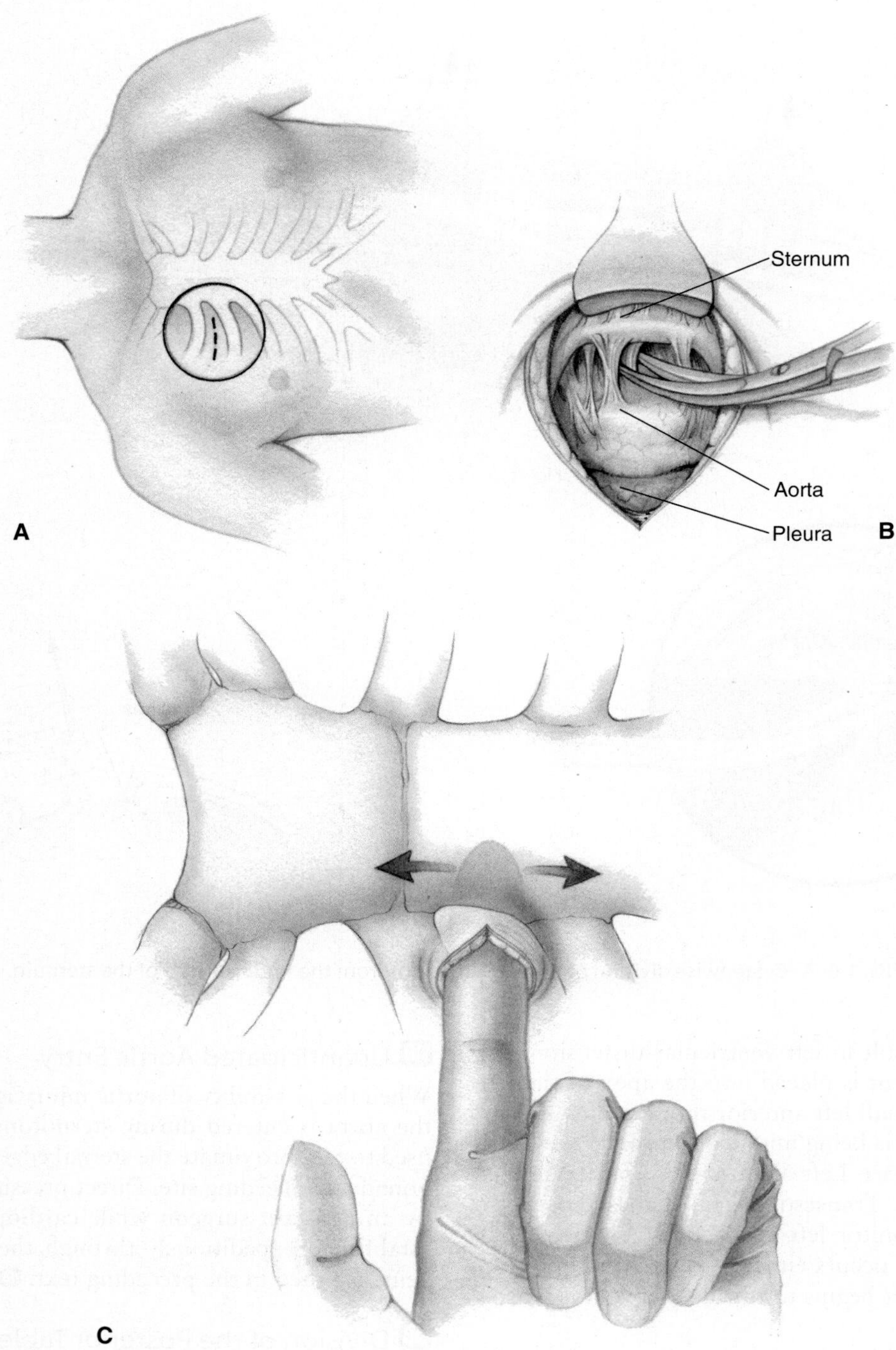

FIG. 1.7 A–C: Stepwise technique for separating the ascending aorta from the sternum in repeat procedures (see text).

dissection is carried out so that the sternal retractor can be safely positioned and slowly opened.

By slow and careful sharp dissection along the right inferior border of the heart, the proper plane can be identified relatively easily. Some surgeons find that the use of the electrocautery blade on a low setting allows this dissection to be accomplished with less bleeding from the pericardial surfaces. The dissection can then be gradually carried upward, exposing the right atrium and aorta for cannulation in preparation for cardiopulmonary bypass.

⊘ Right Ventricular Tear

A small (Himmelstein) chest retractor can now be inserted and must be spread apart only slightly; an overzealous attempt to widen the sternal opening results in stretching of the right ventricular wall. Tearing of the right ventricle

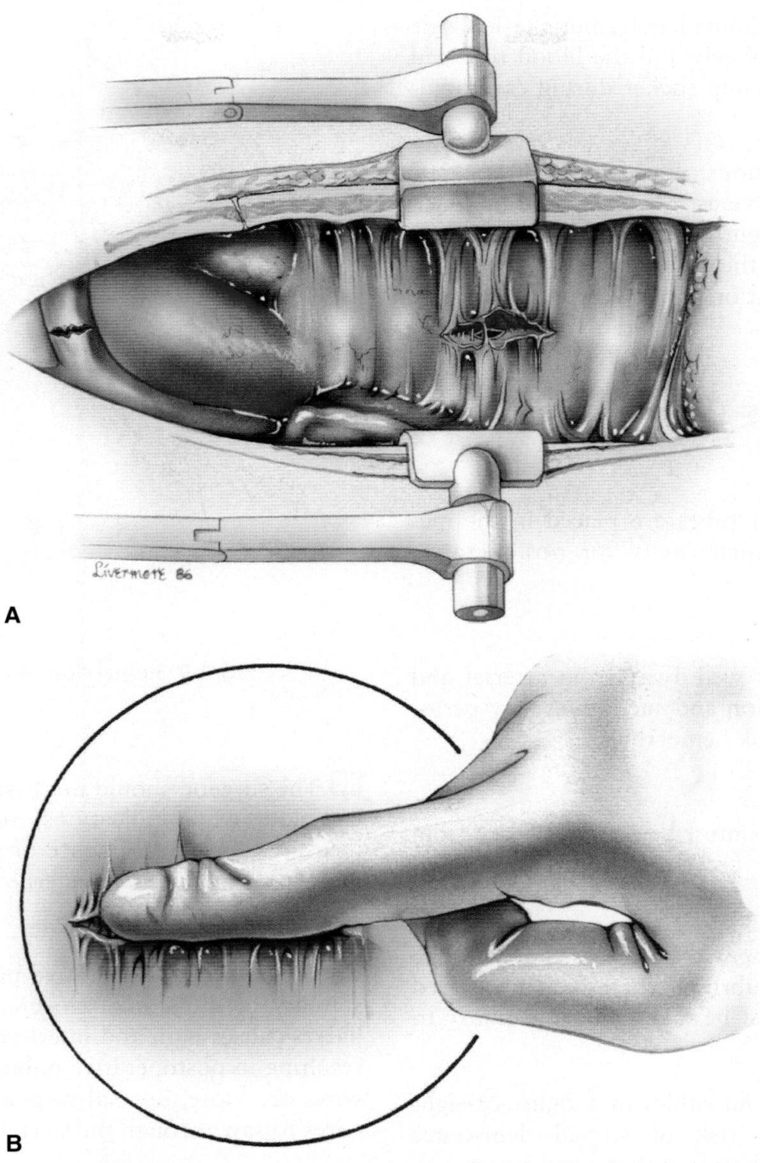

FIG. 1.8 **A:** Mechanism of a tear of the right ventricle and innominate vein in repeat procedures. **B:** Digital control of bleeding from the right ventricle.

because of saw injury or overstretching of the sternotomy is a life-threatening complication. The bleeding should be controlled by direct pressure on the site while cardiopulmonary bypass is initiated as promptly as possible. With the right ventricle totally decompressed, the wound is repaired with multiple, fine pledgeted sutures (Fig. 1.8). In cases of saw injury, pressing the two sternal halves together and toward the heart may tamponade the bleeding while cannulation of the femoral vessels is accomplished. ⊘

⊘ Injury to Innominate Vein

In patients undergoing repeat sternotomies, the innominate vein is often adherent to the undersurface of the manubrium. It may be injured directly with the saw or torn as the sternal halves are being retracted (Fig. 1.8). In most cases, the bleeding can be controlled with digital pressure on the opening in the vein while the vein is carefully dissected free from the posterior aspect of both sides of the manubrium. If control of the bleeding cannot be rapidly secured, the two sternal halves should be pushed together with slight downward pressure by the assistant surgeon to minimize blood loss. Blood should be transfused as necessary and femoral arterial and venous cannulation obtained as quickly as possible. The innominate vein can then be dissected free and repaired with 5-0 Prolene suture on cardiopulmonary bypass. ⊘

If the innominate vein injury is a complex tear or transection, repair may not be feasible. Then, the right side of the vein may be oversewn immediately, but the left side should be allowed to bleed freely and the blood returned to the bypass circuit by a pump sucker during cardiopulmonary bypass.

NB Acute occlusion of venous drainage from the left subclavian and jugular veins during cardiopulmonary bypass may lead to central nervous system injury. The left-sided opening of the innominate vein may be closed just before separation from cardiopulmonary bypass. NB

STERNAL CLOSURE

Technique

Before sternal closure, chest tubes are placed in the mediastinal space and pericardial cavity for postoperative drainage.

⊘ Graft Injury

Chest tubes must be placed well away from arterial and vein grafts. Constant irritation and suctioning may perforate the grafts and cause brisk hemorrhage. ⊘

⊘ Myocardial Injury

The holes on the chest tubes must be oriented away from the myocardial surface to prevent suction injury and bleeding. ⊘

The sternum is reapproximated with six to eight stainless steel wires. Generally, the wires are passed around the sternum except for the manubrium where they are passed through the bone. Care must be taken to avoid injury to the internal thoracic vessels.

NB Alternating steel wires and cables in a figure-of-eight fashion can minimize the risk of sternal dehiscence (Fig. 1.9). However, it must be noted that when emergency opening of the chest in the intensive care setting is required, the removal of figure-of-eight wires and cables is more tedious and may delay resuscitative efforts. NB

In very ill patients who have difficulty being weaned from cardiopulmonary bypass, the heart and lungs become swollen and edematous. This is encountered more frequently in infants and young children. Closing the sternum in this subgroup of patients compresses the heart and compromises cardiac function. The chest is left open in such cases and covered with Ioban (3M Healthcare, St. Paul, MN), which allows visualization of the anterior mediastinum and rapid reentry, if needed. In children, a silastic patch is sewn to the skin edges. When hemodynamics become stable, the patient is returned to the operating room and the sternotomy is closed in the customary manner. Chest closure may be accomplished under sterile conditions in the intensive care unit.

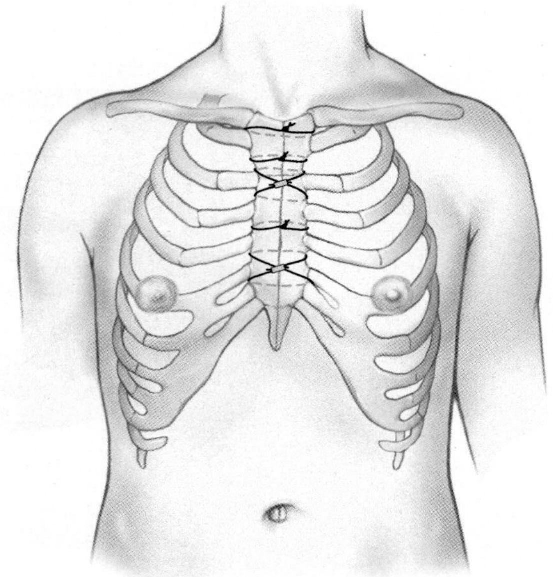

FIG. 1.9 Sternal closure with wires and cables.

NB The surgeon should not hesitate to use this very simple technique when indications are clear. This is a lifesaving measure, and the incidence of sternal infection is surprisingly low when rigorous sterile technique is maintained. NB

⊘ Loose Wires

The degree of postoperative pain is partly related to the stability of the sternal closure. Movement of the sternal halves causes pain and interferes with normal respiration, resulting in postoperative pulmonary complications. If the wires are loose, normal respiratory movements allow the wires to saw through the sternum (Fig. 1.10). ⊘

⊘ Robicsek Modification

When the sternum is osteoporotic and friable or the previous sternal closure has disrupted, Robicsek modification is successful in most patients. Running wire sutures are placed parasternally on both sides, followed by six to eight interrupted horizontal wire sutures that are placed outside the longitudinal parasternal wires and tightened in the usual manner (Fig. 1.11). ⊘

⊘ Fracture of the Sternum

Approximation of fractured sternal edges is a difficult task. Wires are passed parasternally above and below the fracture site, with the costal cartilages intervening. They are twisted tightly in the parasternal area to stabilize the fracture. These wires are then once again twisted horizontally across the sternum to close it in the usual manner (Fig. 1.12). ⊘

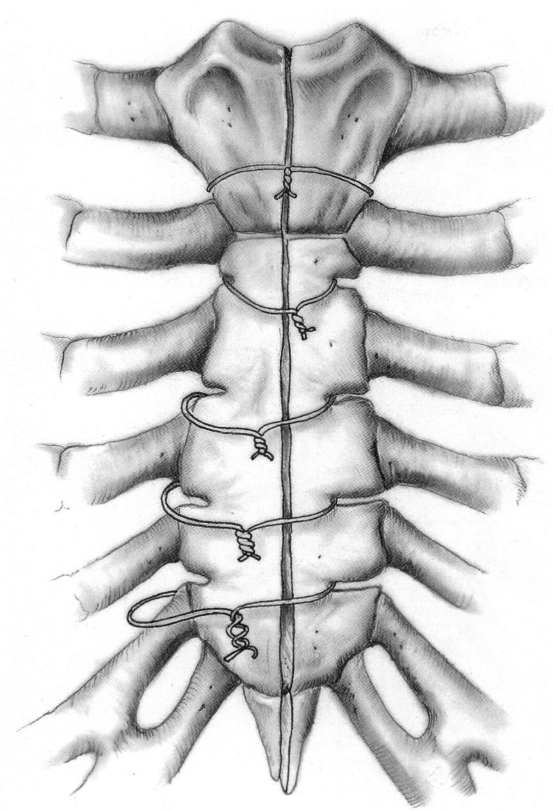

FIG. 1.10 Loose wires sawing through the sternum.

POSTOPERATIVE STERNAL WOUND INFECTION

Sternal wound infection occurs in 1% to 2% of patients undergoing cardiac surgery and carries a very high rate of morbidity and mortality.

General Considerations

General systemic factors such as malnutrition, cardiac cachexia, renal failure, chronic obstructive pulmonary disease, obesity, diabetes, and use of corticosteroids predispose the patient to postoperative sternal wound infection. Every attempt should be made to optimize the patient's state of health before surgery. This may require a period of nutritional supplementation or an aggressive therapeutic regimen to improve cardiac function. Pulmonary toilet and breathing exercises can be beneficial in patients with a history of chronic lung dysfunction. It is a good practice to recommend weight reduction in the very obese, but not to the extent that it produces negative nitrogen balance in the immediate preoperative period. Patients with insulin-dependent diabetes who undergo bilateral internal thoracic artery dissections are at increased risk of developing postoperative sternal wound complications. It is imperative that patients with diabetes have aggressive control of their blood glucose levels in the perioperative period. Long-term use of corticosteroids is associated with poor healing, and therefore, careful handling of tissue is required during surgery followed by meticulous closure of the wound.

Specific Technical Considerations

Specific technical factors that require consideration include internal thoracic artery dissection, excessive postoperative bleeding, reexploration for bleeding, emergency opening of the wound in the intensive care unit, prolonged cardiopulmonary bypass, profound low cardiac output in the immediate postoperative period, and external cardiac massage. Careful control of bleeding points before heparinization ensures adequate hemostasis. After heparin has been administered, no clotting occurs; all capillary ooze must therefore be electrocoagulated and large vessels occluded with metal clips. In repeat surgeries when the resulting raw surfaces are great, the possibility of excessive bleeding must be contemplated. Only unhurried electrocautery dissection with step-by-step hemostasis can prevent excessive postoperative bleeding. There are times, however, when, despite all the preventive measures taken, postoperative bleeding may require exploration; occasionally, the chest may have to be opened in the intensive care unit to relieve acute tamponade. External cardiac massage may be a lifesaving measure, but it does give rise to sternal wound instability and wound complications and may be relatively ineffective in the early postoperative period. Low cardiac output and long perfusion time also have adverse effects on wound healing. Strict adherence to aseptic surgical technique and attention to detail during the surgery are important measures to prevent wound complications.

Wound drainage, with or without sternal instability, is the first sign of possible sternal wound infection. The patient may be septic and febrile, but often he or she is otherwise asymptomatic. After the diagnosis of infection is made, the patient is promptly taken to the operating room and is placed under general endotracheal anesthesia. Then, the incision is completely opened, and all necrotic tissue is debrided and excised. The sternal edges are trimmed to ensure viable bone. After a specimen is obtained for culture and testing for antibiotic sensitivity, the wound is irrigated with a dilute solution of 0.5% to 1% povidone–iodine (Betadine) or saline solution. If the patient is not septic and the wound appears to be clean, the sternum is closed in the usual manner. Robicsek modification is utilized if the sternum is weakened by wires cutting through it or thinned out due to debridement. Two large chest tubes are left behind the sternum and are connected to a closed drainage system. The drainage tubes should be maintained on low suction for 7 to 10 days. Any pleural tubes are then removed, taking the usual precautions to prevent a pneumothorax.

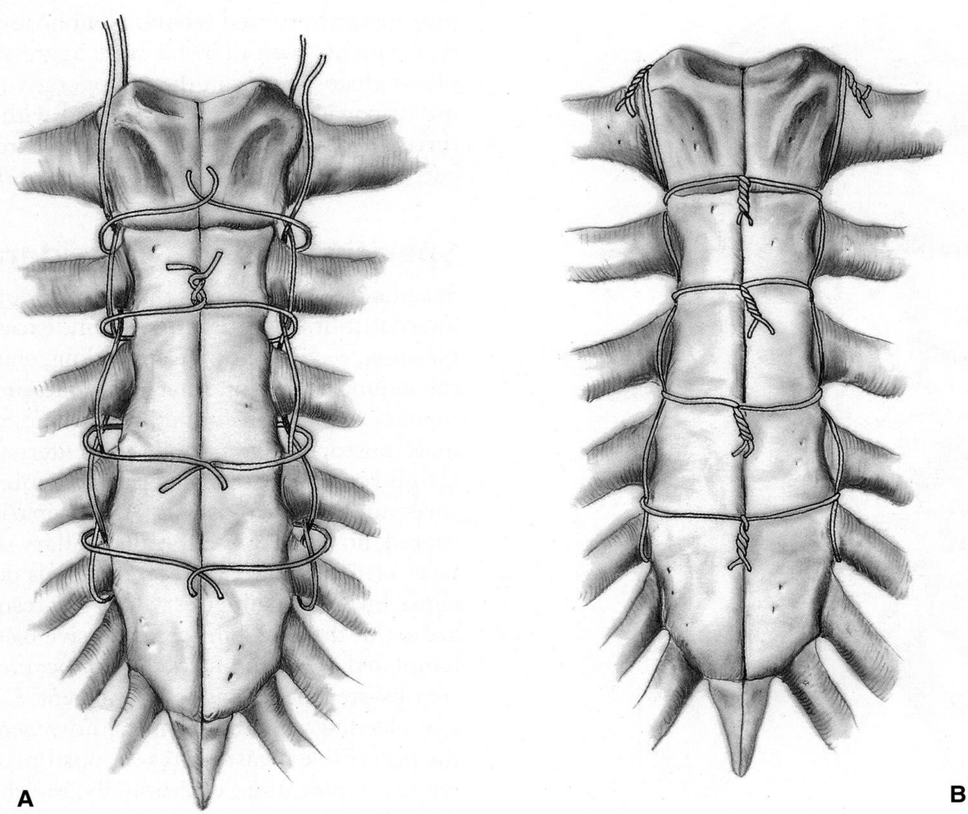

FIG. 1.11 Sternal closure with Robicsek modification.

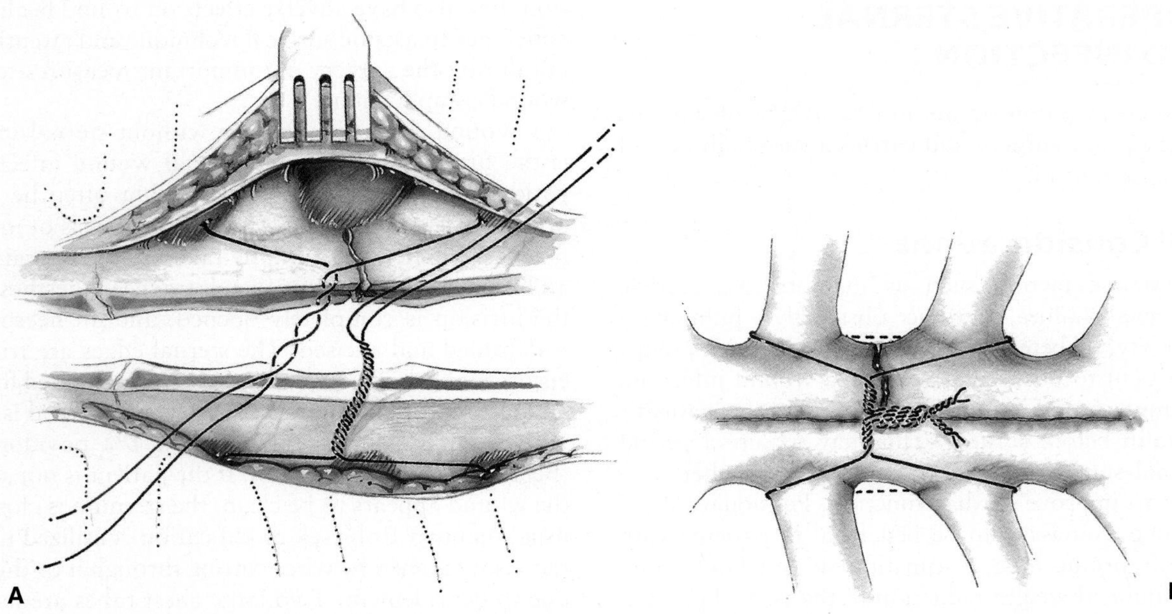

FIG. 1.12 Approximating segments of a fractured sternum.

NB Ischemic Necrosis

Surgeries are now being performed on a much older group of patients, many of whom have multisystem disease. Therefore, surgeons are encountering ischemic wound complications more frequently. In these cases, there is no definite evidence of infection, but necrotic bone and cartilage are present, which require careful debridement. NB

⊘ Placement of Tubes

Tubes should never be in direct contact with the aorta, vein grafts, or thoracic pedicle because they may cause local irritation, erosion, and serious hemorrhage (Fig. 1.13). The holes in the tubes should be oriented so that they are not in contact with the heart or the grafts to avoid suction injury and bleeding. The tubes should be placed on the thymic tissues superiorly or laterally in the gutter between pericardiopleural tissues and the undersurface of the sternum. ⊘

If the infection is massive or there is extensive necrosis, radical debridement is performed. To minimize the risk of reinfection, wide excision of the infected sternum and cartilage is critical. Extensive irrigation of the wound with a power irrigation system will reduce the number of organisms in the wound. When the wound appears to be clean and relatively free of overt infection, pectoralis muscle flaps or myocutaneous flaps are used for secondary closure (see subsequent text). If the quality of the subcutaneous tissues is questionable, the superficial wound should be packed open and delayed closure performed after a few days. In either case, systemic antibiotics should be continued for at least 7 days and for as long as 6 weeks in some patients.

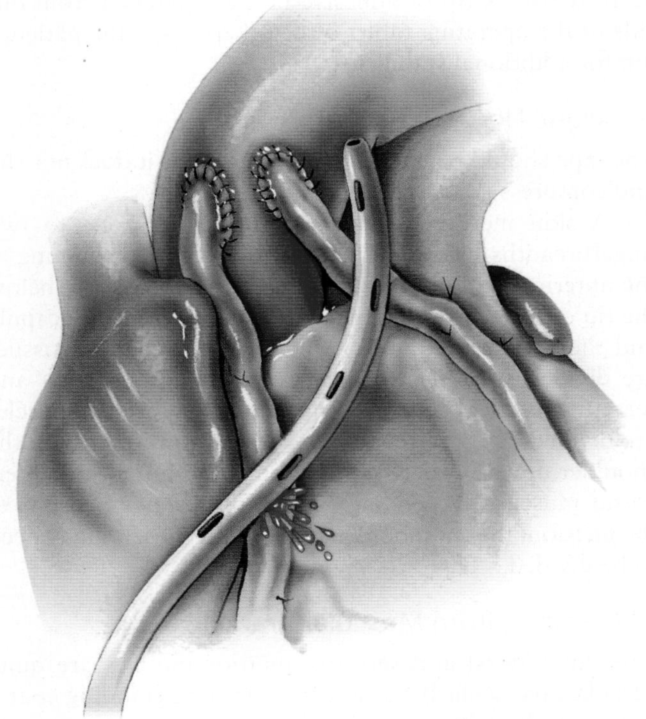

⊘ FIG. 1.13 Improper placement of a drainage tube.

NB Vacuum-Assisted Closure System

A very useful device for delayed closure of sternal or lower mediastinal wounds is the vacuum-assisted closure system (VAC therapy, KCI, San Antonio, TX). It continuously removes fluid and promotes contraction of wound edges, thereby facilitating secondary closure. An advantage of this system is that dressing changes need to occur only once every 2 to 3 days. NB

⊘ Necrotic Cartilage

Costal cartilages that are necrotic and contaminated must be resected because their retention almost certainly leads to chronic draining sinus tracts. ⊘

Pectoralis Muscle Flap

Technique

Through the existing wound, the superficial surface of the pectoralis major muscle is exposed by elevating the overlying skin and subcutaneous tissue proceeding from the midline laterally. Dissection of the muscle off the chest wall is accomplished laterally toward the midline until the parasternal perforator arteries are encountered, usually 2 to 3 cm from the sternal border. The inferior free border of the muscle is identified, and blunt dissection is used to develop the plane deep to the pectoralis major and superficial to the pectoralis minor. A small incision is then made over the muscular insertion, being careful to preserve the cephalic vein for possible future pacemaker insertion. The humeral attachment is then divided, and the flap is advanced medially into the midline wound. The thoracoacromial pedicle must be divided to allow adequate mobility for folding the muscle into the sternotomy wound. When both pectoralis muscles are used, they are sutured together in the midline under slight tension. Occasionally, where one flap is sufficient, the muscle is sutured to the opposite sternal periosteum. The skin flaps are then advanced and closed primarily.

NB Choice of Muscle Flaps

Choice of muscle flaps should be thoroughly analyzed before beginning any procedure. The workhorse of mediastinal reconstruction is the pectoralis major muscle. The maximal bulk of muscle can be obtained using turnover pectoralis flaps based on parasternal perforating arteries from the internal thoracic artery. In most wounds of moderate to large size, bilateral flaps are necessary to fill the midline dead space. Occasionally, in narrower defects, a unilateral flap is sufficient. NB

⊘ Absence of the Internal Thoracic Artery

The internal thoracic artery is often used as a bypass conduit. In these cases, the parasternal perforator arteries have already been sacrificed, and the pectoralis flap should be based on the thoracoacromial pedicle. ⊘

⊘ Wound Coverage of the Lower Mediastinum

Regardless of the pectoralis flap technique, the inferior portion of the wound is most vulnerable. Turnover flaps are not sufficient to cover the lower one-fourth to one-third of the mediastinal structures. The VAC system is effective in promoting contraction of the wound edges. Introducing omentum into the chest wound has also been used to address such problems. Bringing omentum into the mediastinum necessitates entry into the peritoneum. This technique increases the morbidity of the surgery and carries the risk of spreading infection into the abdomen. ⊘

Superior Rectus Flap

An additional and effective technique is covering the lower mediastinal wound with the superior rectus abdominis muscle as a flap.

Technique

The sternotomy incision is extended inferiorly to the umbilicus. The chosen superior rectus abdominis muscle is exposed by elevating skin and subcutaneous tissue to the lateral edge of the muscle down to the level of the umbilicus, where the muscle is divided transversely. During transection of the muscle, the superior epigastric vessels are suture ligated to prevent a donor site hematoma. The muscle is then lifted off the posterior rectus sheath up to the costal margin.

⊘ Absence of the Internal Thoracic Artery

The superior epigastric artery is the continuation of the internal thoracic artery. It is important to know that the internal thoracic artery is intact and patent before mobilizing the superior rectus abdominis muscle. The arteries may have been used as a conduit for myocardial revascularization or been damaged by repeat sternal closure. A selective angiogram is always indicated. ⊘

⊘ Damage to the Epigastric Arteries

Care is taken not to damage the superior epigastric pedicle that emerges from beneath the costal margin to enter the muscle. ⊘

The flap may then be folded superiorly to fill the inferior third of the mediastinum. The rectus is sutured to the pectoralis flaps and the sternal border to maintain its position, and the anterior rectus sheath is repaired with nonabsorbable sutures.

⊘ Hematoma and Seroma

The most common complication is hematoma or seroma at the donor muscle site, whether pectoralis or rectus abdominis. ⊘

Myocutaneous Flap

The pectoralis major muscle is sometimes used as a myocutaneous flap to cover the infected sternal wound.

Technique

The sternal wound is debrided and irrigated with saline and povidone–iodine solution, as described previously. Bilateral musculocutaneous flaps of the pectoralis major muscle are dissected free off the chest wall to the level of the clavicles above, anterior axillary line laterally, and posterior rectus sheath inferiorly. This is accomplished with an electrocautery and blunt dissection. Perforating arteries are sacrificed.

The myocutaneous flaps are now advanced medially and approximated to each other in the midline over two to three closed-system drainage tubes with absorbable sutures. The skin is then closed with interrupted Prolene or in two layers with absorbable sutures.

THORACOTOMY

Posterolateral thoracotomy provides excellent exposure for many closed cardiac procedures, such as repair of coarctation of the aorta, shunting procedures, resection of aneurysms of the thoracic aorta, ductus arteriosus surgery, and closed mitral valve commissurotomy. Anterolateral thoracotomy may be all that is needed for some procedures. In practice, we elect to perform a lateral thoracotomy and extend it anteriorly or posteriorly as needed.

The patient is stabilized securely on the operating table in a lateral position. A small pillow or a roll is placed on both sides of the chest, and a small roll is placed under the axilla. Another pillow is placed between the knees. Often, the upper leg is extended on a pillow over the flexed lower limb. A wide strip of adhesive tape is stretched from one side of the operating table to the other across the patient's hip for additional stability.

⊘ Sciatic Nerve Injury

The tape should be carefully placed so that it does not slip and compress the sciatic nerve. ⊘

A skin incision is made approximately one to two fingerbreadths below the level of the nipple, beginning at the anterior axillary line. It is extended posteriorly below the tip of the scapula, then superiorly between the scapula and the vertebral column. After the subcutaneous tissues are divided with electrocautery, the latissimus dorsi and serratus anterior muscles come into view. These muscles are divided, and the scapula is allowed to retract with the shoulder upward, thereby providing exposure of the intercostal muscles. Depending on the posterior extension of the incision, the rhomboid and trapezius muscles may need to be divided.

⊘ Bleeding from Muscular Branches

Latissimus dorsi and serratus anterior muscles are quite vascular, particularly in patients with long-standing coarctation of the aorta, and therefore, their division may result in substantial blood loss. Therefore, it is essential to identify each blood vessel and ligate it securely. Although cautery coagulation may suffice in many situations, larger vessels should be controlled with suture ligatures. ⊘

NB Muscle Sparing

Often, it may be possible to retract the serratus anterior muscle adequately to provide sufficient exposure for thoracotomy. This is particularly indicated in infants and children. NB

The desired interspace is selected by counting the ribs downward, bearing in mind that the uppermost rib that can be felt is the second rib, not the first. Excellent exposure for patent ductus arteriosus and coarctation of the aorta is provided through the fourth interspace. The intercostal muscle is incised using electrocautery until the parietal pleura comes into view. This, in turn, is opened, taking care not to injure the underlying lung tissue. The intercostal incision is then completed under direct vision.

⊘ Injury to the Lung

The anesthetist should temporarily deflate the lungs to protect the lung parenchyma during entry into the pleural cavity. ⊘

⊘ Injury to the Intercostal Vessels

The neurovascular bundle is protected by the ribs. The dissection must hug the upper border of the rib to avoid injury to the intercostal artery. ⊘

The rib retractor is spread gradually and incrementally to avoid rib fracture. If additional exposure is needed, either the lower or upper rib is resected and removed. Dividing and removing a segment of the rib posteriorly near its angle is equally effective.

NB Postoperative pain owing to rib fracture could be markedly decreased if the affected segment is divided and removed to prevent the fractured bone ends from moving against each other. NB

One or two chest tubes should be placed in the pleural space and brought out anteriorly. The ribs are approximated with four or five interrupted heavy sutures. The serratus anterior and latissimus dorsi muscles anteriorly and the rhomboid and trapezius muscles posteriorly are accurately and meticulously approximated with either interrupted or continuous sutures. The subcutaneous layer and the skin are then closed.

⊘ Needle Injury to the Intercostal Vessels

Care must be exercised when placing the pericostal sutures to avoid injuring the intercostal vessels. ⊘

NB Intercostal nerve block by injection of a long-acting local anesthetic agent near the intercostal nerves in the most posterior part of the incision two to three interspaces above and below the level of the incision is most effective in reducing postoperative pain. NB

ALTERNATIVE SURGICAL APPROACHES

To allow for earlier return of the patient to normal physical activities, achieve a better cosmetic result, and decrease the postoperative pain, many surgeons are utilizing alternative approaches to the heart. In addition to smaller incisions, minimally invasive approaches are being introduced to avoid sternotomy altogether and perform cardiac surgery without cardiopulmonary bypass. The least invasive of these procedures involves cannulation of the femoral artery and vein to provide cardiopulmonary support for performing valve surgeries by endoscopic techniques.

Two of these techniques involve a full sternotomy through more cosmetically acceptable skin incisions. Two minimally invasive approaches include lower or upper ministernotomy and submammary right thoracotomy.

NB Defibrillation

Because access within the pericardial space is limited, all patients undergoing cardiac procedures through a minimally invasive approach should have external defibrillator pads appropriately placed depending on the incision. Alternatively, sterile pediatric internal defibrillator paddles must be available on the operating table. NB

Full Sternotomy through Submammary Incision

A bilateral submammary skin incision results in a cosmetically acceptable scar and is used in girls and young women undergoing more complex cardiac procedures requiring a full sternotomy.

Technique

Skin incisions are made 0.5 cm below and parallel to the lowest contour of both breasts. The incisions are joined in the midline at the level of the junction of the sternum with the xiphoid process (Fig. 1.14).

⊘ Lower Limits of Breast Tissue

The precise limits of breast tissue in preadolescent girls may not be evident. It is important not to make the incision too high as this will result in a scar across the breasts. A transverse incision at the level of the xiphoid process with a slight superior deviation in the midline is a safe option. ⊘

The breasts and skin flaps are dissected off the pectoral muscles with a cautery blade. The skin flaps are then retracted with one or two heavy sutures. Superiorly, it is useful to tie the sutures to a Kerlix gauze roll, which is passed over the anesthesiologist's crossbar and secured to an appropriate weight (usually 5 to 10 lb).

⊘ Injury to Skin

A gauze or lap pad placed behind the heavy sutures protects the skin edges from pressure injury. ⊘

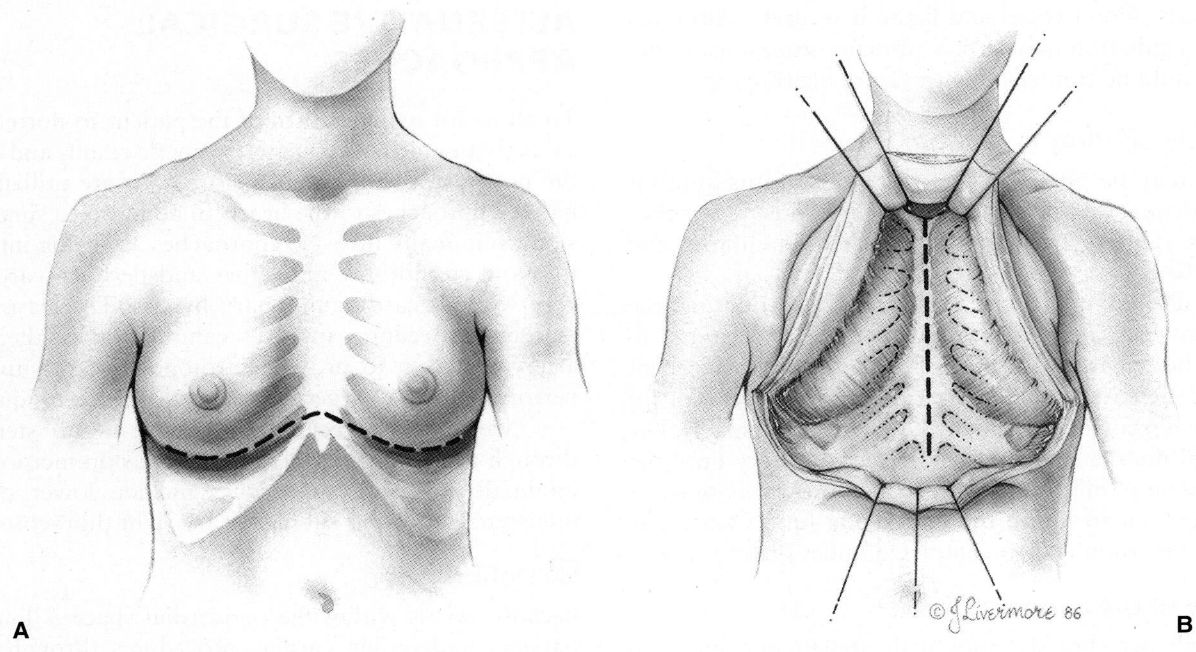

FIG. 1.14 Brom submammary approach.

The sternal opening and closure are performed in the usual manner. The skin flaps are allowed to fall naturally on the pectoral muscles. This position is secured with a few absorbable sutures. Two soft flat drainage catheters are placed behind the skin flaps and brought out through stab wounds at the lateral extremes of the incision. They are connected to a closed suction system.

NB Care must be taken to maintain the normal position of the breasts and alignment of the nipples to ensure satisfactory cosmetic results. NB

NB A single mediastinal chest tube is brought out through a small curvilinear incision just above the umbilicus to avoid an additional scar. NB

Full Sternotomy through a Limited Midline Incision

Full sternotomy allows safe access to the heart and permits performance of most of the cardiac procedures. It has been the approach of choice since the birth of cardiac surgery. Therefore, performing a full median sternotomy through a limited skin incision is most appealing.

Technique

The midline skin incision starts at the level of sternomanubrial junction and extends down toward the xiphoid process for approximately 8 to 12 cm depending on the procedure to be performed and the patient's body habitus (Fig. 1.15). Most mitral valve procedures can be accomplished through

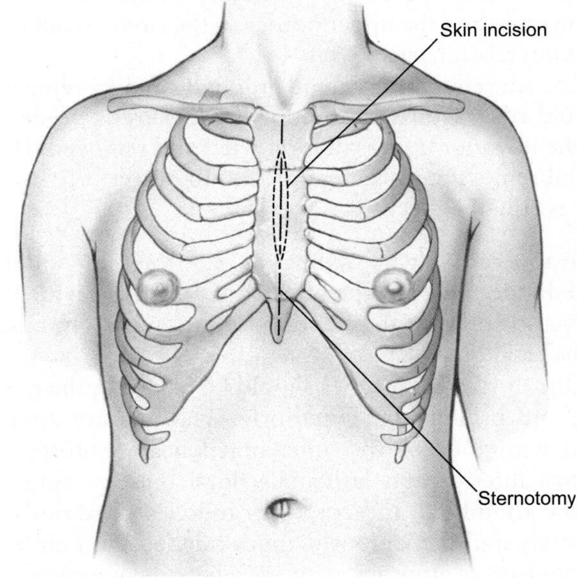

FIG. 1.15 Full sternotomy with limited skin incision.

an 8 to 10 cm opening, but for aortic valve surgery and coronary bypass, grafting up to 15 cm may be required. The subcutaneous tissues are dissected free from the anterior surface of the entire length of the sternum with electrocautery. Often, it may be necessary to extend the dissection for 1 to 2 cm laterally onto the pectoralis muscle on both sides as well as superiorly into the suprasternal notch. It may be possible to place a standard pneumatic sternal saw into the suprasternal notch and divide the sternum from above downward. At times, it may be necessary to use a pediatric or oscillating saw.

⊘ Injury to the Skin

Both ends of the incision must be carefully retracted and protected from an oscillating saw when it is used to open the sternum. The lower end of the incision should be similarly retracted to prevent injury to the skin when the sternum is opened with the standard pneumatic saw from above. ⊘

A pediatric or small Finochietto sternal retractor is then used to spread the two halves of the sternum. The blades are opened very gently and just wide enough to provide adequate exposure. The pericardial edges are suspended from the skin drapes or sternal retractor to elevate the heart maximally into the operative field.

At the conclusion of the procedure, the sternum is closed with at least six wires. It is important to place two wires in the manubrium to assure maximum stability. The skin and subcutaneous tissues are closed in layers. If a significant potential space exists anterior to the sternum, a flat drain connected to closed suction is placed to prevent the accumulation of fluid.

NB This incision is cosmetically pleasing because it cannot be seen when patients wear most V-neck or open-collar tops. NB

NB The internal thoracic arteries and costal cartilages are not prone to injury with this approach. NB

Lower Ministernotomy

We have found the lower sternotomy through a limited skin incision to be an acceptable approach for atrial septal defects and some ventricular septal defects. It may also be used for off-pump coronary artery bypass graft procedures using the left internal thoracic artery.

Technique

The midline skin incision begins at the level of a line drawn between the two nipples and extends to the tip of the xiphoid process (Fig. 1.16). Dissection must be carried up to the level of the third interspace, and the pectoralis muscle is dissected off the sternum to the right or left side. (For congenital heart defects, the right side is dissected, and for left internal thoracic artery harvest, the left side is used.) A saw is used to open the sternum in the midline to the level of the third interspace. Then, an angled bone cutter is used to divide the right or left half of the sternum into the third interspace (Fig. 1.17).

⊘ Injury to the Costal Cartilage

Every effort is made to ensure that the bone cutter divides the sternal half into the interspace between two ribs and not into the costal cartilage. ⊘

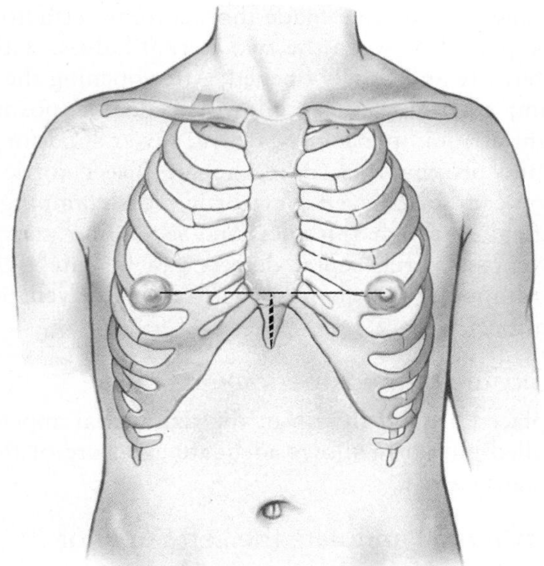

FIG. 1.16 Lower ministernotomy skin incision.

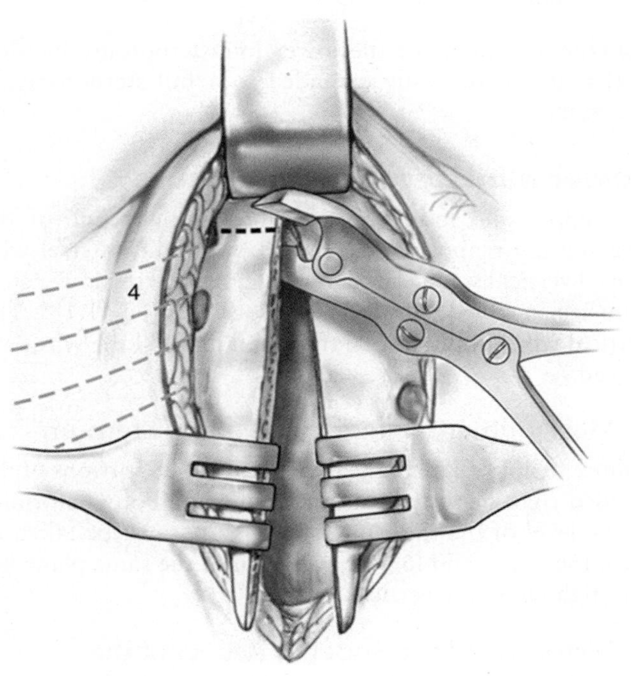

FIG. 1.17 After using a saw to divide the xiphoid and lower sternum, an angled bone cutter is used to divide the right half of the sternum into the third intercostal space.

⊘ Injury to the Skin Incision

The saw may injure the skin edges superiorly. This is avoided by pulling upward with a long narrow retractor on the upper extent of the skin incision to allow the saw to reach the level of the third interspace (Fig. 1.17). ⊘

A single- or double-blade thoracotomy retractor can then be placed between the two sternal halves, with the bar inferiorly and slowly opened. After opening the pericardium, traction sutures allow excellent exposure of the right atrium, inferior vena cava, lower superior vena cava, and proximal ascending aorta. Direct aortic cannulation can be achieved, but aortic cross-clamping may be difficult through this incision. Secundum and most sinus venosus atrial septal defects can be safely closed on cardiopulmonary bypass with induced ventricular fibrillation.

NB Exposure of the Superior Vena Cava

A tie placed around the tip of the right atrial appendage and pulled inferiorly allows adequate exposure of the superior vena cava. NB

⊘ Inability to Cannulate the Left Superior Vena Cava

If a left superior vena cava is present, this approach should not be used. Preoperative transthoracic echocardiography or an intraoperative transesophageal echocardiogram can usually make this diagnosis. ⊘

NB One advantage of the lower ministernotomy incision is that it can be easily extended to a full sternotomy, if necessary. NB

Lower Ministernotomy Closure

The upper and lower portions of the right side of the sternum are reapproximated with one stainless steel wire placed vertically. The left and right halves of the lower sternum are encircled with three or four wires (Fig. 1.18). The vertical wire should not be tightened until all the wires are placed.

⊘ Malalignment of Right Side of the Sternum

Failure to approximate the upper and lower portions of the divided right hemisternum will result in a bony deformity at the level of the third interspace. Care must be taken to push the upper and lower portions into the same plane before tightening the vertical wire. ⊘

⊘ Distortion of the Superior Aspect of the Incision

Tight closure of the muscle layers superiorly will create a dimpling effect. The tissue should be loosely approximated cephalad to the skin opening. ⊘

Upper Ministernotomy

Some surgeons perform aortic procedures through an upper ministernotomy. This incision provides adequate exposure of the aorta and left ventricular outflow tract.

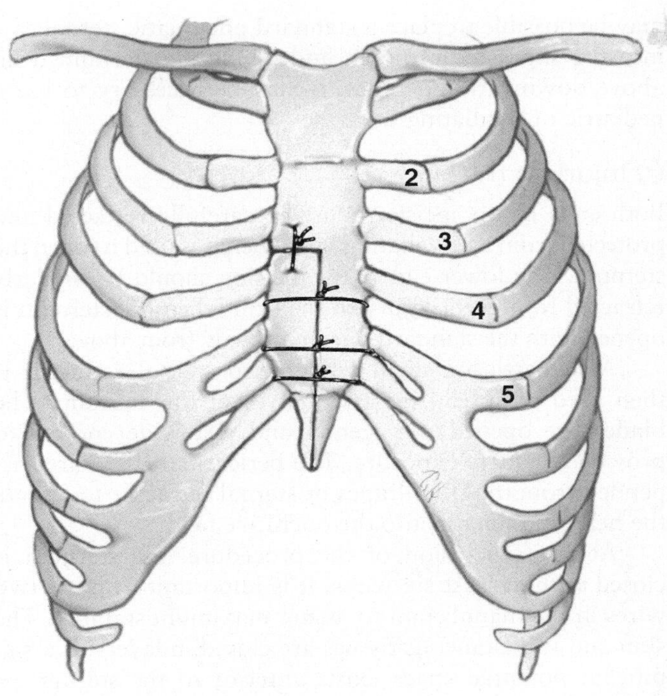

FIG. 1.18 Reapproximation of the lower sternotomy with one vertically placed wire and three horizontal wires.

Technique

A 6- to 8-cm midline skin incision is made starting approximately 2 to 3 cm below the suprasternal notch. Short flaps of subcutaneous tissue are developed both superiorly and inferiorly to expose the sternum. With a pneumatic or a small oscillating saw, the sternum is divided from the suprasternal notch down to the third or fourth interspace. An angled bone cutter is used to divide the sternum into the right, left, or both intercostal spaces. A Finochietto sternal retractor provides good exposure.

⊘ Injury to Internal Thoracic Artery

The retractor blades should be opened carefully to prevent damage to the internal thoracic vessels. Similarly, the bone cutter may injure these vessels. ⊘

⊘ Injury to Costal Cartilages

The bone cutter should divide the sternal half into the intercostal space and not into the costal cartilages. ⊘

⊘ Skin Injury

The upper and lower ends of the skin incision must be protected from saw and traction injuries. ⊘

NB Improving Exposure

Wide excision of the thymic and fatty tissues improves the exposure. NB

NB Use of Retrograde Cardioplegia

Insertion of the retrograde cannula is more easily accomplished before venous cannulation. The cannula is introduced into the right atrium through a purse-string suture below the right atrial appendage. Gentle traction on the right atrial appendage facilitates the cannula placement. It is advanced into the coronary sinus under transesophageal echocardiographic guidance. NB

NB Minimizing Air in Left Ventricle

The usual deairing techniques may not be feasible through this incision (see Chapter 4). Flooding the operative field with CO_2 through an intravenous tubing attached to the edge of the incision will displace air and decrease the possibility of air embolism. NB

At the completion of the procedure, a soft drain is placed in the mediastinum and brought out below the xiphoid process. Placement of this drain is best accomplished when the heart is empty on cardiopulmonary bypass. The sternum is closed with four wires, two of which are placed in the manubrium. The upper and lower portions of the right, left, or both sides of the sternum are reapproximated with a wire placed vertically. The subcutaneous tissues and skin are closed in layers.

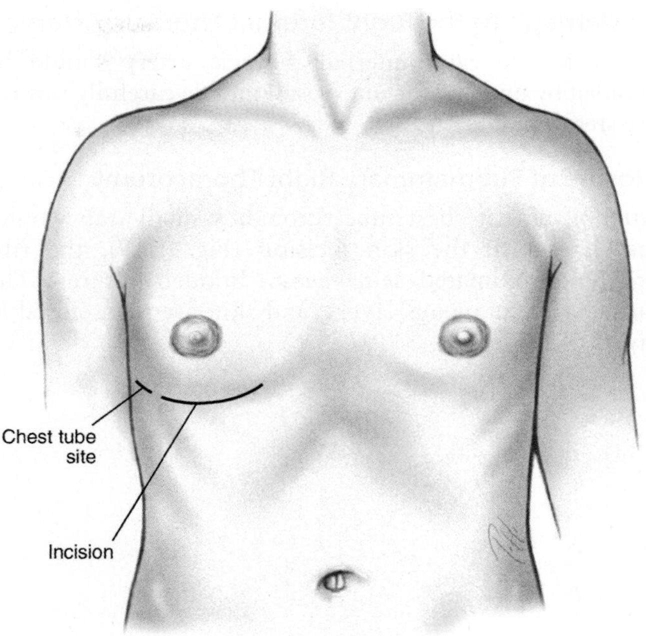

FIG. 1.19 Submammary right thoracotomy skin incision. Note the location of the chest tube.

Submammary Right Thoracotomy

This incision is cosmetically very appealing for young girls and women requiring atrial septal defect closure. It may be used for mitral valve surgeries, although access to the ascending aorta for cross-clamping may be difficult.

Technique

The skin incision is made in the submammary fold of the right breast in an adult or the anticipated future breast fold in a preadolescent girl (Fig. 1.19). This is carried down to the chest wall, and the pectoralis major and pectoralis minor insertions onto the ribs are dissected free up to the fourth interspace. The intercostal muscle is divided just on the upper edge of the 5th rib, and the pleural space is entered.

Two single-blade retractors are placed: one between the ribs and the other at a right angle to the first retractor to spread the subcutaneous tissue and muscle. A lung retractor is then used to hold the right lung laterally (Fig. 1.20).

After opening the pericardium, traction sutures can be placed to allow for exposure of the inferior vena cava, superior vena cava, and proximal ascending aorta. A tie around the tip of the right atrial appendage retracted inferiorly aids in cannulation of the superior vena cava and ascending aorta.

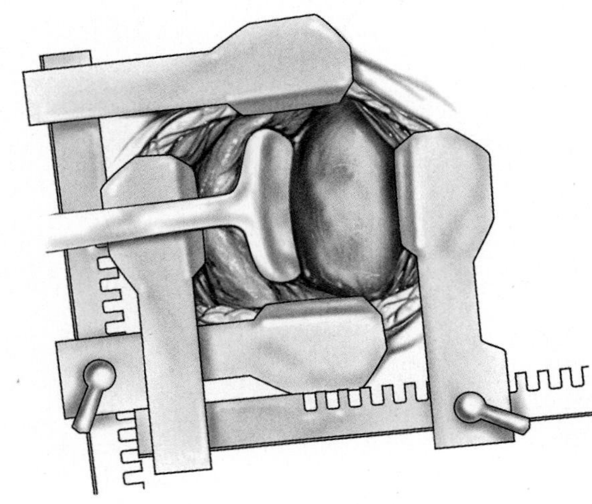

FIG. 1.20 The first single-blade retractor spreads the ribs, the second single-blade retractor retracts the muscle, and a T-shaped retractor holds the lung laterally.

⊘ Inability to Cannulate the Left Superior Vena Cava

A left superior vena cava is not accessible from this approach. ⊘

⊘ Difficult Ascending Aortic Cannulation

The ascending aorta in older children and adults may be difficult to cannulate through this incision. The use of an arterial cannula with a tapered introducer may allow for safe and controlled aortic cannulation when aortic exposure is suboptimal. Femoral arterial cannulation through a small horizontal groin incision may often be required. ⊘

⊘ Damage to the Right Internal Thoracic Artery

Injury to the right internal thoracic artery should be avoided by opening the intercostal muscle carefully toward the sternum. ⊘

Closure of Submammary Right Thoracotomy

After placing a chest tube through a small stab wound just lateral to the skin incision (Fig. 1.19), the ribs are reapproximated with heavy braided sutures. The muscle, subcutaneous layers, and skin are then closed in layers.

NB Correct Chest Tube Placement

The chest tube should be inserted through an incision just lateral to the skin opening. Placement of the chest tube lower than the submammary line creates an unnecessary scar that is not hidden by the usual two-piece bathing suit or tube top. NB

Intercostal nerve blocks with a long-acting local anesthetic in several interspaces can be administered before chest closure from within the pleural space. This decreases the need for parenteral pain medications in the postoperative period.

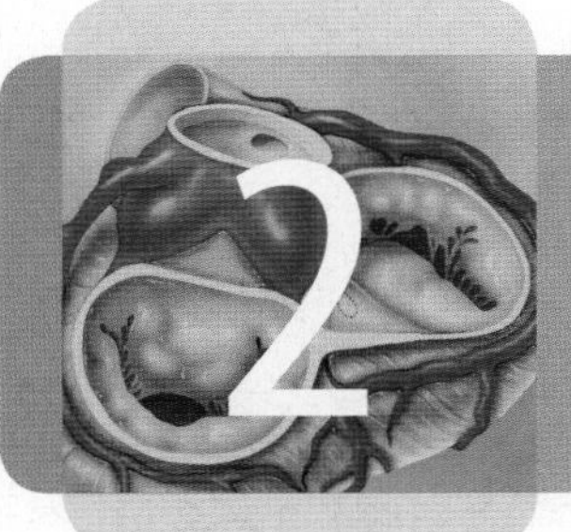

2 Preparation for Cardiopulmonary Bypass

EXPOSURE OF THE HEART

Technique

The remnant of the thymus gland is dissected free from the pericardium. The thymic vessels are all electrocoagulated to prevent the formation of a hematoma or troublesome oozing during the operation. The larger ones should be occluded with metal clips. The pleura is peeled away from the inferior pericardium with a dry sponge, thereby preventing inadvertent entry into the pleural cavities. The electrocautery blade can be used to incise the pericardium and at the same time coagulate the edges. This maneuver may trigger ventricular fibrillation if the cautery blade touches the heart. It is therefore preferable to incise the pericardium with a pair of scissors or a scalpel. The pericardium can then be opened in the usual inverted T fashion and suspended from skin edges or the retractor (Fig. 2.1).

The sternal retractor should be opened gradually without traumatizing the sternal edges. It can be positioned in such a manner that its cross-arm is in the upper part of the wound. This technique helps to prevent entanglement or overcrowding of various pump lines. The blades of the retractor should be placed as low as possible, and the sternum should be opened only to the extent that is essential for adequate exposure. This prevents possible fracture of the first rib and brachial plexus injury (see Fig. 1.2). Many surgeons prefer sternal retractors with three to four blades, which can swivel horizontally and thereby lessen the stress on the sternal edges.

Dissection Around the Aorta

The posterior aspect of the aorta is not always free, and therefore the cross-clamp may not include the entire wall of the aorta (Fig. 2.2). Often, it helps to mobilize the aorta to ensure its complete cross-clamping. In primary cardiac surgeries, the area between the pulmonary artery and aorta is dissected in a limited manner to allow a large curved or right-angled clamp to be passed behind the aorta. In redo surgeries, some sharp dissection behind the aorta must be carried out as well. When a clear passage is created, the clamp is used to pass an umbilical tape around the aorta. Traction on the tape allows the aorta to be lifted out of its bed (Fig. 2.3).

NB Adventitial tissue on arteries and veins is an integral component of the vascular walls. It should not be dissected free but kept intact whenever possible. NB

Incorporation of adequate adventitial tissue in closure of the aortotomy or various cannulation sites, including the superior vena cava and pulmonary artery, is a safe and effective technique. The adventitial component is a natural tissue that acts like a reinforcing pledget, adding strength to the closure.

⊘ Injury to the Aorta

During dissection and passing of the clamp behind the aorta, care must be taken to avoid injury to the posterior wall (Fig. 2.4). If such a complication occurs, it is best to control the bleeding digitally or by packing the area while preparations are made to initiate cardiopulmonary bypass (Fig. 2.5). With the patient on bypass and the aorta cross-clamped, the aorta is opened and the posterior wall is repaired under direct vision (Fig. 2.6). ⊘

⊘ Injury to the Right Pulmonary Artery

On rare occasions when the right pulmonary artery takes a more caudal course, it may be injured during dissection around the aorta. If such a problem arises, it is best to control the bleeding by packing the area and to correct the lesion when the heart is decompressed on full cardiopulmonary bypass. The right pulmonary artery can also be injured during dissection of the superior vena cava, especially when passing a tape around this vessel (Fig. 2.7). ⊘

Dissection Around the Cavae

Dissection required to pass umbilical tapes around the venae cavae in preparation for total cardiopulmonary bypass may be tedious and occasionally may result in injury to the great veins. The parietal pericardium is divided on each side of the vena cava, and a plane is established that allows an appropriate curved clamp to be passed around the cava with ease. The umbilical tapes are then introduced around each vessel with a curved clamp.

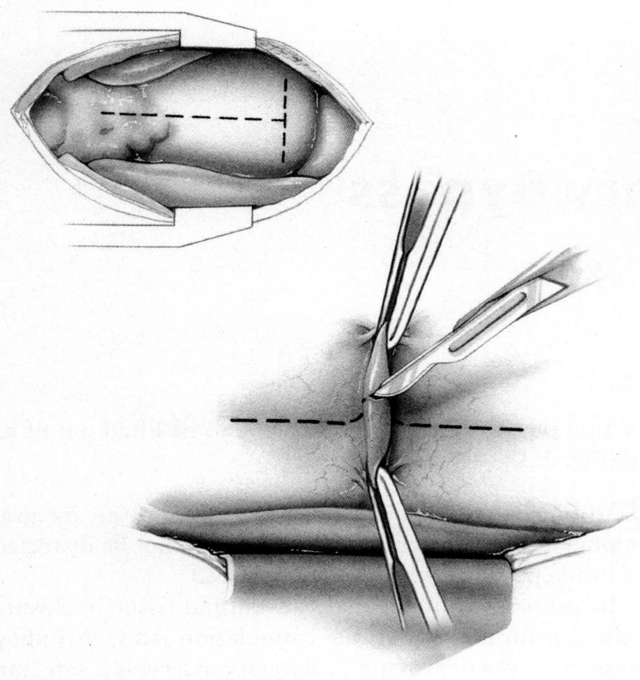

FIG. 2.1 Opening the pericardium.

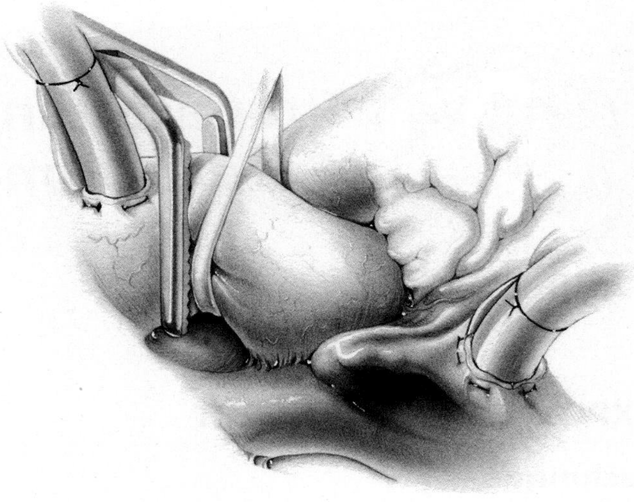

FIG. 2.3 Lifting the aorta from its bed.

⊘ Phrenic Nerve Injury

Dissection around the venae cavae can be cumbersome, particularly if extensive adhesions from previous surgery are present. The right phrenic nerve coursing along the lateral aspect of the cavae and the right atrium on the pleural aspect of the pericardium can easily be injured, either by sharp dissection or injudicious use of cautery. This results in paralysis of the right hemidiaphragm and complicates the ventilatory care of the patient in the postoperative period. The surgeon should therefore attempt to avoid the right phrenic nerve at all costs. ⊘

⊘ Caval Injury

Caval injury is initially controlled digitally. Cardiopulmonary bypass is established, cannulating the aorta and either the inferior vena cava or right atrial appendage, and the problem is managed under direct vision. The site of the tear is brought into view by gently retracting the great vein with an atraumatic tissue forceps, at which time it can be sutured with fine Prolene. On rare occasions when the

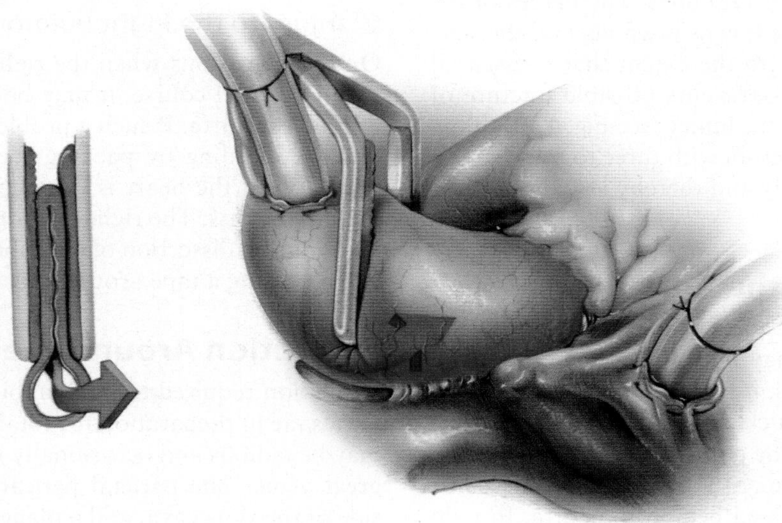

FIG. 2.2 Incomplete cross-clamping of the aorta.

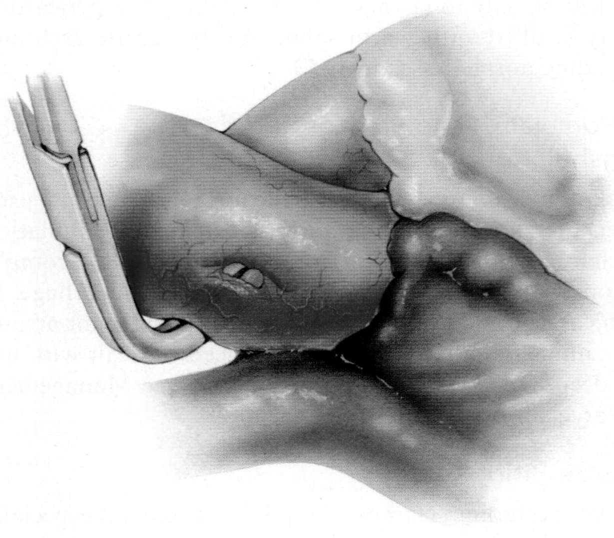

FIG. 2.4 Clamp injury to the aorta.

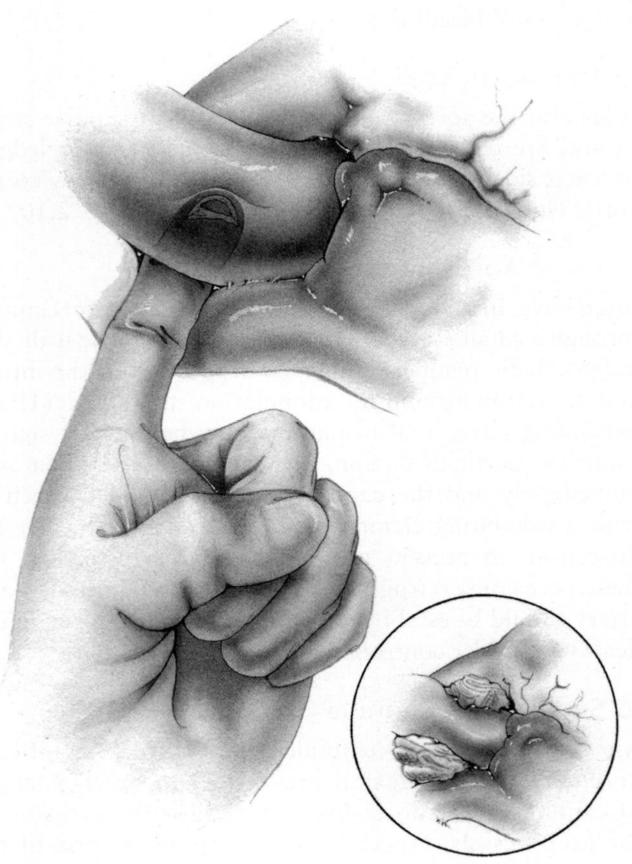

FIG. 2.5 Controlling bleeding after injury to the aorta.

torn caval wall is very friable, the suturing may incorporate an adjacent segment of the intact pericardial wall for buttressing and therefore hemostasis. Tension on the suture

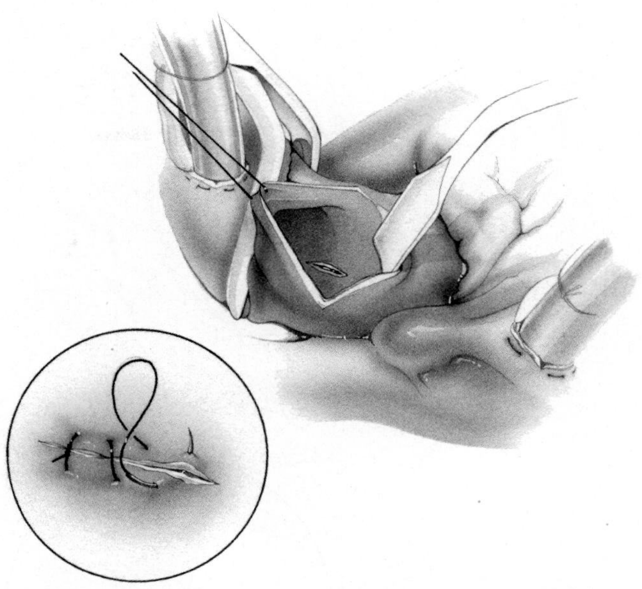

FIG. 2.6 Repair of the posterior wall of the aorta under direct vision.

line is relieved by a curvilinear incision of the pericardium (Fig. 2.8). Alterantively, a patch of autologous or bovine pericardium can be used to repair the vena caval injury. Repair should be done such that there is no hemodynamically significant narrowing of the cavae. ⊘

ARTERIAL CANNULATION

Aortic Cannulation

Technique

Except in a few specific instances, the aorta is directly cannulated for arterial perfusion during cardiopulmonary bypass. Small bites of the adventitia and media as high up on the aorta as feasible are taken with 2-0 or 3-0 Prolene sutures on noncutting needles to form a single or double purse-string. Once the systemic systolic pressure is lowered below 90 mm Hg, a stab wound is made using a 15 blade to scratch the outer layers of the aorta before final entry. The tip of the aortic cannula is then introduced atraumatically into the opening (Fig. 2.9). The sutures can be buttressed with felt or pericardial pledgets to prevent bleeding from the needle holes. The ends of the purse-string sutures, which have passed through a long, narrow rubber or plastic tube, are secured. The tubing is then tied to the aortic cannula and, if desired, further secured to the edges of the wound (Fig. 2.10). The aortic cannula is allowed to fill retrogradely with blood. It is then connected to the arterial line, making sure that all air and foam have been removed from the circuit.

NB In patients undergoing reoperation with scarred aortic walls or pediatric patients, it may be useful to insert an

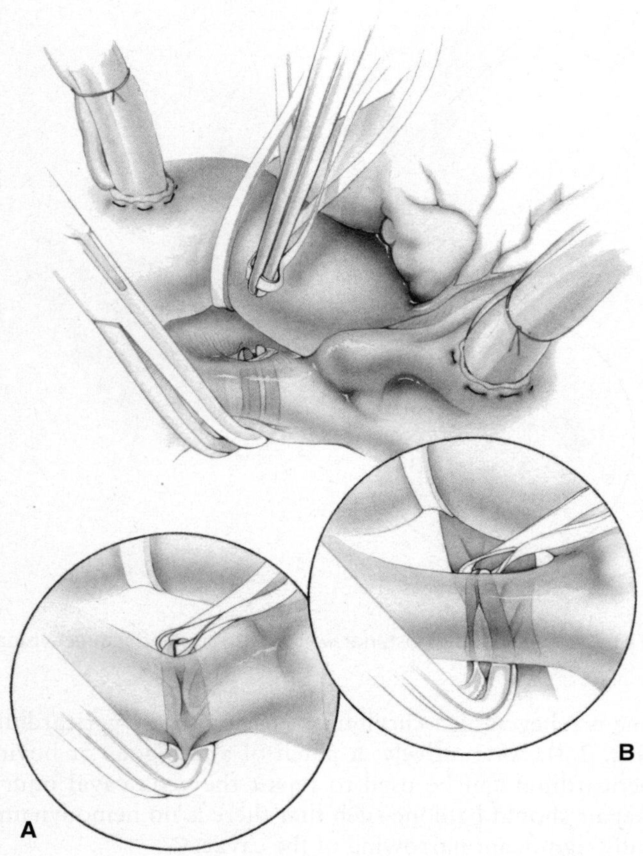

⊘ FIG. 2.7 Injury to the right pulmonary artery and superior vena cava. **A:** The clamp has caught the posterior wall of the superior vena cava. **B:** The clamp has caught the anterior wall of the right pulmonary artery.

appropriately sized Hegar dilator through the stab wound before inserting the aortic cannula. NB

⊘ Aortic Wall Atherosclerosis

Although this technique of aortic cannulation is a generally safe approach, serious vascular complications may nevertheless occur. Transesophageal echocardiography and epiaortic ultrasonographic scan of the ascending aorta are more sensitive for confirmation and localization of atheromatous changes. The aorta should also be routinely palpated for localized thickening and calcific plaques. The site for cannulation should be disease-free if possible. Usually, the anterior aspect of the aorta just proximal to the base of the innominate artery or the segment along the inner curvature of the aorta adjacent to the pulmonary artery is relatively free of calcification. ⊘

NB Epiaortic scanning should be performed before the placement of the purse-string sutures. The transducer is passed into a sterile plastic bag, with the tip coated with lubricating jelly to enhance image quality. The pericardial cavity is filled with warm saline and the aortic arch and ascending aorta are scanned. NB

⊘ Porcelain, Lead Pipe, or Eggshell Aorta

Porcelain, lead pipe, or eggshell aorta is the term used when the entire ascending aorta is calcified. Cannulation or clamping of this kind of aorta has catastrophic complications, namely, stroke and uncontrollable hemorrhage. In such cases, the femoral or axillary artery and right atrium are cannulated and the aorta is replaced or dealt with under deep hypothermic circulatory arrest (see Management of Porcelain Aorta in Chapter 5). ⊘

⊘ Side-Biting Clamps

Partial occluding clamps should be avoided, especially when the aortic pressure is high, unless they are needed to control brisk hemorrhage or other complications. A clamp can crush the diseased wall and give rise to a tear of the intima, resulting in dissection of the aortic wall or disruption with massive bleeding. ⊘

⊘ Thin Aortic Wall

Whenever the aortic wall is thin or friable, the purse-string sutures are reinforced with Teflon or pericardial pledgets on each side of the cannula to prevent any injury to the aortic wall or bleeding from the needle sites (Fig. 2.10). ⊘

⊘ Large Aortic Cannula

Aggressive introduction of too large an aortic cannula through a small aortic opening can tear the aortic wall, dislodge calcific plaques, and cause separation of the intima and dissection around the cannulation site (Fig. 2.11). An expanding adventitial hematoma may be the first sign of traumatic aortic dissection. The cannula must be removed immediately and the cannulation site excluded carefully with a side-biting clamp (which in itself may further the dissection) to prevent progression of the dissection. On these occasions, retrograde perfusion through the femoral artery should be established promptly and the aortic injury dealt with under controlled conditions. ⊘

⊘ Small Aortic Cannula

An excessively small cannula may create a significant gradient in the perfusion pressure. Too great a length of cannula in the aorta may interfere with perfusion of the arch vessels, especially if the tip enters one of the brachiocephalic vessels. The ideal aortic cannula should have a relatively wide but short tip. Although most commercially available cannulas are manufactured with these specifications in mind, the size of the aorta varies in different individuals; therefore, the surgeon must select the appropriate length and width of the cannula judiciously. ⊘

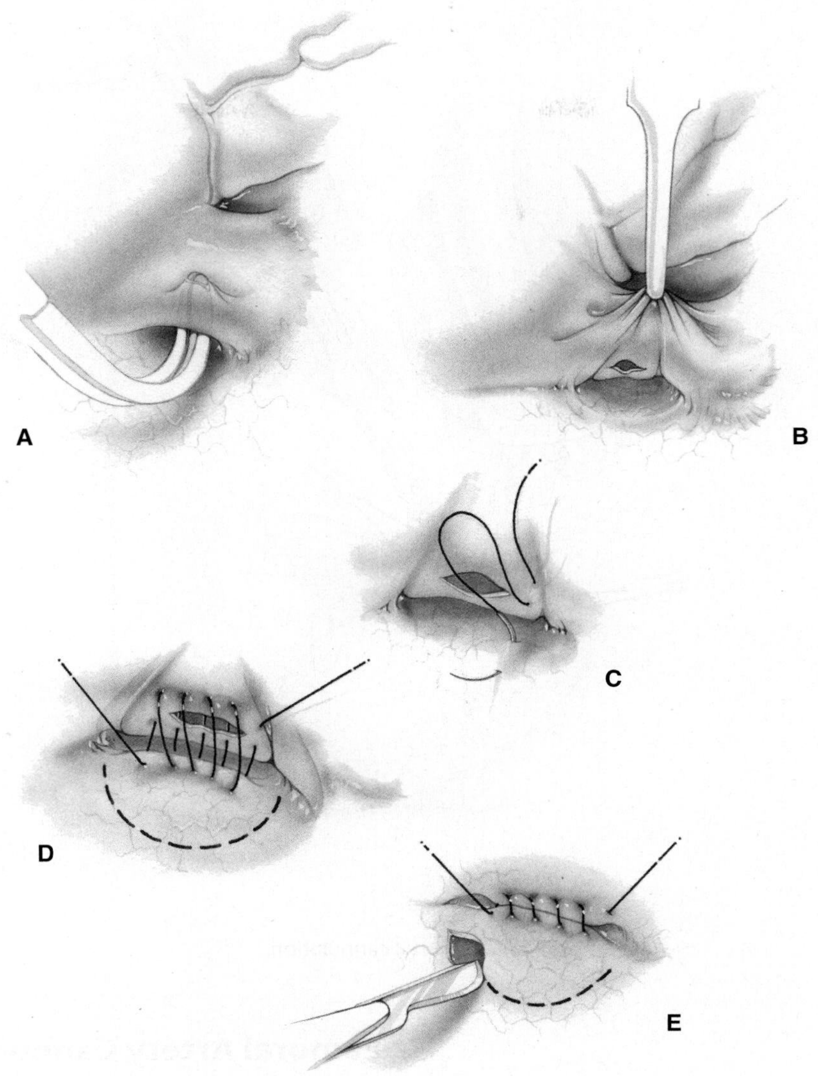

FIG. 2.8 A–E: Technique for repair of vena caval injury.

NB Small-Diameter Aorta

In patients with a relatively small-diameter aorta, the regular cannula may be space occupying, interfering with satisfactory perfusion. Plastic right-angled cannulas have good flow characteristics and will not hit the back wall of the aorta. NB

⊘ Systemic Hypertension

Whenever the systemic pressure is high, aortic decannulation may become hazardous and result in troublesome bleeding. The systemic pressure can be lowered to a satisfactory level by temporarily removing some volume through the venous line. The arterial cannula is then removed and its aortic entry site securely sutured. The arterial line is then connected to the venous cannula, and blood is reinfused as needed. ⊘

A less effective but useful technique is transient lowering of the blood pressure by digital compression of the main pulmonary artery for decannulation purposes. This technique can also be helpful when cannulating the aorta.

NB Repairing Aortic Injury

If the venous lines have already been removed, the cavae can be temporarily clamped, causing the systemic pressure to drop significantly. The aortic cannula is removed, and the now soft, pliable aorta is repaired. The caval clamps are then removed to allow drainage of the venous return into the right atrium. However, it is preferable to recannulate the right atrium and manipulate the blood pressure by adding or removing volume, thereby allowing for safe and controlled aortic repair. NB

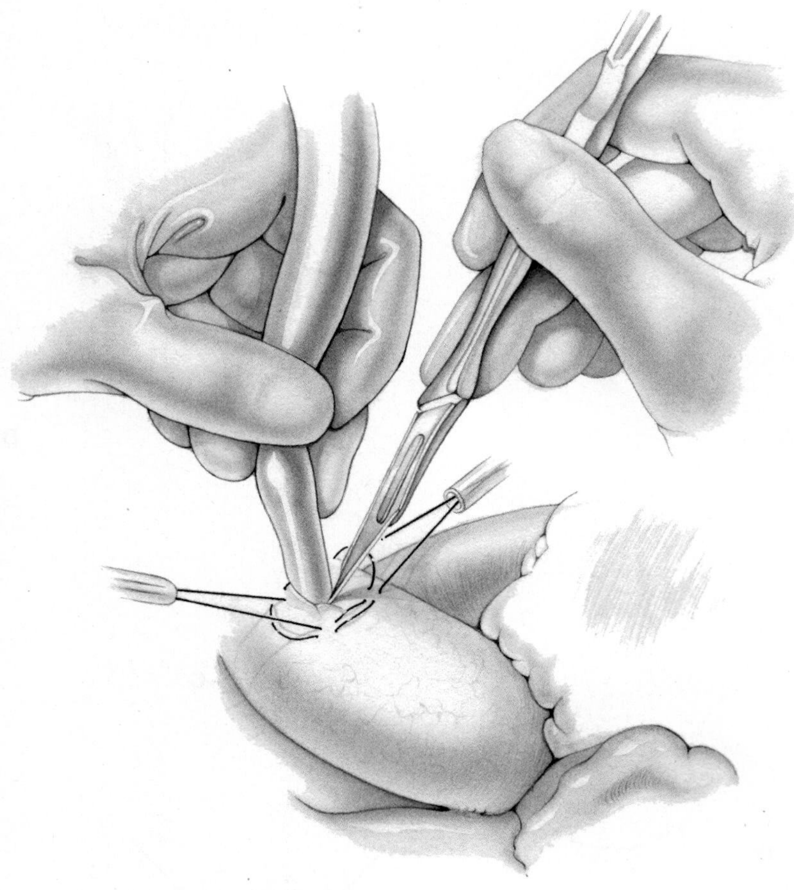

FIG. 2.9 Aortic cannulation.

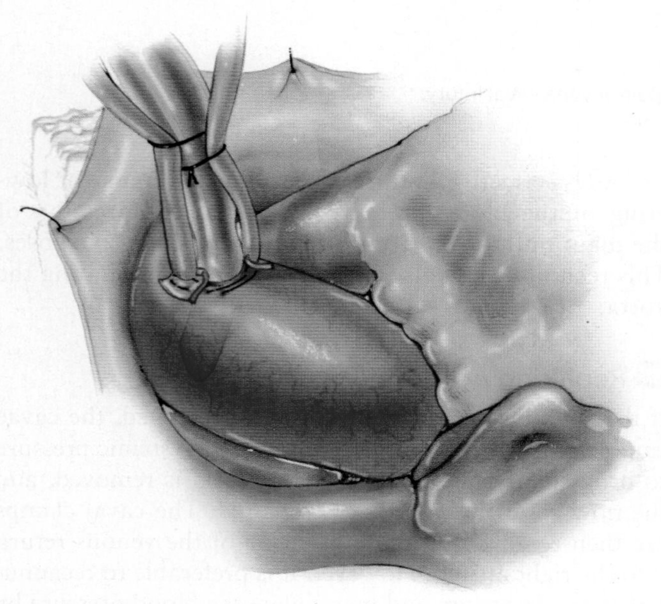

FIG. 2.10 Aortic cannulation, completed.

Femoral Artery Cannulation

Technique

The common femoral artery (or occasionally the external iliac artery) is dissected free for a short distance above the origin of the profunda femoris branch. Umbilical tapes are placed around the common femoral artery above the prospective cannulation site as well as the superficial and profunda arteries distally. Vascular clamps are applied to the femoral artery both above and below the intended arteriotomy site. The profunda artery may be either clamped or snared. A small transverse arteriotomy is made where the arterial wall appears to be relatively normal. A tapered cannula of appropriate size is then gently introduced through a transverse arteriotomy into the arterial lumen and is secured in place (Fig. 2.12A). Alternatively and more commonly, cannulation is performed through a purse-string using the modified Seldinger technique with serial dilations over a semi-stiff wire. The guidewire must be visualized within the descending aorta on echo before any dilation is performed. For closure, proximal and distal clamps are applied and the arteriotomy is closed with interrupted sutures.

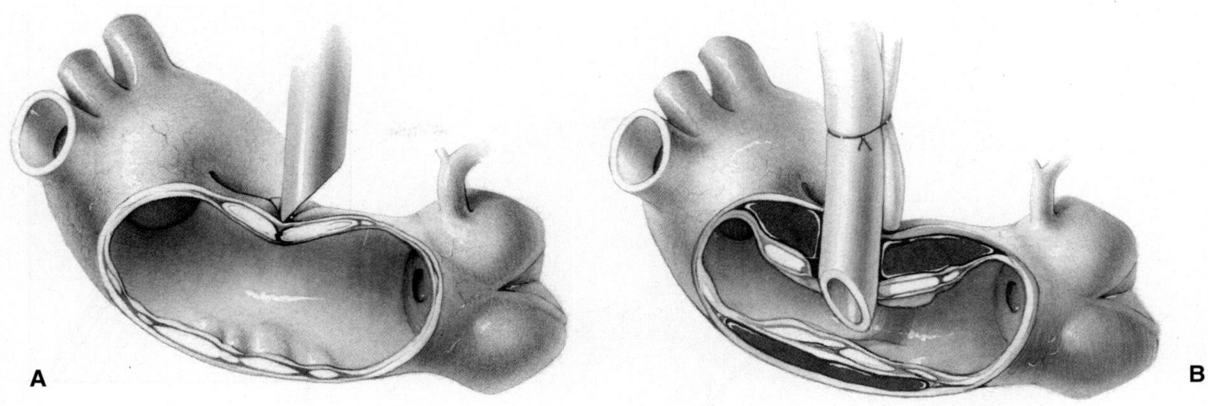

⊘ FIG. 2.11 Traumatic aortic wall dissection during introduction of a cannula.

⊘ Cannula Slippage

The perfusion pressure may cause the cannula to slip out. It should be secured by tying it to the umbilical tape already placed around the artery (Fig. 2.12B). ⊘

⊘ Cannula Injury to the Arterial Wall

The cannula tip may injure the arterial wall and cause separation of intimal plaque, which can result in retrograde aortic dissection (Fig. 2.13). The cannula must never be too large and should be introduced into the arterial lumen in an area that is relatively disease-free. ⊘

⊘ Limb Ischemia Due to Arterial Occlusion

The arterial cannula may occasionally occlude the entire arterial lumen and cause distal malperfusion. This problem is particularly common in younger patients with small arteries and little collateral flow. After cannulation, flow in the distal vessel or the foot should be evaluated using a Doppler. In cases of inadequate flow, a 5 French distal perfusion cannula is inserted distally using Seldinger technique and is attached to the side-arm of the arterial cannula (Fig. 2.14). ⊘

⊘ Injury to the Femoral Artery

A tourniquet or clamp used to tighten the umbilical tape around the proximal femoral artery and cannula may injure the wall of the artery. This can be avoided by placing a peanut sponge under the umbilical tape before tightening it. ⊘

⊘ Femoral Artery Dissection

The surgeon should always look for a column of pulsating blood in the femoral cannula; in the absence of obvious pulsation, it is very likely that the cannula tip is not in the lumen of the vessel. ⊘

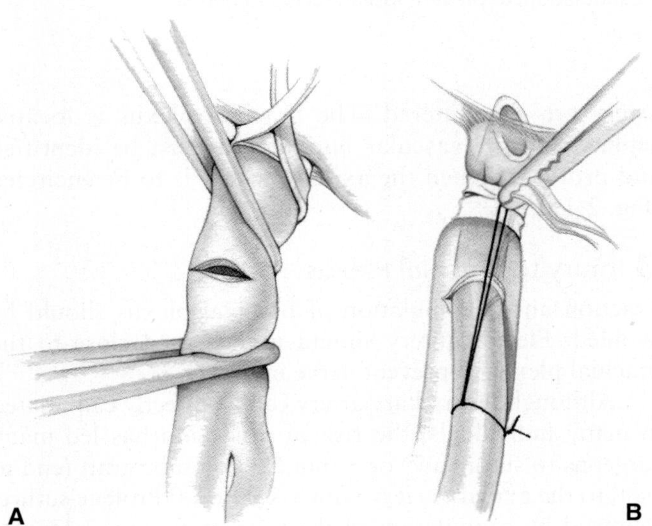

FIG. 2.12 Femoral artery cannulation. **A:** Transverse arteriotomy for introduction of the cannula. **B:** securing the cannula to the umbilical tape.

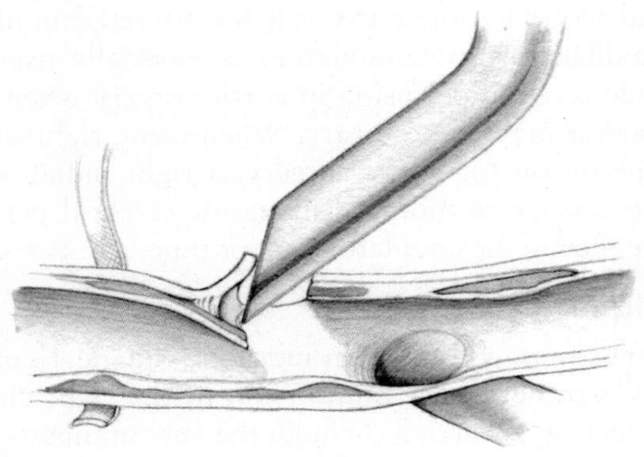

⊘ FIG. 2.13 Cannula injury to the common femoral artery causing retrograde aortic dissection.

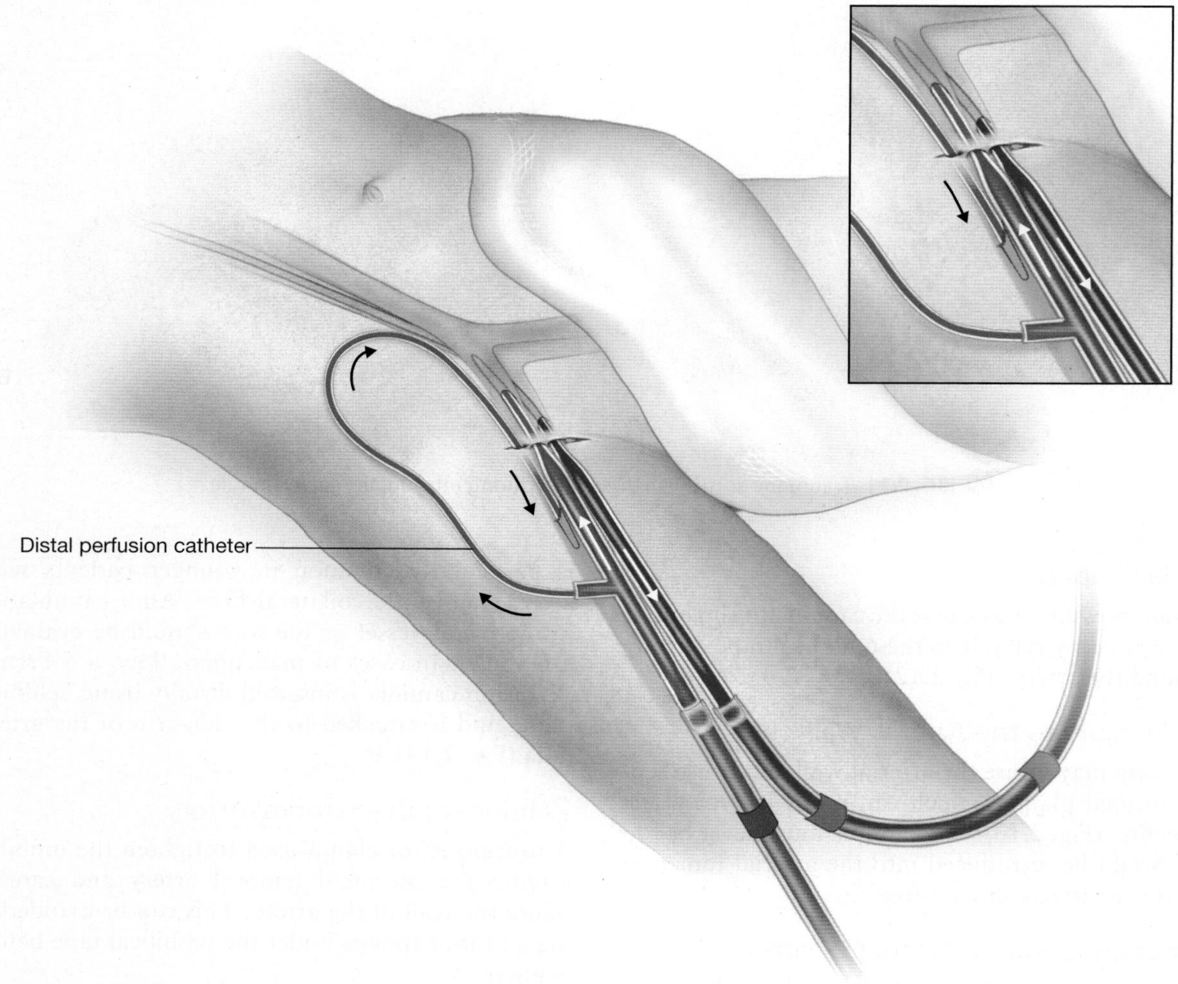

FIG 2.14 Distal perfusion catheter with femoral arterial cannulation, to prevent ipsilateral leg ischemia.

Axillary Artery Cannulation

The axillary artery has emerged as a safe, usually disease-free, and accessible alternative site for arterial cannulation. Right axillary artery cannulation is especially useful for antegrade cerebral perfusion in aortic surgery when circulatory arrest may be necessary. When using right axillary artery perfusion for aortic surgery, a right radial arterial line is necessary to monitor antegrade cerebral perfusion pressure during the circulatory arrest time.

Technique

An approximately 5 to 6 cm incision is made 1 cm inferior and parallel to the midportion of the right clavicle. The dissection is carried through the subcutaneous tissue toward the insertion of the pectoralis minor muscle and the deltopectoral groove. The pectoralis major muscle is dissected and divided along its fibers and the deltopectoral fascia is incised. The axillary vein and then the artery are encountered. The brachial plexus is located cephalad to the vascular bundle and must be identified and protected when the axillary artery is to be encircled (Fig. 2.15).

⊘ Injury to Brachial Plexus

Traction and manipulation of brachial plexus should be avoided. Electrocautery should not be used close to the brachial plexus to prevent nerve injury. ⊘

Although the axillary artery can be directly cannulated in many individuals, the risk of dissection has led many surgeons to suture a 7- or 8-mm Dacron tube graft (end to side) to the axillary artery with a 5-0 or 6-0 Prolene suture, followed by cannulation of the tube graft (Fig. 2.15). At the completion of cardiopulmonary bypass, the base of the tube graft is ligated with two large metal clips flush with the axillary artery wall. The graft is trimmed to 1 cm and the end is oversewn with 5-0 Prolene.

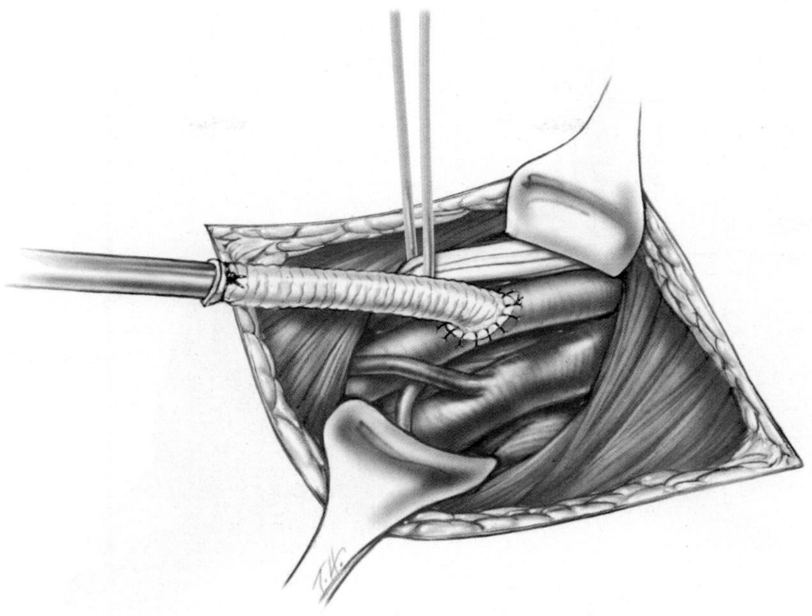

FIG. 2.15 Axillary artery cannulation.

NB Axillary Artery Dissection

In patients with aortic dissection, it is important to ensure that the axillary artery is free of dissection before cannulation. NB

Transapical Aortic Cannulation

In patients with type A aortic dissection, aortic cannulation through the left ventricular apex is another technique that can be utilized.

Technique

A stab incision of 1 cm is made on the anterior wall of left ventricle close to the apex but offset from the LAD. A 22-French aortic cannula with stylet (such as the Edwards Fem-Flex Aortic Cannula) is gently introduced into the left ventricle (Fig. 2.16). It is advanced across the aortic valve into the ascending aorta guided by transesophageal echocardiography. When the cannula is removed, the opening is closed with two or three pledgeted horizontal mattress sutures of 4-0 Prolene.

NB The tip of the cannula must be in the true lumen of the aorta before starting cardiopulmonary bypass. This can be confirmed by transesophageal echocardiography. NB

The cannula is removed from the left ventricle at the beginning of circulatory arrest. Following the anastomosis of the tube graft to the distal aorta, the graft itself is cannulated and cardiopulmonary bypass is resumed.

⊘ Severe Aortic Stenosis

The technique is contraindicated in patients with critical aortic stenosis. The cannula may not pass through the aortic valve. ⊘

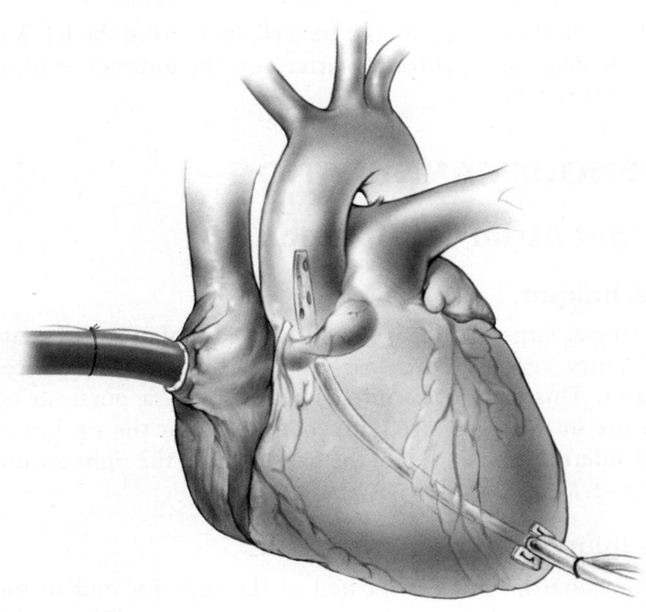

FIG. 2.16 Transapical aortic cannulation; cannula passed across the aortic valve.

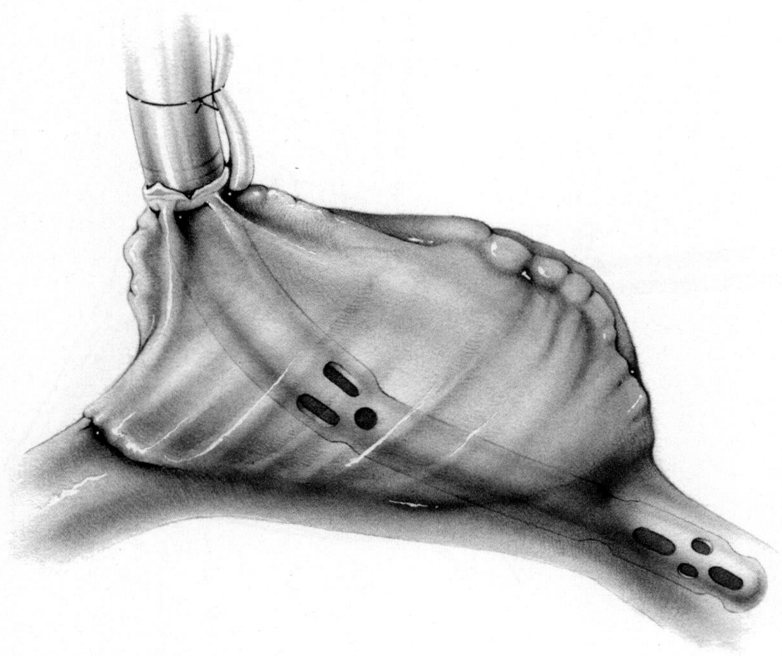

FIG. 2.17 Right atrial cannulation with a single, dual-staged cannula.

⊘ Left Ventricular Wall Bleeding

Purse-string sutures are not required to hold the cannula in place, and may cause troublesome bleeding. ⊘

⊘ Injury to Left Anterior Descending Artery

The cannulation site should be well away from the left anterior descending coronary artery on the anterior wall of the left ventricle. ⊘

VENOUS CANNULATION

Right Atrial Cannulation

Technique

A single, large, dual-stage atriocaval cannula provides satisfactory venous return for most cardiac surgical procedures. This cannula is introduced through a purse-string suture in the right atrial appendage so that the tip lies in the inferior vena cava and the basket lies in the right atrium (Fig. 2.17).

⊘ Injury to the Sinoatrial Node

The sinoatrial node is located at the superior end of the sulcus terminalis near the cavoatrial junction (Fig. 2.18). Injury to the sinoatrial node (Fig. 2.19) may cause temporary conduction disturbances, which can generally be managed with a temporary atrial pacemaker wire and the infusion of isoproterenol or dopamine in the immediate postoperative period. Rarely, it may be necessary to pace the atrium permanently. ⊘

⊘ Injury to the Right Coronary Artery

The right coronary artery follows a course in the right atrioventricular groove. Whenever the right atrial appendage is clamped, usually during cannulation, the sinoatrial node and the right coronary artery are at risk of injury (Fig. 2.20). This is more likely to occur during reoperations. Right coronary artery injury can be treated by bypassing the injured segment with a saphenous vein graft from the aorta to the middle of the right coronary artery (Fig. 2.21). ⊘

⊘ Cannulation Site

When the right atrial appendage is too friable, another site on the atrial wall is selected for cannulation. Bleeding from a tear of the auricle can be controlled with fine Prolene sutures, sometimes reinforced with a small pledget. ⊘

⊘ Atrial Cannulation in Reoperation

In reoperation, the atrial wall is sometimes thin and friable, and its dissection can be tedious and hazardous. It is advantageous to leave a segment of pericardium intact on the atrial wall through which cannulation can be performed safely and securely (Fig. 2.22). ⊘

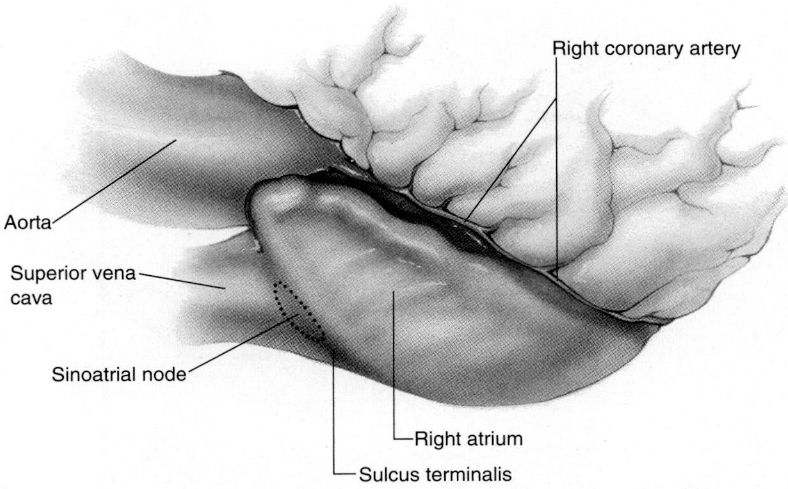

FIG. 2.18 Surgical anatomy of the sinoatrial node and surrounding structures.

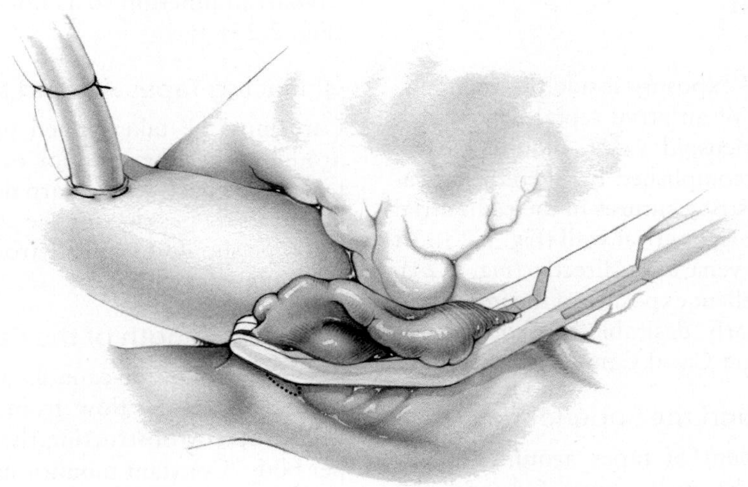

⊘ FIG. 2.19 Clamp injury to the sinoatrial node.

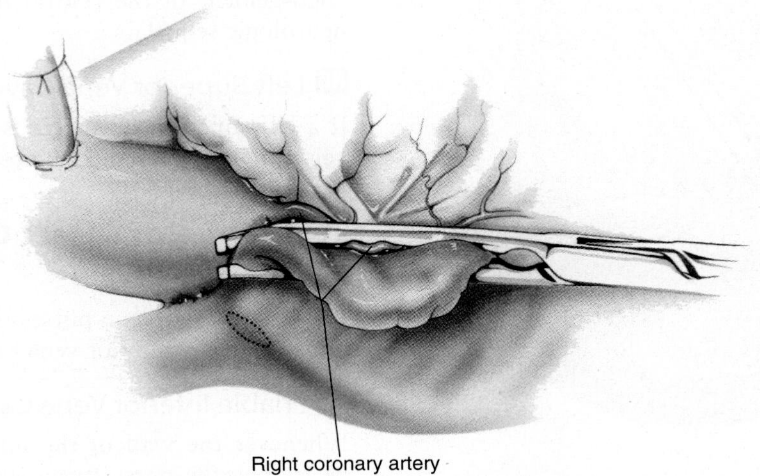

⊘ FIG. 2.20 Clamp injury to the right coronary artery.

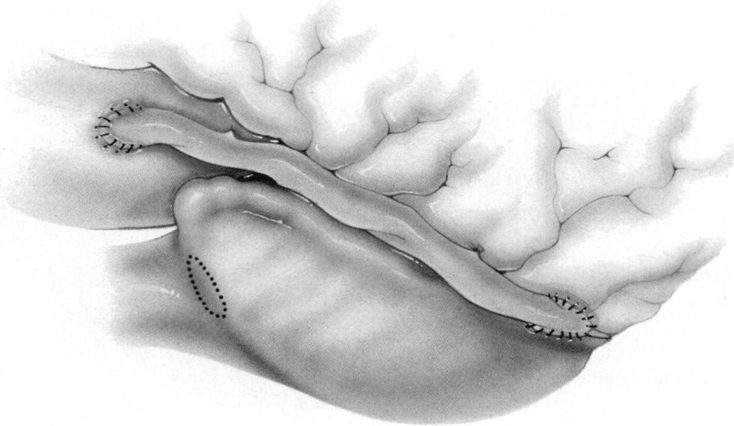

FIG. 2.21 Management of a right coronary artery clamp injury.

Bicaval Cannulation

Technique

Some procedures that entail exposure inside the right side of the heart, such as repair of an atrial septal defect, ventricular septal defect, or tricuspid valve, require bicaval cannulation. This can be accomplished by introducing caval cannulas through purse-string sutures in the right atrial appendage and lower on the right atrial wall (Fig. 2.23). At present, we cannulate each vena cava directly (Fig. 2.24). This technique provides excellent exposure of the intraatrial anatomy, which is particularly desirable in pediatric patients (see Technique of Direct Caval Cannulation section).

⊘ Location of Tape Around the Superior Cava

The actual site for placement of tapes around the superior vena cava should be well above (~1 cm) the cavoatrial junction so as not to injure the sinoatrial node (Fig. 2.23). ⊘

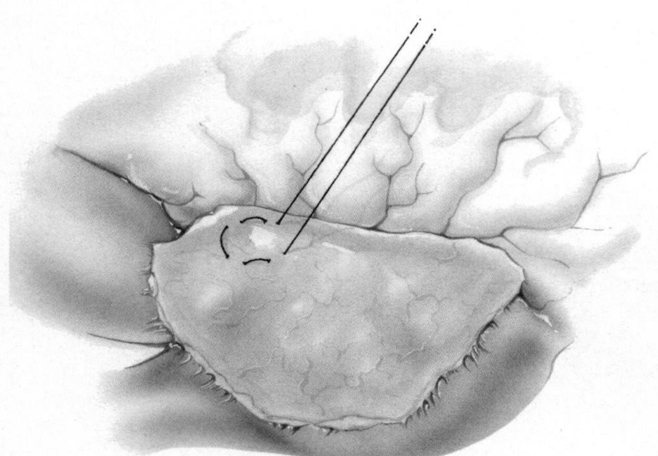

FIG. 2.22 Cannulation through a segment of pericardium left intact on the atrial wall.

⊘ Placing Tapes Around the Cavae

Care must be taken when passing a right-angled clamp around either the superior or inferior vena cava to avoid tearing the back wall. Sharp dissection may be necessary to create a safe passage for the clamp. In addition, the umbilical tape should be pulled around the cava slowly to avoid a sawing injury. ⊘

⊘ Excess Length of the Cannula

Excess length of the cannula in the superior vena cava may interfere with the flow from the azygos and innominate veins, thereby obstructing the venous return from the upper body. Constant monitoring of the pressure in the superior vena cava can reveal any pressure increase and thereby alert the surgical team. Minor manipulation of the cannula usually relieves the obstruction, which can otherwise cause engorgement of the central nervous venous system with neurologic sequela. ⊘

NB Left Superior Vena Cava

If a left superior vena cava is present and no innominate vein is noted, it should be directly cannulated. NB

Technique of Direct Caval Cannulation

Inferior Vena Cava

A 4-0 or 5-0 Prolene purse-string suture is applied at the junction of the inferior vena cava and the right atrium.

NB Friable Inferior Vena Cava Wall

Whenever the wall of the inferior vena cava appears to be friable, the purse-string suture should incorporate the parietal pericardium overlying the diaphragm for added security. However, a curvilinear incision is made on the

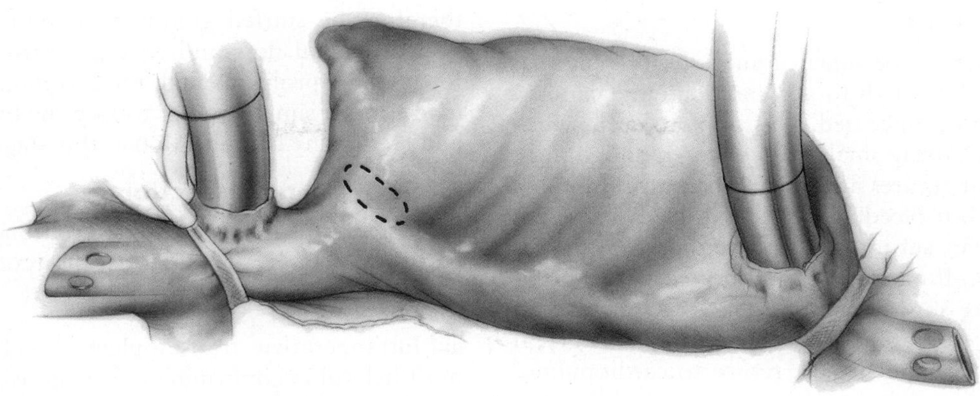

FIG. 2.23 Placement of tapes around the cava in bicaval cannulation.

pericardium 1 to 2 cm from the edge of the suture if it appears to be under tension. NB

A stab wound is made in the center of the purse-string suture. The opening is dilated with a tonsillar clamp. An appropriately sized right-angled cannula is introduced, and the purse-string suture is secured around the cannula.

Superior Vena Cava

The pericardial reflection on the superior vena cava is divided to maximally free up the great vein. A rectangular or oval purse-string suture of 5-0 or 4-0 Prolene is placed in the adventitia of the superior vena cava close to its junction with the innominate vein. The adventitia within the purse-string is divided, and the vein wall is identified and incised with a knife. The opening is enlarged with a tonsillar clamp if necessary. An appropriately sized right-angled cannula is introduced into the lumen, and the purse-string suture is secured. In patients with deep chests, a ringed clamp is used to load the cannula and direct it into the vessel.

Alternatively, with the superior vena caval cannula in place, partial cardiopulmonary bypass is established and the right side of the heart is decompressed. Inferior vena caval cannulation is carried out as just described. This is particularly useful in infants and patients who are hemodynamically unstable.

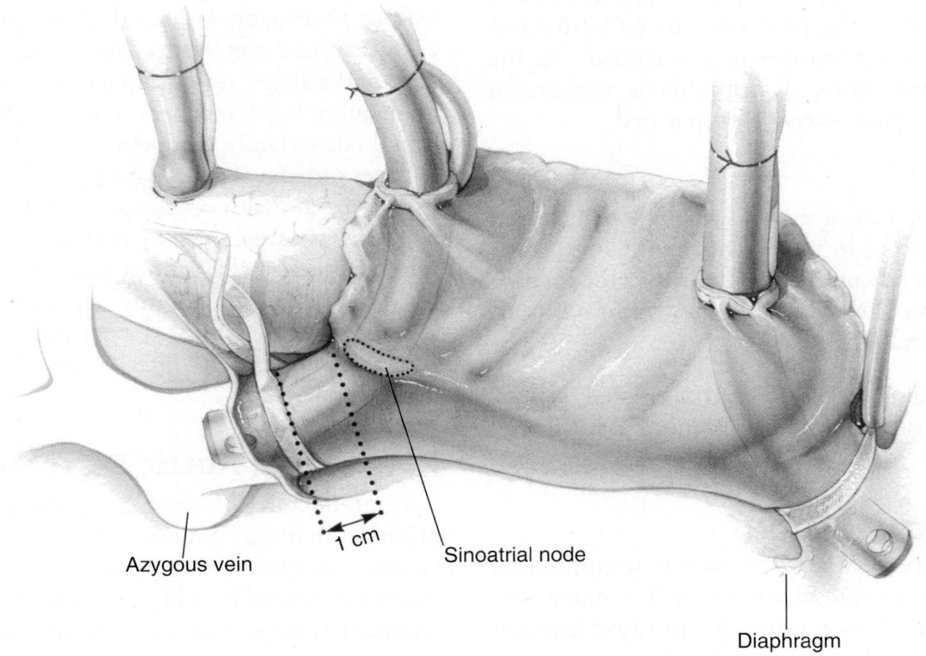

FIG. 2.24 Direct caval cannulation.

⊘ Vena Caval Stenosis

The purse-string suture for superior and inferior venae cavae should be small enough to accommodate the cannula and not cause stenosis once tied. This is apt to occur when the vena cava is relatively small or in children and infants. Occasionally repair sutures are needed to control bleeding once decannulated. If bleeding persists, it is advisable not to place many repair sutures and fix the defect on bypass under direct vision. If narrowing is suspected, direct proximal and distal pressure measurements as well as transesophageal echocardiographic assessment are mandatory. If a significant stenosis is identified, return to cardiopulmonary bypass via direct right atrial cannulation is utilized to repair the caval defect under visualization. ⊘

Femoral Venous Cannulation

If cardiopulmonary bypass is required before or during a redo sternotomy, the venous drainage can be secured by cannulating the femoral vein. This technique is also useful for minimally invasive approaches.

Technique

The femoral vein can be cannulated percutaneously. We prefer to expose the femoral vein through a small incision below the inguinal ligament if simultaneous femoral arterial access is needed. A purse-string suture of 5-0 Prolene is placed on the anterior aspect of the common femoral vein. A long venous cannula with multiple side holes is placed by first passing a guide wire through a needle puncture in the middle of the purse-string stitch. The cannula mounted on a tapered dilator sheath is gently advanced over the guide wire and positioned either in the right atrium or inferior vena cava depending on the procedure to be performed under transesophageal echocardiographic control. At the conclusion of the procedure, the cannula is withdrawn from the vein and the purse-string suture is tied.

⊘ Iliac Vein Injury

Venous cannulas that lack a guidewire often hang up at the pelvic brim, resulting in inadequate venous return. If an attempt is made to advance the cannula into the inferior vena cava, perforation of the iliac vein may occur with catastrophic consequences. ⊘

NB To ensure adequate venous return, assisted venous drainage with a centrifugal pump or vacuum assist is useful. NB

Adequacy of Bypass

Upon initiation of bypass, organ perfusion is compromised by the initial flow of crystalloid volume with minimal oxygen carrying capacity, hypotension due to rapid hemodilution and non-pulsatile flow. This problem is exacerbated when organs including the brain are normothermic at the initiation of bypass. Cardiopulmonary bypass should therefore be started gradually to mitigate this problem. As the arterial flow and venous return increase, a search for possible problems with the cardiopulmonary bypass is made. It is a simple matter to stop the bypass, if necessary, and rectify any complication at this stage of the operation.

Signs of Aortic Dissection

Excessive pressure in the pump line concomitant with low perfusion pressure signals aortic dissection (see Retrograde Aortic Dissection section).

NB Intraoperative transesophageal echocardiography is most helpful in confirming this diagnosis. NB

Only awareness and prompt diagnosis of this complication followed by immediate cessation of cardiopulmonary bypass can ensure patient survival. The cannulation site must be switched from the ascending aorta to one of the femoral arteries, and cardiopulmonary bypass must be reestablished as expeditiously as possible. This permits the continuation of the surgery. The reversal of blood flow into the lumen of the arterial system obliterates the false channel and stops the progression of aortic dissection. The problem of ascending aortic injury is then addressed in a controlled situation (see Traumatic Disruption and Dissection of the Ascending Aorta section).

Improper Positioning of Caval Cannula

A decrease in venous return causes distention of the heart. The decrease can be due to a kink in the venous line, impaction of the basket of the dual-stage atriocaval cannula against the atrial wall, or improper positioning of the caval cannulas. The inferior vena caval cannula can be too far down obstructing the hepatic vein drainage, which can lead to postoperative liver dysfunction. The superior vena caval cannula can be too high, interfering with innominate and azygos vein drainage. As mentioned previously, inadequate head and neck venous return can result in cerebral edema and postoperative neurologic complications. In cases of bicaval cannulation, cardiopulmonary bypass is usually begun with only superior vena caval return, and its adequacy is ascertained by noting the volume of venous return and the central venous pressure. If the central venous pressure remains high, the superior vena caval cannula is moved around until a near-zero central venous pressure is achieved. The inferior vena caval cannula is then unclamped.

Retrograde Aortic Dissection

Retrograde aortic dissection is indeed a catastrophic complication that may follow femoral or external iliac cannulation. A diseased artery, faulty cannulation technique, and trauma produced by a high-velocity perfusion jet are major factors that may cause a tear of the intima with medial separation. It is therefore essential to introduce an adequately sized, beveled, smooth cannula into a relatively normal vessel in an atraumatic manner. The perfusion should be

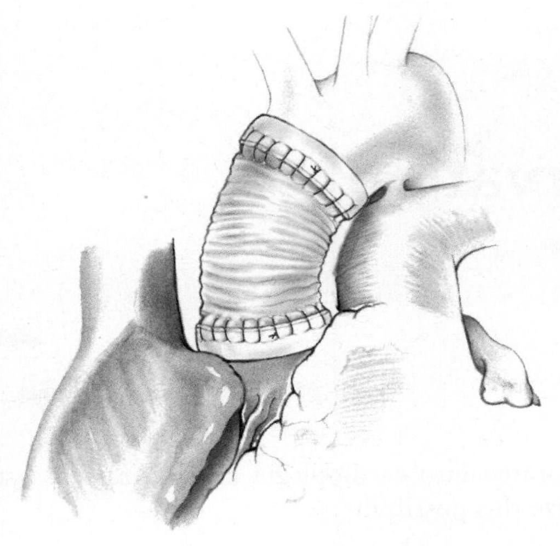

FIG. 2.25 Use of a Hemashield tube graft for aortic disruption.

started gradually, with the surgeon being cognizant at all times of the possible occurrence of aortic dissection. The most significant diagnostic feature is low flow with high arterial line pressure in the circuit. The arterial return into the false lumen is responsible for excessive pressure in the arterial line while the actual perfusion of the patient is inadequate. This leads to a decrease in venous return. If this complication occurs, perfusion should be immediately stopped. The femoral artery or the external iliac artery on the opposite side should then be cannulated if not involved; otherwise, the ascending aorta, the subclavian or axillary artery must be cannulated.

Traumatic Disruption and Dissection of the Ascending Aorta

Intraoperative traumatic dissection or disruption of the ascending aorta is a rare but dramatic complication of open-heart surgery. The areas of aortic cannulation, the proximal anastomosis of an aortocoronary saphenous vein graft, and an aortotomy done for exposure of the aortic valve are the usual sites prone to such a complication. This is especially so in reoperative procedures. Although faulty techniques always predispose a surgical procedure to complications, poor tissue quality and the presence of infection are the most common key precipitating factors in the development of aortic injury. The only preventive measure is awareness of the possibility of such complications and meticulous surgical technique in handling the tissues. In most cases, the torn segment of the aorta will be excised with an arrested heart and replaced with a Hemashield tube graft (Meadox Medicals, Oakland, NJ) (Fig. 2.25).

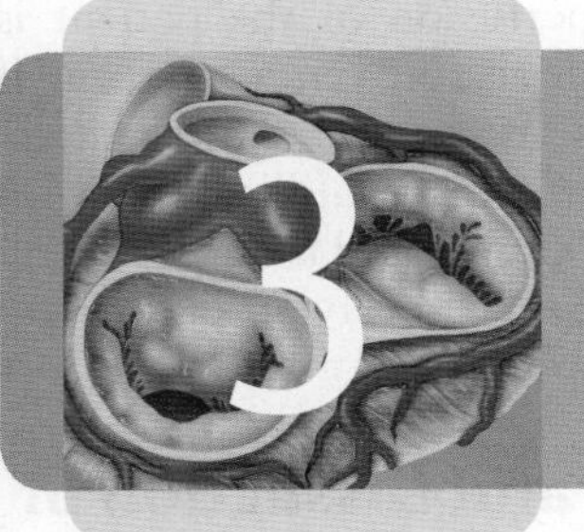

3 Myocardial Preservation

Myocardial protection has clearly made open-heart surgery a safe and reproducible technique. There continues to be many modifications of the chemical composition of the cardioplegic solution, the optimal temperature (cold or warm), and the route of infusion (antegrade or retrograde). As the concepts of myocardial preservation and surgical approaches have evolved, improved cannulas and cardioplegia delivery systems have been introduced.

AORTIC ROOT INFUSION TECHNIQUE

The cannula is introduced into the root of the aorta through a 4-0 Prolene, one-and-a-half-circle purse-string suture that is snugged down and secured to the cannula. Although any large-bore needle or cannula is satisfactory, those with a trocar introducer and a side arm for direct intraaortic pressure monitoring are most useful. The side arm can also be used for venting.

⊘ Insufficient Infusion Pressure

Distortion of, or insufficient pressure in, the aortic root may prevent adequate coaptation of the aortic valve leaflets, as will aortic valve insufficiency. The cardioplegic solution passes through the open valve and overdistends the left ventricle, which can cause direct myocardial injury. Digital pressure on the right ventricular outflow tract at the level of the aortic annulus may produce coaptation of the leaflets and prevent regurgitation of the cardioplegic solution. ⊘

⊘ Excessive Infusion Pressure

Excessive infusion pressure can traumatize the coronary arteries, resulting in ischemic myocardial injury. Accurate monitoring of the infusion pressure in the aortic root can be satisfactorily accomplished from the side arm of specially designed cannulas. ⊘

⊘ Air Embolism

Air embolism to the coronary arteries can cause serious myocardial injury. Every effort must be made to clear the cardioplegic line of any air bubbles. A bubble trap is now incorporated into cardioplegia administration systems to minimize this possibility. ⊘

⊘ Impurities in the Cardioplegic Solution

Impurities and particulate matter may be present in the cardioplegic solution and can occlude terminal coronary arteries, causing myocardial injury. Quality control in the preparation of the cardioplegic solution prevents such complications. ⊘

⊘ Warm Cardioplegic Solution

Between infusions, the cardioplegic solution remaining in the tubing warms up. The warm solution should be flushed out through either the free arm of the Y connecting tube or into the vent before infusion into the coronary system. ⊘

NB Maintaining Uniform Cooling

Uniform cooling of the myocardium by infusion of cold cardioplegic solution is an integral part of myocardial protection. At some institutions, temperature probes in various parts of the septum and ventricular wall are used to monitor myocardial temperature during the course of the surgery. We typically utilize moderate systemic hypothermia, insulating pads, and topical cooling on the right ventricular surface in order to ensure uniform cooling. NB

⊘ Inadequate Protection of the Right Ventricle

Despite all precautions to keep the heart cool, the anterior surface of the heart tends to rewarm because of the ambient air temperature and the heat radiated from the operating room lights. A gauze pad soaked with cold saline and ice placed over the heart provides additional protection for the right ventricle. ⊘

NB Topical Hypothermia

Placement of an insulating pad, a commercially available cooling "jacket," or a cold lap pad behind the heart can minimize rewarming of the heart by the warmer blood in the descending aorta during the cardioplegic arrest. Care must be taken to avoid cold injury to the left phrenic nerve. NB

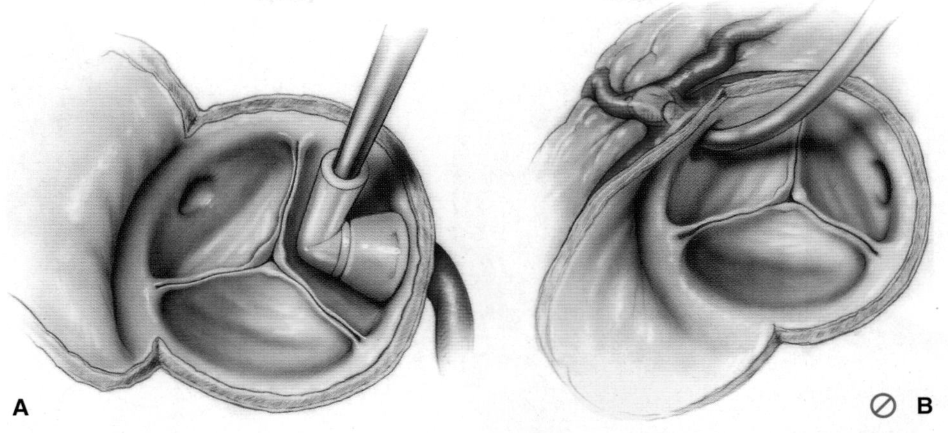

FIG. 3.1 **A:** Hand-held cannula for direct infusion into the coronary artery. **B:** Cannula advanced into the coronary artery causing obstruction at the bifurcation.

DIRECT CORONARY ARTERY PERFUSION

When the aortic root is to be opened, as during aortic valve replacement, cardioplegic solution is administered directly into each coronary ostium with a cannula (Fig. 3.1A). This technique is equally useful in patients who have more than mild insufficiency of the aortic valve.

⊘ Cannula Damage to Coronary Ostium

Excessive pressure from the cannula against the coronary ostium can cause an intimal tear or late ostial stenosis. ⊘

⊘ Size of the Cannula

The cannula must be the correct size, and only a snug fit is necessary to prevent leakage. A cannula head that is too large or excessive pressure on the coronary ostium may not only interfere with satisfactory perfusion of the coronary system but can also traumatize the coronary ostium. ⊘

⊘ Short Left Main Coronary Artery

The cannula can also interfere with satisfactory infusion of cardioplegic solution if the left main coronary artery is short. A branching artery may have its origin very near the ostium of the left main artery and therefore be obstructed by the head of the cannula itself (Fig. 3.1B). Prior knowledge of this anatomy allows the surgeon to take preventive measures. The use of a cannula with side holes prevents this complication. A flexible, hand-held, soft-tipped cannula with a collar around the tip can provide satisfactory infusion of cardioplegic solution directly into the coronary arteries (Fig. 3.1A). The collar presses against the aortic wall and the coronary ostium to prevent spillage of cardioplegic solution into the aorta. ⊘

MYOCARDIAL PRESERVATION BY THE RETROGRADE PERFUSION METHOD

Retrograde infusion of cardioplegic solution into the coronary sinus is very efficient, although its effectiveness in perfusing the right atrium, right ventricle, and inferior wall of the left ventricle may not always be adequate. The technique provides retrograde perfusion of segments of myocardium that may not be equally perfused by the antegrade route in patients with severe coronary artery disease. To ensure optimal myocardial protection, an integrated method of antegrade and retrograde cardioplegia delivery is used in most centers.

Almost all retrograde cannulas are dual lumen to allow infusion of cardioplegic solution and monitoring of pressure in the coronary sinus. A balloon, manually inflatable or self-inflating, surrounds the distal body of the cannula, approximately 1 cm from the tip, proximal to the flow holes. A stylet is provided for ease of proper placement.

Technique

Through a stab incision in the center of a 4-0 Prolene purse-string suture in the mid-atrium, a special retroplegia cannula is introduced and directed into the coronary sinus. The correct position of the cannula is verified by palpation or echocardiography. The stylet is withdrawn when the cannula is in a satisfactory position. The purse-string suture ends are snugged through a tourniquet, which is then tied to the cannula.

NB When difficulty is experienced in placing the retrograde cannula, it is often possible to elevate the decompressed

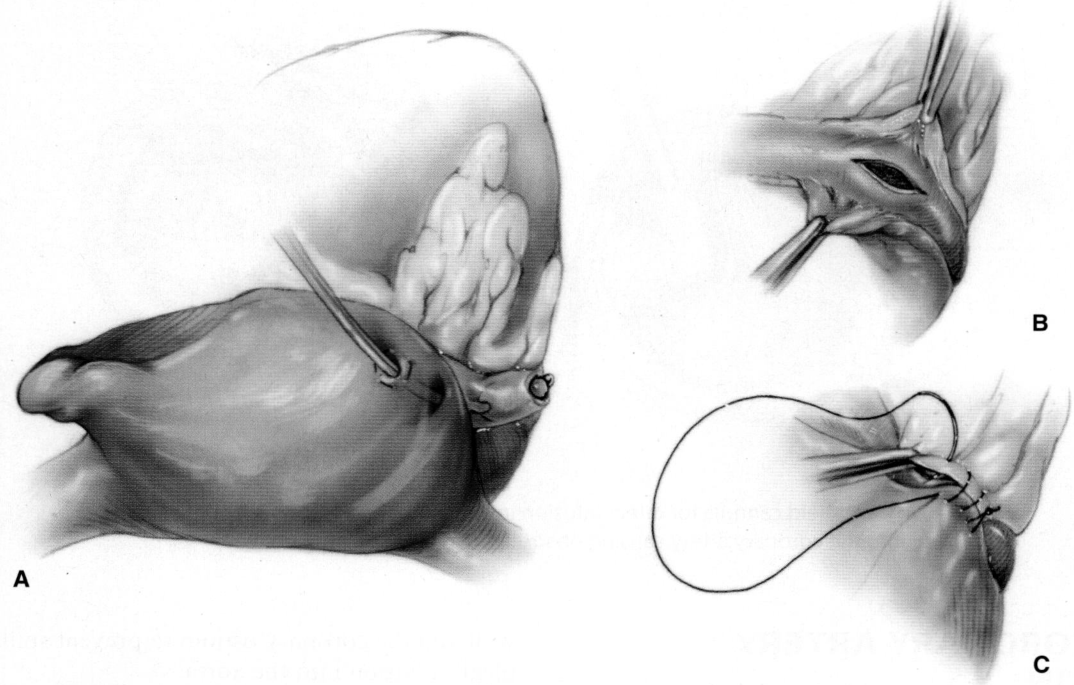

FIG. 3.2 **A:** Perforation of the coronary sinus by a retrograde cannula. **B:** Coronary sinus tear. **C:** Suture closure of the coronary sinus tear using epicardial tissue.

heart while on bypass, visualize the course of coronary sinus, and direct the cannula tip. NB

NB Intraoperative transesophageal echocardiography can often be helpful in directing the cannula along the course of the coronary sinus and verifying the correct position of the cannula. This is particularly important when performing cardiac surgery through minimally invasive incisions. NB

⊘ Perforation of the Coronary Sinus

The stylet and cannula must be guided into the coronary sinus very gently and not be advanced if any resistance is encountered. The coronary sinus wall is very thin and can be perforated by the stylet or the cannula tip. ⊘

A tear in the coronary sinus must be dealt with by closing the epicardium carefully over the tear with a fine Prolene suture (Fig. 3.2). Alternatively, it is patched with a piece of autologous pericardium when the patient is on full cardiopulmonary bypass to prevent stenosis or occlusion of the coronary sinus.

NB Monitoring Infusion Pressure

The infusion pressure must be kept above 20 mm Hg and below 45 mm Hg in order to achieve effective myocardial perfusion and avoid edema and coronary sinus rupture. To accomplish this, the position of the cannula or the flow rate must be adjusted accordingly. NB

NB Monitoring Temperature

The perfusionist monitors the temperature of the cardioplegic solution as it leaves the delivery system. The temperature can also be monitored as the solution enters the coronary sinus through some specially designed retrograde cannulas. NB

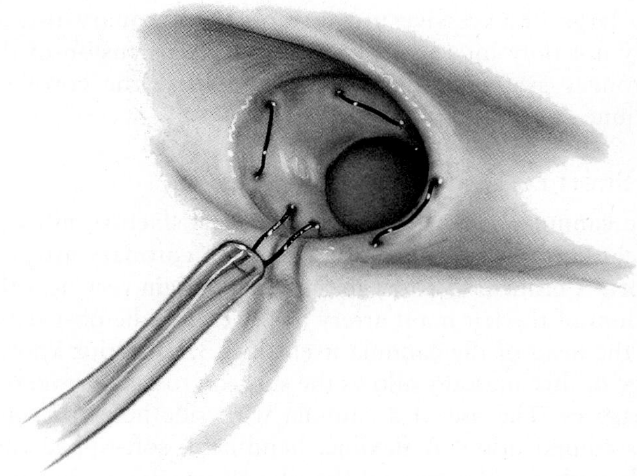

FIG. 3.3 Purse-string suture within the coronary sinus for direct placement of the cannula.

⊘ Spillage of Cardioplegic Solution into the Right Atrium

When the balloon is inflated, it should minimize the amount of cardioplegic solution that enters the right atrium. Cannulas with manually inflatable balloons are usually more effective in preventing backflow. ⊘

⊘ Inadequate Infusion of Cardioplegic Solution into the Right Coronary Vein

If the cannula is advanced too far into the coronary sinus, the inflated balloon may obstruct the right coronary vein–coronary sinus junction, thereby preventing any direct infusion of cardioplegic solution into the distribution of the right coronary vein. ⊘

Retrograde Cardioplegic Infusion by the Open Technique

When bicaval cannulation has been performed and the right atrium is opened, cardioplegic solution can also be administered directly into the coronary sinus. The balloon of the cannula is kept within the ostium of the coronary sinus with a purse-string suture of 4-0 or 5-0 Prolene to prevent leakage of cardioplegic solution into the right atrium (Fig. 3.3). This technique is particularly useful in pediatric cardiac surgery. Alternatively, a catheter with a manually inflatable balloon is used. The balloon is inflated snugly to prevent backflow and to secure it in the appropriate position.

⊘ Injury to the Conduction Tissue

The purse-string suture must be placed on the inside of the coronary sinus ostium to prevent injury to the conduction tissue. ⊘

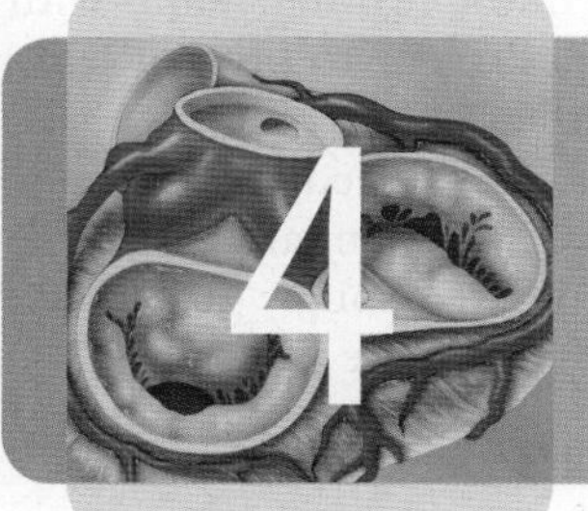

4 Venting and Dearing of the Heart

Venting of the left side of the heart is an effective technique for cardiac decompression and air removal. It is particularly useful when a dry field is desired for precise repair of intracardiac defects.

LEFT VENTRICULAR APICAL VENTING

The apex of the left ventricle provides a satisfactory and accessible site for venting and is particularly effective for removal of air trapped in the ventricular cavity. However, it is rarely used today. Its relevance becomes important when left ventricular venting is necessary before repeat sternotomy (see Repeat Sternotomy section in Chapter 1).

Technique

The region of the left ventricular apex may be thin walled and covered by fat. The site chosen for insertion of the vent must be well away from the branches of the coronary arteries and free of loose myocardial fat. There can be bleeding from this ventricular site after removal of the vent catheter.

A double-armed, 2-0 nonabsorbable suture is passed in a U-shaped fashion through a suitable site near the left ventricular apex buttressed with rectangular Teflon felt pledgets. The distance between the stitches on the Teflon felt should be equal to the diameter of the vent catheter. The suture ends are then passed through a narrow plastic tube as a tourniquet.

With a no. 11 knife blade, a 3- to 4-mm incision is made in the center of the U-shaped stitch. This opening in the left ventricular apex is then dilated with a hemostat so that the vent catheter can be introduced gently into the left ventricle. The tourniquet is then snugged down and secured to the vent catheter. If any catheter side hole remains outside the heart, the vent will be ineffective.

When the heart is beating, gravity siphonage of the vent is usually adequate to decompress the heart and/or remove trapped air bubbles. When the heart is fibrillating or motionless, particularly after the administration of cardioplegia, the vent should be connected to gentle suction with adequate negative pressure to decompress the heart. When the catheter is removed, the U-shaped stitch is tied down snugly and, if necessary, reinforced with a few simple sutures.

⊘ Length of the Catheter

When an excessive length of the catheter is introduced into the left ventricle, its tip may traverse the aortic valve and drain much of the pump flow. This rare problem can occur particularly in infants and small children (Fig. 4.1). ⊘

⊘ Suction Injury

Excessive suction can damage the left ventricular endocardium. For this reason, some vents have a double lumen and the second lumen can be left open to air. Alternatively, and probably a safer technique, the vent tubing can be vented with a one-way valve. ⊘

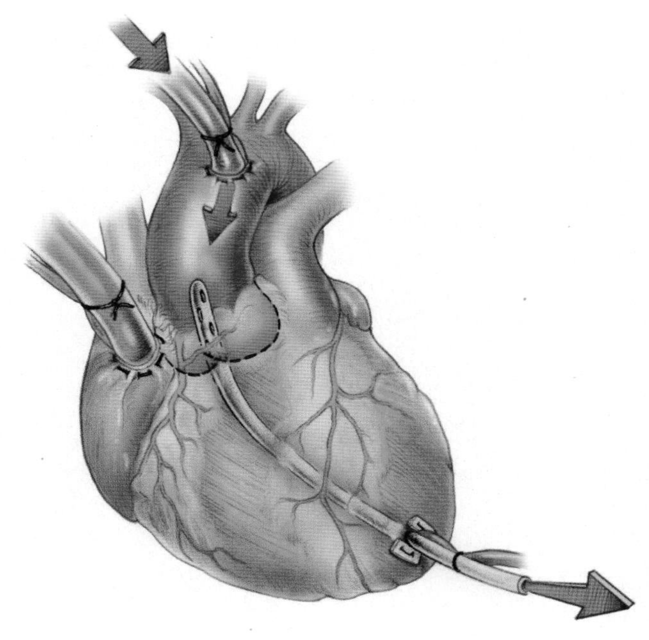

FIG. 4.1 A vent catheter in the left ventricle crossing the aortic valve; pump flow is being suctioned.

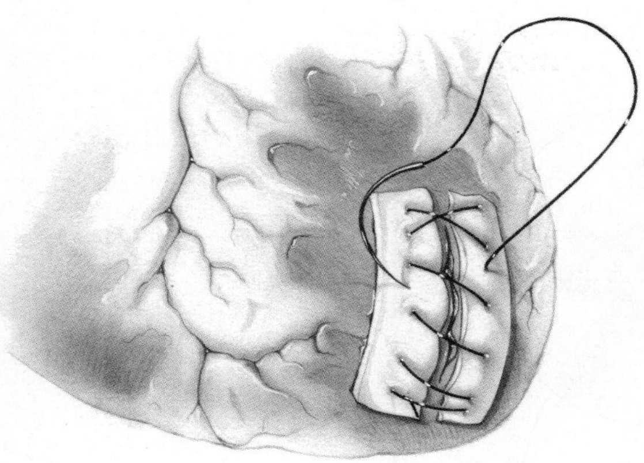

FIG. 4.2 Repair of a tear in the left ventricular apex.

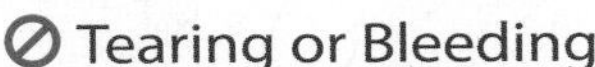

⊘ Tearing or Bleeding

When there is a tear or excessive bleeding from the left ventricular apex, the heart is decompressed. Long strips of Teflon felt with nonabsorbable sutures are used to repair the tear, as in techniques for resection of a left ventricular aneurysm (Fig. 4.2). This is probably most safely accomplished with the heart arrested with cardioplegia. ⊘

⊘ Air in the Ventricular Cavity

If suction is too great or the apical opening is too large, air may be sucked into the left ventricular cavity around the vent site. ⊘

VENTING THROUGH THE RIGHT SUPERIOR PULMONARY VEIN

Venting through the right superior pulmonary vein is convenient, effective, and our technique of choice. After clamping the aorta, through a stab wound in the center of a rectangular or oval purse-string suture on the right superior pulmonary vein, the vent catheter is introduced into the left atrium and through the mitral valve into the left ventricle. The purse-string suture is then passed through a narrow rubber tube and snugged down (Fig. 4.3).

⊘ Dissecting the Adventitia with the Suture

The adventitia within the purse-string suture over the right superior pulmonary vein should be dissected free to prevent any obstruction to the smooth insertion of the vent catheter. ⊘

⊘ Injury to the Phrenic Nerve

When placing sutures on the right superior pulmonary vein, care should be taken to avoid the phrenic nerve, which runs on the parietal pericardium along the anterolateral aspect of the right superior pulmonary vein. This is more likely to occur in reoperations. ⊘

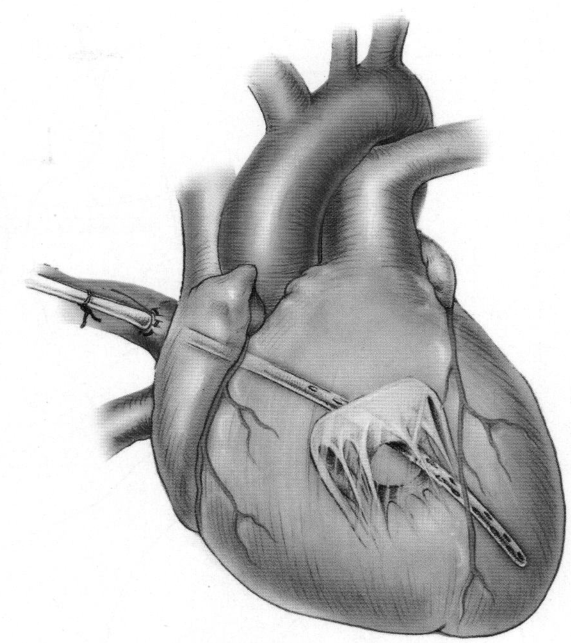

FIG. 4.3 Venting through the right superior pulmonary vein.

NB Reinforcing the Suture

When tissues are thin and friable, the purse-string suture should be reinforced with Teflon felt. NB

⊘ Air Embolism

Air embolism can be eliminated by cross-clamping the aorta or fibrillating the heart before placing the vent catheter. ⊘

⊘ Vent Injury

The catheter should be introduced gently and allowed to cross the mitral valve into the left ventricle without excessive force to prevent injury of the mitral valve or perforation of the left atrium or left ventricle. This complication is more likely when the heart becomes flaccid after infusion of cold cardioplegic solution. An unexplained pooling of blood in the pericardial cavity should herald the occurrence of such a catastrophe. The tear should be located and repaired with pledgeted sutures before continuing with the operation (Fig. 4.4). ⊘

NB Difficulty Introducing Vent into Left Atrium

Sometimes the vent will not pass easily into the left atrium. In these cases, the vent can be positioned after the heart is opened by passing a right-angled clamp through an atrial septal defect or patent foramen ovale

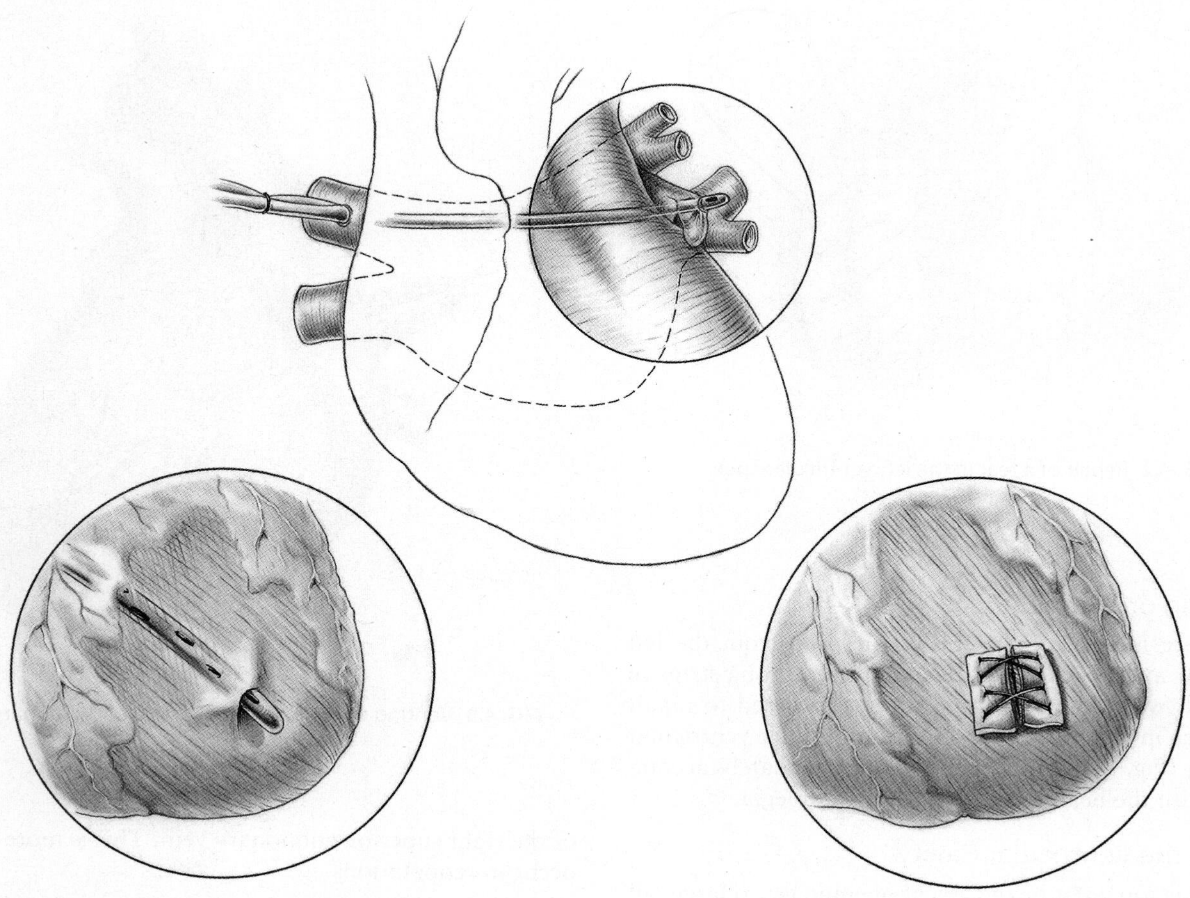

FIG. 4.4 Vent injuries to the left ventricle and left atrium.

into the opening on the right superior pulmonary vein. The vent is then pulled into the left atrium and positioned appropriately. NB

VENTING THROUGH THE SUPERIOR ASPECT OF THE LEFT ATRIUM

The left heart can also be vented through the superior aspect of the left atrium between the aorta and superior vena cava. This technique is similar to that described earlier for the right superior pulmonary vein. It is rarely used because it is cumbersome and control of bleeding from the vent site can be difficult (Fig. 4.5).

PULMONARY ARTERY VENTING

A simple but highly effective method to decompress the heart is to introduce a vent catheter through a purse-string suture on the anterior surface of the pulmonary artery (Fig. 4.6). This technique prevents overdistention of both the right and left sides of the heart without the risk of systemic air embolism.

⊘ Pulmonary Artery Tear

The wall of the pulmonary artery may at times be paper thin and delicate, resulting in a tear at the vent site. This can be prevented by using pledgets on the purse-string suture. The pulmonary artery tear, if it occurs, can easily be repaired with direct suturing reinforced with pledgets. ⊘

VENTING THROUGH THE FORAMEN OVALE

We have found venting the left atrium and left ventricle through the foramen ovale in patients with congenital heart disease very useful. With this technique, a dry field is maintained for precise repair of heart defects.

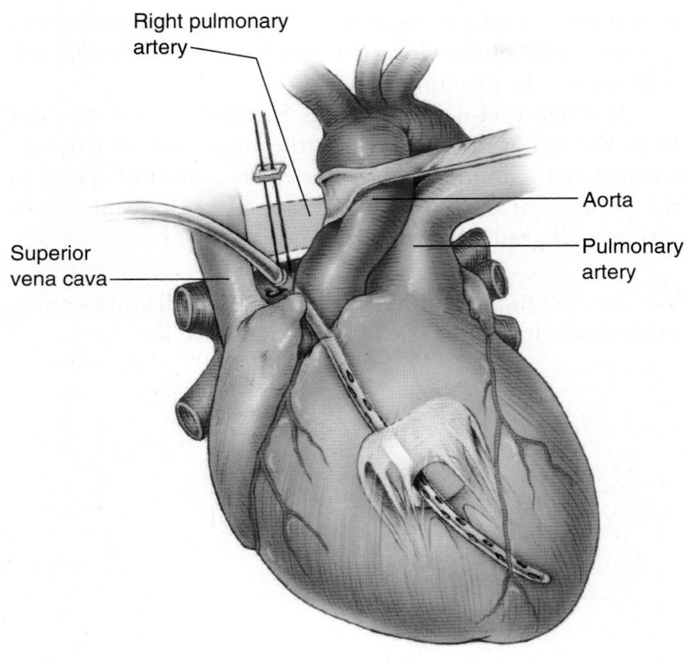

FIG. 4.5 Venting through the superior aspect of the left atrium.

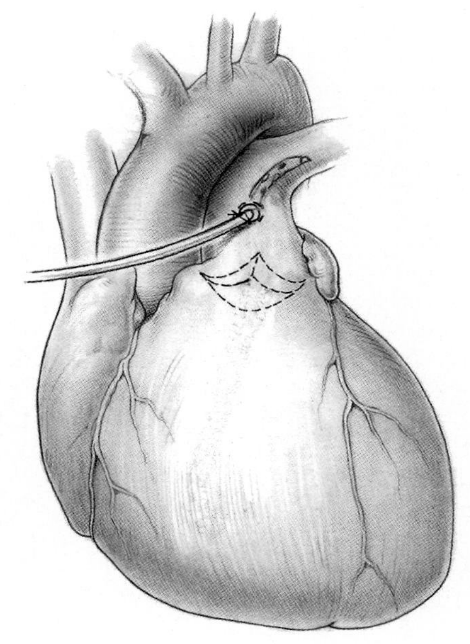

FIG. 4.6 Venting through the pulmonary artery.

Technique

With the right atrium open, a small, right-angled vent is introduced through the foramen ovale and connected to low suction. If the foramen ovale is not patent, a stab wound is made in the fossa ovalis. At the end of the procedure, the vent is removed and the opening is closed with fine suture.

DEAIRING OF THE HEART

Air embolism is indeed a serious complication of cardiac surgery, and every precaution should be taken to minimize its occurrence. A very effective way to minimize air embolism is to flood the operative field with carbon dioxide. This can be achieved by introducing a constant flow of carbon dioxide gas through sterile intravenous tubing anchored to the pericardium. The carbon dioxide displaces air (specifically nitrogen) and will dissolve in the blood when the heart is allowed to fill.

The heart usually starts to beat soon after the aortic cross-clamp is removed. When warm blood is administered in a retrograde fashion as the aortotomy is being closed in patients undergoing aortic valve replacement or as the atriotomy is being closed in patients undergoing mitral valve surgery, the heart may at times begin to beat spontaneously before the removal of the aortic cross-clamp (see Chapter 5). With each beat, the heart ejects free air bubbles that may be trapped inside it. Every cardiac surgery team has its own preference to deair the heart. We use the following technique.

The venting system, if used, is discontinued, and the heart is allowed to fill slowly by reducing the venous return. The cardioplegia administration site on the aorta or a residual opening on the aortotomy site is kept open with the tip of a right-angled clamp to facilitate venting and displacement of blood and air. At times, saline or blood can be injected slowly through the left ventricular vent, if in place, to displace air and blood through the aortic opening. The heart is shaken and the left atrial appendage is carefully invaginated into the left atrium to displace air bubbles.

⊘ Clots and the Left Atrial Appendage

Blood clots have a tendency to lodge in the left atrial appendage, particularly in patients with mitral stenosis and chronic atrial fibrillation. This can easily be detected by transesophageal echocardiography. If present, these clots must be removed. ⊘

Very gentle ventilation is begun. Often the heart has regained spontaneous rhythm and begins to eject blood through the aortic opening. A slotted vent needle is now introduced into the aortic opening and high suction is applied to it. The heart is allowed to fill and the aortic cross-clamp is removed. Transesophageal echocardiography is used routinely to monitor left ventricular function and evaluate the adequacy of valvular repair and function as well as the presence of residual air in the heart. As the left ventricular function improves, good ejection expels residual air. Occasionally, despite all these maneuvers, a pocket of air appears to be trapped in the apex of the left ventricle. Under these circumstances, the patient is placed in the Trendelenburg position, a large-bore needle is introduced into the apex of the left ventricle, and blood and air are aspirated. The right superior pulmonary vein, left atrial appendage, and roof of the left atrium in the gutter between the superior vena cava and aorta may also be subjected to needle aspiration.

⊘ Needle Injury to the Left Ventricle

When the left ventricle appears to be dilated and thin, and the patient's tissues are delicate, needle aspiration of the left ventricle apex may be hazardous and cause bleeding. The needle site may require suture closure. ⊘

A long, 14- or 16-gauge needle passed through the anterior wall of the right ventricle and through the septum into the left ventricle near the apex is a safe and effective technique to aspirate residual air. The right ventricle entry site may need suture closure if bleeding continues after administration of protamine.

Another useful technique is to allow blood to eject from the left ventricle through the open end of left ventricular vent cannula that is buried in a pool of blood in the pericardial cavity. Any air trapped in the ventricle or atrium will gradually be ejected.

NB This technique requires the heart to be full and ejecting; otherwise, air may be sucked into the heart. **NB**

SECTION

II

Surgery for Acquired Heart Disease

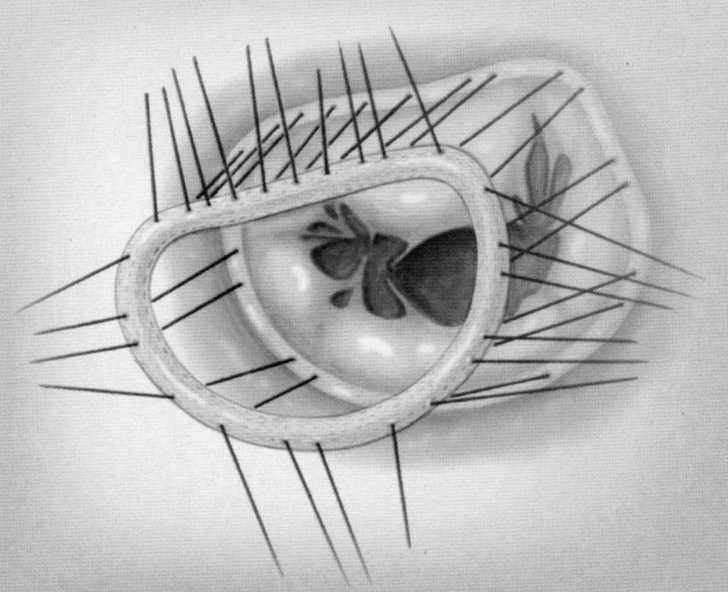

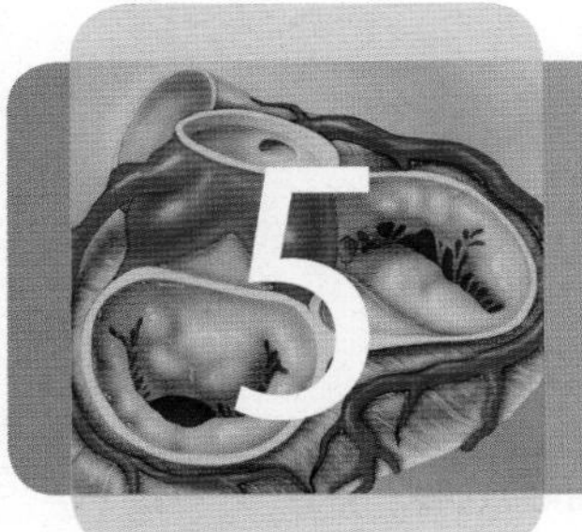

5 Surgery of the Aortic Valve

Aortic stenosis secondary to degenerative calcification, congenital bicuspid aortic valve disease, or rheumatic fever is the most common indication for aortic valve replacement. Acute aortic insufficiency as a result of aortic dissection, endocarditis, or balloon valvuloplasty requires urgent surgical intervention. Chronic aortic valve regurgitation caused by the slow enlargement of the aortic root or dysfunction of the valve cusps is seen with congenital abnormalities, most commonly bicuspid aortic valve, as well as rheumatic disease, endocarditis, calcific cusp degeneration, and degenerative aortic wall disease. The timing of surgery is important to prevent irreversible left ventricular dysfunction.

SURGICAL ANATOMY OF THE AORTIC VALVE

The aortic valve has three cup-shaped leaflets or cusps: the noncoronary cusp, the left cusp, and the right cusp. These spring from three crescent-shaped valvular annuli within the expanded sinuses of Valsalva. The plane of the aortic annuli forms the line of demarcation between the left ventricular cavity and the aorta.

Attachments of the aortic valve to the left ventricular outflow tract are both muscular and membranous (Fig. 5.1). The three fibrous annuli are all associated with somewhat different structures. The noncoronary annulus is singular in that it does not give rise to a coronary artery and is attached to the left ventricle only by membrane. Adjoining halves of the left and noncoronary annuli and the small area beneath the intervening commissure, the fibrous subaortic curtain, are continuous with the anterior leaflet of the mitral valve. Below the noncoronary and right coronary annuli and the intervening commissure lie the central fibrous body and the membranous septum, which are divided into atrioventricular and interventricular segments by the contiguous attachment of the nearby tricuspid valve. This membrane usually circles under the noncoronary annulus and merges with the anterior leaflet of the mitral valve. The bundle of His passes into the muscular ventricular septum just below the membranous septum before dividing into left and right bundle branches. These travel inferiorly and downward along the medial side of the left ventricular outflow tract. This conduction tissue is, therefore, close to portions of the noncoronary and right coronary annuli. Behind the noncoronary sinus, and in direct opposition to it, are the interatrial groove and parts of the left and right atria (thus explaining the rupture of an aneurysm of the noncoronary sinus of Valsalva into these cavities).

Part of the right coronary annulus, as mentioned earlier, is directly attached through the central fibrous body to the muscular septal wall. It courses along the right ventricular outflow tract, merging at its commissure with the left coronary annulus adjacent to the pulmonary valve annulus. The right coronary artery originates from the upper part of the right coronary sinus of Valsalva and courses down the right atrioventricular sulcus. The left or anterior segment of the left coronary annulus underlies the only part of the aortic root not related to any of the cardiac chambers. The right or posterior half of the left coronary annulus is in opposition to the left atrium. The left main coronary artery arises from the upper part of the left sinus and runs a short but variable distance behind it before dividing into its branches.

It is important to understand the functional anatomy of the aortic valve when considering valve repair or valve preserving aortic root procedures. The aortic root consists of four components: the aortic annulus, the aortic cusps, the sinuses of Valsalva, and the sinotubular junction. The aortic annulus is attached to the interventricular septum and fibrous structures along 55% of its circumference, with the remaining 45% being attached to the ventricular myocardium. The aortic cusps have a semilunar shape and the length of the base is normally 1.5 times the length of the free margin. The commissure is the highest point where two cusps meet, which is just below the sinotubular junction. The annulus has a scalloped shape, and the diameter of the annulus in younger individuals is normally 15% to 20% larger than the diameter of the sinotubular junction. In older patients, these two diameters are nearly equal. The average length of the free margin of an aortic cusp is 1.5 times the diameter of the sinotubular junction. In general, the noncoronary cusp is slightly larger than the other two, and the left is the smallest.

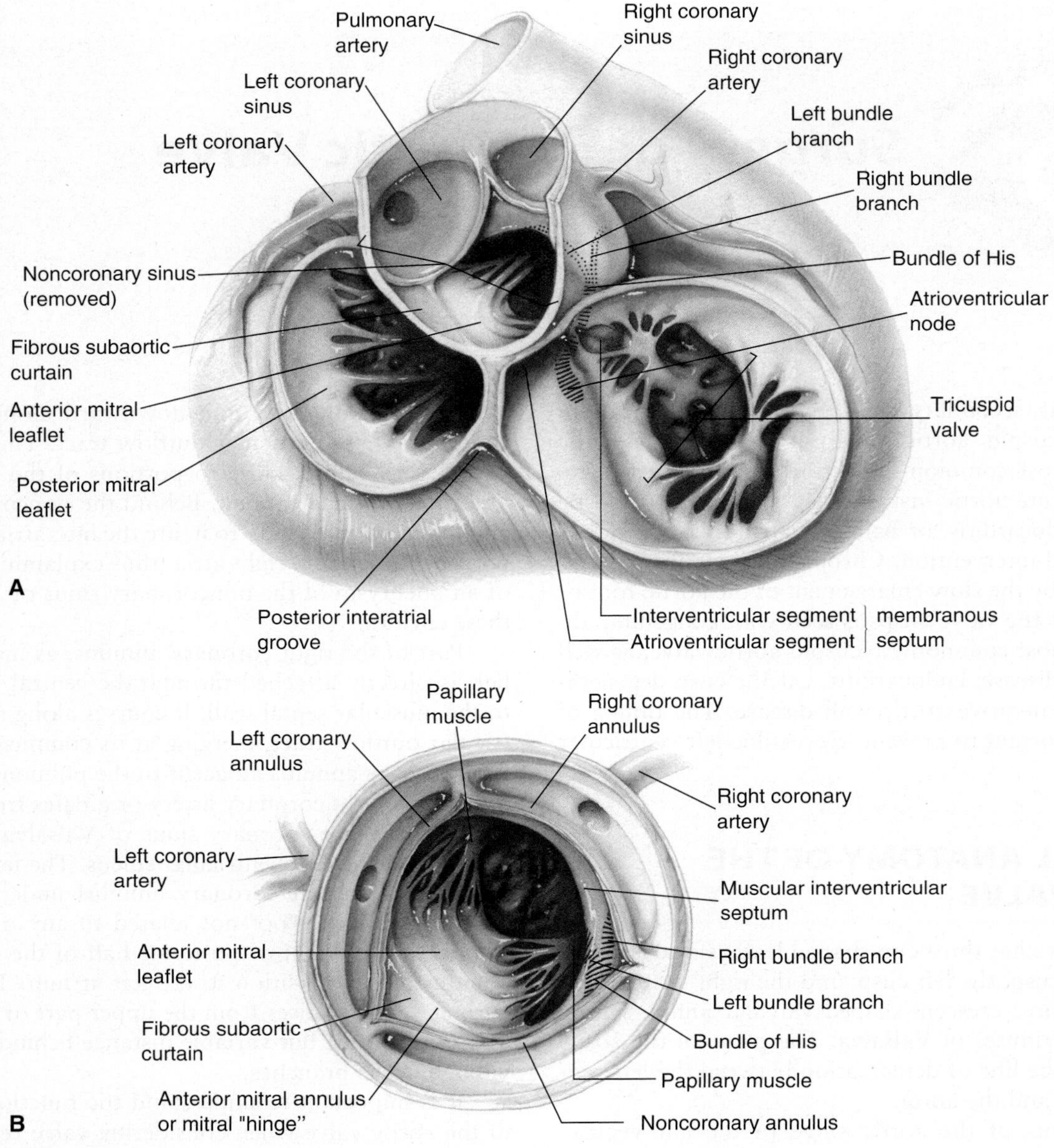

FIG. 5.1 A: Posteroanterior view of the heart with the aorta and pulmonary artery transected above the sinuses. The atria have been removed at the level of the atrioventricular valves. The noncoronary sinus has been excised at the noncoronary annulus and the aortic leaflets have been removed. **B:** Superior view into the aortic root. The leaflets have been excised.

APPROACH TO THE AORTIC VALVE

Aortic valve surgery can be performed through a median sternotomy with a full or limited skin incision, or using an upper ministernotomy (see Chapter 1). The distal ascending aorta is normally cannulated directly and a dual-staged venous cannula is placed into the right atrium. In cases with diffuse calcific or atherosclerotic involvement of the aorta or with aortic dissection, the arterial cannulation may need to be altered, and the conduct of the procedure modified (see Management of Unclampable Aorta).

Myocardial Preservation

Detailed techniques for preservation of the myocardium have already been discussed in Chapter 3. A modified synchronized technique for myocardial protection has been used in our practice for valvular surgery, particularly for aortic valve disease.

Technique

With a retrograde cardioplegic cannula in place in the coronary sinus and an antegrade cannula in the aortic root, cardiopulmonary bypass is initiated and hypothermia (32°C) is achieved. 500 mL of cold blood cardioplegic solution (4°C to 8°C) is administered into the aortic root, followed by an additional 500 mL via coronary sinus. Myocardial activity ceases, and electrocardiographic monitoring reveals a flat line.

⊘ Left Ventricular Distention

Antegrade administration of blood cardioplegic solution into the aortic root can be satisfactorily accomplished only if the aortic valve is relatively competent (see Chapter 3). Presence of significant aortic valve insufficiency results in backflow of the cardioplegic solution into the noncontracting left ventricular cavity. This causes left ventricular distention and possible myocardial injury. Therefore, when the aortic valve is incompetent, the blood cardioplegic solution should be administered using a retrograde technique to achieve complete cardiac standstill. In addition, a left ventricular vent should be placed through the right superior pulmonary vein. Myocardial protection can be augmented by administering cardioplegic solution into the coronary ostia after the aorta has been opened. ⊘

⊘ Difficulty in Cannulation of Coronary Sinus

Rarely, the retrograde cannula cannot be introduced safely into the coronary sinus. Bicaval cannulation is performed, and the retrograde cannula in placed in the coronary sinus under direct vision (see Chapter 3). ⊘

⊘ Cardioplegic Arrest with Retrograde Cardioplegia

Cardioplegic arrest of the heart using a retrograde technique alone may at times be slow, particularly when the heart is enlarged. In these cases, aortotomy should be performed and cardioplegic solution administered directly into the coronary arteries. ⊘

⊘ Calcium Deposits

The aortic leaflets may become so deformed because of calcific deposits that they physically obstruct cannulation of the coronary arteries and prevent satisfactory administration of blood cardioplegic solution. In this case, the left coronary cusp should be quickly excised to facilitate direct cannulation and infusion of blood cardioplegic solution into the left coronary ostium. Infusion into the right coronary artery can be performed when the heart has been arrested and the diseased aortic valve has been excised. ⊘

Cold blood cardioplegia is administered (usually every 10 minutes) in a retrograde manner to ensure the complete cessation of electrical activity of the myocardium. Between cardioplegia doses, cold oxygenated blood is continuously infused through the retrograde cannula whenever clear visualization of the aortic root is not required (such as placement of valve sutures in the sewing ring of the prosthetic valve). For optimal protection of the right ventricle, direct infusion of blood cardioplegic solution into the right coronary artery is carried out every 20 minutes, and ice wrapped with gauze is placed topically on the heart to minimize surface rewarming.

When the aortic valve has been seated and the valve sutures are being tied, the patient is rewarmed. Retrograde infusion of cold blood or cold blood cardioplegic solution through the coronary sinus is continued to ensure a complete cessation of myocardial activity. When the aortotomy closure is started, warm blood is infused retrogradely through the coronary sinus. Often concurrent with closure of the aortotomy, normal cardiac activity is observed. If the patient has undergone concomitant coronary artery bypass grafting, blood cardioplegia or cold blood can be infused simultaneously antegradely through the vein grafts and retrogradely through the coronary sinus.

⊘ Right Coronary Artery Air Embolism

Infusion of warm blood using the retrograde technique is continued for several minutes after the cross-clamp is removed to minimize the risk of air bubbles trapped in the aortic root entering the right coronary artery. ⊘

Exposure of the Aortic Valve by Transverse Aortotomy

A low transverse incision is perhaps most commonly used and is preferred by many surgeons (Fig. 5.2). The epicardial fat and adventitial tissue from the right ventricular outflow tract and pulmonary artery may overlie the desired line of aortic incision. These can be dissected free and retracted with a few pledgeted sutures (Fig. 5.2A). Fine Prolene sutures are inserted in the adventitia of the aortic wall on each side of the proposed incision line, which should be 10 to 15 mm above the origin of the right coronary artery. When the ascending aorta has been cross-clamped, the aortic wall is incised for a short distance between these sutures. A small leaflet retractor is introduced into the lumen of the aorta to expose the aortic valve.

⊘ Retractor Injury

Often the aortic wall is dilated and thinned out, particularly in elderly patients with poststenotic dilation. Aggressive traction may result in a transverse tear of the wall of the aortic root (Fig. 5.3). This may necessitate replacement of the ascending aorta or patch repair of the aortic wall. ⊘

Under direct vision, the opening is then extended on both sides; care must be taken to stay approximately 10 mm above the aortic commissures (Fig. 5.2B). Alternatively, the incision can be extended obliquely upward and/or downward, converting it to an oblique incision or tailoring it to provide optimal exposure (Fig. 5.2C, dashed line).

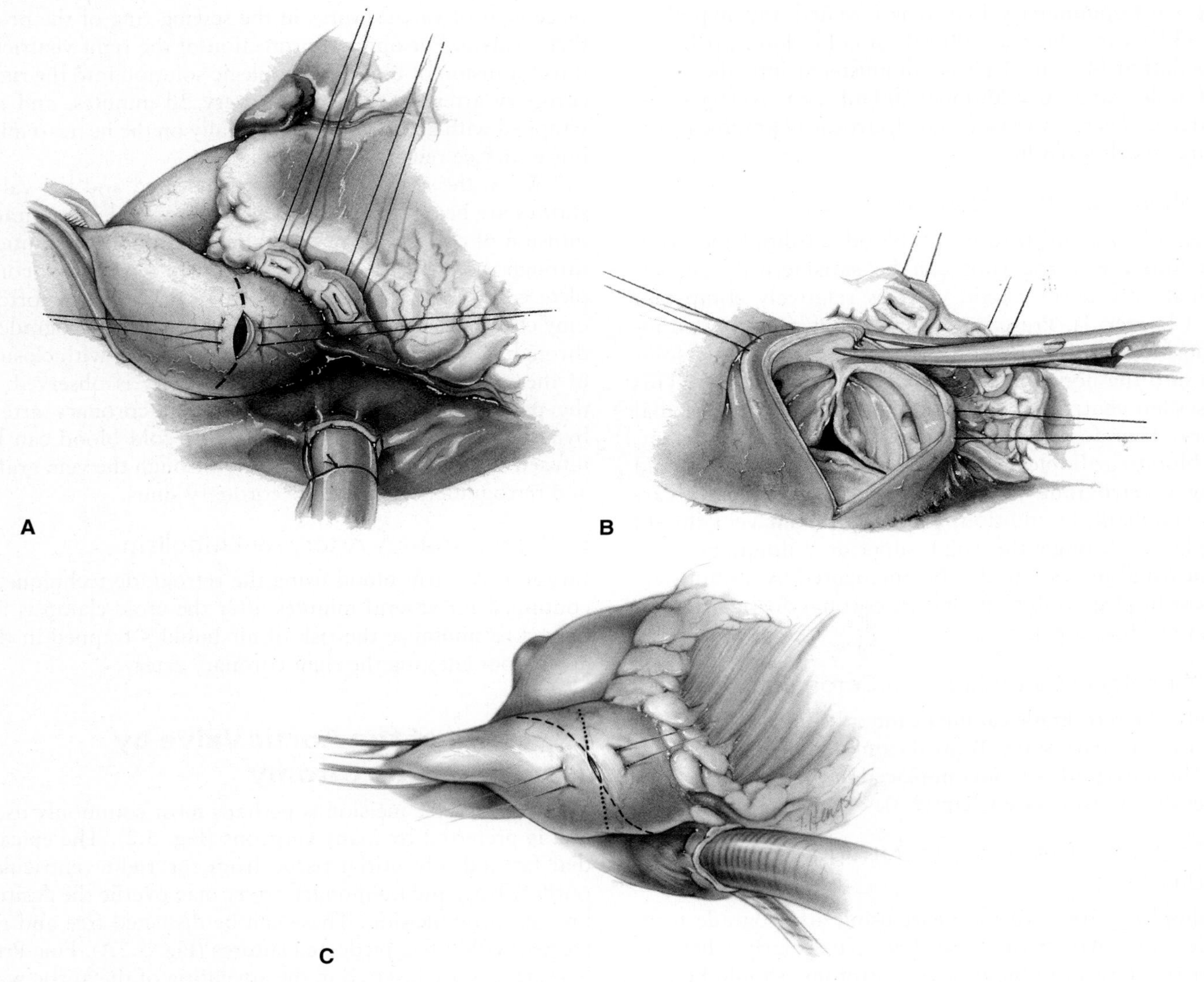

FIG. 5.2 **A:** A low transverse incision to expose the aortic valve. **B:** Extension of transverse incision. **C:** Initial small transverse aortotomy may be extended transversely or obliquely.

⊘ Aortotomy too Close to the Right Coronary Ostium

Poststenotic dilation, which is commonly seen in patients with aortic stenosis and congenital bicuspid aortic valve, may distort the aortic root and cause upward displacement of the ostium of the right coronary artery. The usual transverse aortotomy may then be too low and impinge on the right coronary ostium. Care must be exercised in these patients to identify the origin of the right coronary artery before opening the aorta. ⊘

Exposure of the Aortic Valve by Oblique Aortotomy

An oblique or hockey-stick incision is started high on the medial aspect of the aorta and is then continued diagonally downward into the noncoronary sinus stopping 10 mm above the aortic annulus. The aortic walls are then retracted on each side (Fig. 5.4). This incision is particularly useful in patients with small aortic roots.

⊘ Excessive Inferior Extension of the Aortotomy

The lower limit of the incision should be well above the aortic annulus to avoid difficulty in placing sutures in the annulus for insertion of the prosthesis. This will also facilitate the aortic closure. ⊘

⊘ Right Ventricular Hematoma

Epicardial fat overlying the right ventricle is very friable and if traumatized can develop into a large hematoma in heparinized patients. The epicardial fat can be gently retracted away from the operative field with pledgeted traction sutures (Fig. 5.2A). ⊘

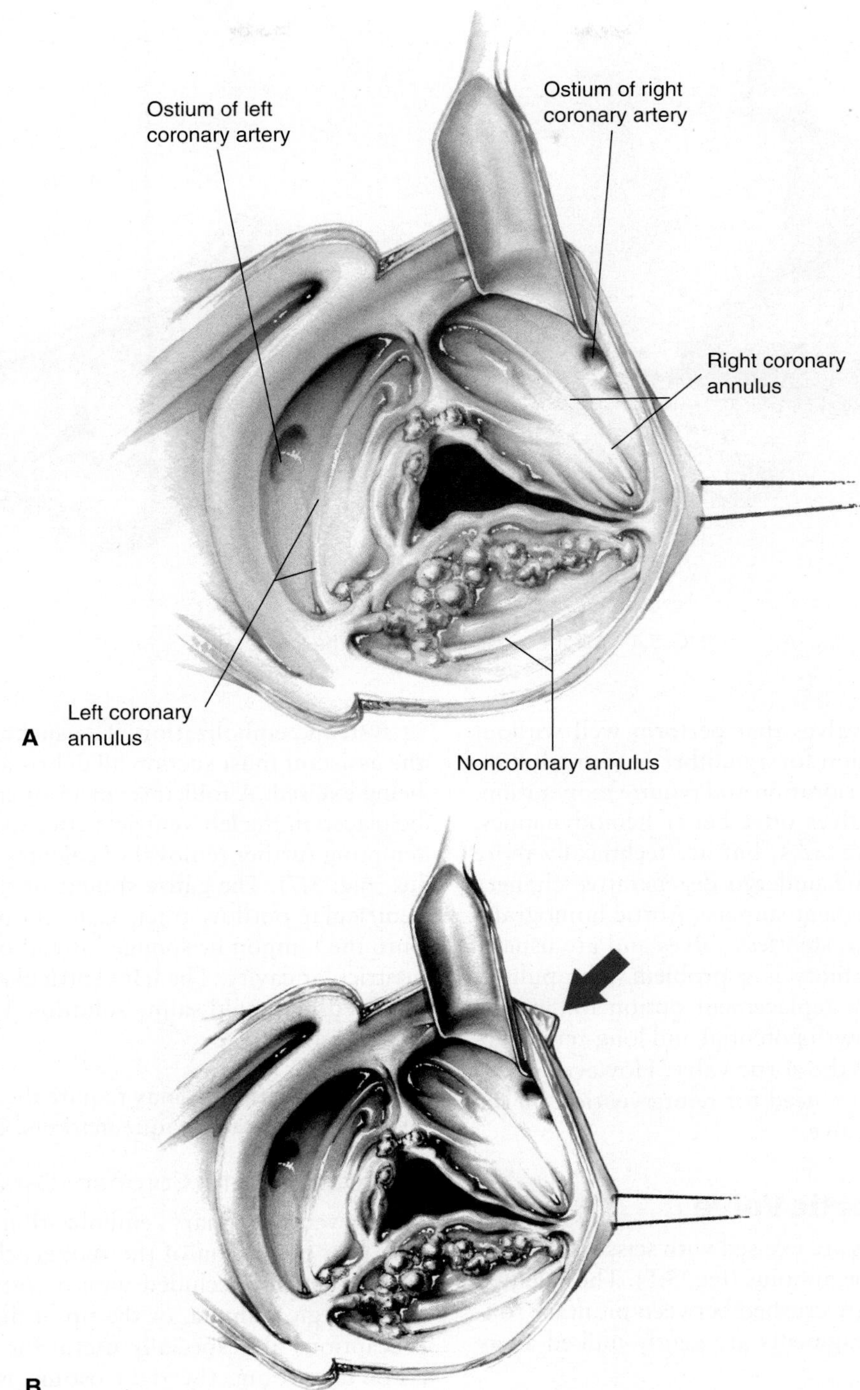

FIG. 5.3 **A:** Surgical view of a diseased aortic valve. Note that the aortotomy is approximately 10 mm above the commissures. **B:** Retractor injury to the aortic wall.

AORTIC VALVE REPLACEMENT

Valve replacement is required in nearly all patients with aortic stenosis and many patients with aortic insufficiency. The choice of replacement valve depends on the patient's age, concomitant disease, lifestyle, and anatomic factors. Contemporary mechanical valves include bileaflet and, which normally do not require rereplacement, but do require anticoagulation and have a higher risk of thromboembolic events. Stented bioprostheses include bovine

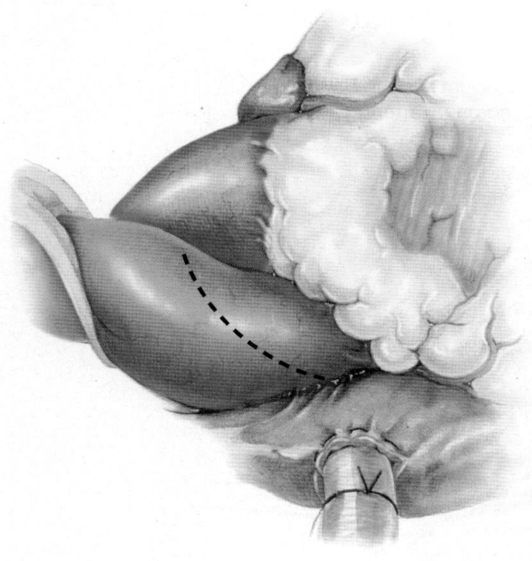

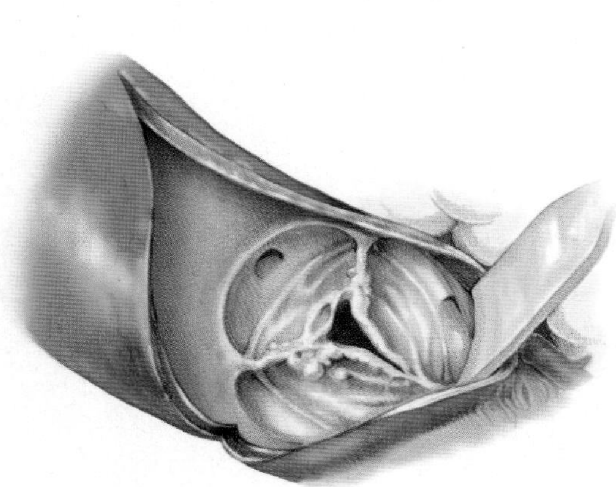

FIG. 5.4 Oblique incision to expose the aortic valve.

pericardial and porcine valves that perform well without the need for anticoagulation for a number of years, but do experience structural deterioration and require reoperation. Stentless bioprosthetic valves offer better hemodynamics, especially in smaller valve sizes, but are technically more demanding to implant and undergo degenerative changes leading to valve rereplacement surgery. Aortic homografts have advantages similar to stentless valves and are usually more durable, but availability is a problem. The pulmonary autograft is the best replacement option for infants and children, offering growth potential and long-term freedom from reoperation on the aortic valve. However, it is a two-valve procedure with a need for reintervention on the pulmonary replacement valve.

Excision of the Aortic Valve

The diseased valve leaflets are excised with scissors, leaving a 1- to 2-mm margin at the annulus (Fig. 5.5). The calcified segments of the annulus are crushed between pituitary rongeurs, and the calcium fragments are gently milked away or excised (Fig. 5.6).

⊘ Limits of Excision

Excision of the aortic valve too close to the annulus may disrupt the annulus and leave little tissue to hold the sutures securely. Therefore, a margin of valve leaflet should be left behind and may be trimmed away subsequently if it is deemed necessary. ⊘

⊘ Detachment of Calcium Particles

Care must be taken to not allow fragments of calcium to fall into the left ventricular cavity because they can result in systemic embolization. The sucker tip is detached, and the assistant must suction all debris as the valve leaflets are being excised. A folded segment of sponge or tampon may be placed in the left ventricle after valve excision before attempting further removal of calcium from the aortic annulus (Fig. 5.7). The gauze sponge or tampon guards the left ventricular outflow tract. Calcium particles or debris fall onto the tampon or sponge instead of being lost in the left ventricular cavity. The left ventricular cavity is flushed and irrigated with cold saline solution. The tampon or sponge is then removed. ⊘

NB Some institutions may require the tampon or the sponge to incorporate radiopaque markers. NB

⊘ Protecting the Coronary Ostia

To prevent coronary embolization during calcium removal or extraction of the sponge, the coronary ostia can be temporarily occluded with a cotton swab, a handheld cardioplegic cannula, or the tip of the suction head. These precautions are especially useful for protection of the left coronary ostium; the right ostium is less likely to be exposed to calcium particles because of its anterior position and the fact that it is often covered by the blade of a retractor. ⊘

⊘ Anterior Mitral Leaflet Detachment

Because of the continuity of portions of the aortic and mitral valves, the anterior mitral leaflet can become detached from its annulus during excision of the aortic valve leaflets. The surgeon should also be aware of this possibility during the removal of calcium and the trimming of the aortic annulus near the left and noncoronary cusps (Fig. 5.8). The

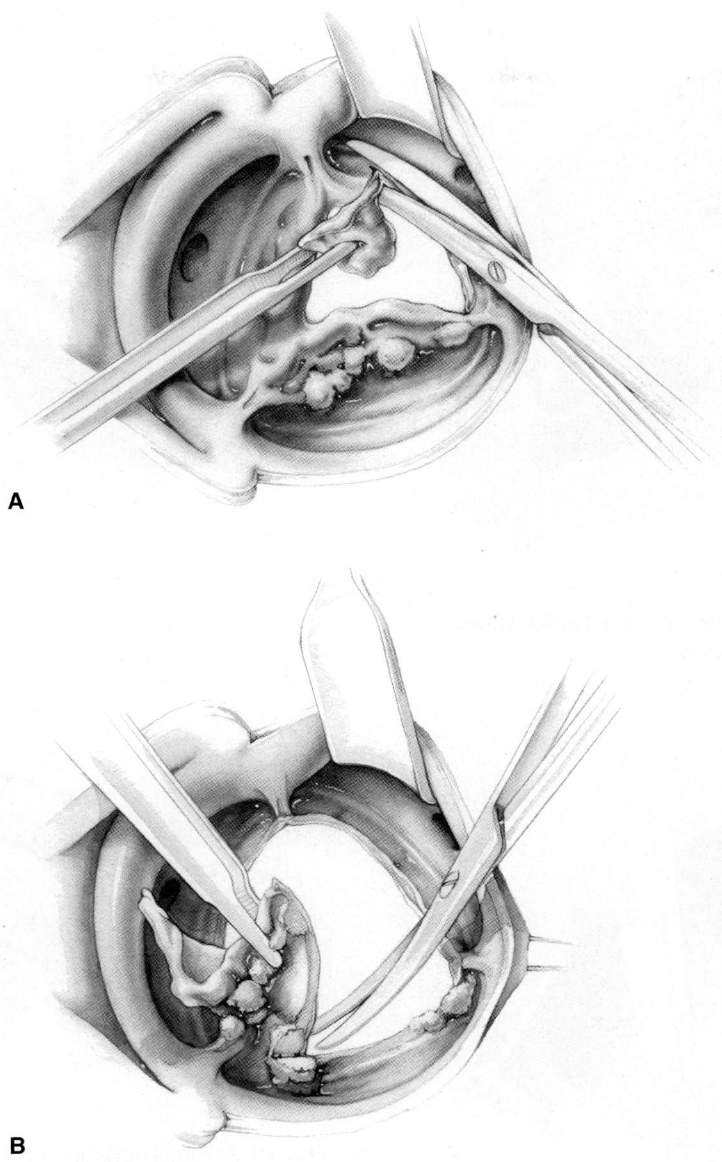

FIG. 5.5 Excising the diseased aortic valve. **A:** Right coronary leaflet. **B:** Noncoronary leaflet.

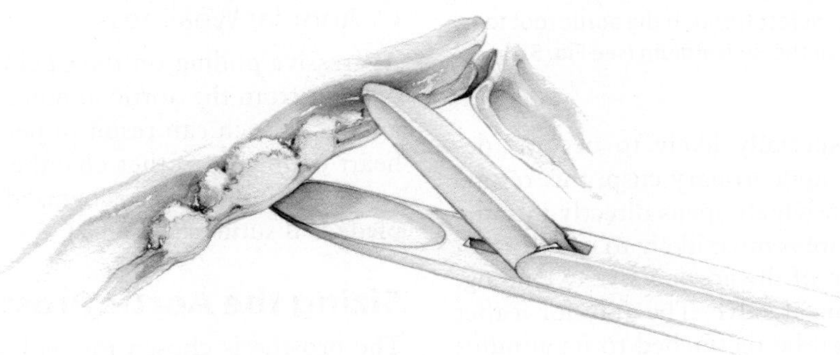

FIG. 5.6 Crushing and removing calcium fragments from a diseased annulus.

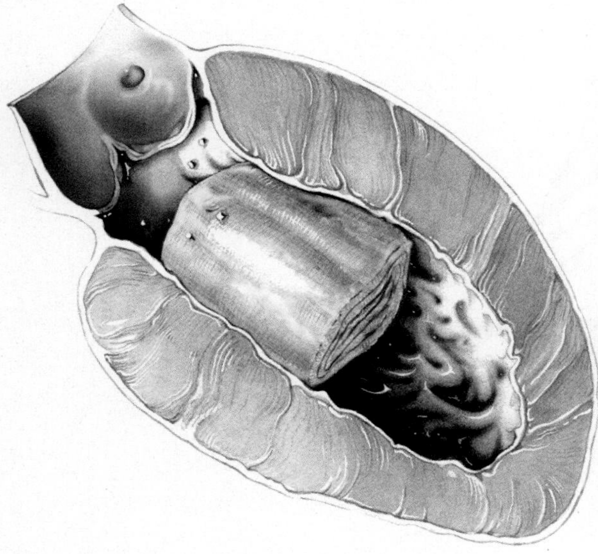

FIG. 5.7 Use of a sponge to prevent calcium particles from falling into the left ventricular cavity.

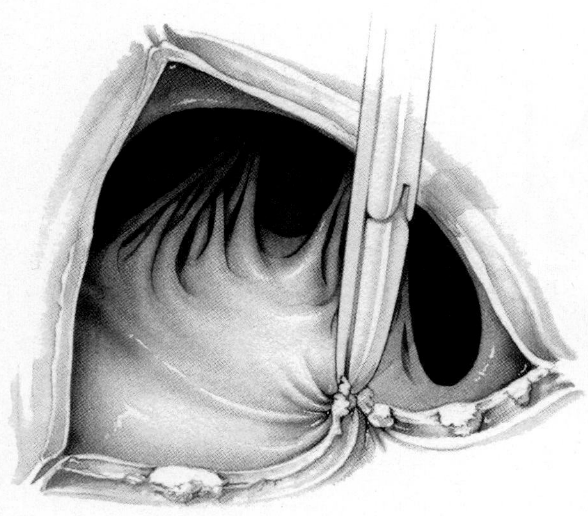

FIG. 5.8 Injudicious pulling on the calcium embedded in the aortic annulus, creating a defect through the aortic root to other chambers of the heart or the pericardium (see Fig. 5.4).

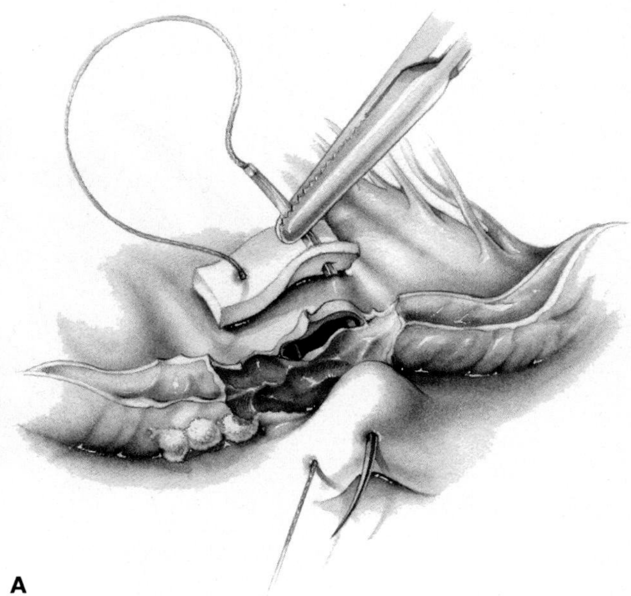

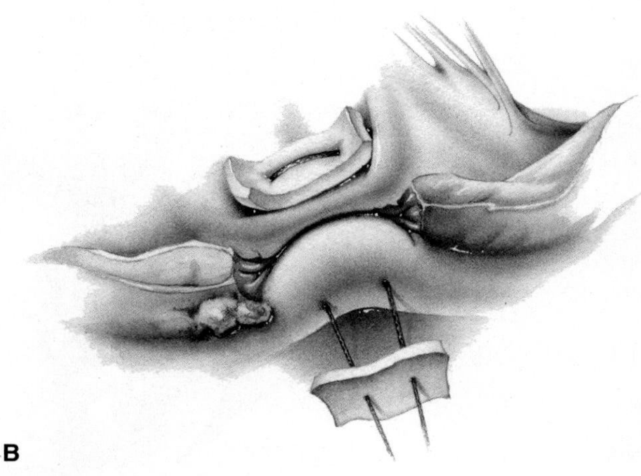

FIG. 5.9 **A:** Partial detachment of the anterior mitral leaflet, creating a defect in the left atrium. **B:** The defect is closed with pledgeted sutures, which can also be used to anchor the prosthesis.

anterior mitral leaflet is especially likely to become detached with the removal of noncoronary cusp; this results in a defect in the aortic root, which opens directly into the left atrium. This misadventure is most likely to occur when there is massive calcification of the aortic valve extending, as it often does, onto the mitral valve. The anterior leaflet of the mitral valve must then be reattached to its annulus by means of interrupted pledgeted suture(s) incorporating the torn peripheral edge of the mitral valve and the annulus (Fig. 5.9). ⊘

⊘ Annular Weakness

Aggressive pulling on the calcium while attempting to remove it from the aortic annulus may occasionally weaken an area, which can result in perforation either outside the heart or into the other chambers of the heart. The weakened area must be recognized and approximated with pledgeted sutures (Fig. 5.9). ⊘

Sizing the Aortic Prosthesis

The prosthesis chosen for replacement of the aortic valve must fit snugly in the annulus. Three simple sutures are inserted, one in each commissure (Fig. 5.10A) or in the annulus near each commissure (Fig. 5.10B). The aortic

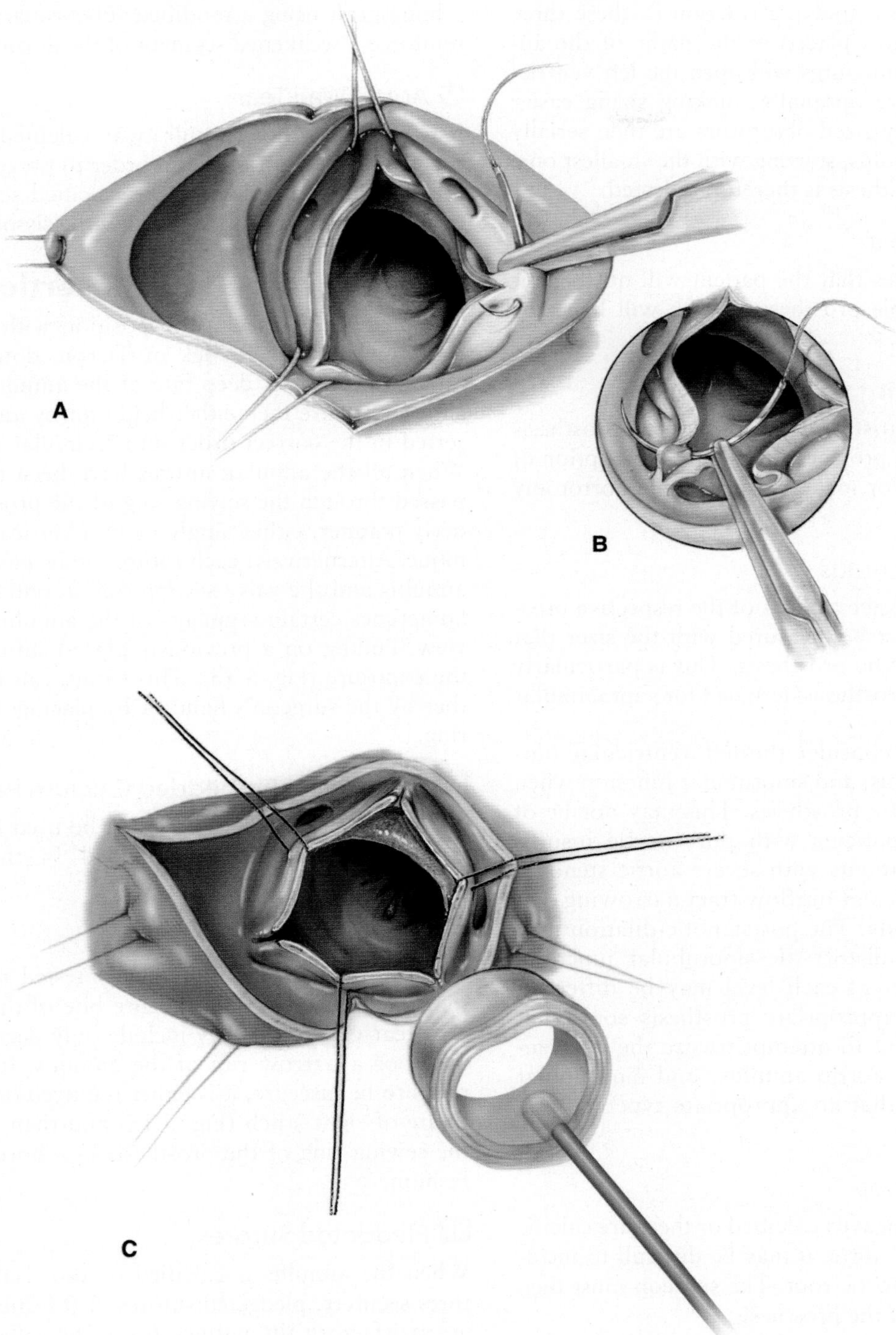

FIG. 5.10 A: Three simple sutures being inserted in the aortic valve annulus, one in each commissure. B: Sutures can be alternatively placed through the annulus near each commissure. C: Sutures placed in the nadir of the annulus for optimal sizing.

orifice can be opened by applying traction to these three sutures. At times, sutures placed in the nadir of the annulus between the commissures will open the left ventricular outflow tract more optimally, making sizing easier (Fig. 5.10C). Differently sized obturators are then serially introduced into the annulus, starting with the smallest one. The correctly sized prosthesis is therefore selected.

⊘ Loose Prosthetic Fit

A very loose fit indicates that the patient will not benefit from the largest possible prosthesis, which will have the optimal hemodynamics. ⊘

⊘ Tight Prosthetic Fit

A tight fit may make satisfactory seating of the prosthesis difficult. Oversizing the prosthesis may cause disruption of the aortic annulus and/or make closure of the aortotomy difficult. ⊘

⊘ Measuring the Annulus

Because the sizers are exact replicas of the respective prostheses, the annulus must be measured with the sizer that corresponds to the specific prosthesis. This is particularly relevant when using a prosthesis designed for supraannular implantation. ⊘

It is important to consider the left ventricular outflow tract, aortic annulus, and sinotubular junction when sizing for an appropriate prosthesis. This may not be of much significance in patients with pure aortic insufficiency. However, in patients with severe aortic stenosis, there may be left ventricular outflow tract narrowing owing to septal hypertrophy. The poststenotic dilation may sometimes obscure or distort the sinotubular junction. Therefore, the diameter at each level may be different, making sizing for an appropriate prosthesis somewhat demanding. It is prudent to attempt to size the left ventricular outflow tract, aortic annulus, and sinotubular junction separately so that an appropriate type of prosthesis can be selected.

⊘ Calcified Aortic Root

When the aortic root is heavily calcified or there are calcific ridges in the wall of the aorta, it may be difficult to introduce the sizer into the aortic root. The surgeon must then visually judge the size of the prosthesis. ⊘

NB Decalcification of the Aortic Root

Often there is calcification in the aortic root involving the sinuses and extending into the coronary artery ostia. With experience, it is possible to decalcify the aortic root wall in specific locations to facilitate implantation of an appropriately sized prosthesis. The technique consists of gently crushing segments of calcified intima with a rongeur and then removing them from the aortic wall to facilitate the surgery. Implantation of a stentless aortic bioprosthesis or a homograft using a modified subcoronary technique will reinforce a weakened segment of the aortic wall. NB

⊘ Aortic Wall Tear

It is important not to pull away calcified segments from the wall of the aortic root in order to prevent a buttonhole injury. The connection of the calcified segment with the intima must be sharply divided with scissors. ⊘

Technique for Suture Insertion

The prosthesis is sewn into position with interrupted sutures such as 2-0 Tevdek or Ticron, double-armed with tapered needles. A deep bite of the annulus is taken. The suture ends are then either held taut by an assistant or inserted in the correct order into a circular ring (Fig. 5.11). When all the annular sutures have been placed, they are passed through the sewing ring of the prosthesis in an orderly manner, either singly or in a vertical mattress technique. Alternatively, each suture can be passed through the annulus and the valve-sewing ring in one step (Fig. 5.12). Sometimes certain segments of the annulus are not in full view. Pulling on a previously placed suture will improve the exposure (Fig. 5.13). This suture can be held taut, either by the surgeon's hand or by placing it in the circular ring.

NB Removal of Embedded Calcium Particles

The tip of the suture needle can be used to dislodge calcium particles deeply embedded in the myocardium (Fig. 5.14). NB

⊘ Suture Security

The sutures must be individually tested to make certain that they include a good, secure bite of the annulus; they may tear through if they include only degenerative leaflet tissue or a narrow rim of the annulus. If the suture appears to be insecure, it is either removed or converted to a figure-of-eight stitch (Fig. 5.15) and then passed through the sewing ring of the prosthesis in a horizontal mattress fashion. ⊘

NB Pledgeted Sutures

When the annulus is calcified or too friable to hold sutures securely, pledgeted sutures (2-0 Ethibond or Ticron) are satisfactory alternatives. It is technically easier to insert the sutures in an everted manner, with the pledgets lying above the annulus in the aorta (Fig. 5.16A). The alternative technique of placing sutures from below, which allows the pledgets to remain subannular, provides a secure and satisfactory buttressing effect (Fig. 5.16C). This technique is used for supraannular insertion of a prosthetic valve. If utilized with a disc valve, the surgeon must ensure that no pledgets interfere with the normal movement of the disc. Also, if a suture breaks while being tied, the loose pledget must be retrieved. The prosthesis often must be removed in

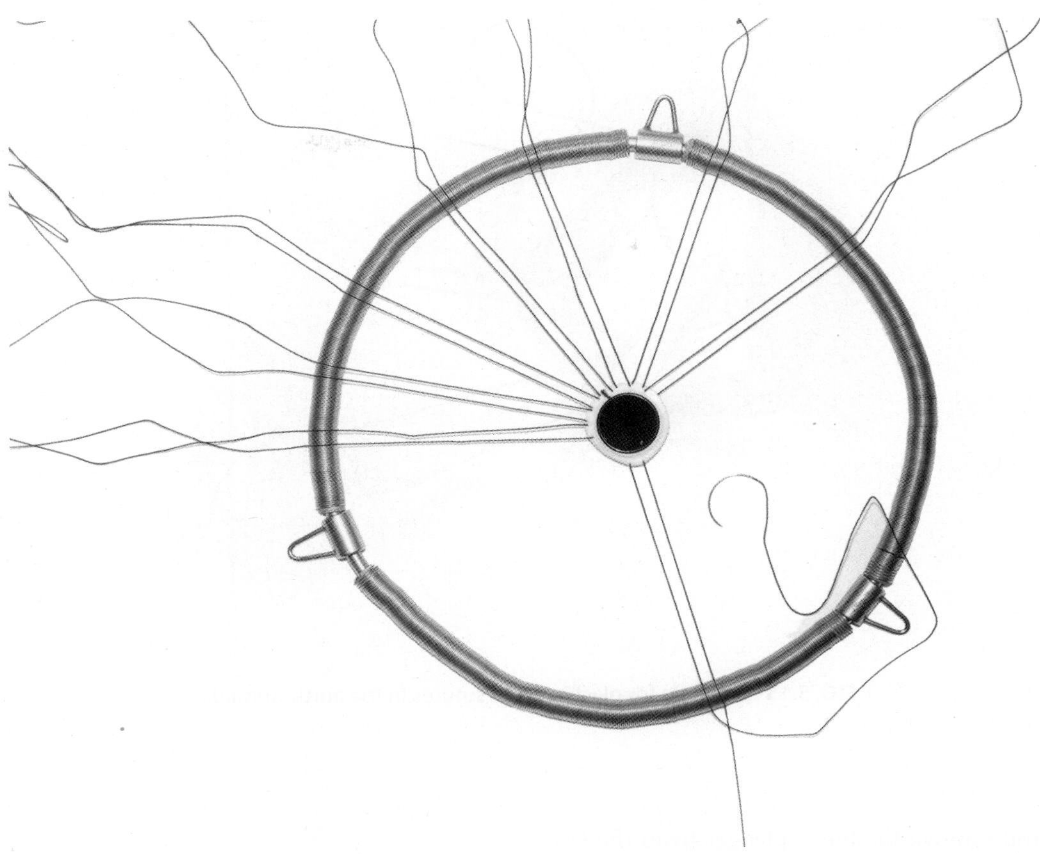

FIG. 5.11 Ring for placement of sutures in sequence.

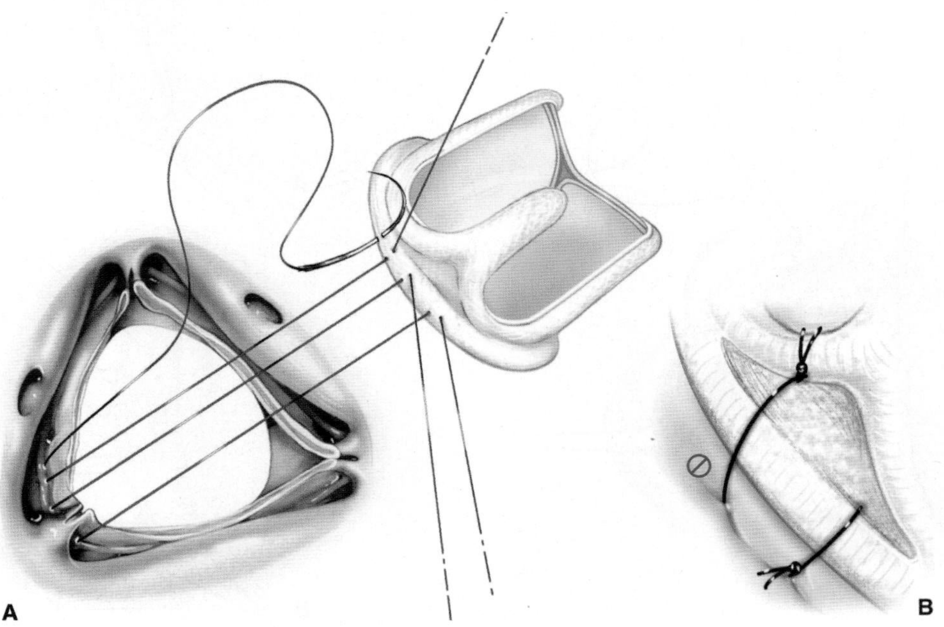

FIG. 5.12 **A:** Passing sutures directly from the annulus to the prosthetic sewing ring. **B:** Proper placement of sutures in the sewing ring to place the knot away from the valve itself.

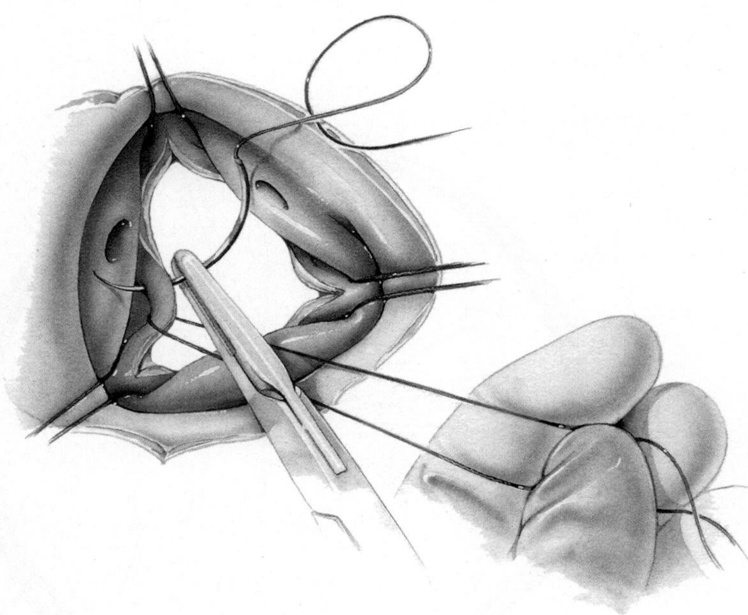

FIG. 5.13 Exposure for placement of sutures in the aortic annulus.

order to locate and remove the loose pledget from the left ventricle. Whether the pledgeted sutures are placed from below or above the annulus, they are inserted into the sewing ring of the prothesis in a horizontal mattress fashion (Fig. 5.17). The routine use of pledgets has markedly reduced the occurrence of paravalvular leaks.

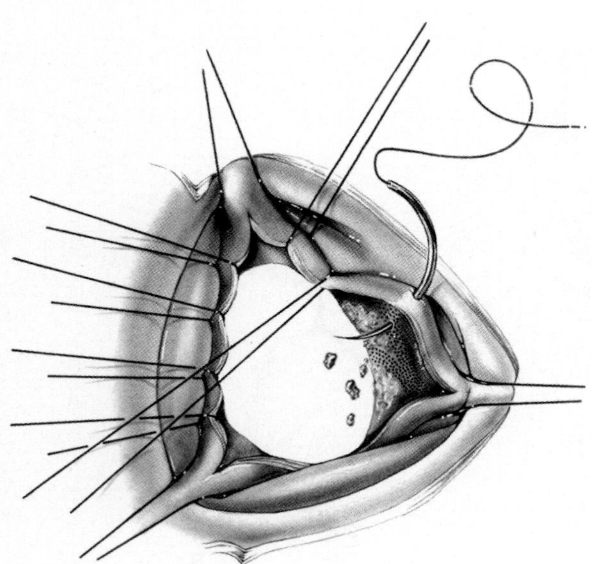

FIG. 5.14 Using the tip of the needle to dislodge calcium embedded in the myocardium.

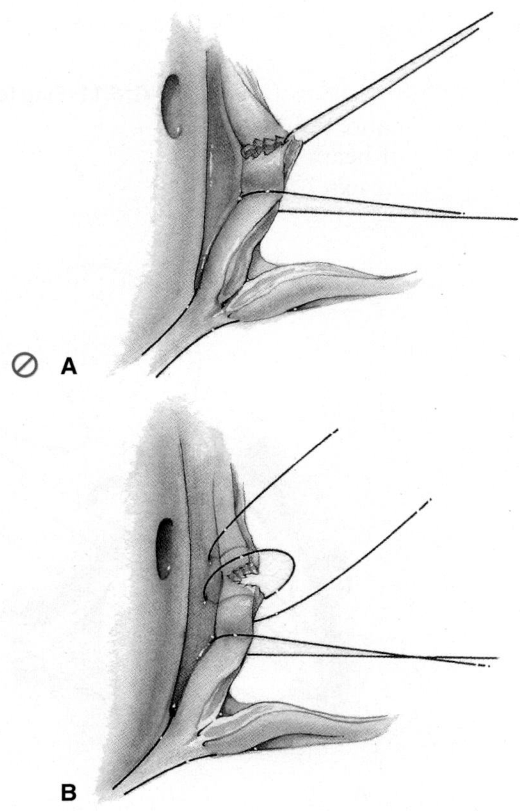

FIG. 5.15 Converting an insecure suture **(A)** to a figure-of-eight suture **(B)**.

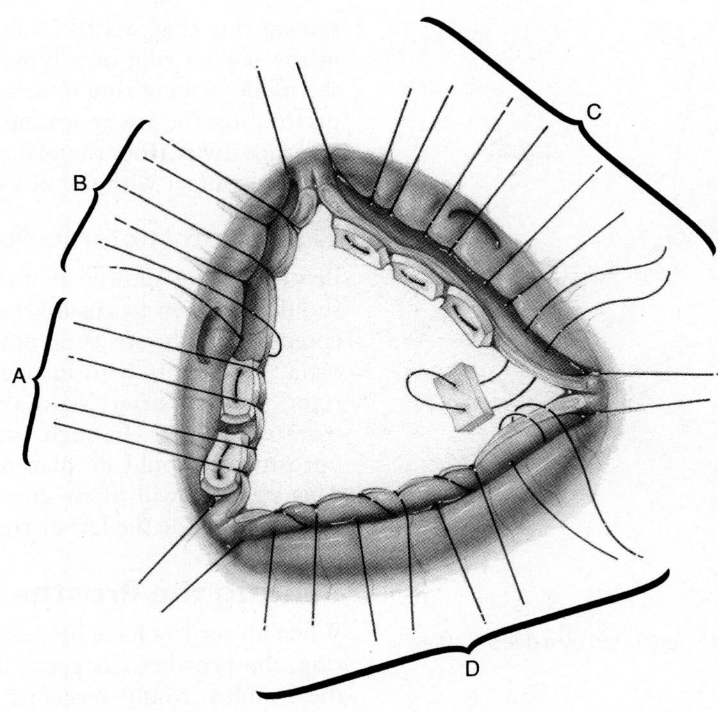

FIG. 5.16 **A:** Inserting the sutures in an everted manner, with the pledgets lying above the annulus in the aorta. **B:** Simple sutures. **C:** Inserting the sutures from below allows the pledgets to remain subannular. **D:** Figure-of-eight sutures.

⊘ Heart Block

Deeply placed sutures near the noncoronary and right coronary annuli can injure the conduction tissues and give rise to various forms of heart block (Fig. 5.18). When there is massive calcification extending onto the ventricular septum or when the tissues are friable because of endocarditis or abscess formation, this complication may be inevitable. Temporary ventricular wires are recommended for all patients undergoing aortic valve surgery. If the patient is still in complete heart block at the completion of the procedure,

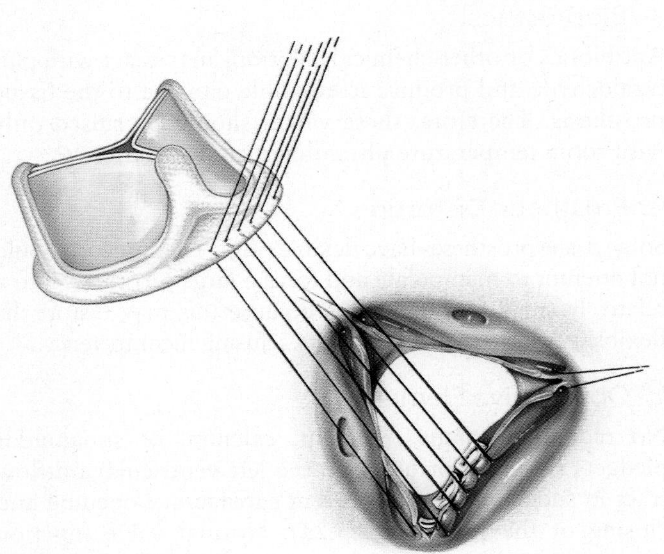

FIG. 5.17 Horizontal mattress sutures, with pledgets below the annuli, placed in a horizontal mattress fashion in the prosthetic ring.

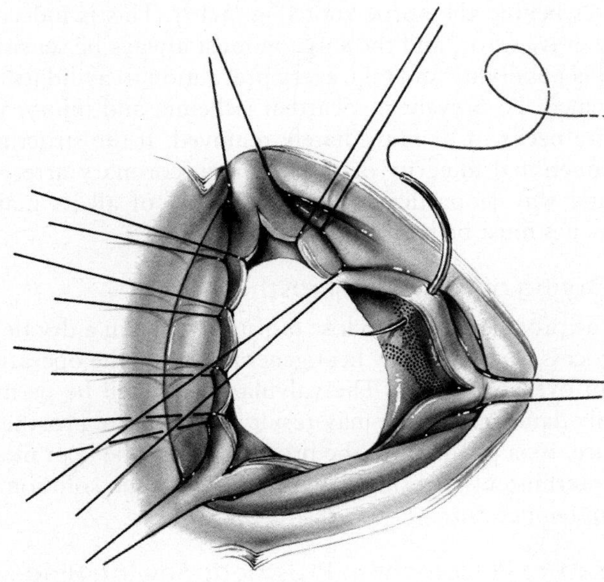

FIG. 5.18 Injury to the conduction tissues caused by deeply placed sutures.

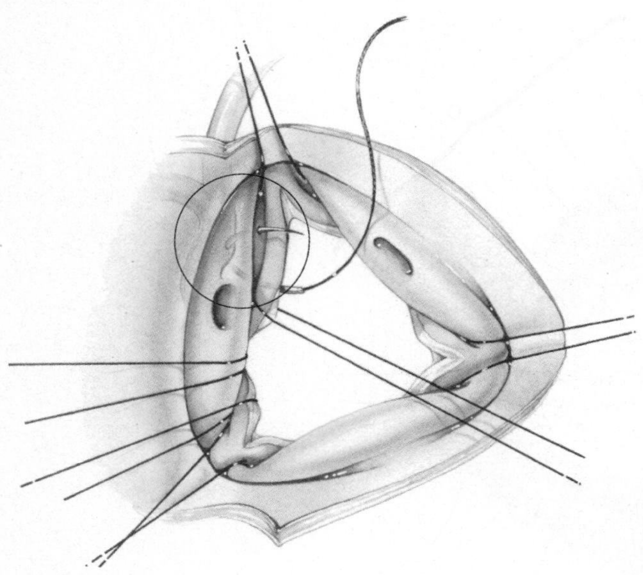

FIG. 5.19 Left main coronary artery punctured by a deep suture near the left coronary annulus.

temporary atrial wires should be placed to allow for atrioventricular sequential pacing. A permanent pacemaker may need to be implanted before the patient's discharge if atrioventricular conduction has not been reestablished. ⊘

⊘ Injury to the Left Coronary Artery

The precise site of suture placement in the aortic annulus is often obscured by pathologic changes, calcifications, and deformities. Deep sutures placed near the left coronary annulus may puncture the left main coronary artery as it passes behind the aortic root (Fig. 5.19). This is indeed a very grave error, and the surgeon must always be sensitive to this possibility and take every precaution to avoid its occurrence. To prevent myocardial ischemia and injury, the suture needs to be immediately removed. If the structural or functional integrity of the left main coronary artery is in any way jeopardized, bypass grafting of all its major branches must be performed. ⊘

⊘ Drying of the Tissue Prosthesis

Tissue prostheses tend to lose moisture when in a dry field, a process accelerated by heat generated from the operating room overhead lights. The valvular tissue will be permanently damaged, which may result in premature prosthetic failure. As a precaution, the prosthesis must be kept moist by intermittently rinsing it with normal saline solution at room temperature. ⊘

⊘ Suture Placement in Prosthetic Sewing Ring

Suture needles are passed through the prosthetic sewing ring from below upward, with the needle exiting at the junction of the outside half with the inside half of the sewing ring (Fig. 5.12B). Sutures placed in such a manner in the sewing ring of a bioprosthesis are well away from the tissue–sewing ring interface and avoid traumatizing or perforating the tissue leaflets. Similarly, the suture knots will face away from the orifice of a mechanical valve, preventing contact with the disc or leaflets. ⊘

⊘ Bioprosthetic Struts Position

Before placing sutures in the prosthesis, every precaution should be taken to ensure that the tissue prosthesis is oriented so that the struts do not obstruct the coronary artery ostia. In patients with bicuspid aortic valves, the left and right coronary artery's ostia are usually displaced farther from each other. In such situations, one strut of the bioprosthesis should be placed midway between the ostia. This strategy will likely ensure that the other two struts will not occlude the left or right coronary ostia. ⊘

Seating the Prosthesis

When all sutures have been accurately placed in the sewing ring, the prosthesis is gently lowered and fitted snugly in the annulus. Many surgeons rinse the sutures with saline solution for its lubricating effect, allowing the sutures to be pulled through the sewing ring more smoothly.

⊘ Narrow Sinotubular Junction

When the sinotubular junction of the ascending aorta is narrower than the aortic annulus, the appropriate size prosthesis will be too large to pass through it. In such situations, the holder is removed and the prosthetic low-profile valve is turned on end, then lowered and seated safely in the aortic annulus (Fig. 5.20). ⊘

⊘ Chemical or Thermal Injury to a Bioprosthesis

Antibiotics or other chemical solutions may react with glutaraldehyde and produce irreversible damage to the tissue prosthesis. Therefore, these valves should be rinsed only with room temperature physiologic saline solution. ⊘

⊘ Prosthetic Distortion

Some tissue prostheses have flexible rings. The surgeon should not attempt to manipulate and force a large prosthesis into a relatively small aortic annulus because this may distort the flexible ring and the valve leaflets, causing incompetence. ⊘

⊘ Obstructive Elements

No redundant tissue fragment, calcium, or subannular pledgets should protrude into the left ventricular outflow tract in such a way as to prevent satisfactory opening and closing of the valve (Fig. 5.21). Normal valve function must be ensured and any obstructing element removed before final anchoring of the prosthesis. ⊘

After the prosthesis has been satisfactorily seated, the sutures are tied down securely and cut short.

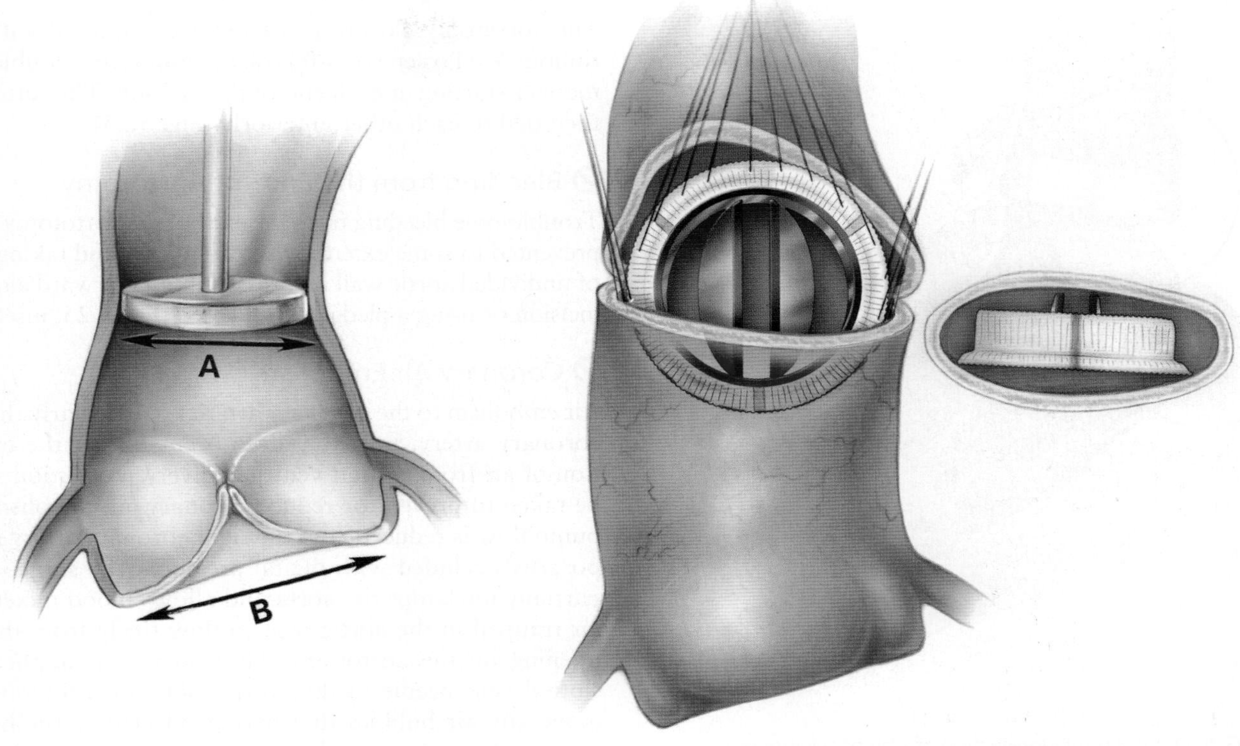

FIG. 5.20 Technique for implantation of the optimal size prosthesis through a narrow ascending aorta. **A:** Sinotubular diameter. **B:** Annular diameter.

⊘ Direction of Tying

The direction of tying the sutures should always be parallel to the curve of the sewing ring (Fig. 5.22). Any deviation from this principle may traumatize the leaflet tissue or the prosthetic valve through contact with the suture material or the surgeon's fingertip. ⊘

⊘ Long Suture Ends

Sutures, when tied, must be cut short, and the direction of the knot must be leaning toward the periphery of the sewing ring of the prosthesis. A long suture end will scratch the leaflet tissue, resulting in chronic irritation, injury, and, finally, perforation of the tissue leaflets. A long suture end can also protrude into the prosthetic orifice and interfere with the normal closure of the occluding mechanism of a mechanical valve. ⊘

⊘ Abnormal Location of the Coronary Artery Ostium

Occasionally, the orifice of the left main coronary artery is located next to the commissure of the aortic annulus. It is important to orient a bioprosthesis so that the struts do not face the coronary ostium (Fig. 5.23). ⊘

⊘ Unobstructed Prosthesis Function

Before closure of the aortotomy, it is imperative that normal, unobstructed opening and closing of a mechanical prosthesis be visually verified. ⊘

⊘ Septal Hypertrophy

Patients with long-standing aortic stenosis and/or hypertensive heart disease may have marked septal as well as concentric hypertrophy of the left ventricle. The surgeon must be cognizant of any discrepancy in size between the left ventricular outflow tract and the aortic annulus. Special technical details should be considered when implanting prostheses of different design. ⊘

The single-disc group of prostheses, exemplified by the Medtronic-Hall mechanical valve, can be rotated after implantation to ensure free movement of the disc. The smaller part of the disc that descends into the left ventricle must be positioned away from the septum. Most of the bileaflet prostheses can also be rotated and are subject to the same principle of free movement of the leaflets. The leaflets are often positioned parallel to the septum. In cases of extreme septal hypertrophy, there may be relatively decreased flow across the leaflet

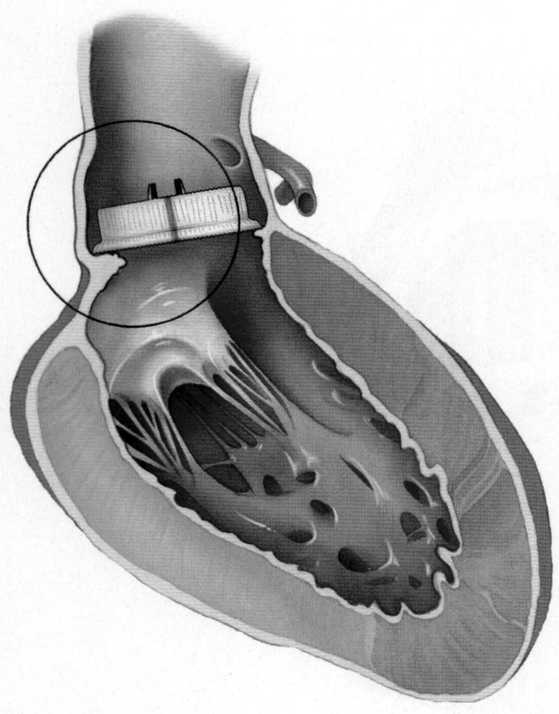

FIG. 5.21 Subannular projection of a bit of calcium or a pledget, which may limit motion of the valve.

close to and parallel with the septum. This possible theoretical disadvantage probably has no hemodynamic consequence.

When the left ventricular outflow is markedly limited by septal hypertrophy, some septal muscle mass can be excised (Fig. 5.24). Alternatively, multiple vertical myotomies may allow the left ventricular outflow tract to open up.

Aortotomy Closure

The aortotomy closure is usually accomplished with continuous 4-0 Prolene or 5-0 Prolene sutures in a double-layer manner starting at each end of the incision. The sutures are then tied to each other anteriorly (Fig. 5.25).

⊘ Bleeding from the Ends of Aortotomy

Troublesome bleeding from the ends of the aortotomy can be prevented to some extent by suturing back and taking a bite of undivided aortic wall before continuing forward along the incision or using a pledget at each end (Fig. 5.25, inset). ⊘

⊘ Coronary Air Embolism

Air embolism to the coronary arteries, particularly the right coronary artery, probably does occur during the evacuation of air from the left ventricle. Every precaution should be taken to prevent or reduce coronary air embolism. The pump flow is reduced, and the right coronary artery is temporarily occluded with digital pressure. The surgeon then partially unclamps the aorta and allows blood mixed with air trapped in the aortic root to flow freely from the vent opening on the aortotomy. High suction is applied to a slotted vent needle in the aortic root to continuously remove any air bubbles that may be ejected as the heart is filled and ventilation is begun (see Chapter 4). Only when all air has been evacuated can the vent needle be removed and the vent suture tied down. ⊘

⊘ Friable Aortic Wall

A friable aortic wall may necessitate the placement of additional reinforcing pledgeted sutures. Occasionally, when the aortic wall has been denuded of its adventitia or if the aorta is thin walled or friable, the aortotomy suture line can be reinforced with strips of autologous pericardium (Fig. 5.26). ⊘

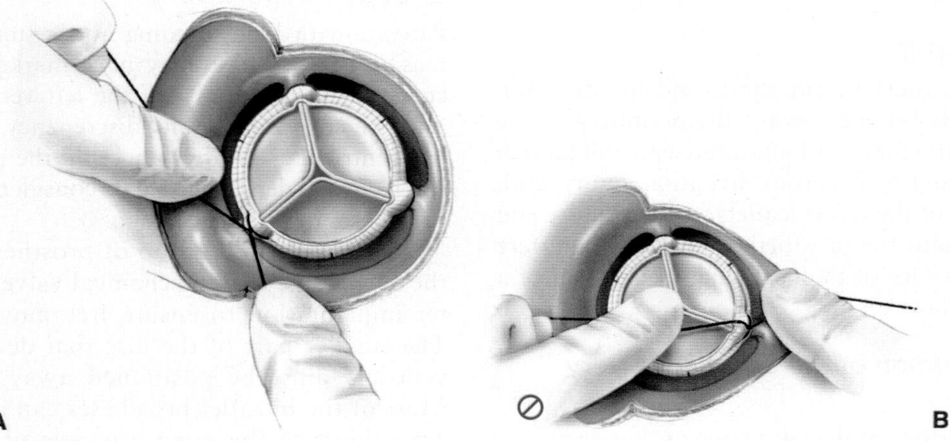

FIG. 5.22 Tying sutures down parallel with the direction of the sewing ring **(A)**, not across the prosthetic leaflets **(B)**.

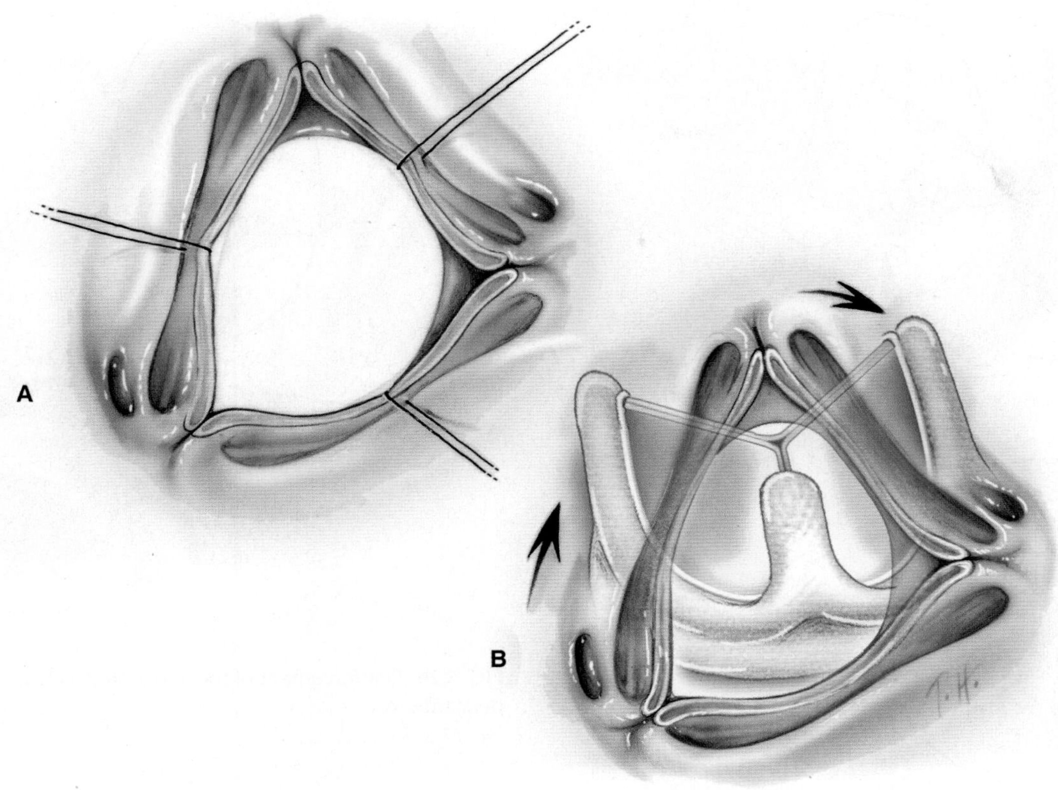

FIG. 5.23 **A:** Aberrant location of coronary artery ostia at the commissures. **B:** Rotation of the bioprosthesis to prevent coronary artery flow interference by the struts.

⊘ Controlling Bleeding from the Aortotomy Ends

To control bleeding from either end of the aortotomy, it is prudent to cross-clamp the aorta temporarily or to reduce the perfusion flow considerably; this will provide good exposure of the bleeding sites and facilitate satisfactory placement of pledgeted sutures to obtain absolute control of bleeding. ⊘

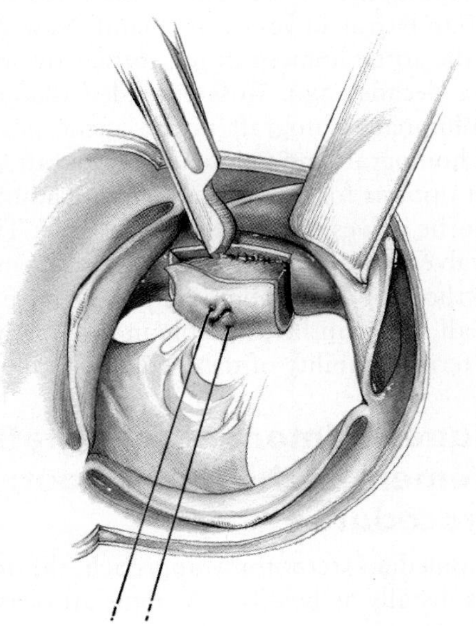

FIG. 5.24 Myectomy to open left ventricular outflow tract.

NB Closure of Oblique Aortotomy

Before seating the prosthesis, the closing aortotomy suture is started at the inferior extent of the opening, well into the noncoronary sinus, and tied. The suture line is continued for five or six bites and is left loose and tagged. The prosthesis is then seated and the valve sutures securely tied. The aortotomy closure suture is tightened with a nerve hook and continued to completion. NB

NB Augmentation of the Aortotomy

Sometimes the struts of the tissue prosthesis protrude into the aortotomy and could result in tension along the suture line. Patch enlargement of the aortotomy with a Hemashield Dacron patch allows ample room for the prosthetic struts and ensures a safe closure (Fig. 5.27) NB.

⊘ Aortic Wall Injury

Rarely the strut of a bioprosthesis may perforate the aortic root during closure of the aortotomy secondary to tenting

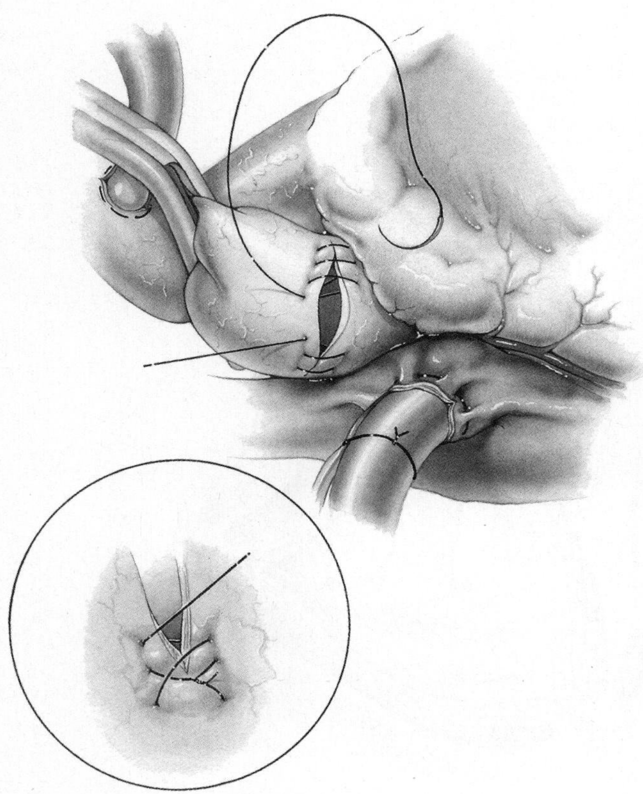

FIG. 5.25 Aortotomy closure with a special precaution to prevent bleeding from the ends of the incision.

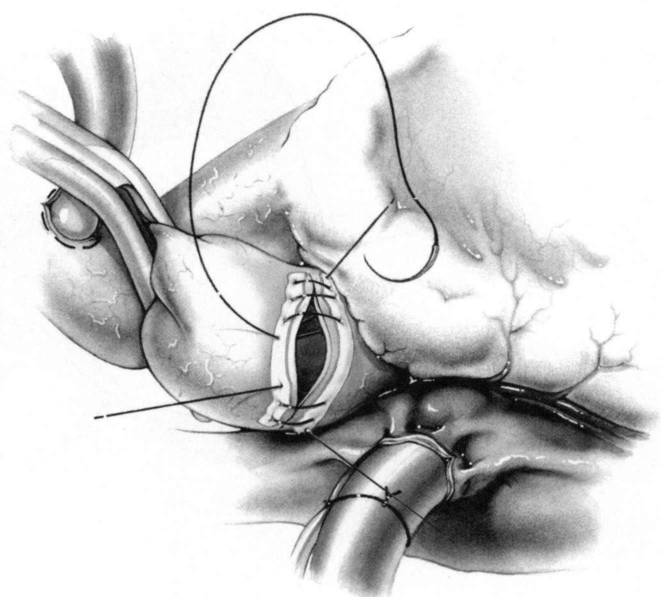

FIG. 5.26 Reinforcement of the aortotomy with strips of pericardium.

of the anterior aorta over the strut (Fig. 5.28). This may necessitate resection of the damaged ascending aorta and replacement with an interposition tube graft. It is important to ensure that the aortic suture does not catch the strut of the bioprosthesis during closure. This error may not only lead to prosthetic regurgitation, but will also weaken the suture line. ⊘

Technique

The aorta is cross-clamped as high as possible, retrograde cold blood cardioplegic solution is administered, and cardioplegic arrest of the heart is established. A right superior pulmonary vein vent is placed (see Chapter 4), and the heart is decompressed. The torn and diseased aorta is resected. If the quality of the aortic wall is good, the defect can be closed with a patch of glutaraldehyde-treated pericardium or Hemashield Dacron. Conversely, if the aortic wall is very thin, dilated, and friable, then the aorta is dissected free from pulmonary artery and transected just above the commissures. The aortic wall is reinforced with a strip of felt and anastomosed to an appropriately sized tube graft (see Chapter 8). The distal end of the tube graft is then sewn to the distal aorta in a similar manner.

HOMOGRAFT, AUTOGRAFT, AND PORCINE STENTLESS AORTIC ROOT IN AORTIC VALVE REPLACEMENT

The mechanical and bioprosthetic valves used in clinical practice have proved to be effective valve substitutes. Nevertheless, the inconvenience and risk of lifelong anticoagulation therapy for mechanical valves and limited longevity of bioprostheses are of concern. Donald Ross of London and Sir Brian Barrat-Boyes of Auckland, New Zealand, introduced the aortic homograft for aortic valve replacement nearly five decades ago. Ross extended the concept and used a pulmonary autograft in the aortic position. Both the aortic homograft and pulmonary autograft are good replacement options for children and young adults. Stentless porcine aortic valves have become available. The stentless porcine valves have been shown to have hemodynamics similar to those of aortic homografts, and have the advantage that all sizes can be available in the operating room. The long-term durability of these valves is still not known.

Technique: Pulmonary Autograft Replacement of the Aortic Root: the Ross Procedure

Through a median sternotomy approach, the aorta is cannulated as distally as possible. A single atriocaval cannula is usually sufficient, but bicaval cannulation is equally satisfactory. A left ventricular vent through the right superior pulmonary vein will decompress the heart and keep

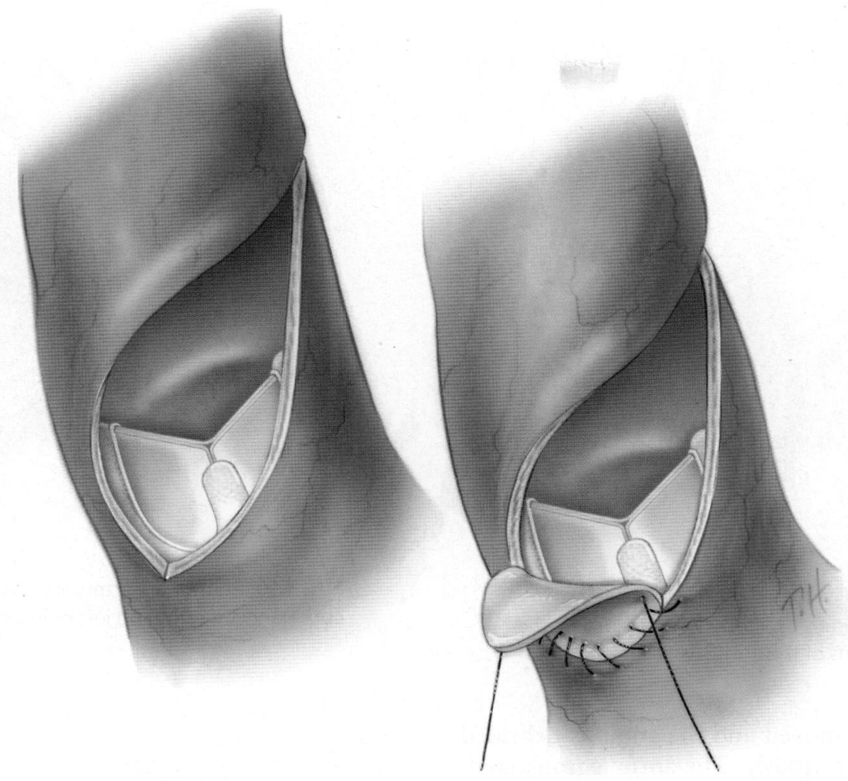

FIG. 5.27 Patch enlargement of the aortotomy.

the field relatively dry. After initiation of cardiopulmonary bypass, systemic cooling is started. The aorta is clamped, and antegrade blood cardioplegic solution is administered. This is complemented by continuous retrograde cold blood followed by cold blood cardioplegic solution (see Myocardial Preservation earlier).

Of course it is of paramount importance that the pulmonary valve be normal. All patients who are considered to be candidates for aortic valve replacement with a pulmonary autograft undergo extensive evaluation preoperatively. Nevertheless, it is necessary for the surgeon to

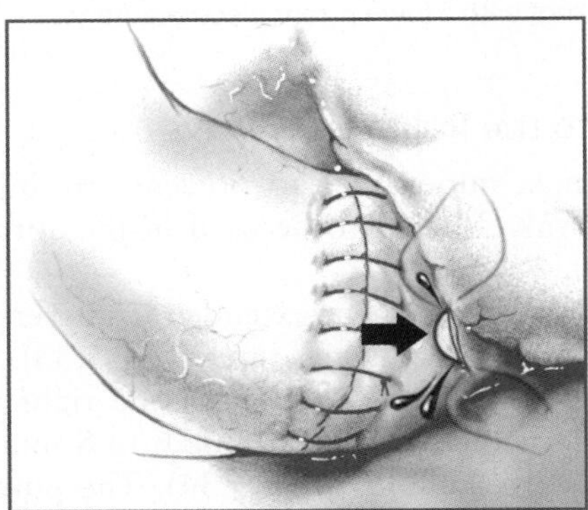

FIG. 5.28 Perforation of the aortic wall by a bioprosthetic strut.

visualize and ascertain the normality of the pulmonary valve at the outset before committing to this procedure.

A transverse incision is made on the anterior aspect of the pulmonary artery near the confluence of the right and left pulmonary arteries. The pulmonary valve is visualized. It must be a normal-appearing trileaflet valve, free of any disease.

⊘ Abnormal Pulmonary Valve

If there is any evidence of pulmonary valve disease, such as previous endocarditis, bicuspid leaflets, or the presence of perforations in the leaflet, the valve is left intact and the pulmonary artery opening is closed with 4-0 Prolene suture. The aortic valve should then be replaced with another alternative such as a homograft or any other appropriate prosthetic valve. ⊘

After satisfactory inspection of the pulmonary valve, a low transverse aortotomy is made. Cold blood cardioplegia is administered directly into the coronary ostia, in particular the right coronary artery, for better protection of the right ventricle.

⊘ Congenital Anomaly of the Coronary Arteries

Abnormal origin of the coronary arteries from the aortic root may complicate the procedure and requires some technical modifications. ⊘

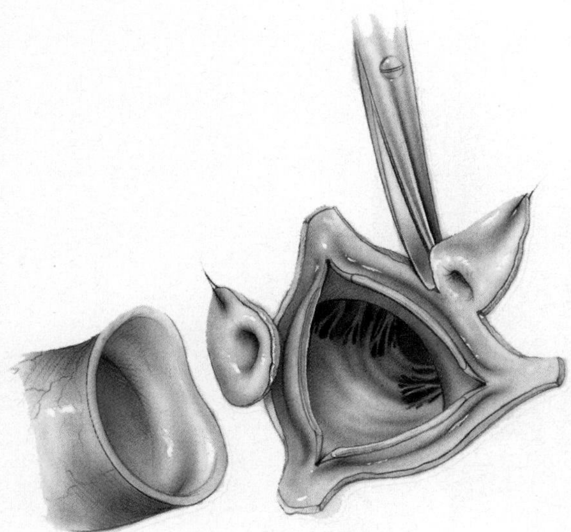

FIG. 5.29 Aorta has been transected. Coronary ostia are removed as large buttons of the aortic wall.

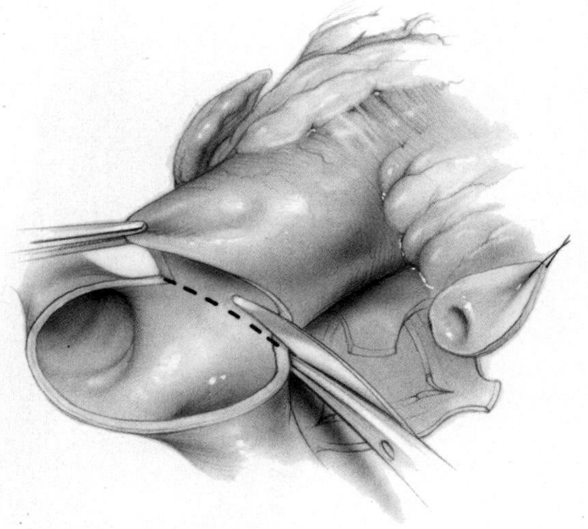

FIG. 5.30 Pulmonary artery is transected at the confluence of right and left pulmonary arteries.

The aortic valve is removed and the annulus debrided of calcium as described previously. The aorta is transected, and the left and the right coronary artery ostia are both removed with a large button of aortic wall. The buttons are dissected free along the course of the coronary arteries to ensure their full mobility (Fig. 5.29).

⊘ Aberrant Branches of Coronary Arteries

Special care must be exercised not to injure any aberrant coronary arteries. ⊘

The pulmonary artery is now completely transected at the confluence of its branches (Fig. 5.30). The dissection is continued with a low-current electrocautery, freeing the pulmonary artery and its root from the root of the aorta down to right ventricular muscle (Fig. 5.31). All small bleeding vessels are electrocoagulated.

⊘ Injury to the Left Main Coronary Artery

The course of the left main coronary artery is intimately related to the pulmonary artery and its root. Dissection in this area must be carried out with utmost care. ⊘

NB Retrograde perfusion of blood through the coronary sinus identifies small bleeding vessels that otherwise would have gone unnoticed. Hemostasis at this stage of the surgery is important, as bleeding from this area is difficult to control once the procedure is completed and the aortic clamp removed. NB

When the pulmonary artery is well mobilized, a right-angled clamp is introduced into the right ventricle through the pulmonary valve. An incision is made on the right ventricular outflow tract down onto the right-angled clamp 6 to 8 mm below the pulmonary valve annulus (Fig. 5.32A).

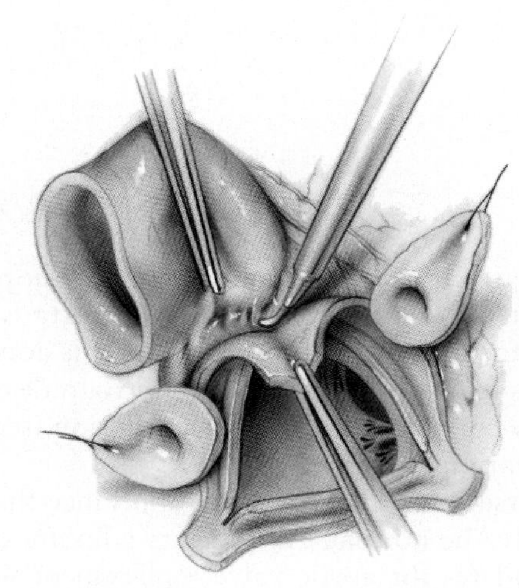

FIG. 5.31 Pulmonary artery is dissected free of the aortic root with a low-current electrocautery.

⊘ Injury to the Pulmonary Valve

It is of utmost importance to prevent any injury to the pulmonary valve that is to be used in the aortic position (Fig. 5.32B). ⊘

This incision is then extended transversely across the right ventricular outflow tract (Fig. 5.33). The endocardium on the posterior aspect of the right ventricular outflow tract is incised with a knife 6 to 8 mm below the pulmonary valve annulus (Fig. 5.34). The pulmonary artery is now enucleated using Metzenbaum scissors with the blade angled in such a way as to not injure the first septal branch of the left anterior descending coronary artery (Fig. 5.35).

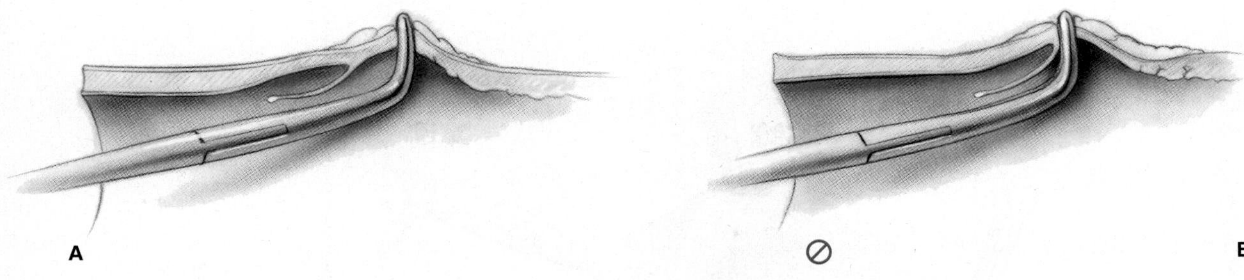

FIG. 5.32 Tip of the right angle should be 6 to 8 mm below the pulmonary annulus. **A:** The optimal site for detachment of the pulmonary root from the right ventricle. **B:** Pulmonary valve can be injured if the ventriculotomy is too high.

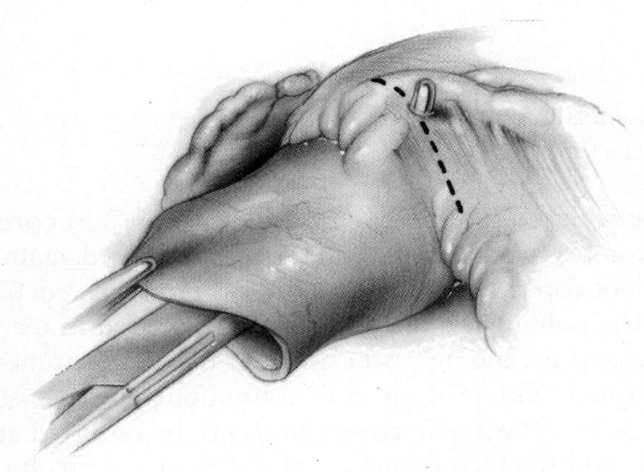

FIG. 5.33 The tip of the right-angled clamp and right ventricular incision along the dashed line.

⊘ Injury to the First Septal Coronary Artery

The first septal branch of the left anterior descending coronary artery has a variable course and may at times be very large. The enucleating technique allows detachment of the pulmonary artery root without injury to this branch, which can lead to massive septal infarction. Some surgeons require patients who are candidates for the Ross procedure to undergo coronary angiography preoperatively for the specific delineation of coronary artery anatomy. If the first septal artery takeoff is very high and its size is significant, the Ross procedure may be contraindicated. If the septal artery is severed, both ends should be oversewn to prevent fistulous runoff into the right ventricle. ⊘

The pulmonary autograft is freed from the right ventricular outflow tract and is trimmed of excess fatty tissue. It is then placed in a pool of blood alongside the right atrium.

⊘ Buttonhole in the Pulmonary Artery

To prevent buttonhole injury to the pulmonary artery wall, a finger is carefully placed inside it across the pulmonary valve while removing epicardial fatty tissue. ⊘

Simple interrupted 4-0 Ticron sutures are now placed very closely together at the level of the annulus and below the level of the commissures to create a circle of stitches in a single plane (Fig. 5.36). This entails taking bites of the subaortic curtain, the membranous, and muscular segments of the left ventricular outflow tract. The aortic annular sutures are now passed through the pulmonary autograft just below its annulus.

Alternatively, the pulmonary autograft can be anastomosed to the aortic root with a continuous suture of 4-0 Prolene. The suture line should begin at the commissure between the left and right coronary sinuses, passing the needle inside out on the aortic annulus and outside in on the pulmonary autograft. The posterior suture line is completed, and then the second needle is used to complete the anterior anastomosis. A nerve hook may be used to ensure that the suture line is tight before tying the two ends together.

⊘ Orientation of the Pulmonary Autograft

The correct orientation of the pulmonary autograft is of great importance. It should be placed in such a manner so that its sinuses overlie the sinuses of the native aorta to facilitate left main coronary artery implantation. ⊘

⊘ Injury to the Pulmonary Autograft Leaflet

When placing sutures in the pulmonary autograft, care must be taken not to pass the needle through the pulmonary valve leaflet. ⊘

The pulmonary autograft is lowered into position, and the sutures are tied over a strip of autologous pericardium (Fig. 5.37). With the continuous suture technique, a strip of pericardium may be incorporated into the anastomosis.

An incision is then made in the area of the proposed implantation of the left main coronary artery button. A

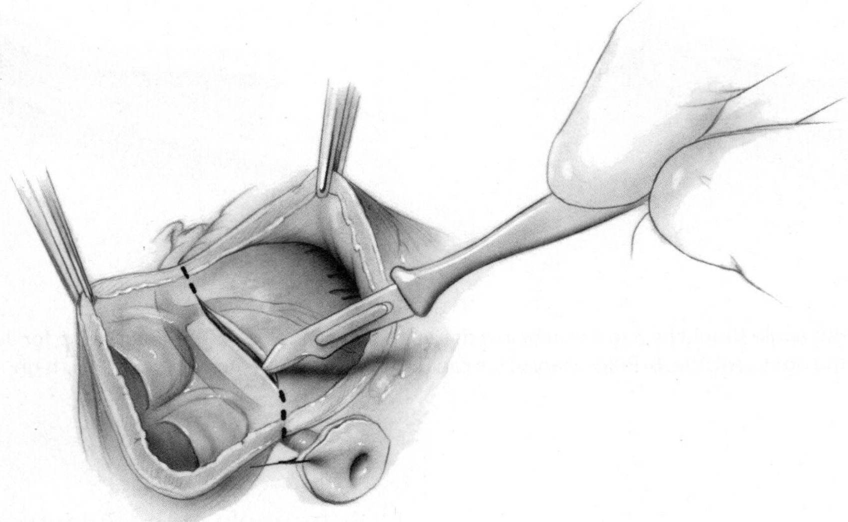

FIG. 5.34 The endocardium on the posterior right ventricular outflow tract is incised 6 to 8 mm below the pulmonary annulus.

4.0-mm punch is used to enlarge the opening. The left main coronary button is attached to the pulmonary autograft with 5-0 or 6-0 continuous Prolene suture (Fig. 5.38). The right coronary button is attached to the pulmonary autograft in the same manner.

⊘ Kinking of the Left Main Coronary Artery

There should be no kinking of the left main coronary artery. An appropriately sized probe must be passed into the left main coronary artery to ensure its unobstructed course. ⊘

NB It is often prudent to perform the right coronary attachment after completion of the distal aortic anastomosis. The aortic clamp can be removed for a moment to distend the aortic root and the precise location of the right coronary anastomosis can be noted. The aorta is clamped again, and the right coronary artery anastomosis is completed. NB

The pulmonary autograft is now trimmed to meet the transected ascending aorta and the distal anastomosis is performed with 4-0 or 5-0 continuous Prolene suture (Fig. 5.39). The aortic cross-clamp can be removed at this point, and the reconstruction of the right ventricular outflow tract completed while the patient is being rewarmed.

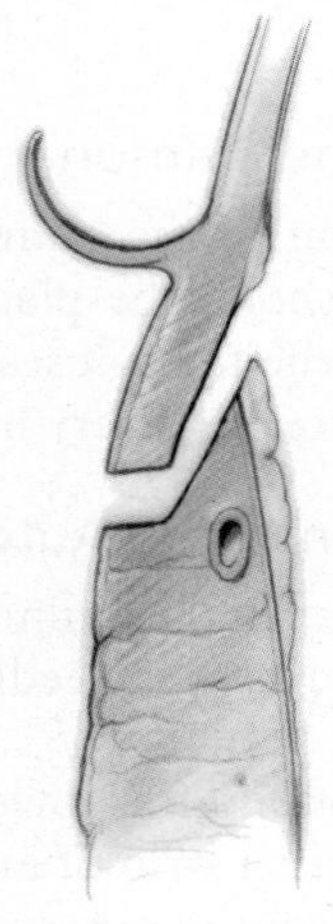

FIG. 5.35 Pulmonary root is enucleated without injury to the first septal coronary artery.

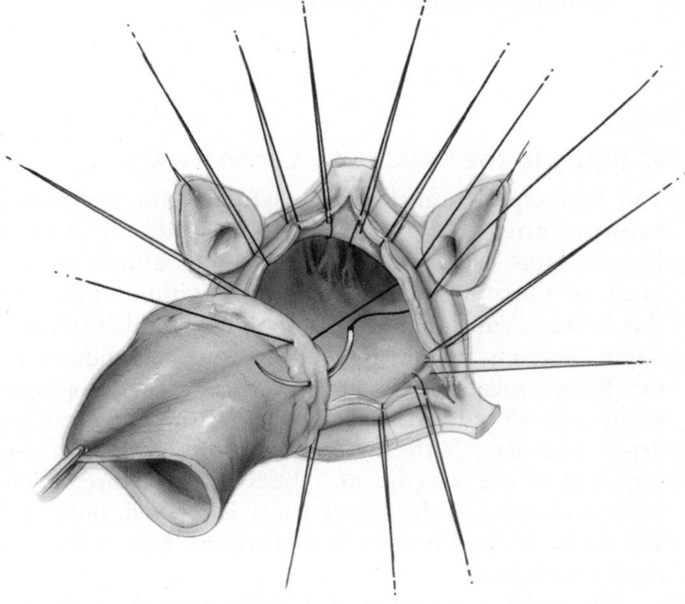

FIG. 5.36 Interrupted sutures are placed in the annulus and pulmonary autograft (see text).

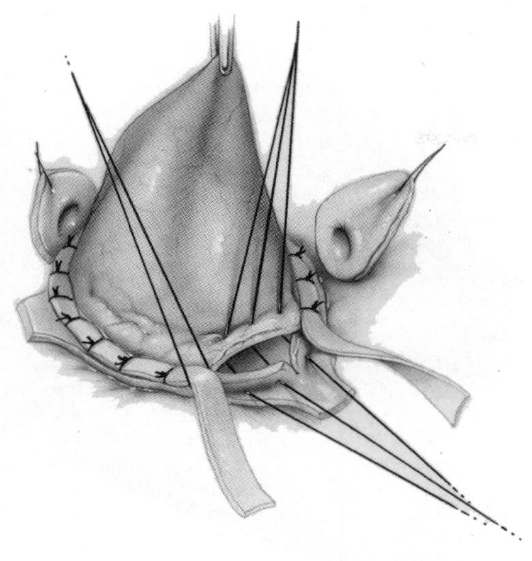

FIG. 5.37 Sutures are tied over a strip of pericardium.

An appropriately sized, cryopreserved pulmonary homograft is selected and oriented with one sinus posteriorly and two sinuses anteriorly in an anatomic manner. It is trimmed appropriately, and the distal anastomosis is carried out with 4-0 or 5-0 Prolene suture.

⊘ Kinking of the Pulmonary Homograft

Leaving the pulmonary homograft too long may result in kinking of the distal suture line when the heart is filled with blood. ⊘

⊘ Gradient across Distal Suture Line

There is a tendency for a gradient to develop across the distal anastomosis. This may be secondary to an immune reaction with subsequent fibrosis. It may also be due to the purse-string effect of a continuous suture line. To prevent this complication, sutures should be spaced close together. Additionally, the pulmonary homograft should be oversized to minimize the gradient even if some narrowing of the anastomosis occurs. ⊘

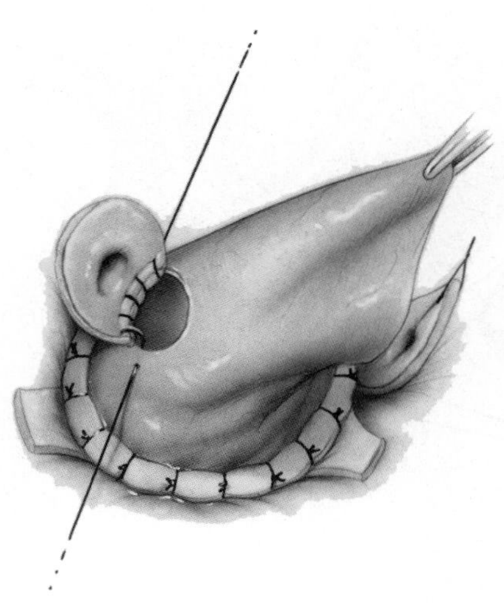

FIG. 5.38 Anastomosing the left coronary button to the pulmonary autograft.

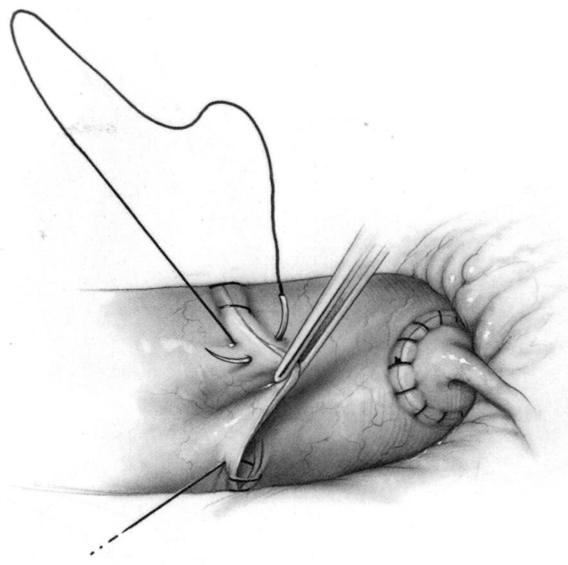

FIG. 5.39 Attachment of the pulmonary autograft to the aorta.

Using 4-0 Prolene, the proximal anastomosis is started on the posterior aspect of the incision on the right ventricular outflow tract. After completing the suture line medially, the lateral aspect of the posterior suture line is accomplished, taking shallow bites of the endocardium to avoid the septal branches of the left anterior descending coronary artery (Fig. 5.40B). The remainder of the suture line anteriorly is completed (Fig. 5.41). The heart is filled, deairing performed, and the patient is weaned from cardiopulmonary bypass.

⊘ Septal Artery Injury

Full-thickness bites on the right ventricle posteriorly risks injury to high septal coronary branches. ⊘

NB The surgeon may elect to complete the right ventricle to pulmonary artery connection with a pulmonary homograft before implanting the pulmonary autograft in the aortic root. NB

NB Dilation of Autograft

In infants and young children, implantation of the pulmonary autograft as a complete root has been demonstrated to allow somatic growth to occur. The concern is that dilation may also take place, resulting in aortic valve insufficiency. Excising the entire left and right aortic sinuses and using this native aortic tissue to replace the corresponding sinuses of the autograft, and reinforcing the noncoronary portion of the autograft with the retained native aortic wall

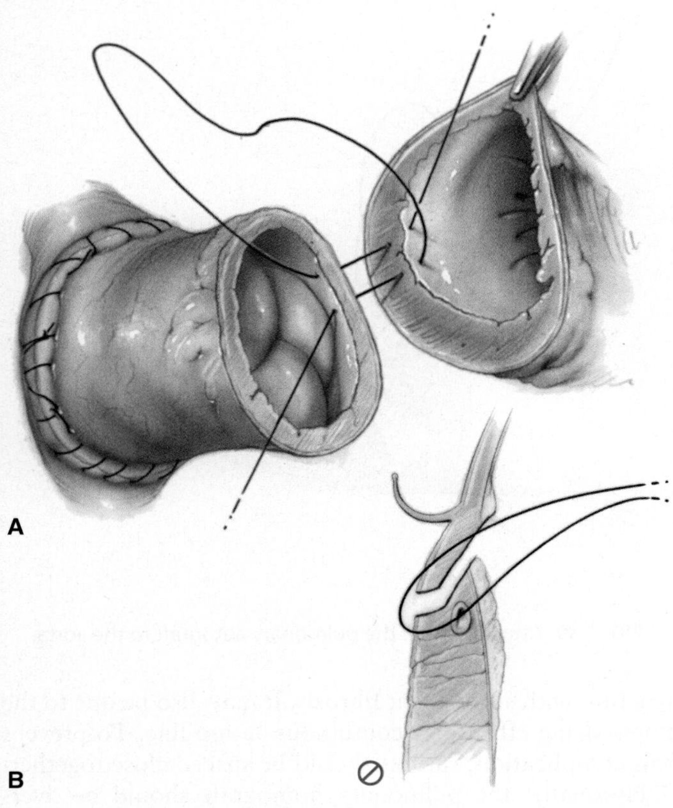

FIG. 5.40 **A:** Approximating the cryopreserved pulmonary artery homograft to the right ventricular outflow tract. **B:** Full-thickness sutures may occlude the septal artery.

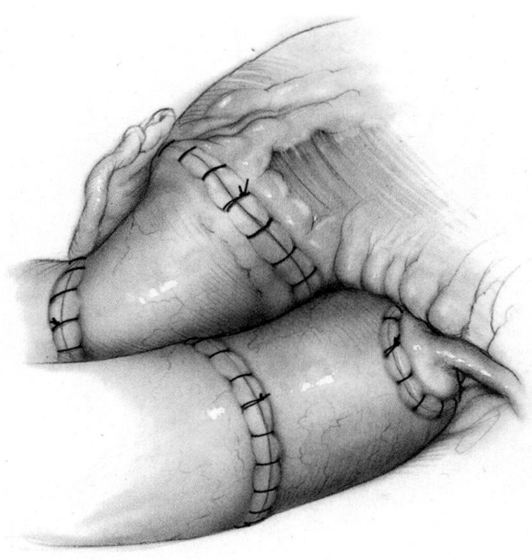

FIG. 5.41 Completed pulmonary autograft replacement of the aortic root.

may help prevent dilation (Fig. 5.42). Another technique to prevent dilation of the pulmonary autograft is to wrap it with Hemashield (Fig. 5.43). In older children and adults, geometric matching of the aortic and pulmonary artery roots is necessary to avoid aortic insufficiency if the root replacement technique is used. This may involve plication of the aortic annulus with pledgeted horizontal mattress sutures at the commissures and/or the use of an interposition tube graft to fix the diameter of the sinotubular junction. Alternatively, many institutions prefer to implant the pulmonary autograft in older children and adults using a modified subcoronary technique, as was originally performed by Ross. The technique is similar to that described for the implantation of a stentless bioprosthesis. NB

Technique: Aortic Valve Replacement Using Stentless Bioprosthesis or Aortic Homograft

It is clear that the normal geometry of the aortic root can be better maintained if the whole root is replaced with an aortic allograft or stentless aortic bioprosthesis. This technique is described in detail in the section on pulmonary autograft replacement of the aortic root (Ross procedure). Nevertheless, a modified subcoronary technique for the replacement of the aortic valve with an aortic homograft has been practiced since its introduction with excellent results. Below, one will find out technique for subcoronary

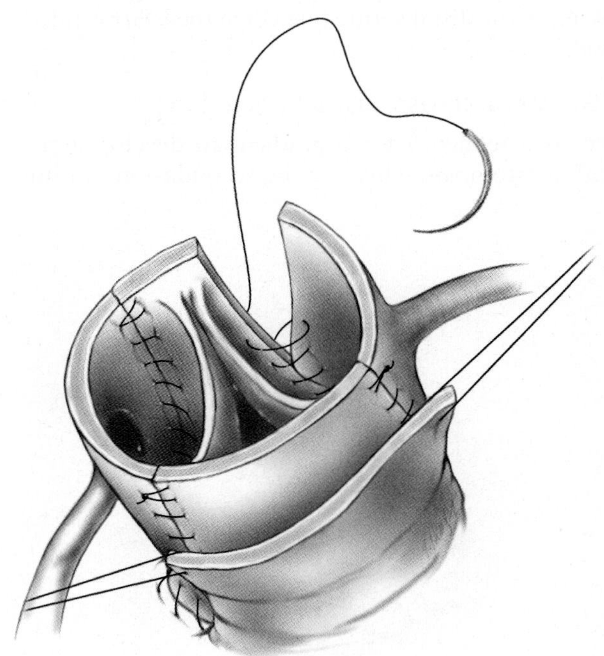

FIG. 5.42 Large coronary buttons completely replace native aortic sinuses. Preserved noncoronary aortic sinus is incorporated in anastomosis of autograft to ascending aorta, thereby reinforcing noncoronary sinus of autograft.

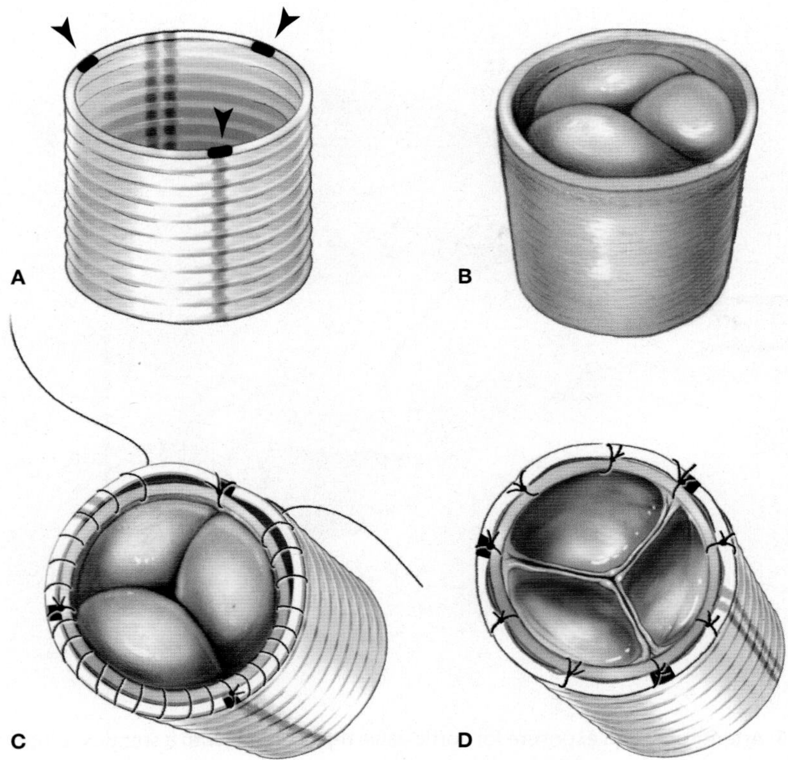

FIG. 5.43 Wrapping of pulmonary autograft with a Hemashield graft.

implanation of stentless aortic root bioprosthesis; however, similar principles apply when using an aortic homograft. We have employed a similar technique when implanting the stentless aortic root bioprosthesis.

Three traction sutures are placed on the anterior surface of the aorta (Fig. 5.44). A small transverse aortotomy is made and then extended both upward and downward under direct vision to provide good exposure of the aortic root. The aortic valve is excised. Three 4-0 Ticron simple sutures are placed in the nadir of each annulus. Traction on these sutures opens the aortic annulus and left ventricular outflow tract maximally, allowing accurate sizing (Fig. 5.45).

⊘ Too Low Aortotomy

If the aortotomy is too proximal, it will be impossible to resuspend the commissures of the prosthetic valve or homograft high enough (see later). A small transverse aortotomy is made initially at least 1 cm above the right coronary ostium. The aortic root should be visualized through this opening. If the incision is too close to the valve commissures, it should be closed and a new incision made more distally on the aorta. ⊘

⊘ Undersizing the Valve

The valve sizer should fit snugly in the aortic annulus. It is advisable to oversize the valve 1 to 3 mm. The larger surface area of the cusps allows greater apposition of the leaflet tissue, thereby reducing the possibility of valvular insufficiency. ⊘

⊘ Discrepancy between the Sinotubular and Aortic Annulus Diameter

If the diameter of the sinotubular junction is more than 2 mm greater than that of the annulus, the modified subcoronary technique should not be used. Some patients with poststenotic dilation of the aorta will demonstrate this finding. Performing a subcoronary implant of a stentless prosthesis or homograft valve in these patients will result in valvular insufficiency when the aortic root is pressurized and the commissures of the implanted valve are pulled outward. Some surgeons have advocated reducing the size of the sinotubular junction in such patients. However, it is probably safer to perform the implant as a root replacement (see previously) or select a stented prosthesis. ⊘

NB Type of Aortotomy

In patients with good-sized aortic roots, the aortotomy should be made transversely several millimeters above the native commissures. This allows precise sizing and resuspension of the prosthetic commissures. In patients with small aortic roots, an oblique aortotomy extended downward into the noncoronary sinus allows better visualization and easier placement of sutures. However, the oblique

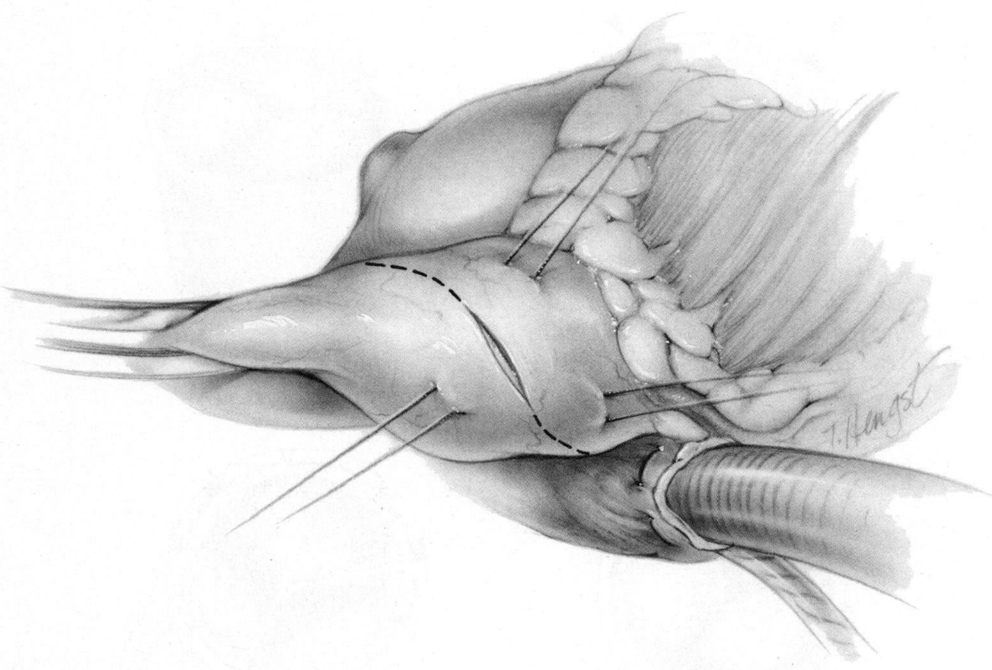

FIG. 5.44 Arteriotomy and exposure for aortic valve replacement with a stentless bioprosthesis.

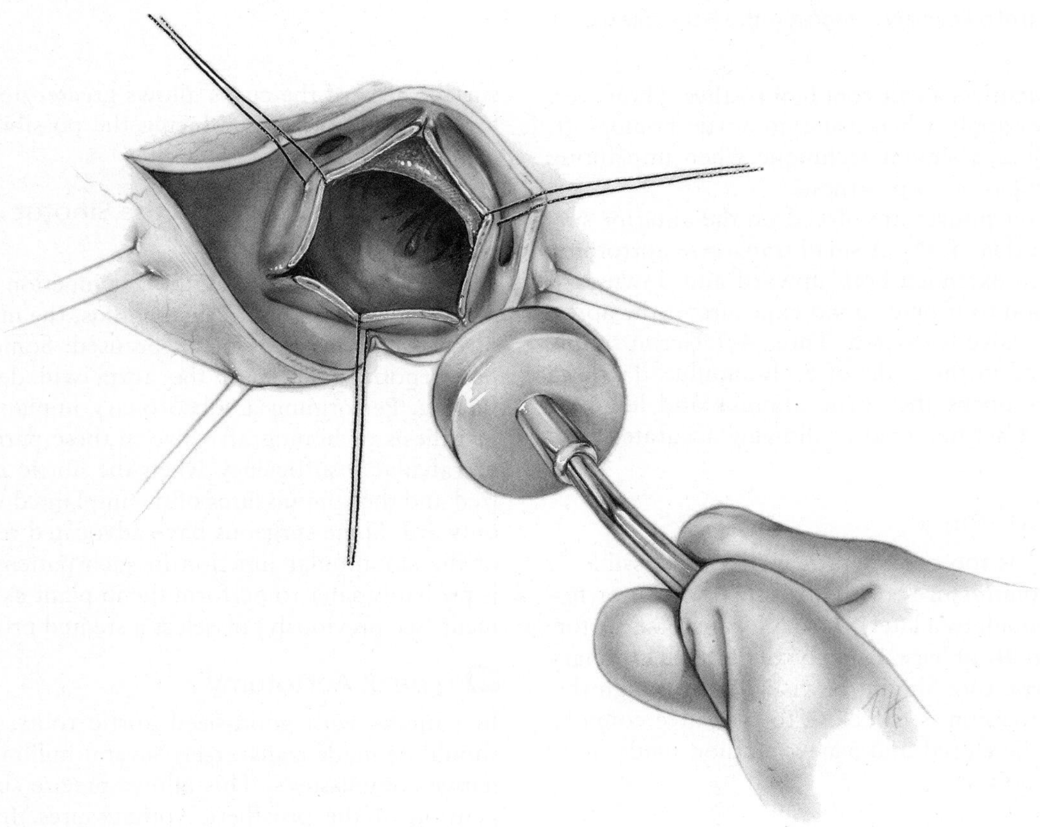

FIG. 5.45 Sizing the left ventricular outflow tract.

incision does distort the anatomy of the aortic root so that resuspending the commissures is more challenging. NB

Simple interrupted sutures of 4-0 Ticron are now placed 2 to 3 mm apart at the level of the annulus and below the level of the commissures to create a circle of stitches in a single plane. This entails taking bites of the subaortic curtain, the membranous, and muscular segment of the left ventricular outflow tract. The three sutures that were originally placed in the nadir of the aortic annulus are now passed through the Dacron skirt of the appropriately sized stentless bioprosthesis just below the lowest aspect of the leaflet cusps (Fig. 5.46).

⊘ Leaflet Injury

It is important to place the needle well away from the margin of the bioprothetic leaflet attachment. Needle perforation of the leaflet tissue of the bioprosthesis results in irreparable injury (Fig. 5.47). ⊘

The remaining sutures are placed in the skirt of the device in a similar manner. The prosthesis is lowered into position, and the sutures are tied snugly and cut short.

NB Many surgeons using homografts prefer to invert the device into the left ventricle and attach the homograft to the annulus with a continuous suture. This technique takes less time and can be accomplished with very good results. However, the porcine aortic root bioprosthesis is not as pliable as a homograft and may be damaged during the process of its inversion into left ventricular outflow tract followed by being pulled up into the aorta. The use of multiple interrupted simple sutures allows a precise proximal suture line without distortion or purse stringing. NB

With the prosthesis seated within the aortic root, the right and left coronary sinus portions of the stentless bioprosthesis are scalloped to fit beneath the patient's own coronary ostia, leaving a 4- to 5-mm rim of prosthetic

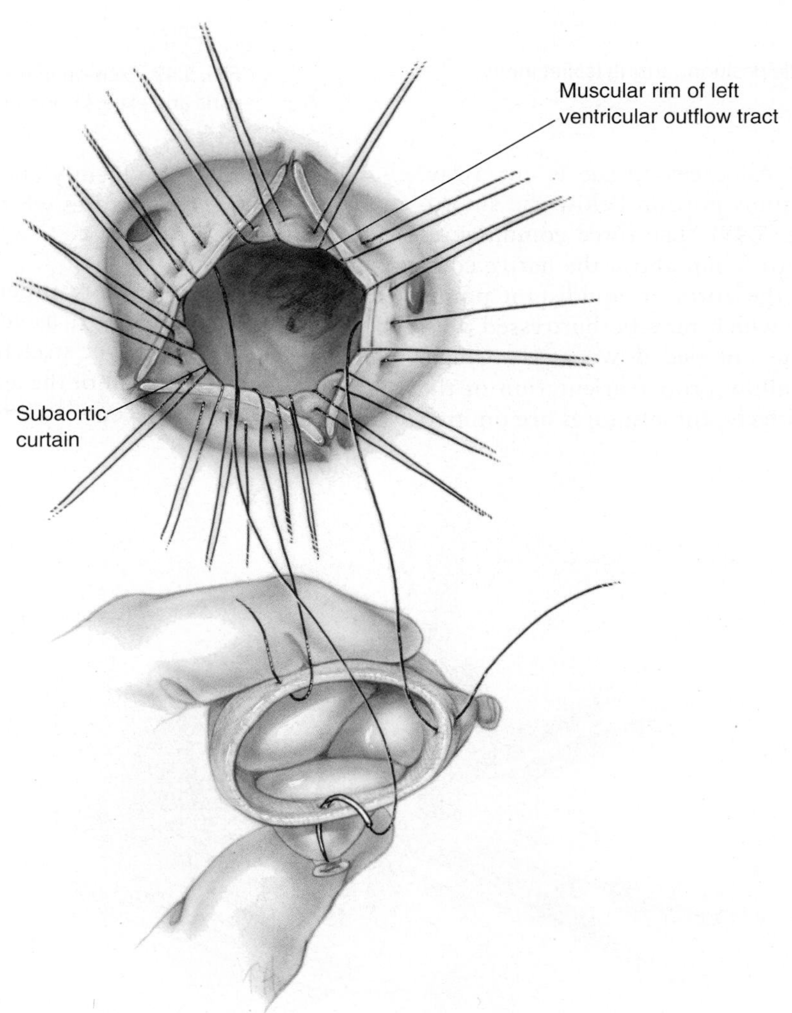

FIG. 5.46 Simple interrupted suture placement in the annulus, subaortic curtain, and muscular segment of the left ventricular outflow tract and bioprosthesis.

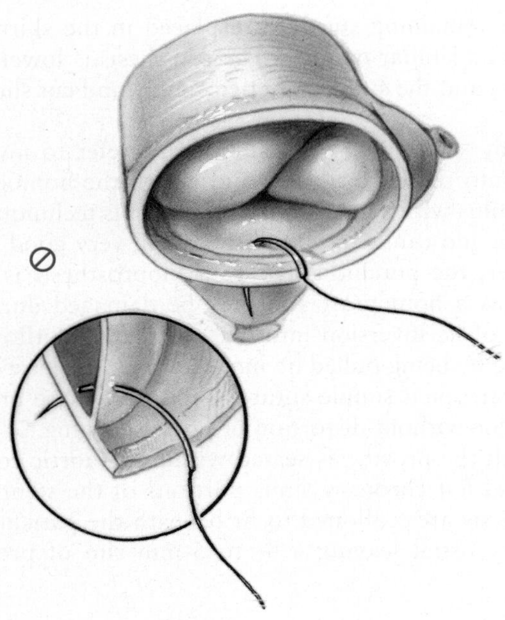

FIG. 5.47 Incorrect needle position causing leaflet injury.

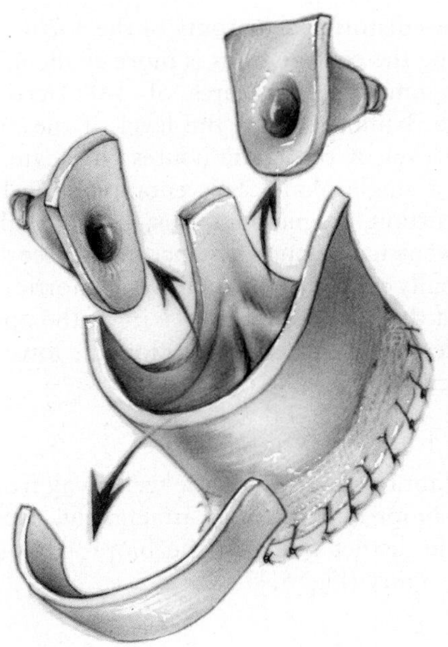

FIG. 5.49 Excision of the coronary artery ostia and excess noncoronary prosthetic wall.

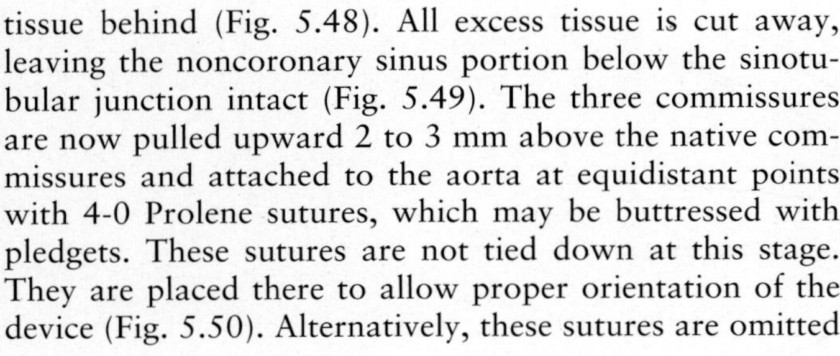

tissue behind (Fig. 5.48). All excess tissue is cut away, leaving the noncoronary sinus portion below the sinotubular junction intact (Fig. 5.49). The three commissures are now pulled upward 2 to 3 mm above the native commissures and attached to the aorta at equidistant points with 4-0 Prolene sutures, which may be buttressed with pledgets. These sutures are not tied down at this stage. They are placed there to allow proper orientation of the device (Fig. 5.50). Alternatively, these sutures are omitted and the surgeon frequently checks the positioning of the bioprosthetic commissures while performing the distal suture line (Fig. 5.51).

NB The importance of resuspending the commissures of the bioprosthesis as high as feasible cannot be overemphasized. This maneuver stretches the device upward and allows a larger segment of the leaflets to coapt during diastole, preventing any central aortic leak. **NB**

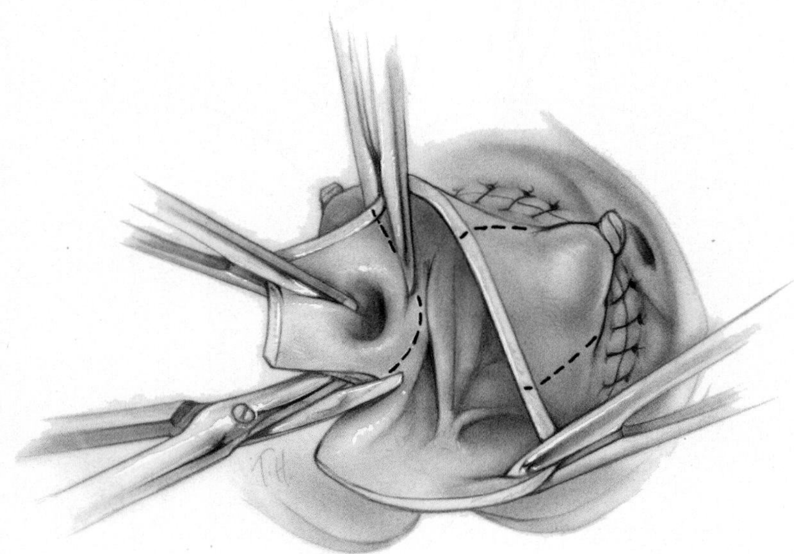

FIG. 5.48 Removal of the coronary sinuses of the prosthesis.

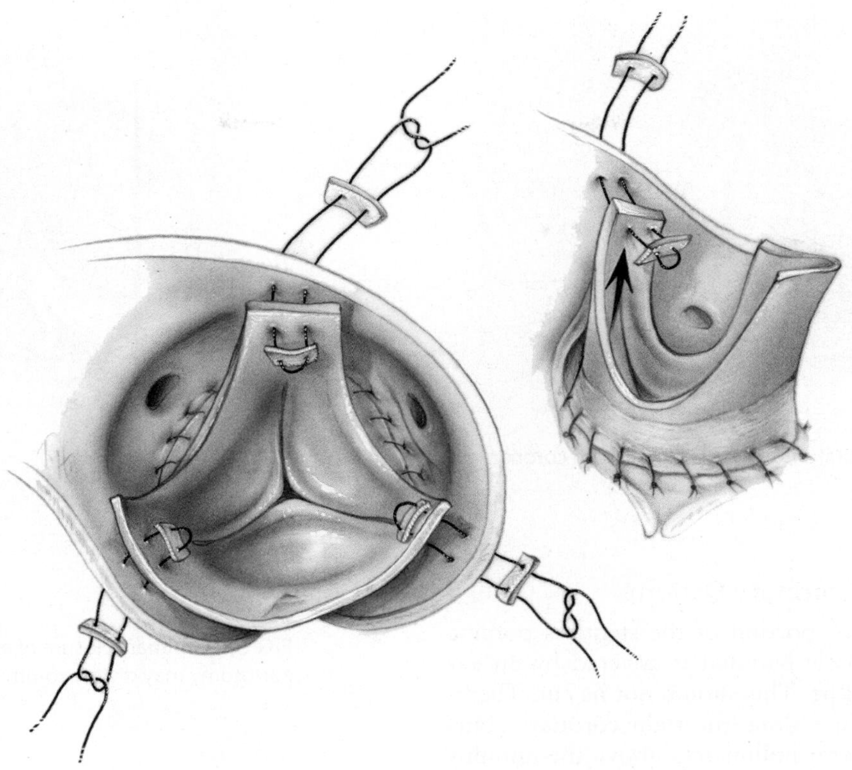

FIG. 5.50 Suspension of the prosthetic commissures above the native aortic commissures.

The scalloped portion of the device is sutured to the native aortic wall parallel with the native annulus. This technique ensures a precise, waterproof suture line well away from the coronary ostia. The suture line starts at the nadir beneath each coronary artery ostium and progresses upward to the top of the commissure on each side (Fig. 5.52). The sutures are tied together at the top of the commissure between the left and right coronary sinus outside the aorta. If commissural sutures have been used, they are now tied outside the aorta and may be buttressed with a pledget.

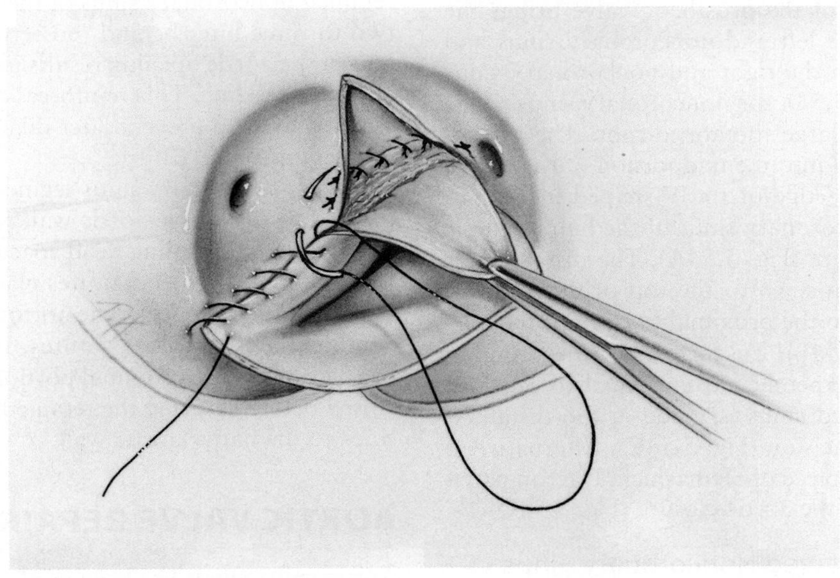

FIG. 5.51 Distal suture line beneath the left coronary ostium with frequent assessment of commissure placement.

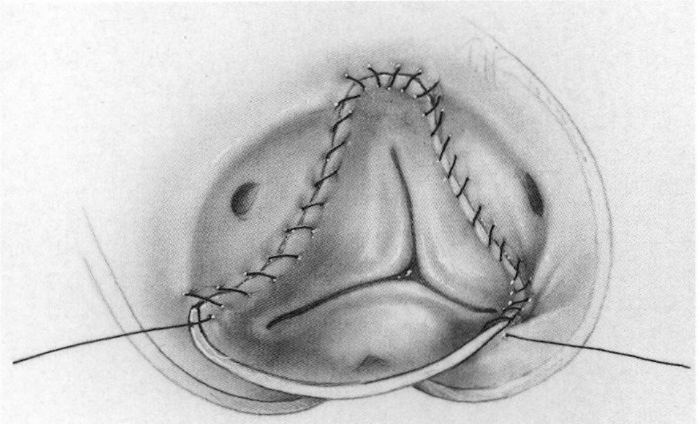

FIG. 5.52 Completed distal suture line beneath both coronary artery ostia.

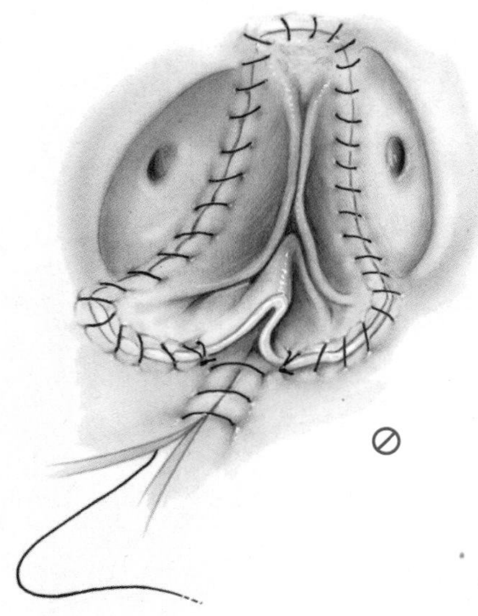

FIG. 5.53 Primary closure of an oblique aortotomy may distort commissural alignment.

⊘ Low-Lying Right Coronary Ostium

The right coronary sinus portion of the stentless porcine bioprosthesis has a muscle bar that is covered by an extension of the Dacron skirt. This should not be cut. Therefore, the distal suture line along the right coronary sinus must be performed several millimeters above the annulus so as not to buckle the muscle bar of the prosthetic valve. If the patient's right coronary ostium is particularly low, the prosthetic valve should be rotated 120 degrees to place the muscle bar in the patient's noncoronary sinus. All three prosthetic sinuses are then scalloped. ⊘

⊘ Distortion of Commissures with Closure of an Oblique Aortotomy

If closure of the native aortic wall over the retained noncoronary sinus portion of the prosthetic valve brings the commissure between the left and noncoronary sinus and the commissure between the right and noncoronary sinus too close together (Fig. 5.53), the noncoronary sinus of the prosthesis is used to enlarge the aortic root. The aortotomy incision is extended into the midportion of the native noncoronary sinus. The edge of the V-shaped incision is sutured to the retained coronary sinus of the bioprosthesis using a 4-0 Prolene suture (Fig. 5.54A). The distal aspect of the aortotomy is then sewn to the top of the retained sinus and continued onto the proximal portion of the aortotomy incision (Fig. 5.54B). To correct for the resulting length discrepancy, a perpendicular cut equal to one-half the width of the retained sinus is made in the distal aspect of the aortotomy incision (Fig. 5.54C). Alternatively, a small, triangle-shaped piece of Hemashield Dacron patch can be used to complete the aortic closure (Fig. 5.54D). ⊘

⊘ Bulging of the Retained Noncoronary Sinus Wall into the Lumen of the Aorta

If closure of the aortotomy results in protrusion of the prosthetic noncoronary sinus into the aorta and the commissures are appropriately located, the noncoronary sinus should be scalloped and reattached to the aortic wall as was done for the right and left coronary sinuses. Alternatively, the bulge, if not excessive, can be approximated to the native aortic wall with separate sutures. ⊘

NB Closure of a Transverse Aortotomy

When a transverse aortotomy has been made, the rightward aspect of the closure will often include the top of the retained noncoronary sinus of the prosthetic valve. Taking two to three bites behind (posterior to) the rightward extent of the aortic opening results in a nearly circumferential aortic suture line. This reinforces the sinotubular junction, which may help prevent later dilation and resultant valvular incompetence. NB

The noncoronary sinus segment of the bioprosthesis is secured to the native aortic wall with another 4-0 Prolene suture. The intervening dead space can be obliterated with one or two 4-0 Prolene sutures placed inside to outside and tied over a felt pledget. The aortotomy is then closed with continuous 4-0 Prolene sutures. If an oblique aortotomy has been used, the proximal portion of the opening must be closed before suturing the retained prosthetic noncoronary sinus to the native aortic wall.

AORTIC VALVE REPAIR

Aortic valve repair has been used successfully in congenital patients with subaortic membranes and/or ventricular septal defects with cusp prolapse (Fig. 5.55). Only select adult patients are candidates for aortic valve repair. Stenotic

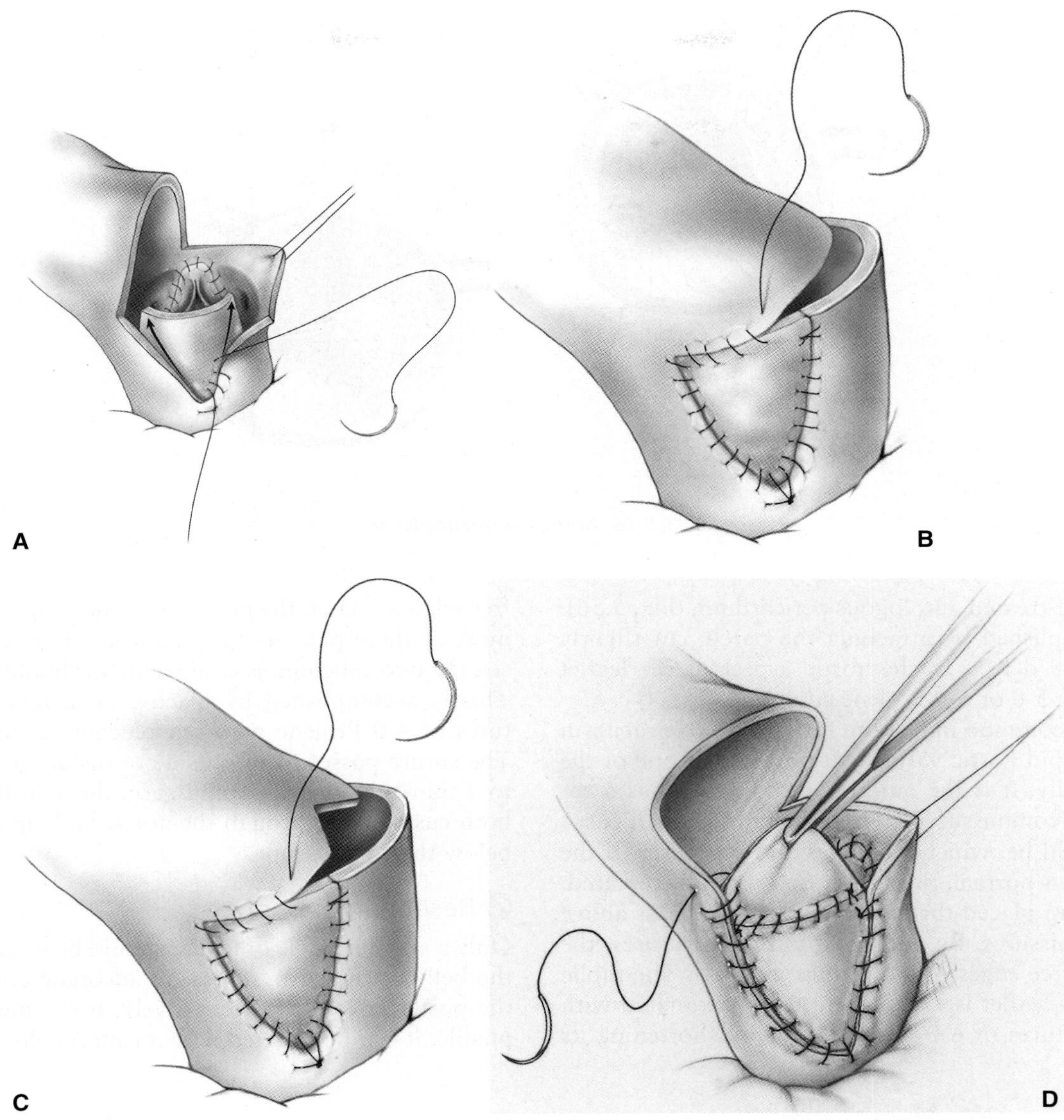

FIG. 5.54 **A:** Using a portion of the noncoronary sinus of a stentless valve to enlarge an aortotomy in such a way as to correctly align commissures. **B and C:** Completing aortic closure with native aortic wall. **D:** Aortic closure completed with a patch of Hemashield.

aortic valves are not amenable to repair. Aortic valve repair may be possible in patients with aortic insufficiency secondary to dilation of one or more components of the aortic root or cusp prolapse only if the cusps are not thickened, have good mobility, and are not calcified

⊘ Ultrasonographic Decalcification

Ultrasonographic decalcification of stenotic aortic valves has been abandoned because of the resultant scarring and retraction of the leaflets. ⊘

NB Prolapse of one cusp in an adult patient with a trileaflet aortic valve is rare. Repair can be achieved with the technique described in Chapter 21. NB

Techniques

A successful and durable aortic valve repair requires a thorough understanding of the mechanism of the aortic valve dysfunction. Transesophageal echocardiography demonstrates the quality, height, and coaptation level of the leaflets, as well as the respective diameters of the annulus, sinuses, sinotubular junction, and ascending aorta (see Surgical Anatomy of the Aortic Valve discussed earlier). Patients with a dilated sinotubular junction or aneurysm of the aortic root with aortic valve insufficiency and normal cusps are candidates for a valve sparing procedure (see Chapter 8).

Perforation of a cusp due to healed endocarditis or iatrogenic injury may be patched with a piece of

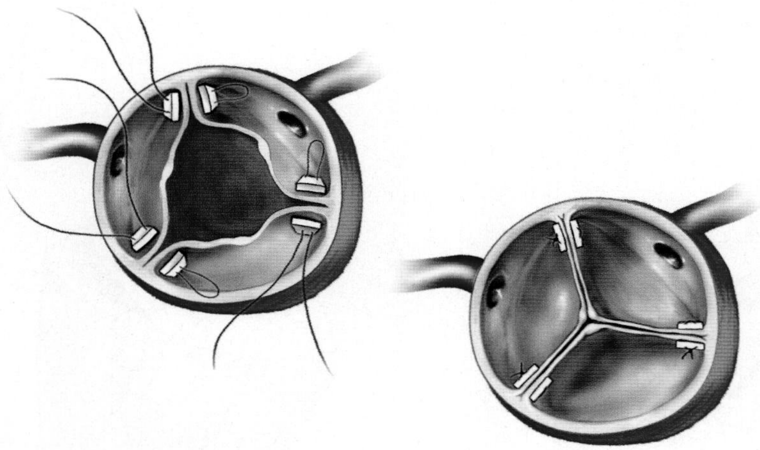

FIG. 5.55 Aortic comissuroplasty.

glutaraldehyde-treated autologous pericardium (Fig. 5.56). This is accomplished by attaching the patch, cut slightly larger than the defect, to the aortic aspect of the leaflet with a running 5-0 or 6-0 Prolene suture.

The most common indication for aortic valve repair in adults is bicuspid aortic valve with prolapse of one of the cusps. Generally, it is the anterior cusp, which has a raphe where the commissure between the right and left cusps normally would be, which elongates and prolapses. If the posterior cusp is normal, the anterior cusp can be repaired. Stay sutures are placed through the aortic wall just above the two commissures. By pulling up on these sutures, the length of the free edges of the leaflets is noted. The raphe of the anterior leaflet is excised and reapproximated with interrupted sutures of 6-0 Prolene, thereby shortening its free edge to match the posterior leaflet (Fig. 5.57). Because most of these patients have associated annuloaortic ectasia, the two subcommissural triangles should be narrowed. This is accomplished by placing horizontal mattress sutures of 4-0 Prolene with felt pledgets outside the aorta. The suture passes from outside to inside the aortic root 2 to 3 mm below each commissure, through the annulus of both cusps, then through the aortic wall again 2 to 3 mm below the commissure.

⊘ Resection of Raphe

Only a small triangle of leaflet should be resected, avoiding the belly of the cusp, to ensure adequate coaptation with the posterior leaflet. Alternatively, if the median raphe is pliable, it can be plicated with a running Prolene suture. ⊘

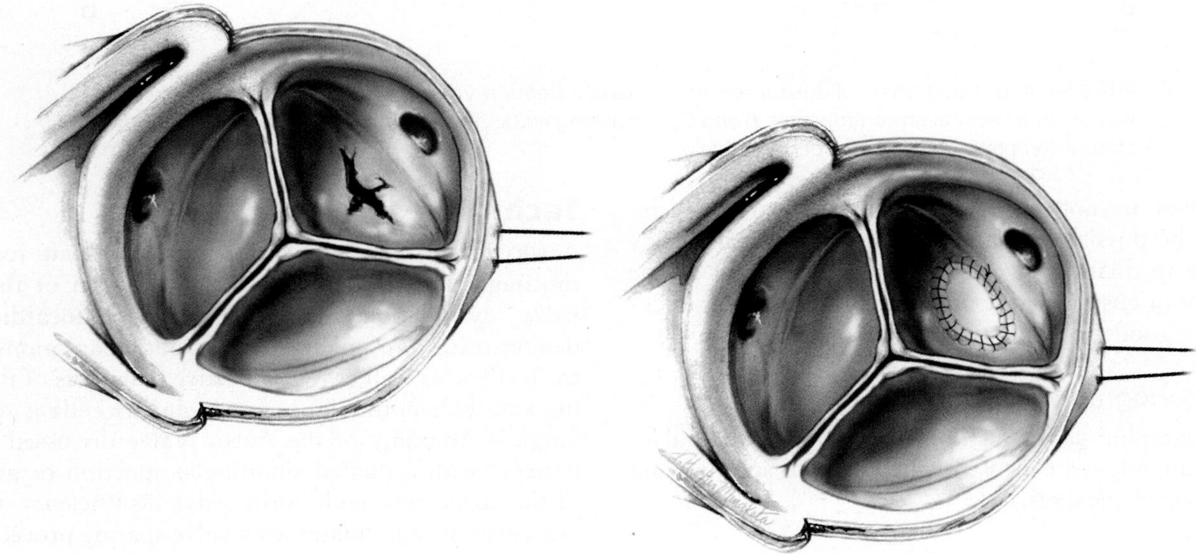

FIG. 5.56 Patch repair of cusp perforation.

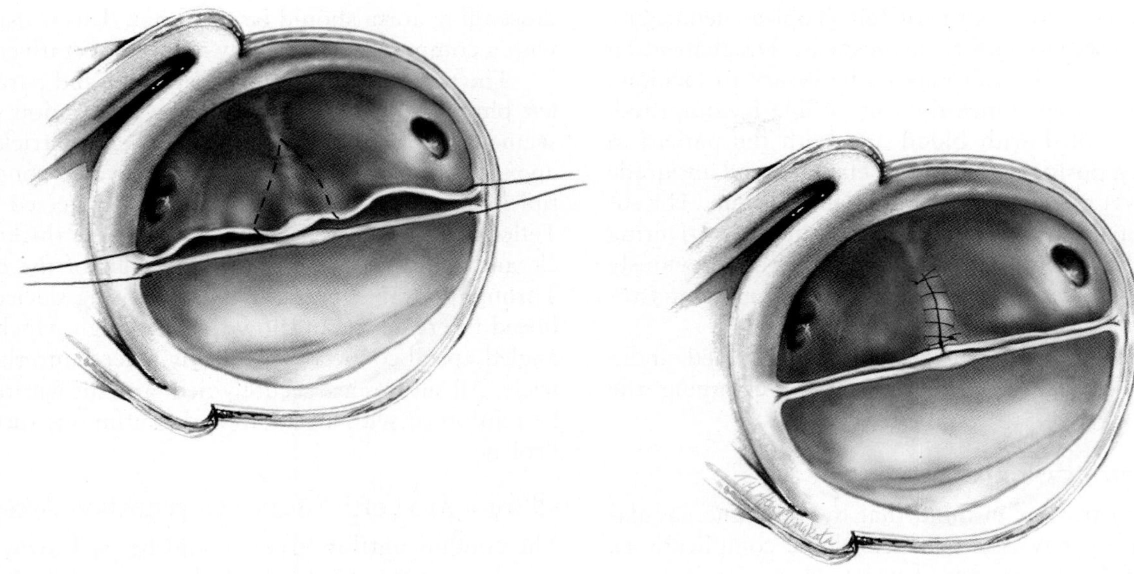

FIG. 5.57 Repair of bicuspid aortic valve: resection of raphe and shortening of free edge of leaflet.

NB Patients with bicuspid valves and aortic roots measuring greater than 45 mm in diameter should undergo aortic root replacement. NB

NB The shortened elongated leaflet edge may be reinforced with a double running suture of 6-0 Gore-Tex tied on the outside of the aorta, taking care to not shorten the free margin too much. NB

⊘ Aortic Stenosis

Overplication of the commissures can lead to functional aortic stenosis. The surgeon may use a valve sizer to ensure the adequacy of the aortic opening. ⊘

PROBLEMATIC CASES

Patients with unclampable aortas, small aortic roots, and aortic valve endocarditis present special challenges for the cardiac surgeon. Alternate surgical approaches and techniques are often required.

Management of Unclampable Aorta

Because people are living longer, cardiac surgeons are encountering an increasing number of patients with atherosclerotic disease of the ascending aorta who require surgical intervention for valvular or coronary disease. The degree of involvement of the aorta ranges from a few isolated atherosclerotic plaques to total calcification of the aorta, often referred to as porcelain aorta. Cannulation and clamping of such diseased aortas can be hazardous, resulting in stroke or even death. The presence of atherosclerosis and/or calcification of the aorta may be detected on preoperative chest x-ray or computed tomography scan. Intraoperative transesophageal echocardiography may demonstrate atherosclerotic changes in the ascending and descending aorta. However, epiaortic ultrasonographic scanning is the most specific diagnostic tool available, allowing the surgeon to map the aorta and locate possible cannulation and clamping sites. The severity and extent of atherosclerosis affecting the aorta will guide the surgeon as to the optimum approach. If both proximal and distal segments of the aorta are heavily calcified, the entire length of the ascending aorta may be replaced with a tube graft (see Chapter 8). Often, the aortic root can be retained and endarterectomized to allow aortic valve replacement to be performed and the proximal aorta to be attached to the tube graft. More often, the disease affects the aorta in a patchy manner. These patients can be managed less aggressively.

Technique

The aorta is cannulated if a safe area is identified by epiaortic ultrasonographic scanning. The axillary artery is usually soft and the preferred site for arterial cannulation (see Chapter 2 for axillary artery cannulation). Alternatively, femoral artery may be used for arterial cannulation (see Chapter 2). A single dual-staged atriocaval cannula is placed through the right atrial appendage. Cardiopulmonary bypass is initiated, and the patient is slowly cooled to 18°C to 24°C. The heart is decompressed with a vent through the right superior pulmonary vein or the pulmonary artery.

When cooling has been completed, the patient is placed in Trendelenberg position and the pump is stopped. The aorta is opened and transected. A hemashield tube graft is anastamosed to the distal aorta. This suture line may need to be reinforced with a strip of felt. Topical hemostatic supplies are used to ensure hemostasis. Decalcification of distal nature aortic wall may be necessary to facilitate placement of sutures. Once this suture line is completed, the tube graft filled with blood and with the patient in Trendelenberg position, the graft is clamped and antigrade pump flow (via axillary artery cannulae) is begun. The suture line is repaired to ensure optimal hemostaisis. During rewarming, the aortic valve is replaced using the previously described techniques and the proximal tube graft anastomosis to the native aorta is completed.,

Rarely aortic valve replacement is performed under hypothermic circulatory arrest to avoid clamping the aorta.

NB Hypothermic Circulatory Arrest

It is important to bear in mind that hypothermic circulatory arrest itself may result in neurologic complications, especially with longer periods of arrest. Therefore, it is usually preferable to limit the arrest time to that required to perform the distal anastomosis of a replacement tube graft or to complete an endarterectomy. NB

A safe option in some elderly patients with unclampable aortas or with internal thoracic arterial conduits located under the sternum is the apico-descending aortic conduit.

Apicoaortic Valve Conduit

Apicoaortic valve conduit is not a new concept. The procedure has been performed in select groups of adult and pediatric patients for many decades. A conduit containing a bioprosthetic valve is interposed between the apex of the left ventricle and the descending thoracic aorta either with or without cardiopulmonary support.

Technique

The use of a double lumen endotracheal tube allows the left lung to be deflated, and facilitates exposure. A left thoracotomy through the fifth or sixth intercostal space provides good access to both the descending aorta and the left ventricle. The inferior pulmonary ligament is ligated and divided to free up the left lung and improve access to the descending aorta. The parietal pleura overlying the lower descending thoracic aorta is incised and retracted. A disease-free segment of the aorta is identified and excluded with a large Satinsky partial occluding clamp. The distal end of the valve conduit is sewn to the aortic opening with 3-0 or 4-0 Prolene. The partial occluding clamp is removed after clamping the conduit.

NB The patient must be heparinized before clamping the aorta. NB

⊘ Calcification of Descending Aorta

If this procedure is contemplated, the presence of severe atherosclerotic disease and/or calcification of the descending aorta should be ruled out. This is usually done with a computed tomography scan preoperatively. ⊘

The pericardium is opened anterior and parallel to the left phrenic nerve and suspended with traction sutures. A segment of the anterior wall of the left ventricle near the apex is selected for placement of the valve conduit. Multiple U-shaped 2-0 Ticron sutures, buttressed with soft Teflon felt, are passed deeply through the thickened muscle and then through the sewing collar of the connector. Through a stab wound, a muscle coring device is introduced to create the outflow tract through which the rigid angled apical connector is quickly placed into the left ventricle. All sutures are securely tied, and the suture line may be reinforced with an additional continuous suture of 3-0 Prolene.

⊘ Injury to Left Anterior Descending Artery

The conduit outflow tract should be well away from the coronary artery and the thinned portion of the left ventricular apex. ⊘

⊘ Clot in Left Ventricle

Detailed echocardiography should be done to detect the presence of blood clot in the left ventricular apex and along the septum. Dislodgement of clot will result in systemic embolization and a potential cerebral vascular accident. ⊘

⊘ Location of Papillary Muscle

Intraoperative transesophageal echocardiography can locate the papillary muscles and ensure that the conduit is placed away from their insertion sites. ⊘

The grafts of the valve conduit and connector are appropriately trimmed and anastomosed with a continuous suture of 3-0 Prolene. Following careful deairing, clamps on the grafts are removed.

NB Biological glue and/or hemostatic products applied on all suture lines help to reduce bleeding. NB

NB The procedure may be more safely accomplished with femoral–femoral bypass support (see Chapter 2). The heart can be lifted and fibrillation induced to facilitate the introduction of the muscle coring device and rigid connector into the left ventricle. NB

NB Although stented porcine valve conduits are most commonly used in these patients, the Freestyle aortic root bioprosthesis (Medtronic, Minneapolis, MN) has been used as an intervening device between the apical prosthesis and tube graft from the descending aorta. NB

Management of the Small Aortic Root

It is clear that no prosthetic valve is hemodynamically equal to the patient's own heart valve. Therefore, whenever valve replacement is done, the patient receives a less optimal valve substitute. Fibrosis, calcification, or simply a very small aortic root can limit the maximal orifice of the aortic annulus. Therefore, a prosthesis that fits in the annulus comfortably may be unacceptable hemodynamically. This is particularly significant in larger patients with small aortic roots. Patient–prosthesis mismatch occurs when the effective orifice area of the implanted prosthetic valve is too small in relation to the patient's body size. This mismatch results in a higher transvalvular gradient and less regression of left ventricular hypertrophy, which may lead to increased cardiac morbidity and mortality. Many techniques have been developed to overcome this mismatch between the patient and prosthesis.

Tilted Prosthesis Technique

Depending on the type of prosthesis, by tilting the plane of implantation by 5 to 10 degrees, it is often possible to implant a larger valve into the aortic root. Simple interrupted sutures are used to attach the prosthesis to the left and right coronary annuli. Starting from either end of the noncoronary annulus and arching upward to a central point 5 to 8 mm above its nadir, sutures, double-armed with needles (2-0 Ticron), are passed first through the sewing ring in a horizontal manner downward from above and then through the aortic wall. The needles are finally passed through small pledgets or strips of Teflon felt outside the aorta (Fig. 5.58). The prosthesis is then lowered in this tilted position, and the sutures are tied. The sutures on the noncoronary side are tied outside the aorta over the Teflon felt pledgets.

NB Location of the Aortotomy

The right margin of the aortotomy should be at a higher level than usual, 1.5 to 2 cm above the noncoronary annulus, to facilitate sewing the prosthesis in a tilted manner and, at the same time, to allow satisfactory closure of the aortotomy. NB

⊘ Buttressing of the Sutures

All sutures anchoring the prosthesis onto the aortic wall above the annulus must be buttressed with Teflon pledgets or a strip of Teflon felt or pericardium. The aortic wall requires reinforcement to be strong enough to hold the prosthetic valve in position. ⊘

⊘ Opening Angles of Disc Prostheses

The opening angles of discs differ by manufacturer. The Medtronic-Hall disc opens maximally to a 75-degree angle. This is an important point of concern. The combined tilting angle and disc opening angle should not be more than 80 to 85 degrees. Otherwise, there is the risk that when the disc opens, it may not close! ⊘

The concept of the tilting technique allows the implantation of a larger prosthesis in the supraannular position along the noncoronary annulus.

⊘ Use of Bileaflet Prostheses

Bileaflet prostheses have excellent hemodynamics and are preferred by many surgeons for use in patients with small aortic roots. When used in the tilted position, the

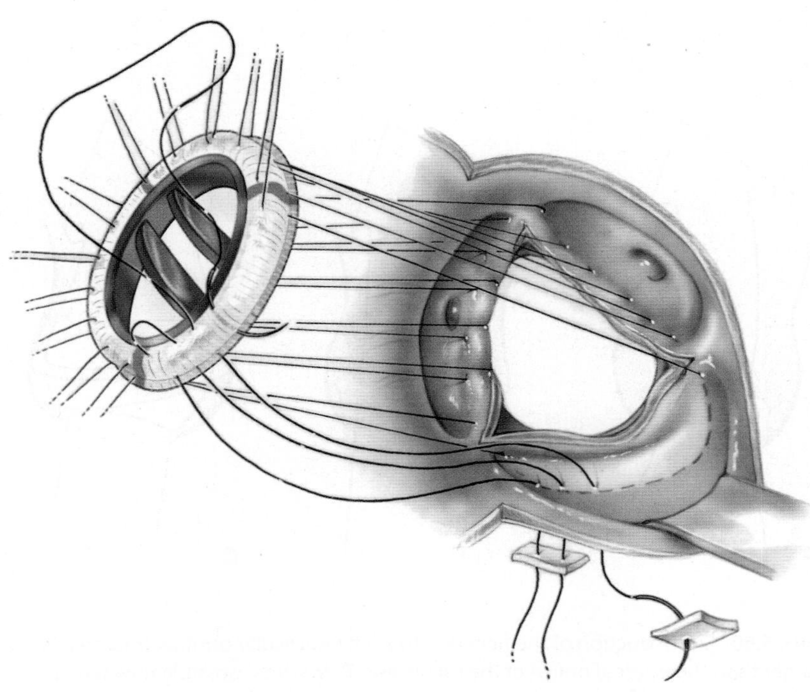

FIG. 5.58 Technique of securing a disc prosthesis (Medtronic-Hall) in the tilted position.

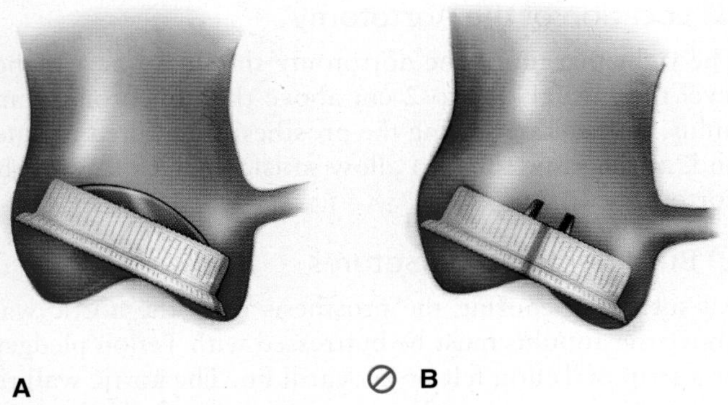

FIG. 5.59 **A:** The aortic bileaflet prosthesis in the tilted position with proper orientation of the leaflets. **B:** Position with possible interference of the leaflet function.

leaflets may impact the aortic wall and not open or close completely (Fig. 5-59A). Free mobility of the leaflets must be ensured by proper orientation of the prosthesis (Fig. 5.59B). ⊘

⊘ Inappropriate Size of the Prosthesis

It is pointless to attempt to insert a prosthesis whose internal orifice is larger than the orifice of the left ventricular outflow tract or aortic annulus. If the left ventricular outflow tract is too narrow, the tilting technique of valve replacement obviously will not be very rewarding (Fig. 5.60). ⊘

NB Septal Myectomy

Septal hypertrophy may be significant in patients with severe aortic stenosis. At times, the left ventricular outflow tract may become narrower than the aortic root. The hypertrophied septal mass may interfere with the normal function of mechanical prosthetic valves. A limited myectomy or shaving off excess septal muscle bulging into the left ventricular outflow tract may allow for a wider lumen and ensure the normal function of the valvular prosthesis (Fig. 5.24). NB

Patch Enlargement Technique

It is always preferable to use the largest possible prosthesis whenever valve replacement is contemplated. A prosthesis larger than the aortic annulus, however, does not abolish the obstructive gradient across the left ventricle and the aorta (Fig. 5.60). Therefore, if the aortic annulus is a dominant obstructive factor, it must be enlarged to accept a larger prosthesis. Often the subaortic curtain is long enough to allow satisfactory enlargement of the aortic root. The oblique aortotomy is extended downward through the commissure between the noncoronary and the left coronary aortic annuli onto the subaortic fibrous curtain up to, but not including, the mitral annulus (Fig. 5.61A). A patch of glutaraldehyde-treated autologous pericardium or bovine pericardium is cut in the appropriate shape and size and sewn into place with a continuous 3-0 Prolene suture (Fig. 5.61B).

When further enlargement is warranted, the incision is extended across the subaortic curtain, through

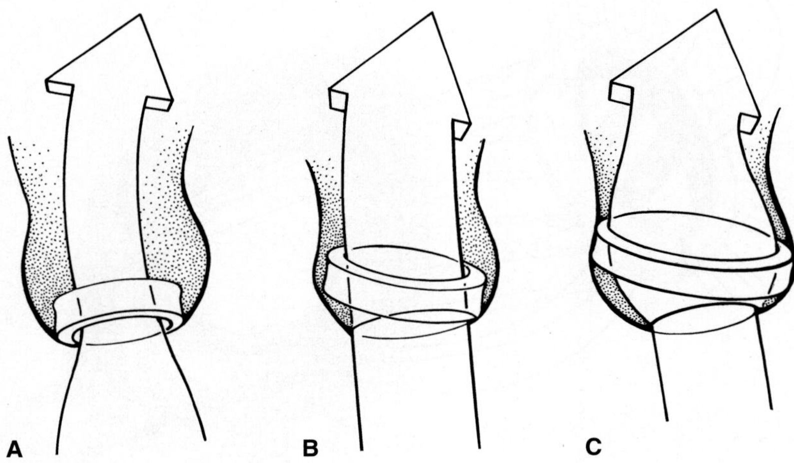

FIG. 5.60 **A:** Obstruction of the flow due to a left ventricular outflow tract that is larger than the internal orifice of the prosthesis. **B:** Maximal possible flow when left ventricular outflow tract is same size as the internal orifice of the prosthesis. **C:** No increase of flow with a left ventricular outflow tract that is smaller than the internal orifice of the prosthesis.

the mitral annulus, and for a variable distance onto the anterior leaflet of the mitral valve. This necessarily entails incision of the left atrial wall to a similar extent from the mitral annulus (Fig. 5.62A). A patch of glutaraldehyde-treated autologous pericardium or bovine pericardium of appropriate size and shape is then sewn into place with 3-0 continuous Prolene suture, incorporating the left atrial wall and the anterior mitral leaflet (Fig. 5.62B). Rarely, this approach may distort the mitral valve, particularly in patients with a small left atrium. The atrial opening may be enlarged by incorporating a second patch of pericardium (Fig. 5.62C). These techniques of aortic root enlargement have the added advantage that the left ventricular outflow tract, as well as the aortic annulus, can be enlarged considerably. The aortic prosthesis of choice is then inserted using the technique described previously (Fig. 5.63).

NB Tilting the Prosthesis

The prosthesis should be sewn in with a slight tilt, as described earlier, so that the anchoring sutures that cross the patch can be tied on the outside wall of the patch 4 or 5 mm above the annulus. This patch is then used to augment the aortotomy closure with a continuous 4-0 Prolene suture. If the autologous pericardium appears to be thin and insecure, it can be reinforced by a patch of Gore-Tex. NB

⊘ Hemolysis

If a Gore-Tex patch or Dacron graft is used, it may be lined with autologous pericardium to prevent possible hemolysis in the postoperative period. ⊘

⊘ Narrow Left Ventricular Outflow Tract

The previously discussed techniques enlarge the aortic annulus quite effectively. If the left ventricular outflow tract is too narrow, however, it remains a limiting factor. Placement of a larger prosthesis or enlargement of the aortic annulus will not relieve the basic hemodynamic problem. ⊘

NB Use of Aortic Homograft or Stentless Valves

The excellent hemodynamics of aortic homografts and stentless bioprotheses in smaller valve sizes may provide satisfactory results without the need for a root enlargement procedure. NB

The obstruction associated with a small aortic root can be satisfactorily relieved in most patients using one of these techniques. The Rastan-Konno aortoventricular septoplasty is rarely indicated in adult patients (see Chapter 24).

Endocarditis

Infective endocarditis is a debilitating disease and is associated with a very high mortality. The native aortic valve leaflets become infected, and the infection may extend into the annulus and the surrounding tissues, resulting in paravalvular and root abscesses. In patients with prosthetic aortic valves, the infection affects the leaflets and the sewing ring of the pericardial and porcine valves. The mechanical valve sewing ring is always involved. Homografts and pulmonary autografts follow the same pattern of infection as the native aortic valve. Often, vegetations form on the valve leaflets and cause systemic embolization with serious consequences.

NB It is important to bear in mind that anticoagulation does not prevent the embolization of vegetations. NB

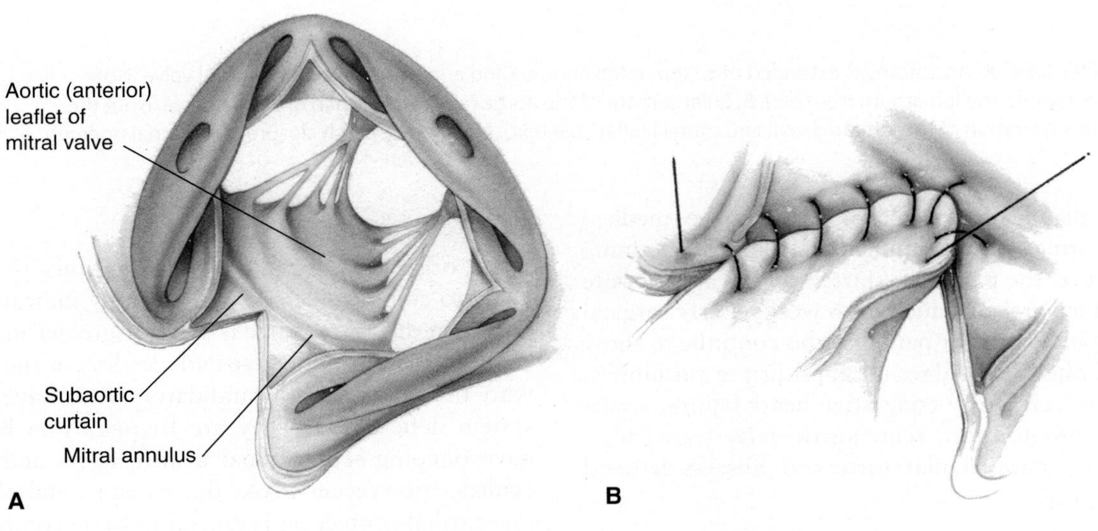

FIG. 5.61 A: Aortotomy is extended onto the subaortic curtain. **B:** Enlargement of the aortic root with a patch of pericardium.

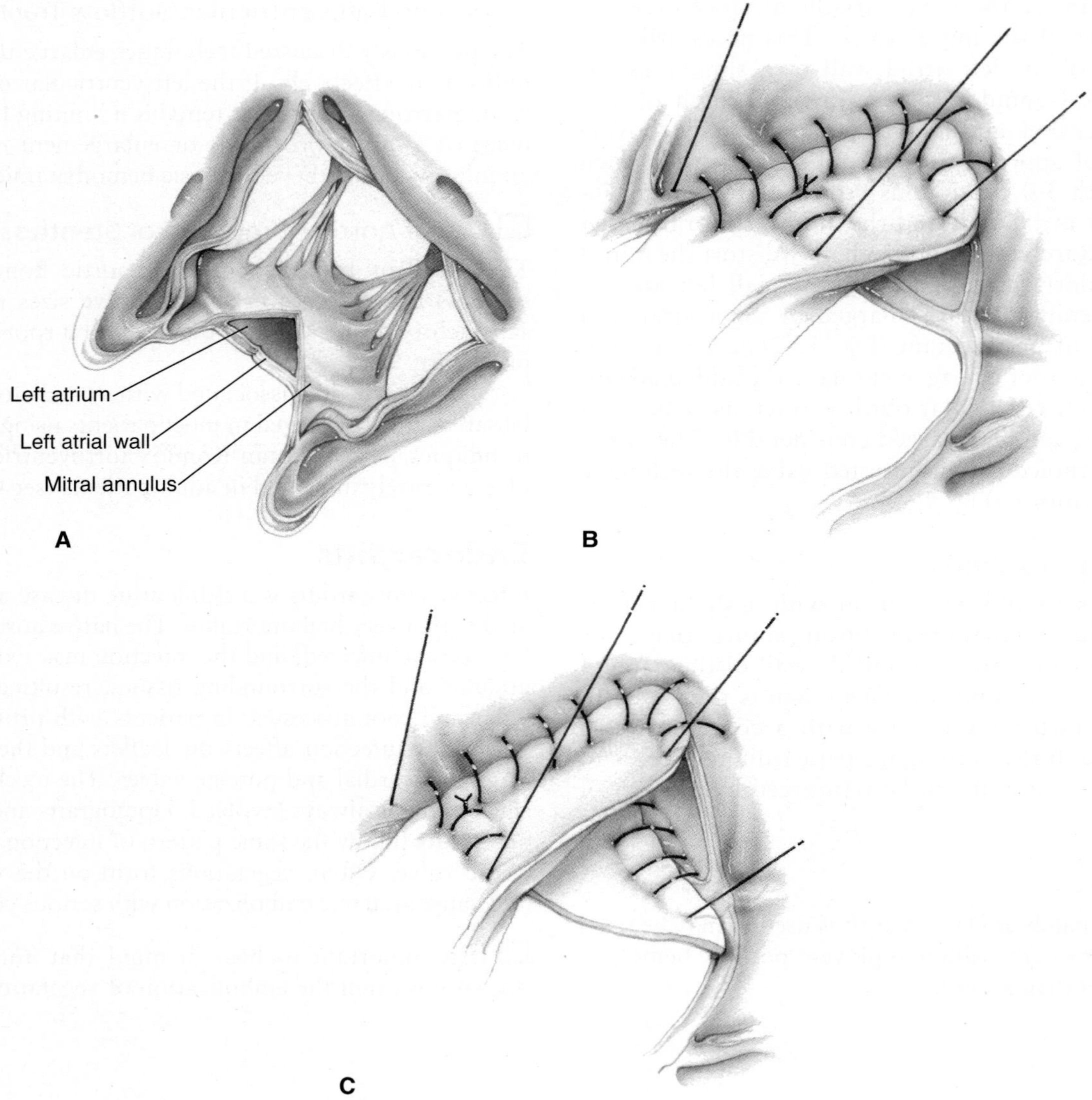

FIG. 5.62 **A:** Aortotomy is extended onto the mitral annulus and anterior leaflet of the mitral valve. Note entry into the left atrium (see text). **B:** Enlargement of the aortic root with a patch of pericardium. Note the incorporation of the left atrial wall and mitral leaflet (see text). **C:** Separate patch closure of left atrial opening.

Accurate diagnosis and prompt aggressive medical management are essential. Immediately after obtaining blood for culture, the patient is started on the appropriate antibiotics, which are continued for 6 weeks. Early surgical intervention is indicated for patients who continue to show signs of sepsis after 3 to 4 days on appropriate antibiotics. The presence of refractory congestive heart failure, recurrent systemic embolization, acute aortic valve leaflet tear, and evidence of a paravalvular aortic root abscess demand immediate surgery.

NB *Staphylococcus aureus* endocarditis is very virulent and causes aggressive tissue destruction. Therefore, early surgical intervention is indicated when this organism is involved. NB

NB Size of Vegetations

Some organisms form bulky vegetations that are more likely to embolize. Surgery is generally indicated if a vegetation on the aortic valve is 1 cm or greater in diameter. NB

Patients with infective endocarditis of the aortic valve who become surgical candidates often have multiorgan system deficiencies. They are frequently in heart failure, have ongoing sepsis, renal insufficiency, and many have evidence of a recent stroke due to septic emboli. Optimum myocardial protection is crucial in these compromised patients to allow for adequate time to completely remove all infected material, reconstruct the aortic root, and achieve a competent aortic valve.

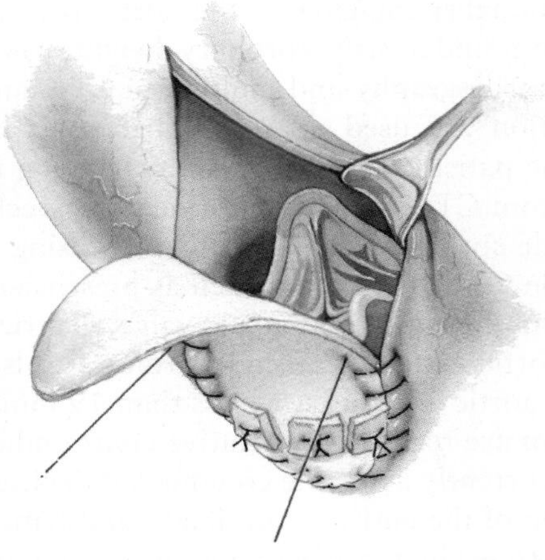

FIG. 5.63 Insertion of the prosthesis into the enlarged aortic root.

⊘ Dislodgement of Vegetations

The antegrade infusion of cardioplegia into the aortic root under high pressure may dislodge and break up large vegetations that can embolize into the coronary arteries. In these cases, retrograde cardioplegia is infused until cardiac contraction ceases. The aorta is opened and cardioplegic solution is administered into the coronary arteries under direct vision. ⊘

⊘ Cross Contamination

To reduce the possibility of recurrence of endocarditis, every effort should be made to prevent cross contamination. This entails changing gloves, local drapes, and surgical instruments used to remove the infected material from the operative field. ⊘

NB Complete Debridement

The most crucial aspect of the procedure is the complete debridement of all the infected tissues, even if that entails the resection of the entire aortic root and adjacent tissues. NB

In areas where the aortic annulus is destroyed, the left ventricular outflow tract and the aorta are reapproximated with a patch of glutaraldehyde-treated autologous pericardium or bovine pericardium. At times, it may be necessary to create a new annulus by sandwiching the aorta and left ventricular outflow tract with two strips of pericardium. The aortic valve is replaced using the standard techniques described in the preceding text.

⊘ Subannular Necrotic Cavities

Removal of necrotic tissue from the subannular area can create small cavities. The surrounding friable tissue will not hold sutures well. Deep bites with pericardial pledgeted sutures are taken to occlude these cavities. When tied, the sutures may later be used to anchor the new prosthesis into position. ⊘

Extensive infection and abscess formation involving the aortic annulus is a serious condition. Following radical debridement, it may be difficult to reestablish continuity between the aorta and left ventricular outflow tract. An effective technique is to replace the aortic root with either an aortic homograft or a stentless bioprosthesis as described in the preceding text.

NB Use of Pulmonary Autograft

Although many surgeons are reluctant to perform a Ross procedure in the face of aortic endocarditis for fear of introducing infection into the right ventricular outflow tract, the pulmonary autograft is another replacement option in younger patients with endocarditis. NB

PARAVALVULAR LEAKS

In most patients, paravalvular dehiscence resulting in leaks around the aortic prosthesis is secondary to imperfect surgical technique. Some of the predisposing factors, such as a calcified or infected annulus (which allows the sutures to cut through the tissues), have been discussed previously. Paravalvular leaks tend to occur more commonly along the noncoronary annulus and the adjacent half of the left coronary annulus. Massive calcification affecting the aortomitral leaflet continuity may obscure the annulus and interfere with correct placement of anchoring stitches. In addition, the exposure of the noncoronary annulus is sometimes difficult from the surgeon's side (patient's right side). Often, the annular sutures are inadvertently placed in the less ideal aortic wall above the annulus. In time, these sutures may cut through the aortic wall and produce a paravalvular leak. Attention to these details when performing aortic valve replacement helps prevent late paravalvular leaks.

Technique for Repair

The paravalvular defect is identified under direct vision. The tissue margin of the defect commonly becomes fibrous after 2 to 3 months. Pledgeted sutures are passed deeply through the tissue margin of the defect and then through the sewing ring of the prosthesis before tying (Fig. 5.64).

When the integrity of the tissue margin of the defect is not satisfactory, sutures are passed through the sewing ring of the prosthesis before taking a deep bite near the annulus through the full thickness of the aortic wall to the outside of the aorta. The sutures are then tied over Teflon felt pledgets (Fig. 5.64).

When there are multiple paravalvular leaks or the site of the leak is not obvious, it is necessary to explant the prosthesis and implant a new one, ensuring that all the valve sutures bites incorporate healthy tissues.

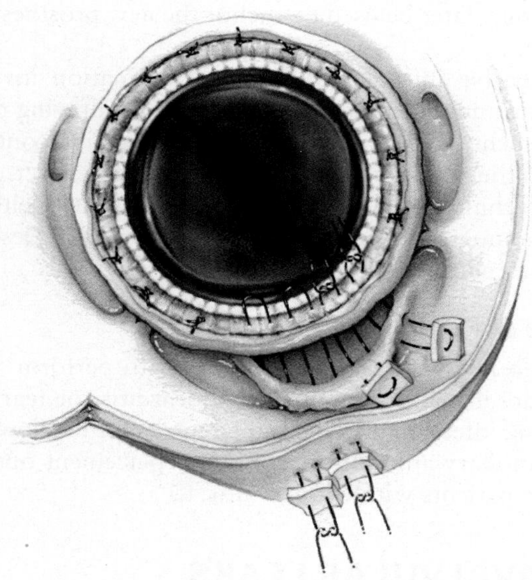

FIG. 5.64 Technique for repair of a paravalvular leak (see text).

NB Interventional Closure of Periprosthetic Leaks

Recently, some institutions have closed paravalvular defects with an atrial septal defect or ductal occluder device in the catheterization laboratory. This procedure may be useful in elderly or critically ill patients to avoid a reoperation. NB

TRANSCATHETER AORTIC VALVE REPLACEMENT

Despite ever-improving results of surgical aortic valve replacement in the setting of symptomatic aortic stenosis, some elderly frail patients are at high risk of mortality and morbidities after surgical aortic valve replacement. Transcatheter Aortic Valve Replacement (TAVR) technologies have evolved to meet the needs of these high-risk patients. Currently, TAVR technology is approved in the United States for patients with a calculated mortality risk of 7.5% (Society of Thoracic Surgeons Risk Calculator), or for those who have other major confounding conditions such as frailty, liver disease, and calcified ascending aortas, among others.

Patient Selection

Much like traditional cardiac surgery, many patient factors and data must be evaluated to deem a patient appropriate for TAVR. Patients must have severe calcific aortic stenosis (regardless of pressure gradients), have a life expectancy of at least one year, and be high risk for surgical valve replacement.

Multimodality imaging of the aortic root is required to evaluate annular size, coronary height, and calcification. Echocardiography and multi-slice CT scans with 3D reconstruction are used in a complementary fashion to evaluate the patient for TAVR. Annular sizing is typically obtained from CT scan and confirmed using echocardiography, while coronary height is obtained using center-line distances on CT. Other issues such as presence of left ventricular thrombus, bicuspid aortic valve, ventricular aneurysm, subaortic stenosis, and endocarditis are also assessed. In general, aortic annulus sizes less than 19 mm or greater than 31 mm are regarded as relative contraindications for the use of currently available commercial devices.

Imaging of the entire aorta, iliacs, and femoral vessels is required to evaluate the vascular access required for delivery sheath insertion. While first-generation devices were 24 French and required large caliber, newer expandable sheaths (14 French) now accommodate vessels as small as 6 mm depending on the extent of calcification. A detailed assessment of the patient's vasculature is essential to choosing the appropriate access site with the least risk of complications. Given the size of the delivery systems for the current commercially available TAVR prostheses, groin vascular complications remain a major risk occurring in 12% to 19% of patients. These involve dissection of the iliac and femoral arteries and less commonly, avulsion and massive hemorrhage. While the recommended minimal luminal diameter for the femoral vessels is 7-8 mm depending on valve size, the extent of vascular calcification and tortuosity impact the incidence of these complications.

Operative Technique

TAVR is best performed in a hybrid suite capable of both surgical and interventional procedures. A temporary ventricular pacemaker is advanced into the right ventricle under fluoroscopy and tested. Femoral arterial access is obtained in both groins and the larger artery is used to insert the delivery sheath (18 to 24 French), while the other is accessed with a 5 French sheath for delivery of the pigtail catheter. These vessels can be accessed with a surgical cut-down or percutaneously in most cases. Usually, two preclosure devices are deployed before the introduction of the large sheath. After the introduction of a long sheath into the descending aorta, a stiff wire with a floppy tip is used to enter the ascending aorta and the root. Now the valve is crossed and the stiff wire is inserted into the left ventricle through the long sheath. The patient should be heparinized. Now a contralateral pigtail is also advanced and left in one of the aortic sinuses. A balloon valvuloplasty is performed under rapid ventricular pacing. At this point, an appropriately sized valve is mounted on the delivery system and advanced over the stiff wire with the end in the left ventricle. Appropriate images of the aortic root are critical with the nadir of all sinuses being visible during a root injection through the pigtail (Fig. 5.65). These measurements along with valve dimensions are reviewed to ensure

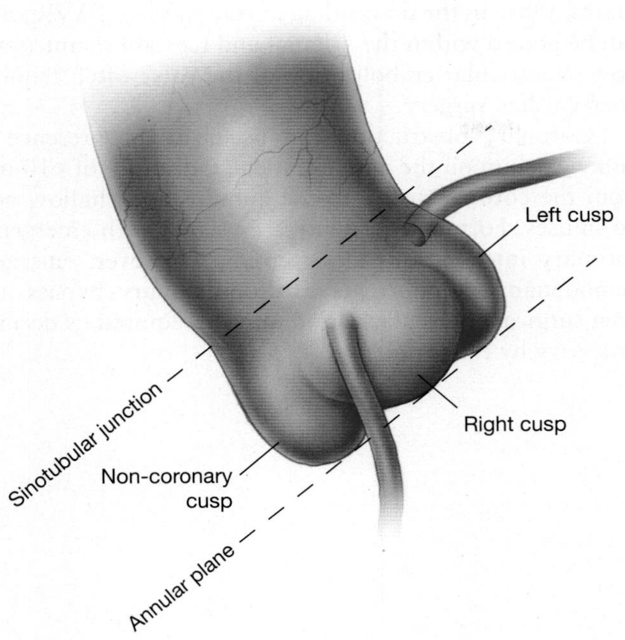

FIG. 5.65 Optimal alignment of the fluoroscopic imaging plane to align the nadir of all three aortic cusps.

that the valve will not obstruct the coronary ostia. Now the valve is carefully positioned and inflated under rapid ventricular pacing (Fig. 5.66). An aortogram combined with echocardiography and hemodynamic measurements should be used to assess the function of the valve with particular attention to paravalvular leaks. Once satisfactory function of the valve is confirmed, wires are withdrawn and the femoral vessels closed as appropriate.

NB Sheath Removal

Removal of the large sheath should be done over a wire that is retained and in the presence of contralateral access in case of a vascular injury. NB

For the transapical technique, it is important to identify a safe area of cannulation lateral to the true apex of the heart. This avoids disruption of the LAD while providing a more secure area for cannulation. Generally, a limited anterior left thoracotomy is used to access the pericardium. Finger pressure and echocardiography are used to identify a suitable are that is in line with the aortic valve for deployment. Two concentric purse-strings with large felt pledgets are used to secure the myocardium around a 26 French sheath that is introduced after serial dilations. The remainder of the procedure is performed as above. Sheath removal should be performed under hemodynamic control and rapid ventricular pacing.

NB Weak Myocardial tissue

In cases of a fragile myocardium or redo operations, the ventricular purse-strings should incorporate the native pericardium to provide more structural support. NB

NB Cardioplumonary support

In patients with significant pulmonary hypertension, poor ventricular function or those with untreated significant coronary arterial lesions, rapid access to cardiopulmonary bypass and circulatory support through the femoral vessels should be available. NB

The stiff and yet fragile nature of the aortic annulus in TAVR candidates can predispose these patients to annular rupture upon aggressive balloon valvuloplasty or valve expansion. This complication often presents with cardiac tamponade.

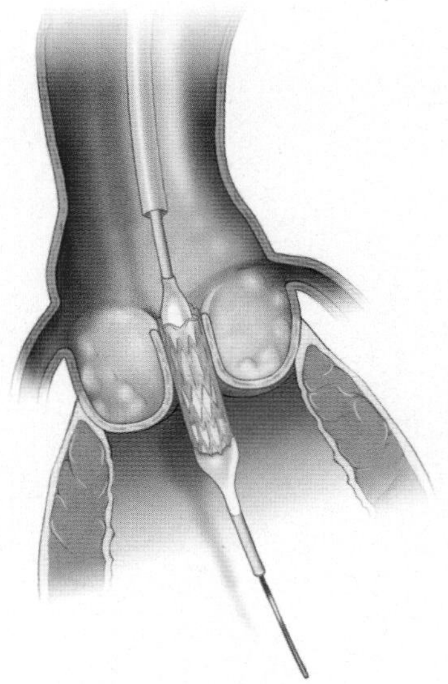

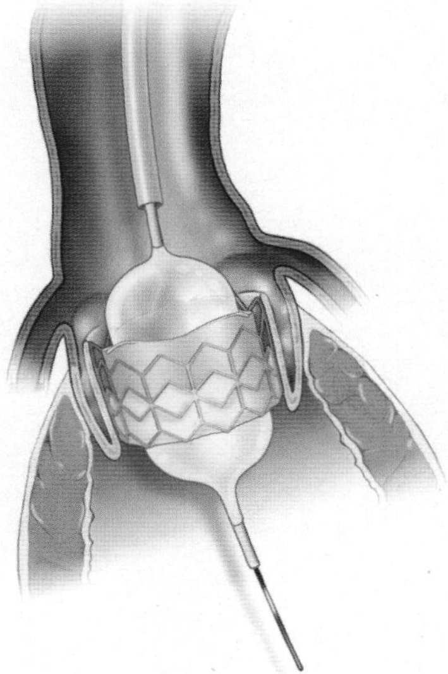

FIG. 5.66 Alignment of the valve to avoid occlusion of the coronary ostia after inflation.

Pericardial tamponade may occur in a minority of patients and may be due to wire perforation of either the atria or the ventricles, bleeding from the transapical access site, annular rupture, or aortic dissection. These complications may be managed by percutaneous drains and reversal of coagulopathy but may eventually require open surgical repair. Annular rupture and dissection requiring surgery carry a dismal prognosis.

Valve embolization or poor deployment occurs in about 1% of patients undergoing TAVR. The strategy to rectify a malpositioned valve depends on the site, hemodynamic stability of the patient, and overall risk. Often the valves can be pulled back into the aorta using intravascular snares. Once in the descending aorta, another TAVR valve can be placed within the original and reestablish antegrade flow. Ventricular embolization of the valve often requires open cardiac surgery.

Coronary obstruction can occur in the presence of bulky calcium on the native leaflets, a distance of <10 mm from the coronary ostia to the annulus and shallow aortic sinuses. Fortunately, many are treated with emergency coronary interventions and stenting. However, emergent hemodynamic support via cardiopulmonary bypass and even surgical revascularization may be required as deemed necessary by the team.

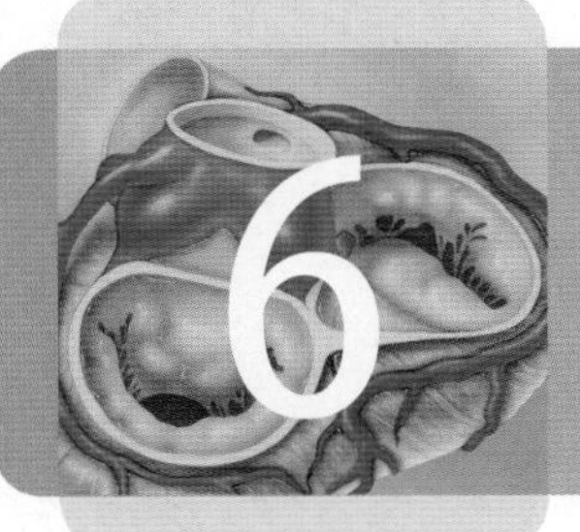

6 Surgery of the Mitral Valve

Degenerative and myxomatous changes are the most common cause of mitral valve disease in North America and Western Europe today. These changes affect the leaflets and subvalvular apparatus, leading to mitral regurgitation. As the population ages, surgeons are seeing more patients with mitral insufficiency secondary to calcific mitral valve diseases.

Rheumatic fever continues to be the major cause of acquired valve disease worldwide. Rheumatic fever results in pancarditis, but the pathologic effects are noted predominantly on the endocardium and cardiac valves, particularly the mitral valve. During the acute phase of myocarditis, the left ventricle dilates, which causes stretching of the annulus of the mitral valve. The mitral insufficiency thus produced is temporary and disappears when the left ventricle regains its normal function. Rheumatic heart disease is a chronic and progressive condition. The earliest permanent change is the fusion of the commissures, followed by thickening and fibrosis of the valve leaflets. These pathologic events are responsible for the creation of the turbulent flow that, together with the continuing rheumatic process, further enhances the progression of the disease and eventual involvement of the subvalvular apparatus. The chords and papillary muscles become thickened, shortened, and fused to each other and to the mitral leaflets. A continuous cycle of progression of pathologic changes and increasingly disturbed flow is therefore created, eventually leading to severe mitral valve disease, notably mitral stenosis or mixed stenosis and insufficiency with or without calcification.

Functional mitral regurgitation may be caused by ischemic or nonischemic cardiomyopathies. The leaflets and subvavular structures are normal but leaflet coaptation is prevented by annular dilation, left ventricular wall motion abnormalities or generalized cavity dilation, and/or papillary muscle dysfunction. Ischemic heart disease and myocardial infarction may also lead to ischemic mitral valve prolapse due to papillary muscle or chordal injury.

Bacterial endocarditis can affect both normal and abnormal heart valve leaflets. The infection may burrow through and invade the mitral valve annulus. Infrequently, the endocarditis extends to the aortic valve and/or the subvalvular apparatus of the mitral valve. It can destroy the mitral valve leaflet configuration, resulting in gross mitral valve insufficiency.

SURGICAL ANATOMY OF THE MITRAL VALVE

The mitral valve forms the inlet of the left ventricle. It consists of two leaflets: the anterior (aortic) and posterior (mural) leaflets, which are attached directly to the mitral annulus and to the papillary muscles by primary and secondary chordae tendineae. A series of chordae tendineae originates from the fibrous tips of the papillary muscles and inserts into the free edges and the undersurfaces of the mitral leaflets, thereby preventing the prolapse of the leaflets into the left atrium during systole and contributing to the competency of the mitral valve. The attachments of the leaflets to the annulus meet at the anterolateral and posteromedial commissures. One-third of the mitral valve annulus provides attachment for the anterior leaflet, and the posterior leaflet arises from the remaining two-thirds of the annulus. Although from the strict anatomic point of view the mitral valve consists of two leaflets, there are multiple clefts within the posterior leaflet. These slits give rise to scallops of leaflet that may prolapse and give rise to valvular insufficiency. Most surgeons and echocardiographers have adopted the classification of Carpentier, which divides both the anterior and posterior leaflets into three functional segments (Fig. 6.1).

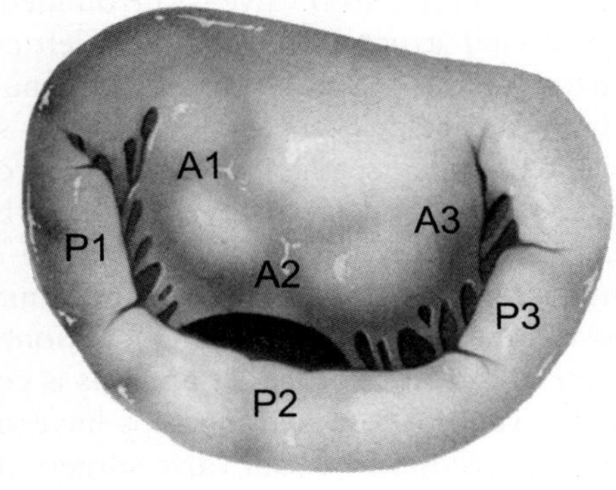

FIG. 6.1 Carpentier functional mitral valve components.

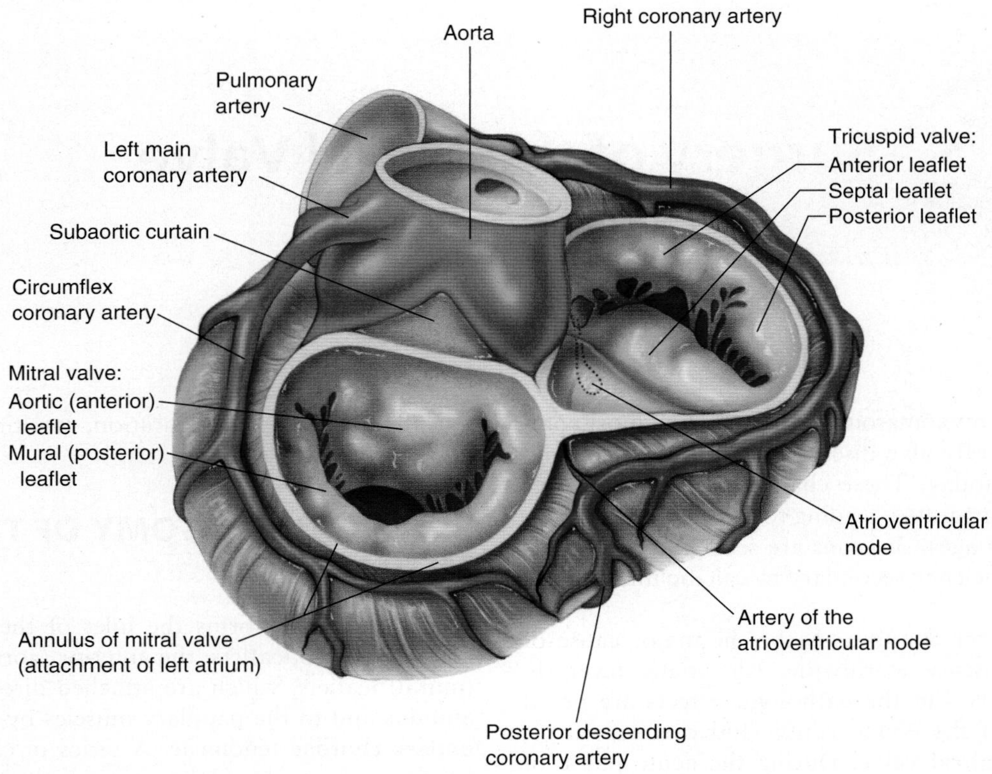

FIG. 6.2 Surgical anatomy of the mitral valve.

When the posterior annulus is studied from a strictly anatomic standpoint, it is attached to the left ventricular myocardium through the interposition of a narrow membrane and is therefore actually slightly elevated above the opening of the left ventricle. This subannular membrane extends underneath the posterior annulus to the region of both commissures and merges with the fibrous skeleton of the heart. The anterior leaflet is continuous with the adjoining halves of the left and noncoronary annuli of the aortic valve and also with the fibrous subaortic curtain located beneath the commissure between the left and noncoronary aortic sinuses (Fig. 6.2).

The annulus of the mitral valve is surrounded by many important and vital structures. The nearby left circumflex coronary artery traverses around the mitral annulus in the posterior atrioventricular groove. The coronary sinus also runs in the more medial segment of the same groove. The atrioventricular node and its artery, usually a branch of the right coronary artery, run a course parallel and close to the annulus of the anterior leaflet of the mitral valve near the posteromedial commissure. As mentioned earlier, the remainder of the anterior leaflet annulus is contiguous with the aortic valve. These relationships have significant clinical implications during mitral valve surgery (Fig. 6.3).

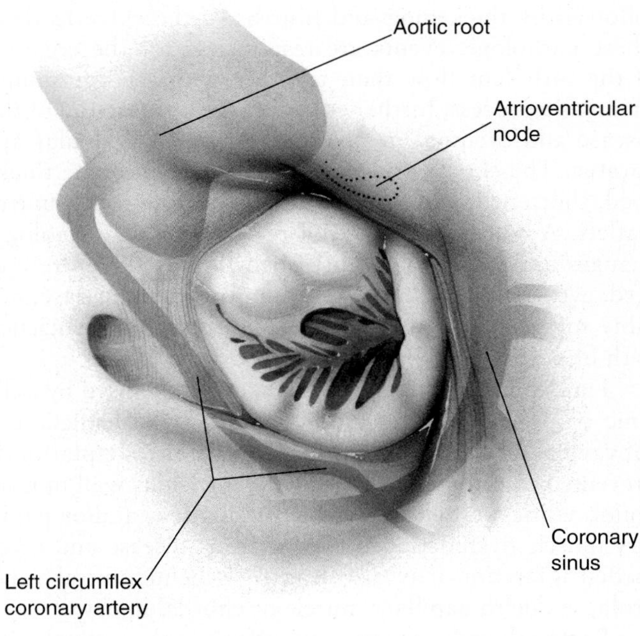

FIG. 6.3 Vital structures surrounding the mitral annulus.

Functional mitral regurgitation occurs secondary to annular or left ventricular changes with anatomically normal leaflets and subvalvular structures. One etiology is simple annular dilation due to left ventricular enlargement. In this case, the leaflet motion is normal, but the leaflets are pulled apart, preventing normal coaptation. Localized left ventricular wall motion abnormalities result in displacement of the papillary muscles. This results in apical tethering of the leaflets with restricted mitral leaflet motion in systole. In some patients, both mechanisms contribute to functional mitral regurgitation.

Technical Considerations

Incision

A median sternotomy is the incision most commonly used. Standard aortic and bicaval cannulation is performed. A right anterior thoracotomy with femoral cannulation affords good access to the mitral valve and spares the midline sternotomy incision.

Myocardial Preservation

When satisfactory cardiopulmonary bypass has been established, the aorta is cross-clamped and cold blood cardioplegic solution is administered into the aortic root to bring about prompt diastolic cardiac arrest. Further administration of blood cardioplegic solution is often administered by the retrograde method (see Chapter 3).

⊘ Aortic Insufficiency

Satisfactory administration of cardioplegic solution into the aortic root can only be accomplished if the aortic valve is competent. Aortic insufficiency, if present, directs the cardioplegic solution into the left ventricular cavity, causing distension and stretch injury to the myocardium. This can be prevented by administering cardioplegic solution using the retrograde technique alone (see Chapter 3). ⊘

Exposure of the Mitral Valve

There are many different approaches for entering the left atrium to provide good exposure of the mitral valve.

Interatrial Groove Approach

The left atrium is opened with an incision just posterior to the interatrial groove (Fig. 6.4). The opening can be extended inferiorly onto the posterior wall of the left atrium.

⊘ Fatty Fragments

There is always a variable amount of loose fatty tissue in the interatrial groove. Fragments of fat and loose tissue may enter the left atrial cavity during the atriotomy. Similarly, when the atriotomy is being closed, fatty fragments may invaginate through the closure into the left atrium. ⊘

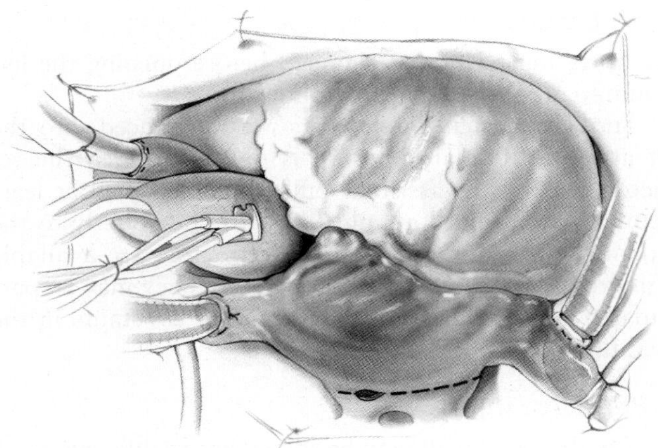

FIG. 6.4 Surgical approach to the mitral valve.

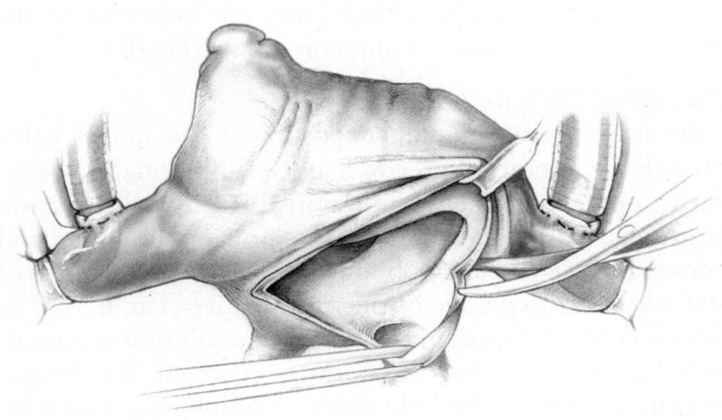

FIG. 6.5 Extension of the incision inferiorly to the back of the heart.

⊘ Extension of the Incision

Upward extension of the incision behind the superior vena cava should be avoided because subsequent closure may be difficult. Generous inferior extension to the back of the heart provides satisfactory exposure of the mitral valve in most cases (Fig. 6.5). Closure of this posterior extension of the incision is facilitated by suturing from inside the left atrial cavity under direct vision. ⊘

⊘ Drainage of Cardioplegic Solution

At least one of the caval snares must be loosened during administration of cardioplegic solution to allow the venous return from the coronary sinus to drain into the oxygenator. If both snares are down, cardioplegia may distend the right heart. If the right atrium is not opened at any time, the cavae do not necessarily require snares around them because venous drainage may be adequate. ⊘

⊘ Air Embolism

The aorta must be cross-clamped before opening the left atrium to avoid systemic air embolism. ⊘

Specially designed retractors are introduced into the left atrium. Optimal exposure is obtained when the retractor held by the assistant pulls the atrial wall at least 1 cm from the mitral annulus upward and slightly to the patient's left. Many self-retaining retractors are available to improve exposure of the mitral valve. They may be particularly helpful if there is a shortage of assistants in the operating room.

⊘ Retractor Injury

Because the atrial wall may be somewhat friable, excessive pull on the retractor may produce a shearing tear of the atrial wall edges, thereby complicating closure. On many occasions, two smaller retractors provide better and safer exposure than a single large one because the assistant is able to divert the pulling force from one retractor to the other to accommodate the surgeon's view (Fig. 6.6). ⊘

Transatrial Oblique Approach

If the left atrium is small, exposure of the mitral valve through the interatrial groove may be suboptimal. In reoperative procedures, dense adhesions may make dissection hazardous, particularly near the region of the interatrial groove. In such cases, an oblique transatrial approach provides excellent exposure of the mitral valve (Fig. 6.7). The aorta is cross-clamped, and cardioplegic solution is administered as before. After the aorta is clamped, an oblique incision is made on the right superior pulmonary vein with a long-handled no. 15 blade. Warm blood will gush out to decompress the left atrium. This will allow expeditious cooling and arrest of the heart.

The vena caval snares are secured. The opening in the right superior pulmonary vein is extended obliquely across the right atrial wall. By gently retracting the right atrial wall edges, the incision can now be extended across the interatrial septum and through the fossa ovalis just inferior to the limbus (Fig. 6.7B). At this time, a retrograde cardioplegic cannula can be introduced into the coronary sinus under direct vision. It can be secured with a fine purse-string suture of Prolene placed on the inside of the coronary sinus ostium, away from the conduction tissues (see Chapter 3). In this manner, retrograde infusion of cardioplegic solution can supplement the antegrade technique.

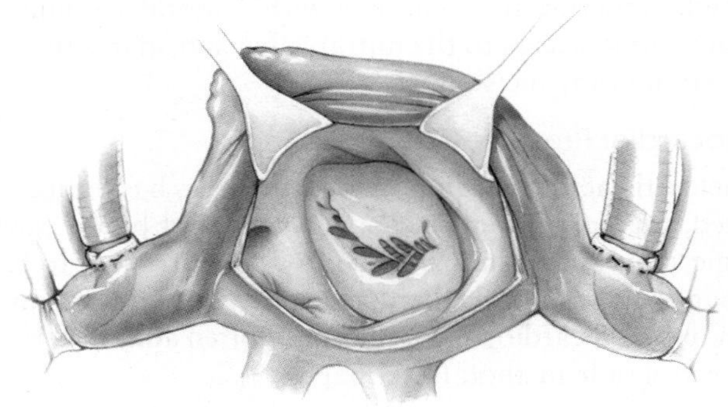

FIG. 6.6 Use of two small retractors to avoid tearing the atrial wall edges.

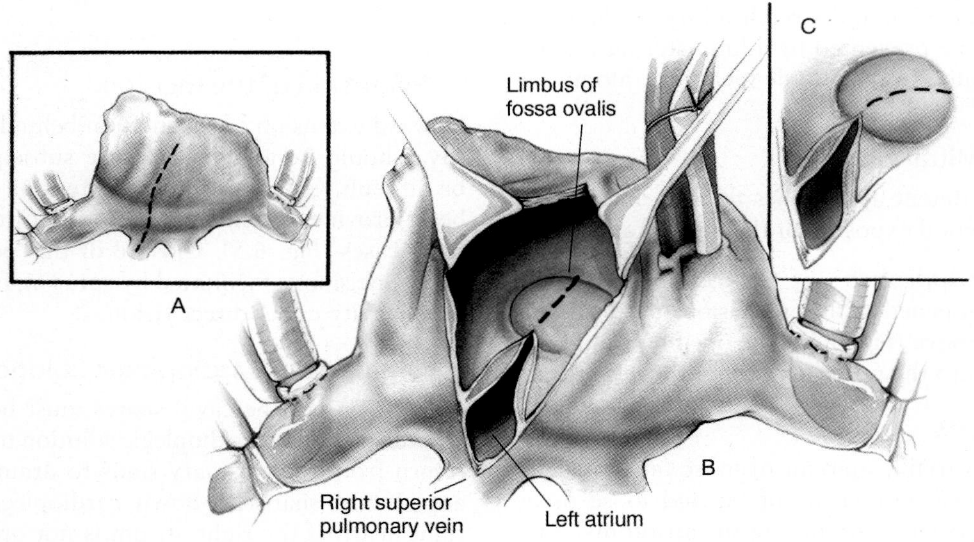

FIG. 6.7 A: Incision on the right superior pulmonary vein extends across the right atrium. **B:** Transatrial incision. Extension of the incision across the interatrial septum just to the limbus of the fossa ovalis. **C:** For additional exposure, the septal incision is extended along the fossa ovalis.

⊘ Overextended Septal Incision

Extension of the septal incision far beyond the anterior limbus of the fossa ovalis may divide the mitral valve annulus, making mitral valve replacement insecure. It could also create a passage outside the atrium into the transverse sinus. The septal incision should therefore terminate just distal to the anterior margin of the fossa ovalis. The septal incision can be extended inferiorly on the fossa ovalis if additional exposure is required (Fig. 6.7C). ⊘

The septal edges are retracted with two small retractors. This provides excellent exposure of the mitral valve without distorting it, an important advantage when mitral valve reconstruction is being contemplated (Fig. 6.8).

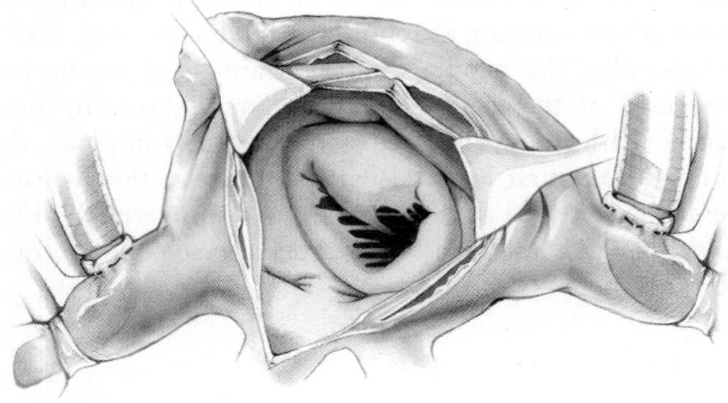

FIG. 6.8 Retraction of the septal edges to provide exposure of the mitral valve without distorting it.

Transatrial Longitudinal Septal Approach

When there are excessive adhesions from previous surgery, excellent exposure of the mitral valve can be obtained through a longitudinal septal approach. Depending on the size of the right atrium, an oblique or longitudinal incision is made on the right atrial wall. Excellent exposure of the right atrial cavity and interatrial septum is thus obtained. A longitudinal incision is made along the posterior margin of the fossa ovalis and extended both superiorly and inferiorly to provide good exposure of the mitral valve (Fig. 6.9A). The right atriotomy incision can be extended across the base of SVC, onto the roof of the left atrium (Fig. 6.9B). This way, the transatrial septal incision can also be extended into the roof of the left atrium (as far as the left atrial appendage base) to provide excellent exposure of the left atrium (especially when left atrium is not dilated (Fig. 6.9C).

⊘ Extension of right atriotomy beyond the base of SVC (transection of SVC) will likely divide the SA nodal artery. Post-operatively, many patients develop junctional rhythm for a few days until the sinus rhythm returns. Few patients may require a permanent pacemaker if there is not a return of sinus rhythm after 7 to 10 days. ⊘

⊘ Proximity to the Mitral Annulus

The annulus of the mitral valve is at the muscular septal wall most anterior to the fossa ovalis. Therefore, the longitudinal septal incision should be made posterior to the fossa ovalis, leaving a good margin of septal wall between

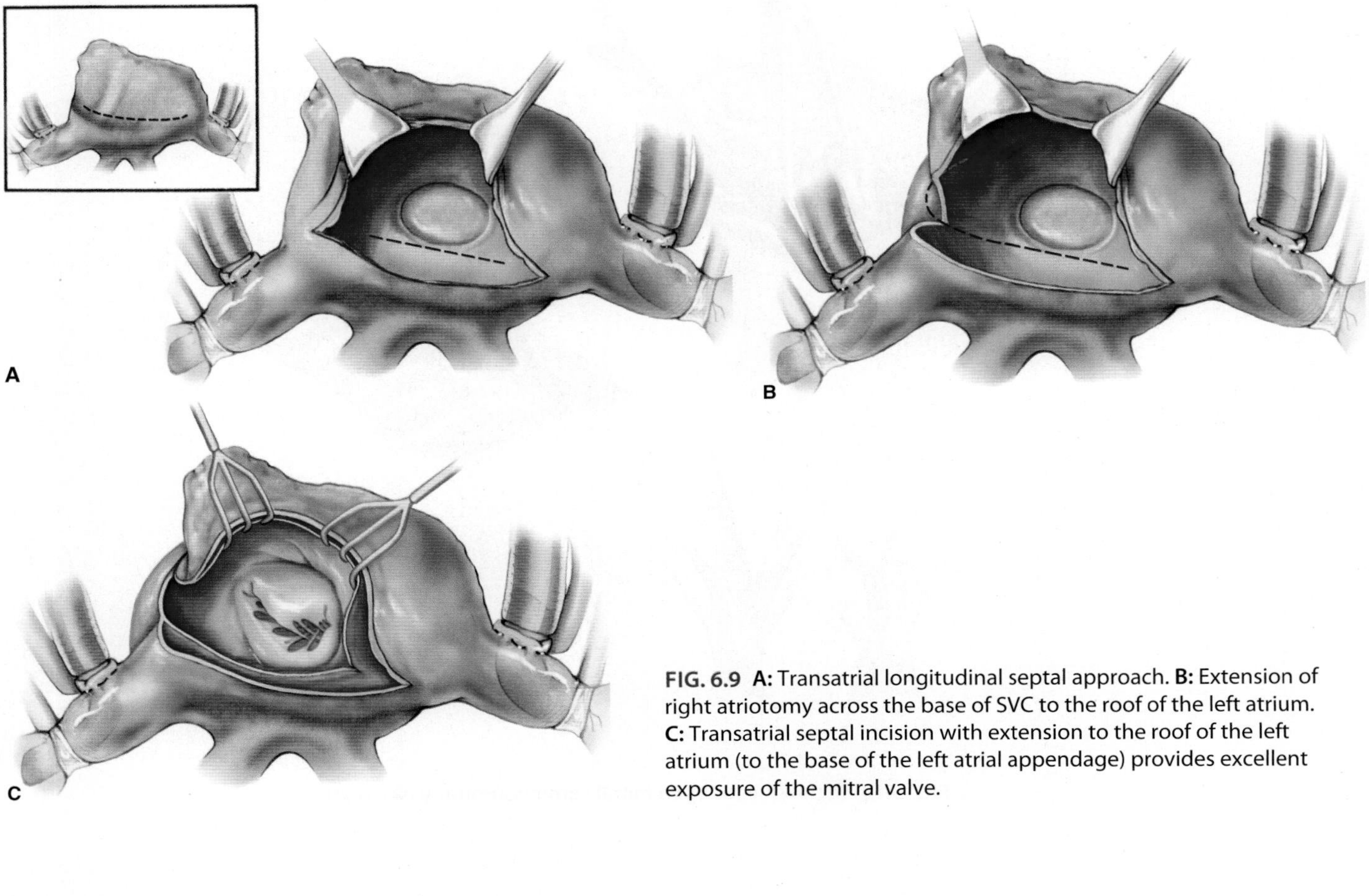

A

B

C

FIG. 6.9 **A:** Transatrial longitudinal septal approach. **B:** Extension of right atriotomy across the base of SVC to the roof of the left atrium. **C:** Transatrial septal incision with extension to the roof of the left atrium (to the base of the left atrial appendage) provides excellent exposure of the mitral valve.

the opening and the mitral annulus. This segment of the septum is retracted to provide excellent exposure of the mitral valve. ⊘

OPEN MITRAL COMMISSUROTOMY FOR MITRAL STENOSIS

Mitral stenosis secondary to longstanding rheumatic fever has continued to be the dominant mitral valve disease affecting large populations worldwide. The disease is now being seen with increasing frequency among immigrants coming to the United States and Western Europe, where rheumatic heart disease had become uncommon.

Mitral commissurotomy can be accomplished safely and precisely under direct vision. With the availability of cardiopulmonary bypass, the closed technique is rarely used today except in third world countries.

A median sternotomy is the incision of choice, although the mitral valve can be approached through either a right or left thoracotomy.

The left atrium is incised by one of the techniques described in the preceding text to expose the mitral valve. The mitral leaflets are identified and, by means of two fine Prolene traction sutures, gently pulled upward toward the left atrial cavity. At times, use of nerve hooks can also provide the same effect. Often this maneuver will stretch the valve leaflets apart and show the line of commissural fusion as a furrow extending between them. If visibility through the valve ostium is adequate, the chords and papillary muscles are examined for evidence of shortening and fusion to each other and, especially, fusion to the undersurfaces of the valvular leaflets.

A right-angled clamp is introduced through the mitral valve opening and placed directly below the fused commissures. It is then opened gently beneath the leaflets to facilitate incision with a no. 15 blade onto the commissures without severing the chordal attachments (Fig. 6.10). Occasionally, the papillary muscles are fused to the undersurface of the leaflet, making commissurotomy hazardous. With the opened right-angled clamp in place, the commissure is first incised near the annulus; this incision is extended inward over the clamp, cutting vertically into the papillary muscle and the thickened, fused chords for a short distance.

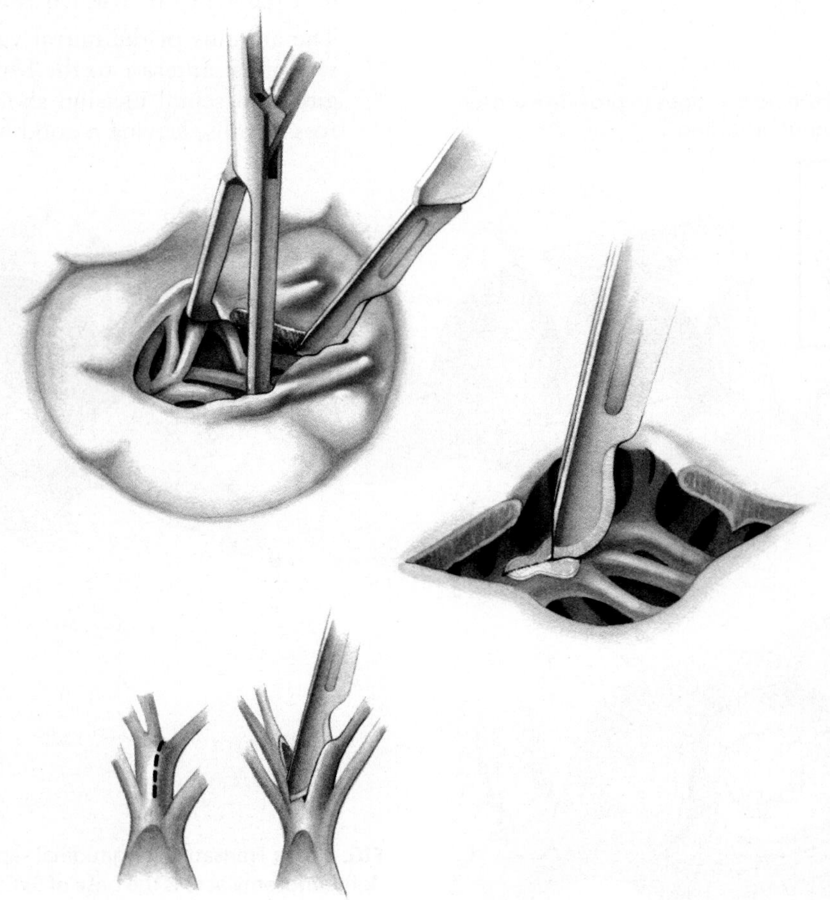

FIG. 6.10 Technique for open mitral commissurotomy (see text).

⊘ Injury to Papillary Muscle

Care must be taken to divide the head of the papillary muscle fused to the undersurface of mitral leaflets straight along its long axis. Oblique division may weaken or even result in a partial division of the papillary muscle, necessitating its repair or reimplantation or even requiring mitral valve replacement. ⊘

⊘ Overextension of Commissurotomy

The extent of commissurotomy must be as complete as possible without producing valvular incompetence. If the incision is extended too far toward the annulus, annuloplasty may become necessary (see Mitral Valve Reconstruction section). ⊘

CLOSED MITRAL COMMISSUROTOMY FOR MITRAL STENOSIS

Closed mitral commissurotomy is now rarely performed in most Western countries. Consequently, only a few of the current generation of cardiac surgeons have had adequate experience with this technique. Nevertheless, closed mitral valvotomy remains a good operation in selected subgroups of patients, and the long-term results have been consistently satisfactory. In third world countries, closed valvotomy continues to be the preferred form of therapy because of its simplicity and low cost compared with open-heart procedures.

Technique

A left posterolateral or anterolateral thoracotomy is made through the bed of the fifth rib. The lung is retracted posteroinferiorly, and a long incision is made anterior and parallel to the left phrenic nerve. The pericardium is then suspended with traction sutures. The left atrial appendage is identified and excluded with a side-biting clamp. A purse-string suture of 2-0 Prolene is placed around the left appendage. Another purse-string suture, reinforced with pledgets, is then placed into the apex of the left ventricle. The left atrial appendage is incised within the purse-string suture, and the surgeon's right index finger is introduced into the left atrium. The mitral valve is palpated to detect calcification, the degree of mitral stenosis, or the presence of insufficiency (Fig. 6.11).

⊘ Tear in the Atrial Appendage

The index finger should be introduced gently, without undue pressure. If the atrial appendage tears, it will result in brisk bleeding. ⊘

⊘ Blood Clot

Preoperative echocardiography is always performed to study the mitral valve pathology and to detect the presence of a blood clot in the left atrial appendage. Nevertheless, before applying clamps to the appendage or introducing a finger into the atrial cavity, the left atrial appendage should be palpated carefully to detect a blood clot. If thrombus is suspected, it should be excluded by clamping the base of

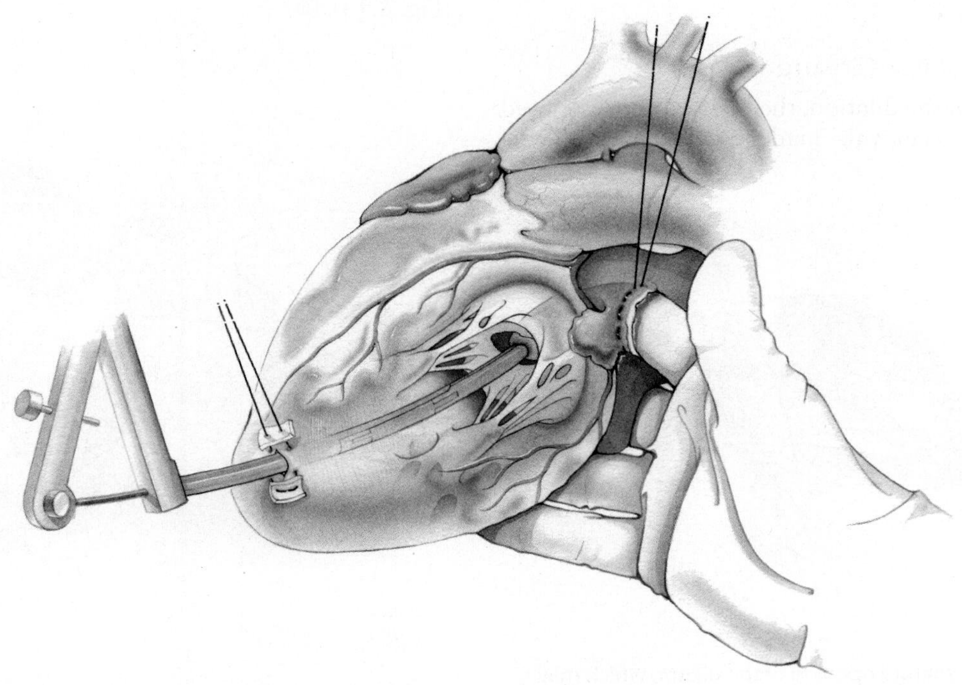

FIG. 6.11 Technique for closed mitral commissurotomy.

the appendage and then removed. If this is not possible, the closed procedure should be abandoned, and the operation converted to an open valvotomy with the use of extracorporeal circulation. ⊘

⊘ Mitral Orifice Occlusion

The index finger should not occlude the mitral orifice for more than two or three cardiac cycles to avoid precipitating dysrhythmia and possible cardiac arrest. ⊘

When the right index finger is in the left atrium, the heart is elevated with the remaining three fingers and palm of the right hand to bring the left ventricular apex into view. With a no. 11 blade held in the left hand, the surgeon makes a small ventriculotomy within the previously placed apical purse-string suture. This can also be performed by the surgeon's assistant if desired. This opening is now enlarged with a series of Hegar dilators until it accommodates the diameter of the Tubb valvulotome. The Tubb dilator is then introduced into the left ventricle with the surgeon's left hand and advanced through the mitral valve into the left atrium. It is then opened quickly to the preset limiting extent of 3.5 to 4.5 cm, closed, and removed. The surgeon's finger is then removed, and the purse-string suture on the left ventricular apex is snugged down and tied over pledgets.

⊘ Premature Opening of the Dilator

It is most important not to open the dilator until the surgeon can feel its tip with the right index finger in the left atrial cavity. Premature opening of the dilator may injure or tear the subvalvular structures and result in mitral insufficiency (Fig. 6.12). ⊘

⊘ Inadequate Dilator Closure

After completion of the dilation, the dilator must be closed completely before removal. Inadequate closure of the dilator will cause tearing of the left ventricular opening during withdrawal. ⊘

⊘ Valvotomy Adequacy

Adequacy of the valvotomy and any evidence of a mitral insufficiency jet must be ascertained with the surgeon's index finger while it is still in the left atrium. ⊘

⊘ Air Embolism

Every precaution should be taken to prevent air from entering the left atrium or left ventricle during the procedure. ⊘

Conversion of a Closed Mitral Valvotomy to the Open Technique

In young adults, the mitral lesion may be fibrotic but elastic and without calcification. The surgeon may find it possible to stretch the orifice maximally with a Tubb dilator only to note that the orifice resumes its previous stenotic size on removal of the dilator. Such patients must be treated with open mitral commissurotomy.

NB Standby Cardiopulmonary Bypass

It is always a prudent precaution to perform this procedure with a heart–lung machine available on standby so that the surgeon will have the option of using cardiopulmonary bypass if it becomes necessary. Venous drainage can be accomplished through a cannula placed in the main pulmonary artery. Arterial return may be through a cannula either in the descending aorta or femoral artery. A left atriotomy will give excellent exposure of the mitral valve (Fig. 6.13). NB

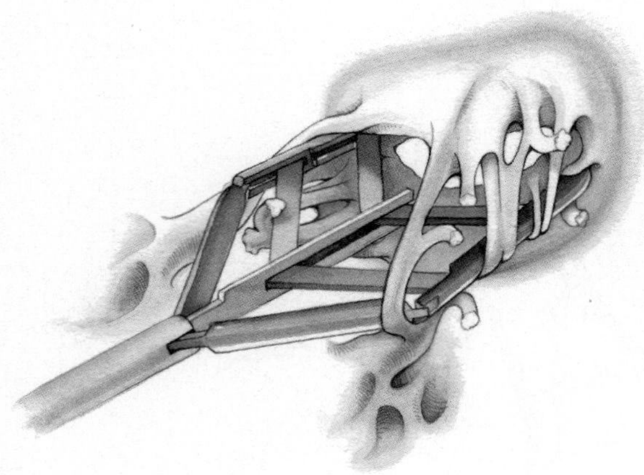

⊘ **FIG. 6.12** Premature opening of the dilator, which may injure or tear the subvalvular structures and result in mitral insufficiency.

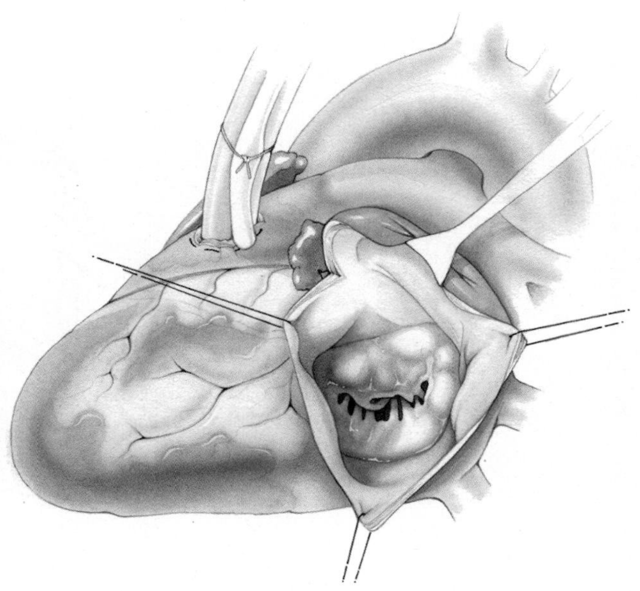

FIG. 6.13 Left atriotomy for exposure of the mitral valve if cardiopulmonary bypass becomes necessary.

MITRAL VALVE RECONSTRUCTION

The mitral apparatus includes the leaflets, annulus, chordae tendinae, papillary muscles, and the left ventricle. Mitral valve incompetence can be the result of annular dilation, leaflet abnormalities, chordal elongation or rupture, papillary muscle injury or displacement, and/or alterations of left ventricular size, shape, or wall motion. For this reason, it is necessary to examine and evaluate every aspect of the mitral valve complex in detail so that efforts at valvular reconstruction will be fruitful. The shape and size of the annulus is noted. Nerve hooks or forceps are used to determine the pliability and motion of the leaflets. The leaflet motion is classified as normal (type I), prolapsed (type II), or restricted (type III). The chords and papillary muscles are then assessed. Mitral valve reconstructive strategies may address any of the components that maintain the valvular competence (annulus, leaflets, chordae, papillary muscles, or the ventricle). Most contemporary techniques have focused on the annulus, the leaflets and the chordae.

All techniques described previously for approaching the mitral valve provide excellent exposure. The transseptal approach, however, has the added advantage of allowing the valve to be evaluated in its normal anatomic configuration without being distorted by excessive retraction. This is a point of importance when contemplating reconstructive procedures (Fig. 6.8).

Reconstruction of the Mitral Valve Leaflets

Mild asymptomatic mitral valve prolapse may progress to clinically significant mitral insufficiency. It is most often the result of myxomatous and degenerative changes of the chords with varying degrees of leaflet abnormality. The P2 segment is most commonly involved, and is managed surgically with a quadrangular resection and annuloplasty. Some surgeons use a triangular resection of the involved leaflet segment to avoid annular reapproximation and to simplify the procedure. Alternatively, the prolapsing segment may be supported with neochordae.

Quadrangular or Triangular Resection

A quadrangular or triangular portion of the posterior leaflet that encompasses the prolapsed segment of leaflet is resected. The posterior annulus in the area of the quadrangular resection is reduced with two to three interrupted sutures of 2-0 Ticron. This step may be unnecessary in triangular resection technique. The leaflets edges are reapproximated with 5-0 Prolene sutures tied on the ventricular or atrial aspect of the leaflets (Fig. 6.14). The posterior annulus is always reinforced with one of the annuloplasty support systems (see below).

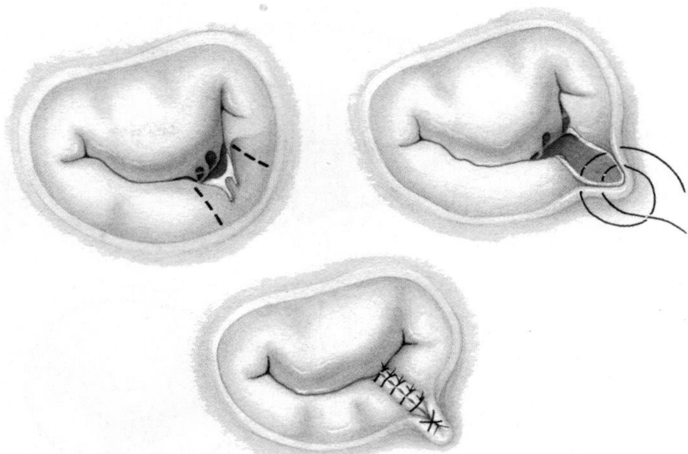

FIG. 6.14 Leaflet resection with an annuloplasty

⊘ Excessive Excision of Leaflet Tissue

Good judgment is needed when excising redundant prolapsed leaflet tissue. Too large an excision may compromise adequate repair. In cases in which a relatively large segment has been removed, leaflet approximation may be facilitated by sliding the remaining leaflet segments toward each other. This can be accomplished by detaching the remaining posterior leaflet segments from the annulus, commissure to commissure, and reattaching them back to the annulus after reduction annuloplasty. The posterior annulus must be reinforced with one of the annuloplasty systems to avoid any tension on the repair (see below) (Fig. 6.15). ⊘

⊘ Mitral Insufficiency from Improper Leaflet Apposition

Taking too wide a bite in the posterior mitral leaflet for reapproximation may decrease the surface area and produce mitral insufficiency by preventing proper coaptation of the leaflets. ⊘

⊘ Thin Leaflet Tissue

The leaflet tissue may be very thin and friable and sutures may cut through it, resulting in the recurrence of mitral valve insufficiency. Pledgets of pericardium can be used to buttress the sutures; care must be taken to avoid deforming the leaflet. ⊘

⊘ Suture Untying

Fine Prolene sutures may come untied if they have not been tied securely. This can result in disruption of the repair and significant valvular regurgitation. In this context, it should be borne in mind that fine Gore-Tex sutures have a greater tendency to untie, and therefore should be avoided in leaflet repair. ⊘

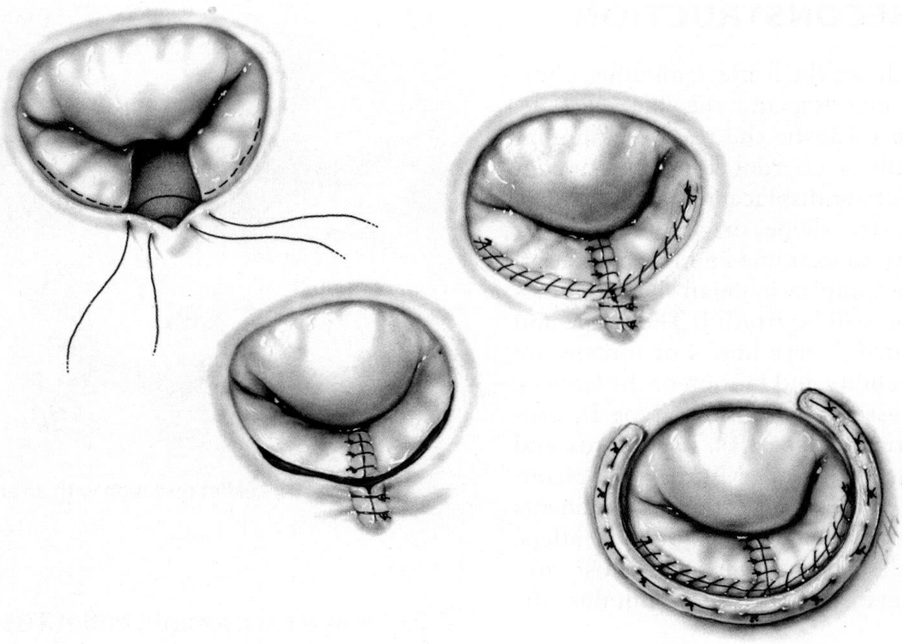

FIG. 6.15 Sliding technique for posterior leaflet repair with reinforcement of the posterior annulus.

⊘ Coexistent Mitral Annular Dilation

There is nearly always coexistent mitral annular dilation. It is therefore prudent to reinforce the posterior annulus with one of the annuloplasty support systems as described later. ⊘

Creation of Artificial Chordae

An alternative to the resection of the prolapsing segment/ruptured chordae is to resuspend the involved segment with creation of artificial chordae. There are now commercially available neochordae that can be used readily to recreate chordae (W.L Gore & Assoc, Inc., Flagstaff, AZ).

Gore-Tex Chordal Replacement

Technique

A 5-0 Gore-Tex suture, double armed with a tapered needle, is used to replace the ruptured or elongated chord of the anterior leaflet. The needle is passed through the tip of the papillary muscle from which the diseased chord originates. The suture is then locked on itself.

One of the needles of the Gore-Tex suture is then passed through the mitral leaflet at the site of attachment of the ruptured chord. The involved leaflet is then pulled upward into the left atrium with the aid of nerve hooks, placing tension on the rest of the chords. The length of the Gore-Tex suture is adjusted to approximate the length of the other normal chords. The Gore-Tex suture is then locked on itself. This will fix the length of the replaced (Gore-Tex) chord. The other arm of the Gore-Tex suture follows precisely the same route, its length similarly adjusted, and locked on itself. The two arms are then tied together (Fig. 6.16).

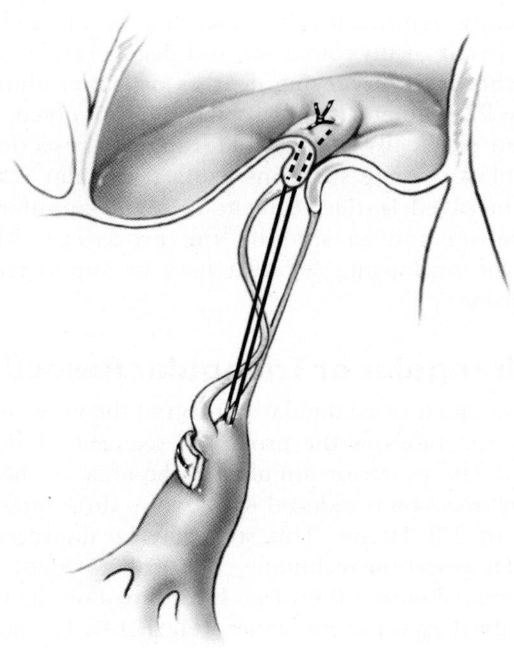

FIG. 6.16 Replacement of elongated or ruptured chords with a Gore-Tex chord.

⊘ Papillary Muscle

The tip of the papillary muscle is usually fibrotic and quite strong. The Gore-Tex suture is buttressed with pericardial pledgets for added security when the papillary muscle tip is muscular. ⊘

NB Importance of Locking

It is absolutely essential for the Gore-Tex suture to be locked on itself, both at the tip of the papillary muscle and at the leaflet attachment, to ensure that the correct length of the replaced (Gore-Tex) chord is fixed. NB

NB Securing Gore-Tex Suture

The Gore-Tex suture may become untied if too few knots are placed. At least 10 or 11 knots are required when securing a Gore-Tex suture. NB

⊘ Shortened Artificial Chord

If the Gore-Tex suture is not securely locked on itself, it will be pulled up while being tied. This will result in a shortened new artificial chord tethering the anterior mitral leaflet and creating valvular incompetence. ⊘

This technique can be modified and applied in the management of elongated as well as ruptured chords.

Edge-to-Edge Mitral Valve Repair

Complex lesions of the mitral valve, prolapse of anterior leaflet, functional mitral insufficiency, and commissural abnormality as well as residual regurgitant jets following mitral valve reconstruction may be satisfactorily repaired utilizing the edge-to-edge repair of Alfieri.

Technique

The free edge of the anterior leaflet, and the corresponding free edge of the posterior leaflet are approximated with 2 or 3 sutures of 4-0 Prolene or 5-0 Prolene if the leaflet tissue is relatively thin. This results in a "double orifice" repair. When the abnormality is near the commissures, the adjacent free edges of the anterior and posterior leaflets are approximated with 4-0 Prolene sutures, resulting in a smaller single orifice.

NB The repair should always be reinforced with an annuloplasty ring. NB

Anterior Mitral Leaflet Abnormalities

Chordal rupture or markedly elongated chords affecting the anterior leaflet of the mitral valve can result in significant mitral valve incompetence. The affected chords can be reinforced by transposing the corresponding posterior leaflet attachment to the anterior leaflet of the mitral valve, often referred to as the flip-over procedure.

Technique

A quadrangular segment of the posterior leaflet, with normal primary chords facing the ruptured or markedly elongated chords of the anterior leaflet, is detached from the posterior leaflet and posterior annulus. It is then flipped over and attached to the anterior leaflet of the mitral valve with multiple interrupted sutures of fine Prolene sutures. All secondary chords from the transposed segment are detached to allow full mobility. The defect in the posterior leaflet is reconstructed as described previously (Fig. 6.14).

A much simpler technique is to replace the ruptured or elongated chord with a Gore-Tex suture without disrupting the posterior leaflet or posterior annulus of the mitral valve.

Reconstruction of the Mitral Valve Annulus

Commissuroplasty

In a small subgroup of patients, the cause of mitral insufficiency is annular dilation only and can be effectively addressed with a commissuroplasty. This can be accomplished by successive figure-of-eight sutures at both commissures, incorporating only the posterior annulus.

The needle of an atraumatic 2-0 Tevdek suture is passed through the annulus at the commissure and then again 1 cm further along on the posterior annulus. The same suture is then placed through the annulus 0.5 cm from the commissure (or midway between the first two stitches). Finally, it is passed through the annulus 1 cm further away before it is tightened and securely tied. If indicated, another figure-of-eight suture, similarly placed, can decrease the annular size even more (Fig. 6.17). Good judgment dictates the appropriate size of each stitch so that a good repair can be accomplished without overcorrection. These sutures may be buttressed with Teflon felt pledgets for added security.

⊘ Symmetric Annulus

It is important to have an anatomically symmetric annulus. Therefore, the procedure should include both the anterolateral and posteromedial commissural aspects of the annulus in exactly the same manner. ⊘

⊘ Residual Mitral Valve Incompetence

Inadequate reduction of the annulus may not correct the valvular insufficiency. The mitral valve must be evaluated after annuloplasty for incompetence by injecting saline into the left ventricle and looking for an insufficient jet. ⊘

⊘ Mitral Stenosis

Overcorrection will result in mitral stenosis. The orifice may be examined digitally, or an appropriately sized obturator may be introduced into the valve to ascertain the presence of an adequately sized orifice. ⊘

⊘ Degenerative Disease

When the pathologic entity is degenerative disease, the tissues are thin and weak, and sutures may tear through. The

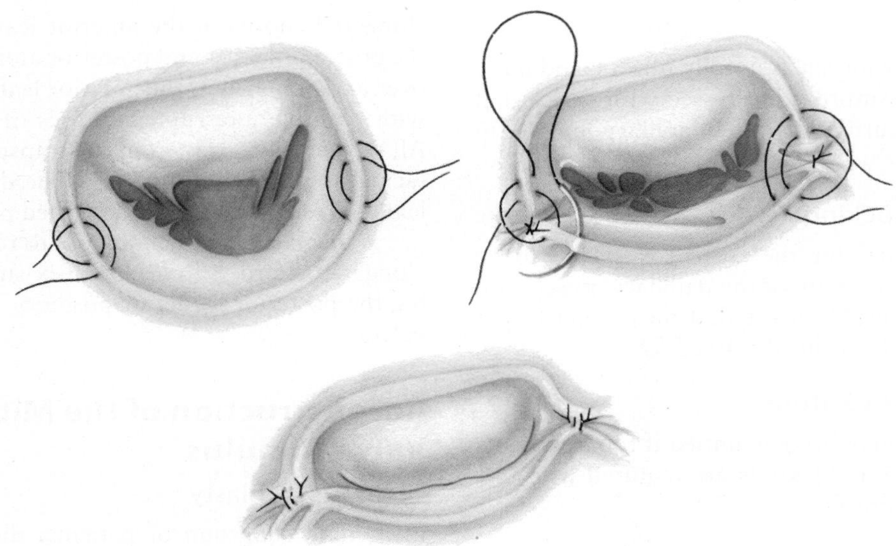

FIG. 6.17 Figure-of-eight technique for a mitral valve annuloplasty.

use of Teflon felt or pericardial pledgets may help prevent this complication. ⊘

⊘ Exclusion of the Anterior Annulus

Annuloplasty should incorporate only the posterior annulus and not the anterior annulus because it is usually the posterior portion that is dilated. Incorporation of the anterior segment of the annulus may distort the mitral configuration and thereby result in valvular insufficiency. ⊘

⊘ Suture Placement

The sutures should be placed in the fibrous annulus, rather than into the leaflet itself, or into the atrial wall beyond the annulus. ⊘

Annuloplasty

Commissuroplasty is useful for a small group of patients who have developed mild mitral insufficiency due to left ventricular and mitral annular dilation. However, the large majority of patients with mitral insufficiency are best served by placement of a complete or partial annuloplasty ring, either as an isolated therapy, or as an adjunct to a leaflet and/or chordal repair.

NB Many rings and bands are commercially available, several of which are specifically designed for different etiologies of mitral regurgitation. The techniques for implanting the complete rings as well as the posterior bands (incomplete rings) are similar regardless of the specific device. NB

Complete Mitral Annuloplasty Ring

Carpentier-Edwards Physio II Annuloplasty ring (Edwards Lifesciences, Irvine, CA) is a semirigid complete ring that is very efficacious in bringing the anterior and posterior

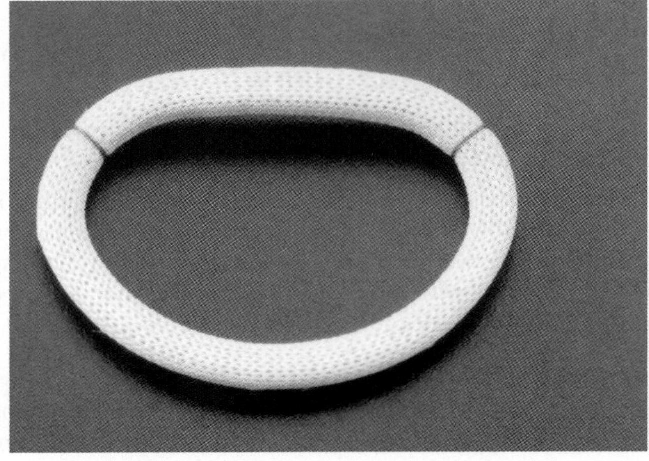

FIG. 6.18 Carpentier-Edwards physio annuloplasty ring (Edwards Lifesciences, Irvine, CA).

annulus closer together, and allows the mitral annuli to regain its normal shape (Fig. 6.18).

Technique

If leaflet or chordal procedures are required, they are accomplished first. The annuloplasty ring is then secured in place. Sutures of 2-0 Ticron are passed through the annulus at each trigone. With the aid of a right-angled clamp placed behind the chords, the anterior leaflet is very gently stretched to expose its surface area. The sizer must correspond to the area of the anterior leaflet and the distance between the trigones. In this manner, the appropriately sized ring is selected. Approximately 7 to 10 simple sutures are placed evenly in the posterior annulus approximately

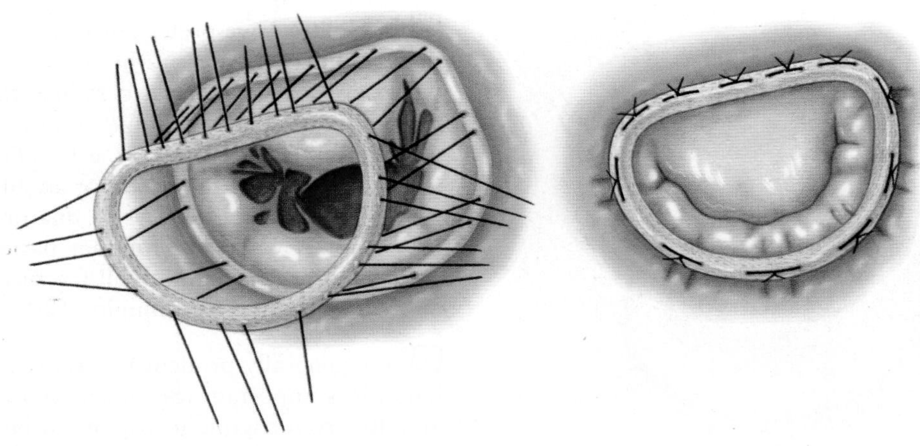

FIG. 6.19 Technique for complete ring annuloplasty

3 to 4 mm apart. Similarly, two to four sutures are placed in the anterior annulus between the trigonal stitches. All sutures are then evenly passed through the ring, which is then lowered into position and the sutures are securely tied (Fig. 6.19).

NB Suture Placement

The sutures should be appropriately spaced on both the annulus and the ring, taking into account their different sizes. This may entail taking wider bites on the posterior annulus to ensure correct seating of the ring. NB

NB Delicate, Friable Tissue

Often, left atrial and annular tissues are edematous and friable. In these cases, horizontal mattress sutures with soft felt pledgets may be used instead of simple sutures. This will prevent tearing of the suture through the tissues. NB

Incomplete Mitral Annuloplasty Ring

The Cosgrove-Edwards Incomplete ring or band (Edwards Lifesciences, Irvine, CA) supports the posterior mitral annulus, in isolation (Fig. 6.20). The choice of annuloplasty ring (complete vs. incomplete) is dependent on surgeon's preferences; in cases of functional mitral regurgitation, most surgeons agree that a complete ring is advisable.

Technique

Sutures of 2-0 Ticron are passed through the annulus at each trigone. The appropriate band size is selected by finding the sizer that corresponds to the area of the anterior leaflet and the distance between the trigones. Approximately seven to nine simple sutures are placed evenly in the posterior annulus approximately 3 to 4 mm apart (Fig. 6.21). All sutures are evenly passed through the band, which is then lowered into position (Fig. 6.22). The sutures are tied securely over the template to allow precise annular reduction. The template is then removed (Fig. 6.23).

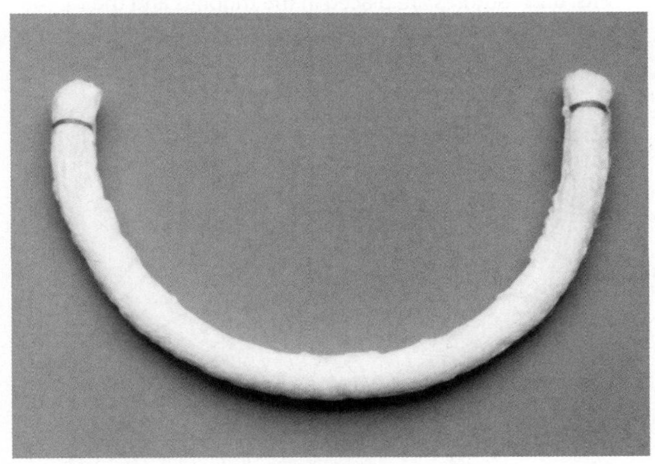

FIG. 6.20 Cosgrove-Edwards Incomplete annuloplasty band (Edwards Lifesciences, Irvine, CA).

NB Sutures must be deep enough to include a substantial bite of good strong annular tissue. At times, sutures can be passed from the ventricle into the atrium through the posterior annulus, taking care not to interfere with the chordal attachments (Fig. 6.21). NB

NB It is important that the distance between the simple sutures be the same on the mitral annulus and annuloplasty band. Redundant posterior annulus is reduced by taking larger simple bites on the annulus than on the band, thereby folding the annulus into the ring. NB

⊘ Hemolysis

An adequate repair may have very mild residual insufficiency. Even a small jet of blood against a foreign material may produce significant hemolysis. The surgeon must take all precautions to prevent this complication. ⊘

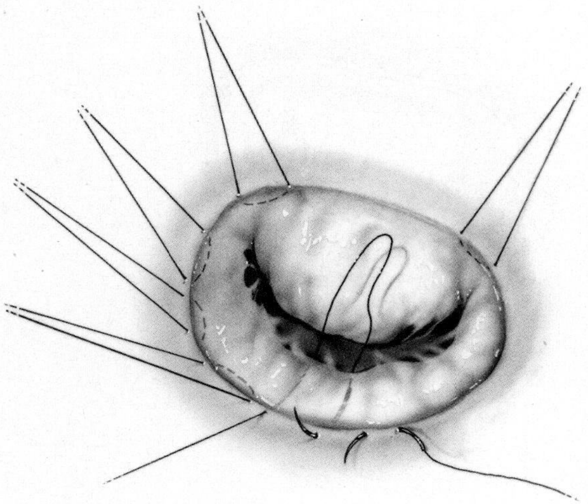

FIG. 6.21 Sutures are placed in the trigones and the posterior annulus.

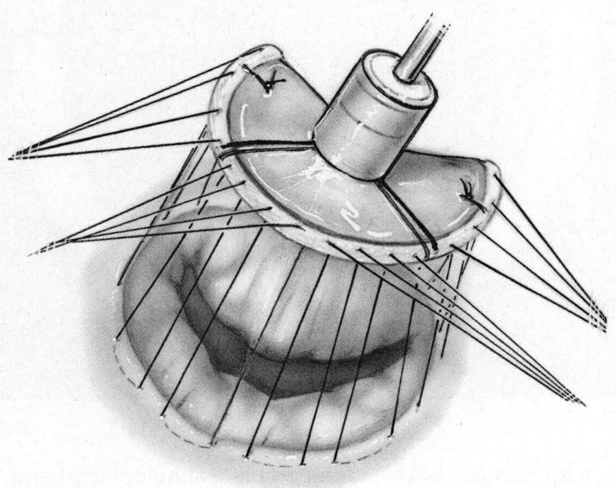

FIG. 6.22 Sutures are placed in the annuloplasty band.

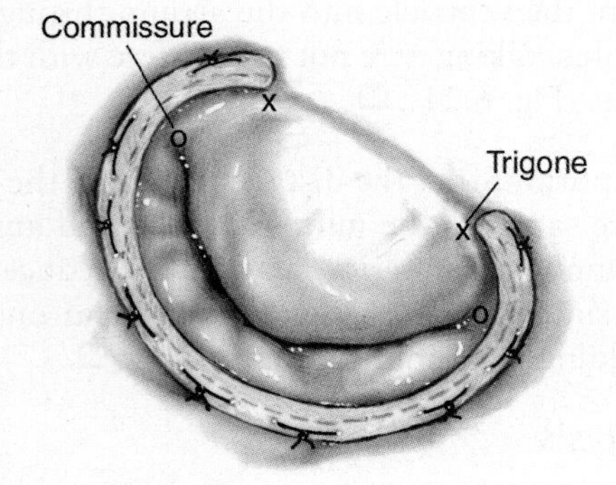

FIG. 6.23 Completed posterior annuloplasty band.

NB In children, we prefer not to use any ring. Instead, we place multiple sutures in the posterior annulus buttressed with pericardial pledgets to reduce the size of the posterior annulus. This technique allows growth of the mitral valve annulus. Alternatively, a fine Prolene double-armed suture is run along the posterior annulus from commissure to commissure and tied over a dilator equal to the appropriate mitral valve size for that patient. The expectation is that the Prolene suture will fracture as the child grows, allowing growth of the annulus. NB

NB It is generally prudent to choose a smaller size ring or band. It is important for the length of the posterior mitral annulus from trigone to trigone to be as short as possible without creating mitral stenosis. In fact, the mitral leaflet should appear redundant and generously fill the mitral orifice when the left ventricle is full for optimal results. NB

Reconstruction of the Chordae Tendineae

The most effective way of repairing a ruptured chorade or elongated chordae is creation of the artificial chordae (see above). Occasionally, chordal shortening may offer an alternative approach. Before chordal shortening can be initiated, the amount of abnormal lengthening must be established. To do this, the leaflets must be pulled gently into the left atrium with two fine Prolene traction sutures or nerve hooks. The degree of elongation of the chords can be closely estimated by measuring the distance between the plane of the mitral valve annulus and the attachment of the lengthened chords to the elevated leaflet (Fig. 6.24). This excess length can be sewn to the undersurface of the leaflet (Fig. 6.25).

Attachment of the Chords to the Mitral Leaflets

A double-armed, 5-0 Prolene suture is used to shorten each elongated chord. The first needle is passed through the chord at or slightly below the plane of the mitral annulus. The second needle is then placed midway between the first suture and the undersurface of the leaflet. Both needles are then passed upward through the leaflet, very close to one another, and tied snugly on the atrial side. This draws up the excess length of chord underneath the leaflet and pulls it down to the level of the plane of the mitral valve to reestablish apposition with the other leaflet (Fig. 6.25).

⊘ Leaflet Tear

The leaflet must be somewhat thickened or fibrous. The chordal-shortening sutures may injure or tear an otherwise normal leaflet, thereby interfering with a satisfactory repair and culminating in leaflet tear. ⊘

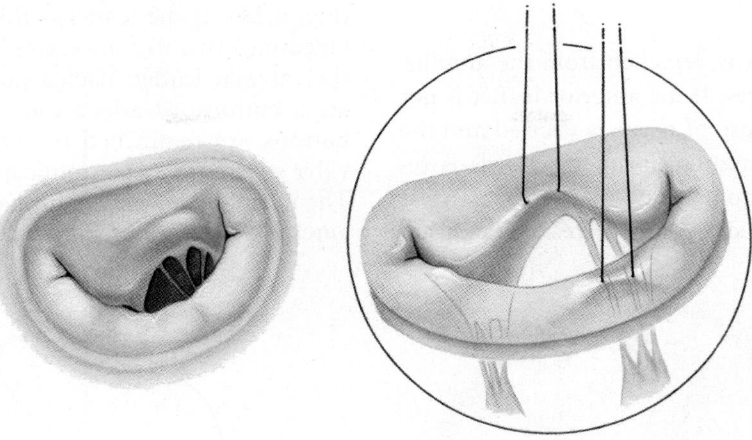

FIG. 6.24 Estimating the degree of elongation of the chords by measuring the distance between the plane of the mitral valve annulus and the attachments of the lengthened chords to the elevated leaflet.

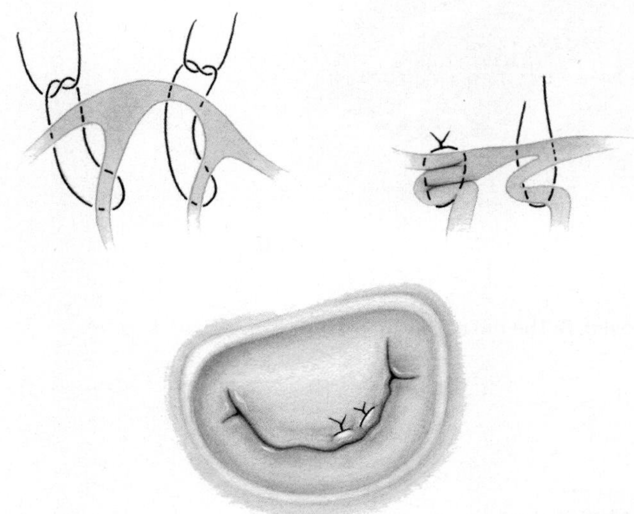

FIG. 6.25 Attachment of the elongated chords to the mitral leaflets.

NB Chordal shortening procedures are mainly performed in children for growth potential possibilities. In adults, we have adopted the simpler technique of using Gore-Tex artificial chords (see subsequent text). NB

Ischemic Mitral Regurgitation

Ischemic mitral valve prolapse may occur following myocardial infarction secondary to injury with elongation or partial or complete rupture of a papillary muscle. Total rupture of a papillary muscle generally requires mitral valve replacement. Incomplete detachment of a single head may be amenable to repair with chordal replacement or transfer and/or resection of a portion of the affected leaflet as described in preceding text.

Most patients with ischemic mitral disease have functional regurgitation due to annular and left ventricular dilation and/or displacement of the papillary muscles. Mitral valve replacement may be the best option in patients with severe ischemic mitral regurgitation who are undergoing coronary revascularization. In patients with moderate ischemic mitral regurgitation and heart failure symptoms, or dilated annulus, or nonviable lateral myocardium, mitral valve repair with an annuloplasty ring may be a good option. Most surgeons use an undersized complete ring annuloplasty in these patients along with revascularization of all ischemic, viable myocardium.

MITRAL VALVE REPLACEMENT

Increasing experience with mitral valve repair has allowed most patients with degenerative mitral valve disease or mitral annular dilation to undergo reconstructive procedures as previously described quite successfully. However, when reparative procedures do not appear to provide a durable successful outcome, mitral valve replacement should be considered.

In recent years, experimental and clinical studies have established the importance of the subvalvular apparatus in retaining the normal geometry of the left ventricle and its function. Therefore, whenever the mitral valve has to be replaced, every attempt should be made to preserve the native subvalvular apparatus or replace native chordal structures with Gore-Tex sutures to maintain the mitral annular–papillary muscle continuity.

Technique

The diseased anterior leaflet is detached from the annulus between the two commissures. If the anterior leaflet is not extensively diseased, an ellipse of tissue is excised and the rim of the leaflet tissue containing primary chords is reattached to the anterior annulus using pledgeted mattress sutures to be used subsequently for valve implantation (Fig. 6.26). If the leaflet is thickened or calcified, it is divided into two to four segments, depending on the size of the valvular leaflet. Each segment is then trimmed to create a button of leaflet tissue with attached chords. These buttons are reattached to the anterior annulus with the valve sutures in an anatomic manner (Figs. 6.27 and 6.28). The normal geometry is probably maintained better if the anterior leaflet is not subdivided.

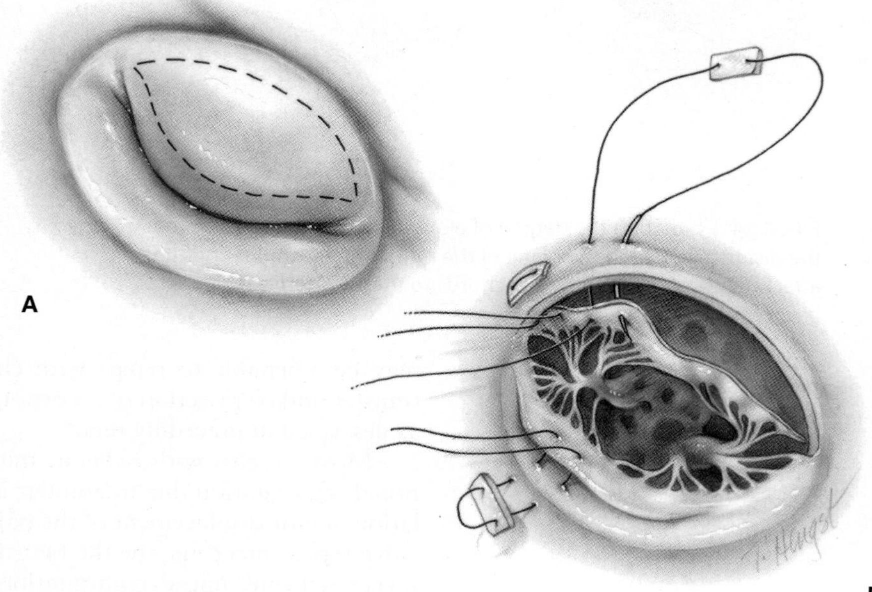

FIG. 6.26 A: An ellipse of the anterior leaflet is removed. **B:** The rim of the anterior leaflet is attached to the anterior annulus.

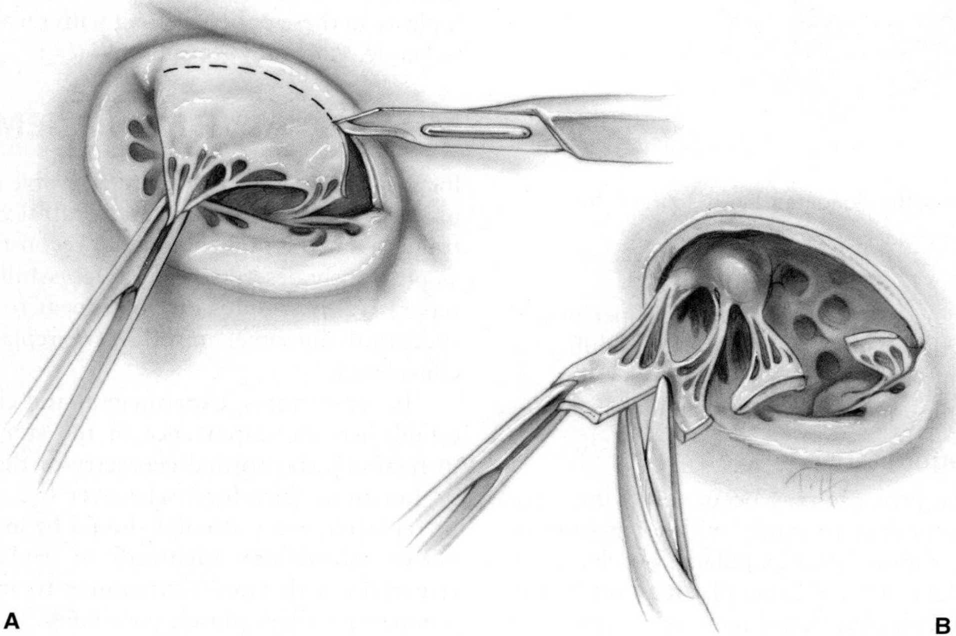

FIG. 6.27 A: Anterior leaflet is detached. **B:** The anterior leaflet is divided into buttons with chordal attachments.

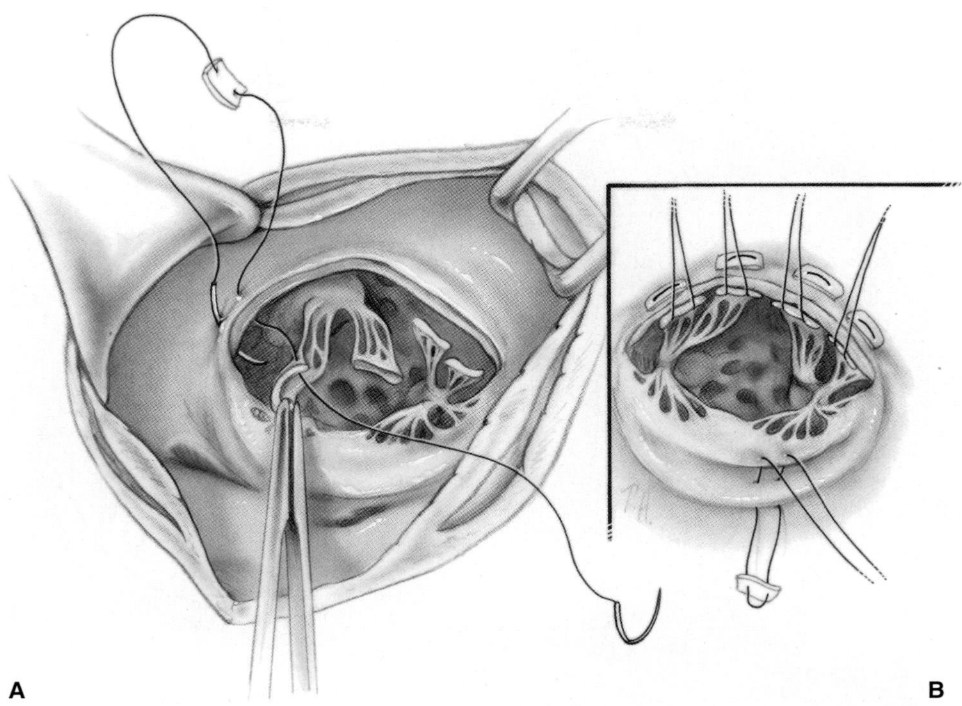

FIG. 6.28 A: Each chordal button is reattached to the anterior annulus, retaining its normal geometric position. **B:** The posterior leaflet is kept intact. Redundant tissue is folded into the left atrium.

The posterior leaflet, when pliable, can usually be retained completely together with the attached chordae tendineae. Redundant leaflet tissue is folded up into the annulus by placing the valve sutures through the annulus and bringing them through the leading edge of the leaflet tissue (Fig. 6.28B). Alternatively, incisions or small wedge resections of leaflet tissue between the chordal attachments are performed if the posterior leaflet is thickened and fibrotic to allow implantation of a larger valve.

At times, the mitral valve leaflet and the subvalvular apparatus are grossly diseased and calcified and must be totally resected. The diseased leaflets are then pulled and stretched slightly with a heavy suture or forceps to bring their annular attachments into view (Fig. 6.29A). With a long-handled no. 15 blade, the mitral leaflets are divided circumferentially 4 to 5 mm from the annulus (Fig. 6.29B). A traction suture in the annulus adjacent to the posteromedial commissure allows better exposure and provides countertraction for the complete removal of the diseased valve (Fig. 6.29C). This suture can subsequently be used in anchoring the prosthesis. The diseased chordae tendineae are then excised with scissors (Fig. 6.29D).

⊘ Excessive Leaflet Excision

A good margin of leaflet tissue should always be left with the annulus to allow secure attachment of sutures for subsequent placement of a prosthesis. Overzealous excision of leaflets may leave a weakened annulus, making valve replacement insecure or even resulting in detachment of the left atrium from the left ventricle. ⊘

⊘ Papillary Muscle Excision

Only the calcified and diseased chords should be excised, leaving the fibrous tips of the papillary muscles untouched. Removal of an excessive amount of papillary muscle may weaken the ventricular wall, which may result in hematoma within the wall and possible rupture (see subsequent text). ⊘

⊘ Excessive Pull on Papillary Muscle

During the process of leaflet excision, the valve tissue should never be pulled overzealously. The heart arrested with cardioplegia is flaccid, and any excessive pull on the papillary muscle may tear a buttonhole defect through the weakened left ventricular wall (Fig. 6.30A, B). If such a catastrophe occurs, it must be detected immediately and repaired with pledgeted mattress sutures (Fig. 6.30C, D). The posterior descending coronary artery is likely to be in close proximity to this type of ventricular wall tear. Precautions must therefore be taken to avoid occluding the coronary artery in the process of repairing the defect. Pledgeted, double-armed, atraumatic sutures are passed deeply, well away from the coronary artery, and tied snugly over another pledget. If bleeding continues after the application of several well-placed sutures, the whole area of the defect should be covered with a patch of

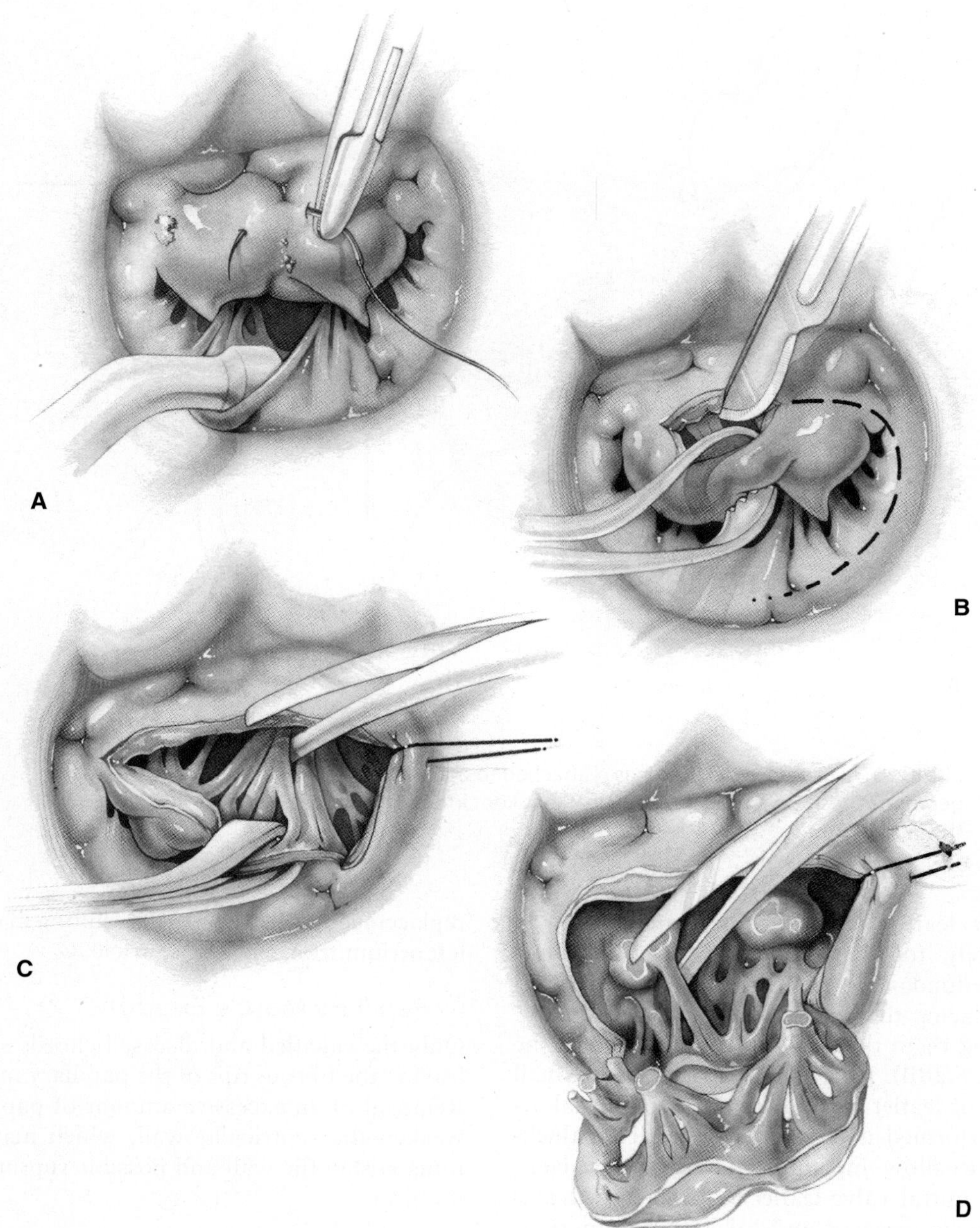

FIG. 6.29 Mitral valve excision. **A:** Diseased leaflets are pulled and stretched with Allis forceps or heavy suture to expose their annular attachments. **B:** The mitral leaflets are divided circumferentially with a long-handled no. 15 blade 4 to 5 mm from the annulus. **C:** A traction suture in the annulus adjacent to the posteromedial commissure allows better exposure and provides countertraction for the complete removal of the diseased valve. **D:** The chordae tendineae and fibrotic tips of the papillary muscles are then removed with scissors.

bovine pericardium, meticulously sewn to the surrounding normal myocardium with continuous 3-0 Prolene sutures. Topical application of Bioglue on the repaired wall is most helpful in controlling the bleeding. Some coronary artery branches may have to be sacrificed within the continuous suturing process. This is inevitable and must be borne in mind when dealing with this potentially lethal problem. ⊘

⊘ Mitral Valve Calcification

Calcification of the mitral valve and annulus is quite common. Care should be taken to remove as much calcium as possible without weakening the annulus. Occasionally, removal of calcium or degenerative material may leave a hollow cavity in the annulus. This should be immediately irrigated and closed securely with soft tailor-made

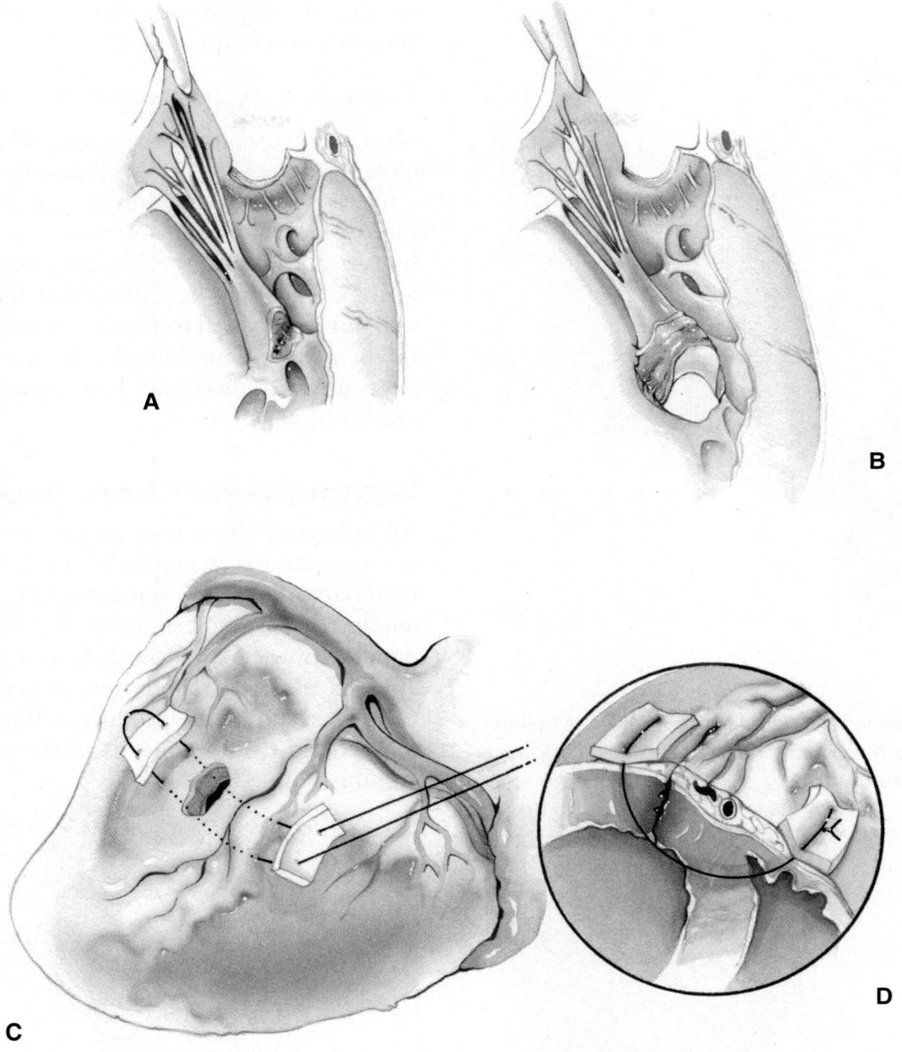

FIG. 6.30 A–D: Mechanism of a buttonhole defect through the left ventricular wall and its surgical repair.

pledgeted sutures. These sutures may or may not be used to help anchor the prosthesis (Fig. 6.31). ⊘

⊘ Annular Calcification

The mural annulus of the mitral valve may become infiltrated with heavily calcified tissue that may extend into and involve the full thickness of the atrioventricular groove and wall. Overzealous removal of this excessive calcium may result in a defect in the atrioventricular groove. Consistency of the surrounding tissues and the location of the circumflex coronary artery in the atrioventricular groove make any attempt to repair this defect most hazardous. ⊘

⊘ Atrioventricular Groove Disruption

Overzealous removal of calcium from the posterior annulus of the mitral valve or forcibly implanting too large a prosthesis may result in disruption of the atrioventricular groove. This catastrophe is often noted as the patient is being weaned off cardiopulmonary bypass when the operative field is flooded with bright red blood. ⊘

NB It is dangerous to attempt to repair this injury from outside the heart. Cardiopulmonary bypass is resumed, and cardioplegic arrest of the heart is once again accomplished. The left atrium is opened and the mitral prosthesis is removed. The extent of the defect is fully evaluated. A large patch of autologous pericardium treated with glutaraldehyde or bovine pericardium is cut to the appropriate size and shape. It is sewn in place, well away from the margin of the defect, to the left ventricular wall, left atrial wall, and left atrioventricular junction. The suture line is reinforced with multiple interrupted sutures buttressed with Teflon felt. A smaller mitral prosthesis is reimplanted in the usual manner except that it is attached to the pericardium

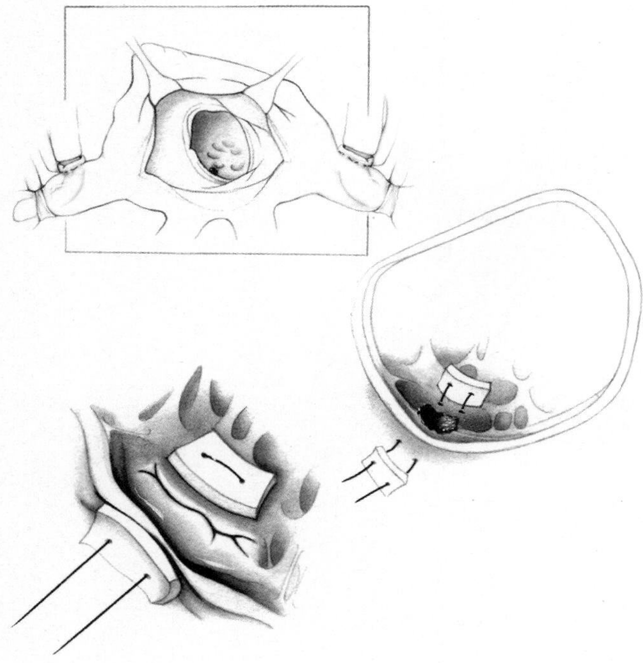

FIG. 6.31 Removal of degenerative calcific material. The hollow cavity in the annulus formed during removal should be irrigated and closed with pledgeted sutures.

instead of the posterior annulus. The surgery is then continued to its completion. NB

⊘ Injury to Posterior Left Atrium

Overzealous removal of organized and/or calcified blood clots from the left atrial wall during mitral valve surgery or a maze procedure may result in a shear injury and serious bleeding. It is always safer to go back on cardiopulmonary bypass and repair the bleeding site from within the left atrium. This may be tedious but the experienced surgeon will not be tempted to repair any bleeding from the back of the heart following mitral valve surgery by displacing the heart upward, no matter how minor the bleeding site may appear to be. ⊘

Technique for Chord Replacement

All the native chordal structures are resected if the subvalvular apparatus is markedly diseased, as in patients with rheumatic disease in whom there is fusion of the chordae tendineae, foreshortening of the chordal apparatus, and papillary muscle thickening. Continuity between the mitral annulus and the papillary muscle is then recreated with 4-0 Gore-Tex sutures to produce artificial chordae tendineae that extend from the heads of the papillary muscle to the annulus (Fig. 6.32).

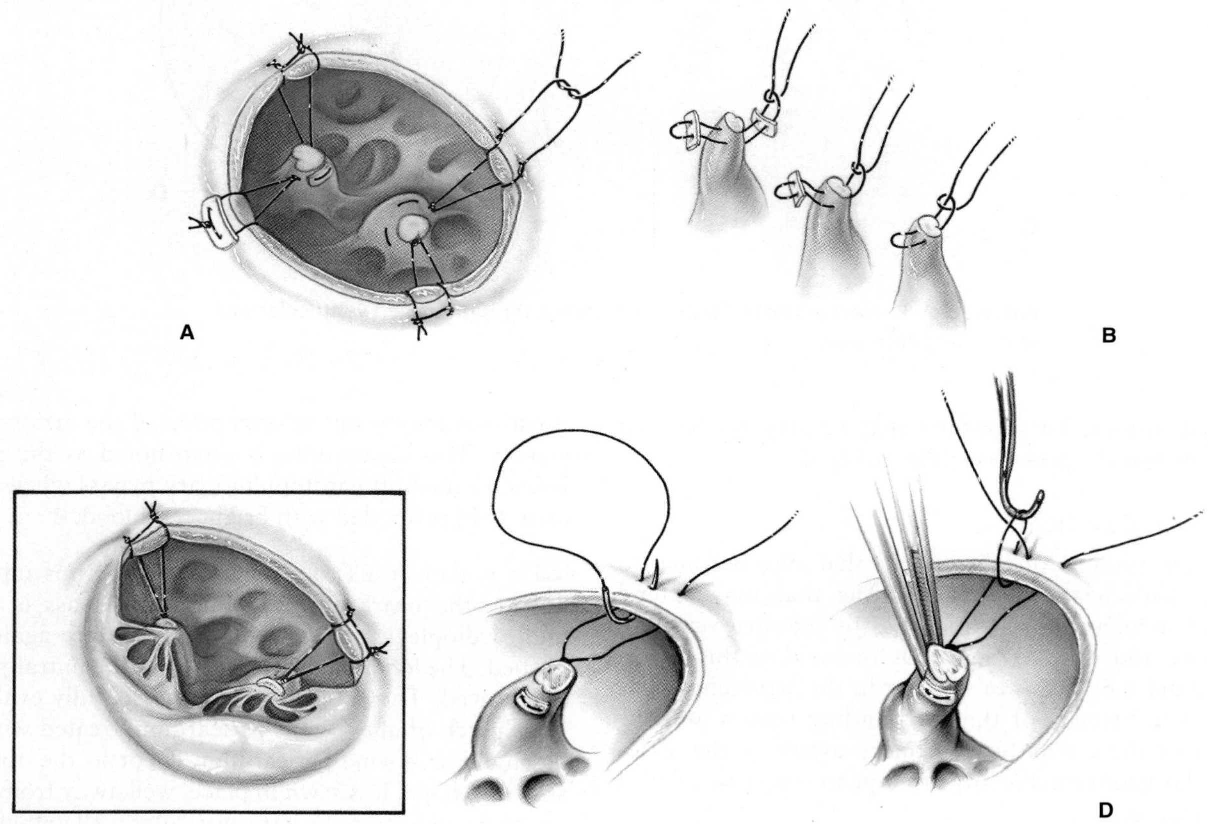

FIG. 6.32 **A:** Papillary muscles are attached to the mitral annulus at the 2, 5, 7, and 10 o'clock positions with Gore-Tex chordal substitutes. **B:** Gore-Tex sutures are attached to the papillary muscles. Teflon felt pledgets may be used to buttress the sutures. **C:** Anterior chordal replacement with retention of the posterior native chordal attachments. **D:** Locking the Gore-Tex suture at the level of the annulus.

A suture of 4-0 Gore-Tex on a double-armed needle is sutured to the fibrous tip of the papillary muscle. If there is no fibrous tissue, the suture is buttressed with a small, soft felt or pericardial pledget and the suture is tied snugly or locked on itself (Fig. 6.32B). Both needles of each suture are passed through the annulus of the mitral valve at approximately the 2, 5, 7, and 10 o'clock positions (Fig. 6.32A). The precise length of the Gore-Tex artificial chord is determined, and each suture is locked on itself and then tied. Locking the stitch prevents any pulling on the Gore-Tex, resulting in shortening of its length. The correct length of the artificial chords allows both the papillary muscle and the Gore-Tex suture to be barely taut, not tight, and certainly not too loose. There should be no "bowing" of the Gore-Tex chord. Often, it is possible to retain the native posterior chordal attachments and replace only the anterior chords with Gore-Tex suture (Fig. 6.32C).

Sizing the Mitral Orifice

The largest possible prosthesis should be chosen for mitral valve replacement. Sizers are introduced sequentially into the annulus until the correct size can be selected. The sizer should fit loosely.

⊘ Injury from the Sizer

It is important not to push the sizer forcefully into the annulus. ⊘

⊘ Combined Mitral and Aortic Valve Replacement

When a double valve replacement is performed, both prostheses should be undersized to ensure proper seating of both valves. ⊘

Valve Choices

Although many prostheses have been successfully used in the past, we believe that technical complications are markedly reduced when a bileaflet mechanical or a low-profile tissue valve is implanted in the mitral position, especially when the subvalvular apparatus is retained.

Technique for Suture Insertion

Simple, figure-of-eight, everting pledgeted mattress, and ventricular pledgeted mattress sutures are commonly used in anchoring the mitral prosthesis. If the annulus is well defined and strong, simple or figure-of-eight sutures of 2-0 Tevdek will be adequate. Conversely, if the annulus is degenerative, pledgeted and horizontal mattress sutures provide added security (Fig. 6.33). Occasionally, a continuous 2-0 Prolene suture may be preferred. The use of everting, pledgeted mattress sutures (Fig. 6.33C) is favored by most surgeons and is the preferred technique in our unit.

Simple sutures can be inserted in the sewing ring of the prosthesis, either singly or in vertical mattress manner.

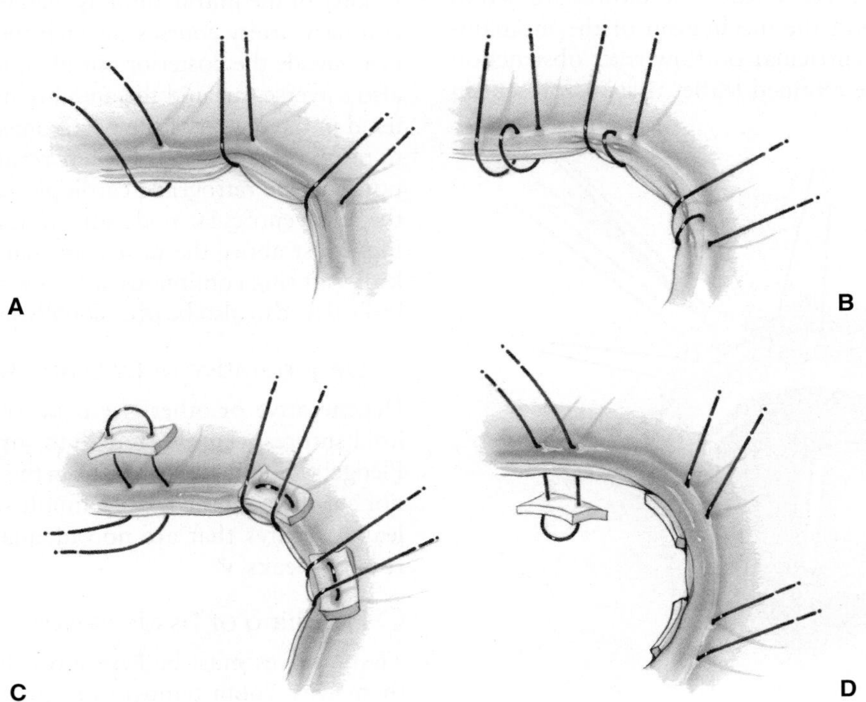

FIG. 6.33 Sutures to anchor the mitral prosthesis. **A:** Simple sutures. **B:** Figure-of-eight sutures. **C:** Everting pledgeted mattress sutures. **D:** Ventricular pledgeted mattress sutures.

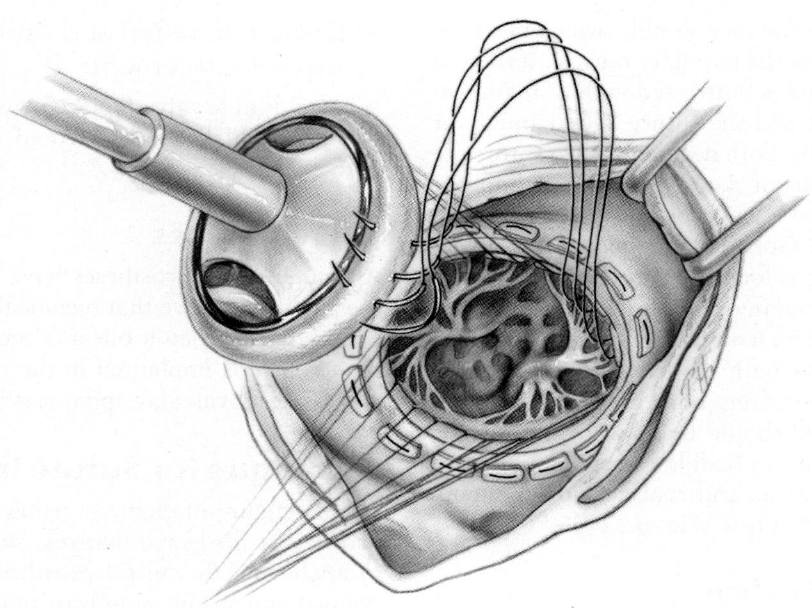

FIG. 6.34 Placement of sutures into the sewing ring of the bileaflet prosthesis (St. Jude Medical, Minneapolis, MN).

Figure-of-eight sutures and mattress sutures are placed into the sewing ring in a horizontal mattress manner (Fig. 6.34). When all the sutures have been passed through both the annulus and the valve sewing ring, the prosthesis is gently lowered into position and the sutures are tied snugly. Any retained redundant subvalvular apparatus must be pulled above the mitral annular plane when the sutures are tied to prevent interference with the mechanism of the mechanical prostheses or left ventricular outflow tract obstruction (Fig. 6.35). If extensive retained leaflet tissue is present in the left atrium, it may be secured away from the prosthetic sewing ring with a 4-0 Prolene suture attaching the leaflet tissue to the left atrial wall.

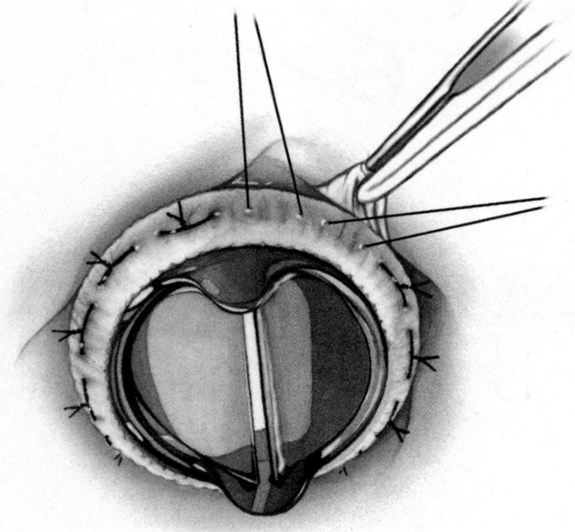

⊘ FIG. 6.35 Pulling retained chordal button tissue above the mitral annular plane as valve sutures are tied.

⊘ Sites of Suture Injury

There are important anatomic structures in the immediate vicinity of the mitral annulus (Fig. 6.36). The left circumflex coronary artery courses through the atrioventricular groove just outside the posterior mitral annulus. The coronary sinus also traverses around the annulus and is likely to be encountered in the region of the posteromedial commissure. Failure to respect this relationship may result in a valve suture incorporating the retrograde cardioplegia cannula. The artery to the atrioventricular node sometimes runs parallel to the annulus just above the posteromedial commissure. The aortic leaflets, being continuous with the anterior leaflet of the mitral valve, can also be occasionally incorporated in a stitch. ⊘

⊘ Degenerative or Delicate Annular Tissue

Degenerative or otherwise delicate annular tissue will not hold sutures securely enough to support a valve prosthesis. Pledgets should always cushion the sutures so that they will not cut through the friable annulus and allow paravalvular leaks. Sutures that are not adequately tightened will also result in leaks. ⊘

⊘ Handling of Tissue Valves

Tissue valves must be kept moist by intermittently rinsing them with room temperature physiologic saline solution. If this vital precaution is not taken, the heat of the operating room lights will soon dry and permanently damage the valve tissue. ⊘

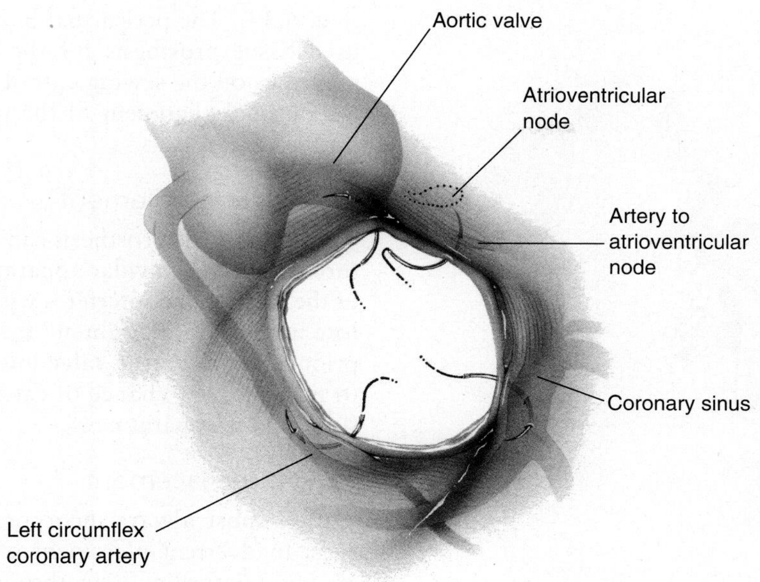

⊘ **FIG. 6.36** Possible sites of suture injuries.

⊘ Antibiotics and Tissue Prosthesis

Tissue prostheses should never be exposed to antibiotic solutions because of possible tissue–chemical interaction, which may result in premature fibrosis and calcification. ⊘

⊘ Interference with the Occluding Mechanism of Mechanical Prostheses

Pledgets on the ventricular aspect may occasionally interfere with the normal function of disc prostheses. ⊘

⊘ Excess Suture Material

The sutures, when tied, should be cut short. Excessive suture material may interfere with the normal occluding mechanism of some prostheses. ⊘

⊘ Excess Retained Chordal Button Tissue

Excess retained chordal and leaflet tissue above the mitral annular plane should be sutured to the atrial wall away from the sewing ring to prevent interference with the prosthetic mechanism. ⊘

⊘ Detached Chords

Unattached chords hanging loose can be drawn into the prosthesis and prevent its normal closure, resulting in incompetence of the prosthesis (Fig. 6.37). ⊘

⊘ Obstructive Calcium Deposits

Calcium in the ventricular wall that protrudes into the ventricular cavity near the annulus can seriously impair normal excursion of the mechanical leaflet mechanism. ⊘

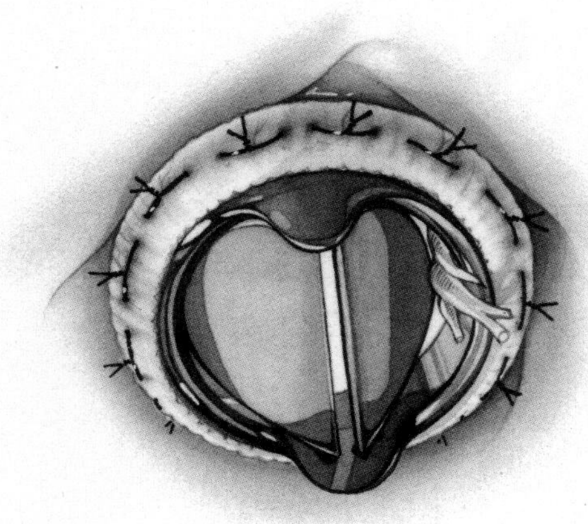

⊘ **FIG. 6.37** Calcium or loose chords impairing the movement of prosthetic disc mechanisms.

⊘ Strut Projection

The struts of the prosthesis must project freely into the left ventricular cavity. Every precaution must be taken to prevent these struts from coming into contact with or becoming embedded in the left ventricular wall. This can result in intractable dysrhythmia and can also interfere with normal prosthetic function (Fig. 6.38). ⊘

⊘ Prosthetic Obstruction of the Left Ventricular Outflow Tract

A bioprosthesis must be placed in such a way that the struts do not obstruct the adjacent left ventricular outflow tract

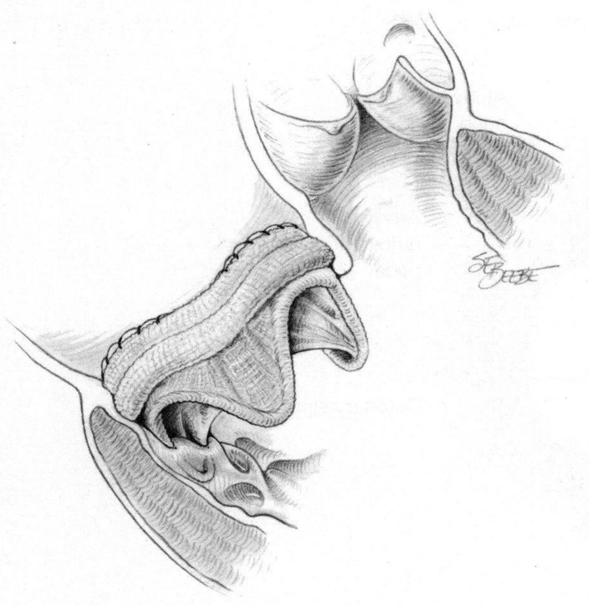

⊘ FIG. 6.38 Strut embedded in the posterior left ventricular wall.

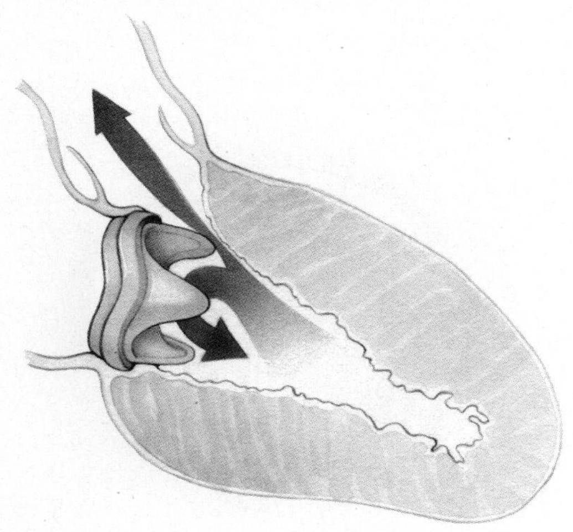

⊘ FIG. 6.39 Prosthetic obstruction of the left ventricular outflow tract.

(Fig. 6.39). The pericardial bioprosthesis is the commonly used tissue prosthesis for the mitral position. There are markings on the sewing cuff of the bioprosthesis to ensure the optimal alignment of the struts in the left ventricular outflow tract. ⊘

⊘ Strut Entanglement

The struts of the prosthesis can become encircled by the sutures or the subvalvular apparatus, which causes distortion of the leaflets and interferes with valve function. It is therefore important to "tighten" the struts of the bioprosthesis, prior to lowering the valve into the left ventricular cavity, to minimize the chance of catching any sutures or part of subvalvular apparatus. ⊘

⊘ Suture Placement

Sutures must always incorporate annular and leaflet tissues. Inadvertent placement of sutures into left ventricular musculature will cut through the left ventricular wall (Fig. 6.40). This can cause a hematoma of the left ventricle, which may enlarge and rupture outside the heart after ventricular contraction resumes. ⊘

⊘ Paravalvular Leak

Weakness or tearing of the posterior annulus may result in disruption of the prosthetic attachment during the surgery as well as postoperatively; consequent paravalvular leak may ensue. Such a complication must be noted and corrected by reinserting the sutures, now reinforced with pledgets, into a stronger part of the posterior annulus. This should allow the prosthesis to be securely reseated. ⊘

NB Exclusion of the Left Atrial Appendage

The left atrial appendage can be closed to prevent blood stasis and subsequent possible thromboembolism. This is especially important when the patient is in atrial fibrillation. Exclusion is accomplished by tying off the auricle or stapling it closed from the outside, or by occluding its orifice from the inside of the left atrium with a purse-string suture (Fig. 6.41). NB

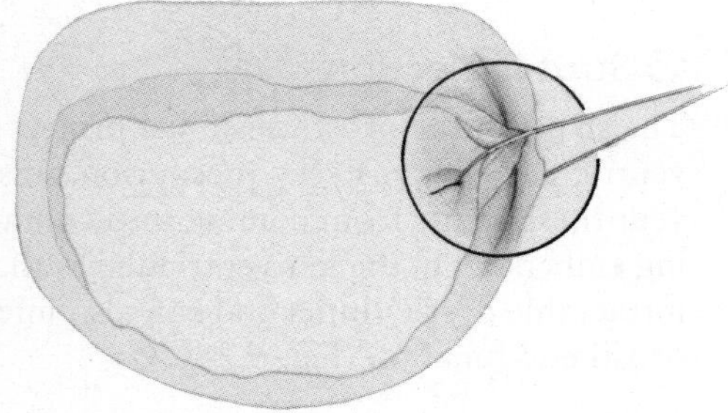

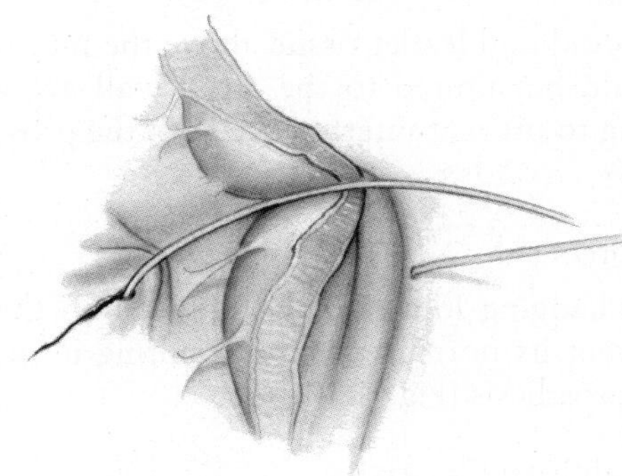

⊘ FIG. 6.40 Deeply placed sutures cutting through the left ventricular wall.

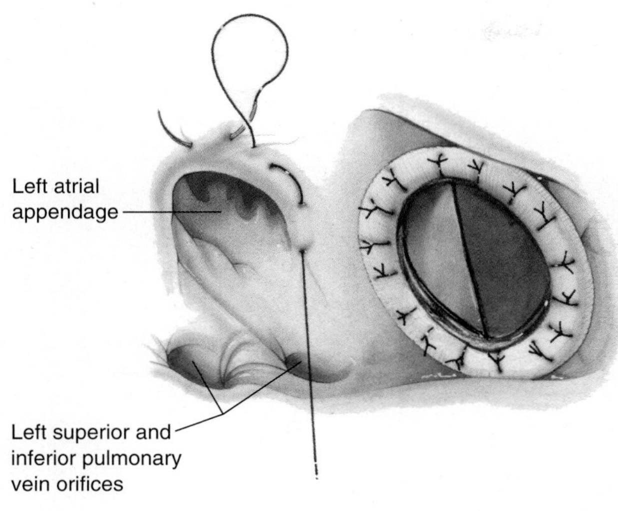

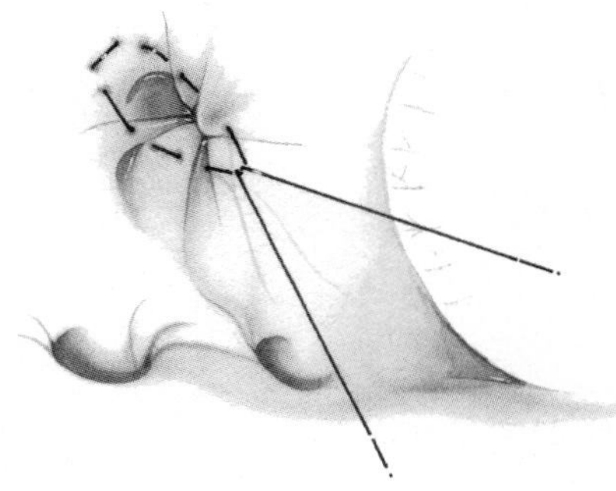

FIG. 6.41 Exclusion of the left atrial appendage.

Mitral Valve Replacement in Children

Selection of an appropriately sized mitral prosthesis in the very young can be challenging. We have found aortic bileaflet mechanical prostheses satisfactory when implanted upside down in the mitral position. In this manner, the leaflets and occluding mechanism will be well above the mitral annulus, sitting entirely in the left atrium, thereby allowing a larger prosthesis to be implanted safely.

This concept can also be used in reoperation for mitral prosthetic malfunction when there has been prosthetic patient mismatch and the mitral annulus is fibrotic or too small for the patient's body surface area.

⊘ Supraannular Bileaflet Aortic Prosthesis

This modification of the bileaflet aortic prosthesis must never be used in an upside-down manner in the mitral position because this would result in the entire valve housing and leaflets residing in the left ventricle itself. ⊘

⊘ Regurgitant Fraction of the Bileaflet Valve

There is an 8% to 10% regurgitant flow across the bileaflet prosthesis. In young hearts with a small left ventricle, the regurgitant fraction may be significant compared with the stroke volume, and the prosthesis may not therefore provide optimal hemodynamics. ⊘

An alternative technique is to implant a tissue prosthesis. The struts are first introduced through the mitral annulus. The sewing ring is then sewn to the atrial wall. Of course, this is a temporary measure because the prosthesis calcifies in children rather rapidly.

⊘ Obstruction to Pulmonary Veins

The sewing ring must be sewn to the atrial wall well away from the orifices of the pulmonary veins to prevent pulmonary venous obstruction. ⊘

LATE ANNULAR COMPLICATIONS

Posterior Subannular Aneurysm

Inadvertent injury to the subvalvular membrane of the posterior mitral annulus (see Surgical Anatomy of the Mitral Valve section) during mitral valve replacement predisposes to the development of a subannular aneurysm. This kind of injury commonly occurs during leaflet excision or an aggressive removal of annular calcific deposits. Patients with this condition require reoperation. The prosthesis is removed so that the edges of the aneurysm can be identified and closed either with horizontal pledgeted mattress sutures or with a Dacron patch (Fig. 6.42). The valve can then be reimplanted placing the posterior annular sutures through the reinforced aneurysm suture closure or the upper edge of the Dacron patch.

Paravalvular Leaks

In most patients, paravalvular dehiscence resulting in leaks around the mitral prosthesis is due to imperfect surgical technique. Some of the predisposing factors, such as calcified or degenerative annulus (which allows the sutures to cut through the tissues), have been referred to previously. Paravalvular leaks tend to occur commonly along the posterior annulus. Massive calcification affecting the aortomitral leaflet continuity may obscure the annulus and interfere with correct placement of anchoring stitches. In addition, exposure of the annulus in the vicinity of the aortic valve may not be ideal. The annulus stitches may be inadvertently placed in the atrial wall or fleshy muscular ventricular wall instead of the annulus. In time, these sutures may cut through the muscular walls and produce paravalvular leaks. It is therefore important for surgeons to be aware of these fine details so that necessary precautions can be taken.

The paravalvular defect is identified under direct vision. The tissue margin of the defect has commonly become fibrous since the time of surgery. Pledgeted sutures are passed deeply through the tissue margin of the defect and then through the sewing ring of the prosthesis before tying.

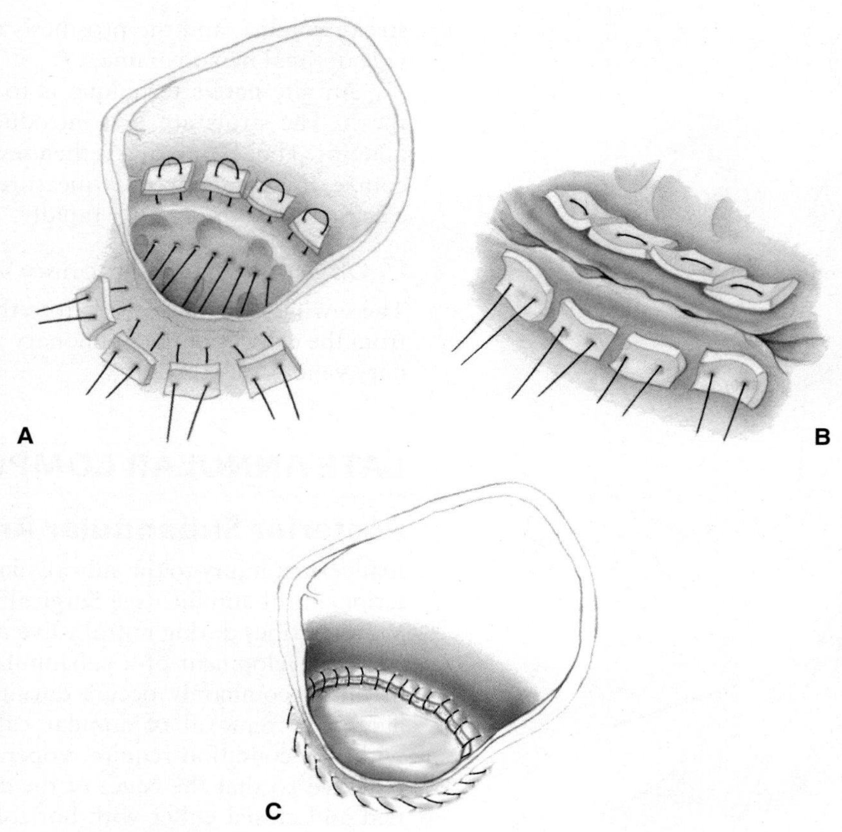

FIG. 6.42 A and B: Primary suture closure of a mitral subannular aneurysm. C: Closure of a mitral subannular aneurysm with a Dacron patch.

When the tissue margin of the defect is not satisfactory, sutures are first passed through the sewing ring of the prosthesis before taking a deep bite in the vicinity of the annulus through the full thickness of the atrial wall. The sutures are then tied over a strip of Teflon felt. If dehiscence of the annular suture line is extensive, the prosthesis may need to be removed. Taking all the aforementioned precautions into consideration, the surgeon must implant a new prosthesis.

⊘ Injury to the Circumflex Artery

Deep sutures may cause injury to the circumflex artery. This will result in myocardial injury, bleeding, and inability to wean the patient from bypass. ⊘

ATRIAL CLOSURE

Interatrial Groove Approach

A double-armed suture of 4-0 Prolene with large half-circle needles is used, starting at each end of the left atriotomy. For a secure closure, the interatrial groove tissue should be included for its buttressing effect (Fig. 6.43). To ensure adequate hemostasis, a bite of tissue beyond the ends of the incision should be taken before continuing the closure (Fig. 6.43, inset). Suturing is continued in both directions. The suture line on each side is then oversewn with the other arm of the suture. Whenever the left atriotomy is extended inferiorly behind the heart, the closure is facilitated if the sewing is begun from the inside of the atrium under direct vision (Fig. 6.43).

NB Atriotomy Closure

Although a single-layer closure is adequate, a second over-and-over suture provides a more secure atriotomy closure. NB

Transatrial Oblique Approach

The divided interatrial septum is approximated with a continuous suture of 4-0 Prolene, starting at the far (anterior) end of the incision and progressing toward the right superior pulmonary vein. Another suture is used to close the right atriotomy. The edges of the right superior pulmonary vein are then approximated with a third suture (Fig. 6.44).

⊘ Injury to the Right Phrenic Nerve

Caution must be exercised in closing the right superior pulmonary vein to avoid incorporating the phrenic nerve in the suture line. ⊘

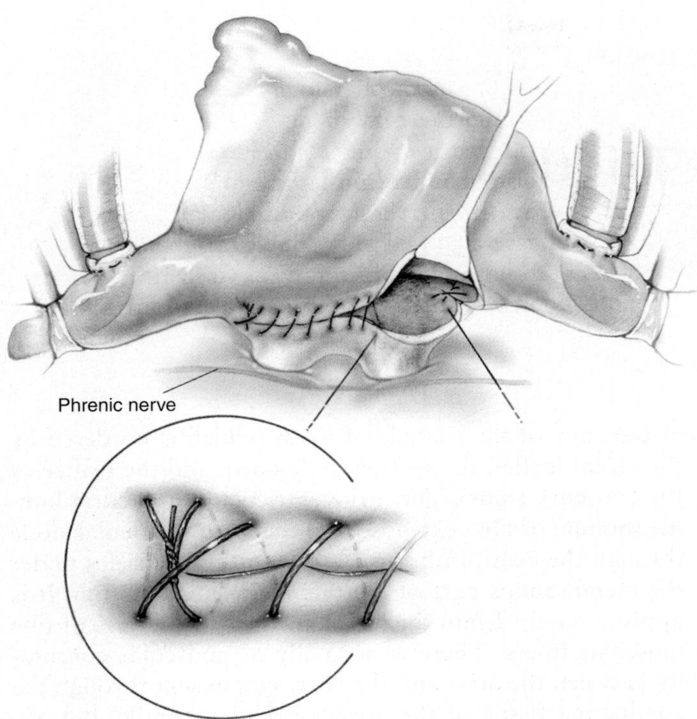

FIG. 6.43 Closure of posterior interatrial groove incision. Inset: Inclusion of tissue beyond the ends of the incision.

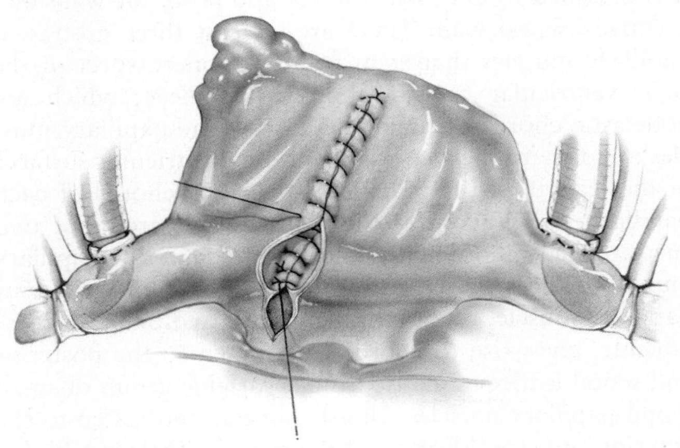

FIG. 6.44 Closure for the transatrial oblique approach.

⊘ Depth of Sutures in the Septum

The septum is quite thick at times; the sutures should incorporate the whole thickness, including the endocardium on both sides of the septum. Otherwise, the suture may tear through the muscular septum, resulting in a septal defect. ⊘

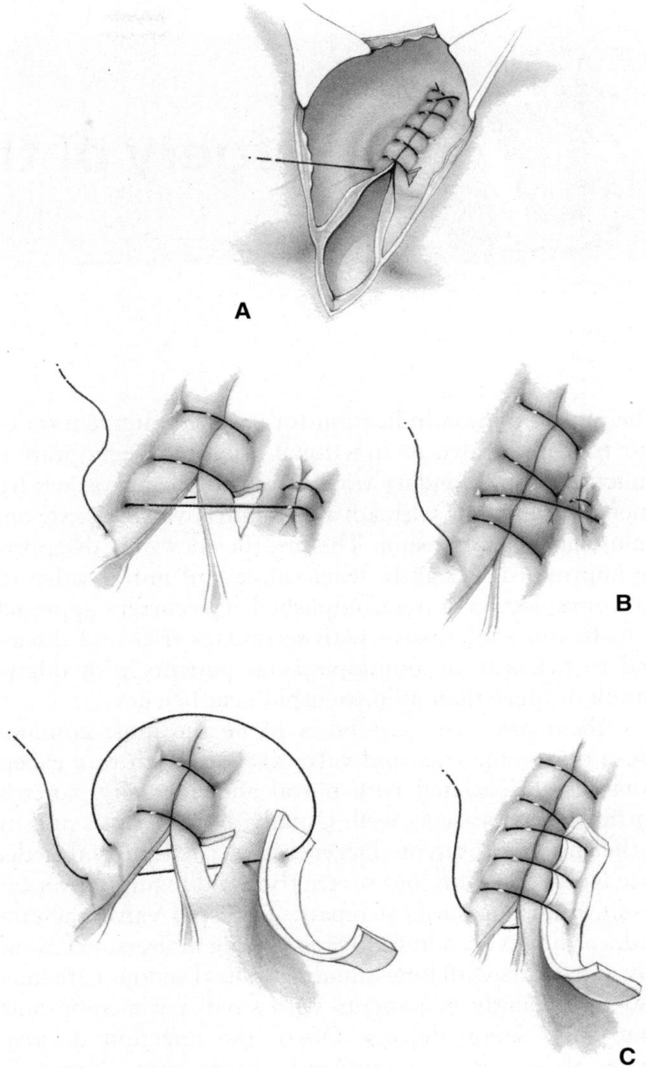

FIG. 6.45 A: Closing tears in the fossa ovalis. B: Buttressing with adjacent fossa tissue. C: Buttressing with Teflon felt.

⊘ Buttressing the Sutures

At times, fossa ovalis tissue can be friable and may not hold sutures well (Fig. 6.45A). The adjacent fossa tissue may be used to buttress the sutures (Fig. 6.45B). Alternatively, pericardial strips may be used to reinforce the suture line (Fig. 6.45C). ⊘

Transatrial Longitudinal Septal Approach

After completion of the procedure, the septum is reapproximated with a continuous 4-0 Prolene suture. The right atrial wall is closed with a second 4-0 Prolene suture line.

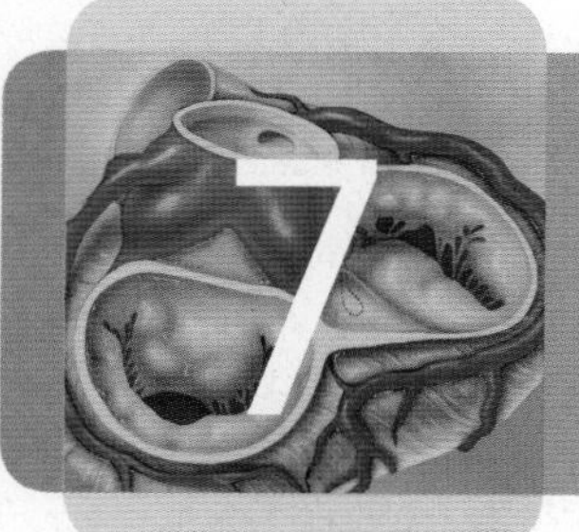

7 Surgery of the Tricuspid Valve

The most common indication for surgical intervention on the tricuspid valve is functional tricuspid regurgitation. Functional or secondary tricuspid insufficiency occurs frequently in patients with advanced mitral valve disease and pulmonary hypertension. The insufficiency may disappear or improve significantly when successful mitral valve repair or replacement is accomplished. The current approach is to be more aggressive with secondary tricuspid disease and to perform an annuloplasty in patients with dilated annuli or more than mild tricuspid insufficiency.

Rheumatic fever continues to be the most common cause of organic tricuspid valve disease. With rare exceptions, it is associated with mitral and, in many patients, aortic valve disease as well. Usually, both stenosis and insufficiency are present. Degenerative tricuspid valve disease is less common, but severe tricuspid regurgitation can result, requiring surgical repair. Tricuspid valve bacterial endocarditis is seen in intravenous drug abusers, occasionally in patients with long-standing central venous catheters, and infrequently in patients with small perimembranous ventricular septal defects. Often, the infection destroys leaflet tissue, causing tricuspid insufficiency. Iatrogenic causes of tricuspid valve dysfunction include pacemaker lead–induced tricuspid regurgitation and radiation therapy, which may result in retracted, calcified valve leaflets. Carcinoid affects the tricuspid and frequently the pulmonic valve, causing stenosis as well as insufficiency.

TECHNICAL CONSIDERATIONS

Surgical Anatomy of the Tricuspid Valve and the Right Ventricle

The tricuspid valve guards the right ventricular orifice. It consists of a septal leaflet, a large anterior leaflet, and a small posterior leaflet, all three of which are attached to and continuous with the tricuspid ring. These valve leaflets are folds of endocardium strengthened by fibrous tissue. Small accessory leaflets are often present in the angles between the major leaflets. The atrioventricular node lies in the atrial septum adjacent to the septal leaflet, just anterior to the coronary sinus. Its location can be pinpointed at the apex of the triangle of Koch (which is bordered by the septal leaflet, the tendon of Todaro, and the orifice of the coronary sinus). The atrioventricular conduction bundle (bundle of His) extends from the atrioventricular node through the central fibrous body into the ventricles under the membranous part of the interventricular septum. It is approximately 2-mm thick and consists of bundles of fine muscular fibers. There is normally no muscular continuity between the atria and the ventricles except through the conducting tissue of the atrioventricular bundle, but aberrations may exist, which can give rise to rhythm disturbances (Fig. 7.1).

The right ventricular cavity is tubular and triangular in contrast with that of the left ventricle, which is conical. It is bounded by concave anterior and posterior walls and a convex septal wall. There are at least three groups of papillary muscles that stem from the inner aspect of the right ventricular cavity. Chordae tendineae, which are nonelastic chords of tissue, arise from the papillary muscles and fuse to the free edges and the ventricular surfaces of the leaflets of the tricuspid valve. The chords of each papillary muscle control the contiguous margins of two cusps. Hence, chords pass from a large anterior papillary muscle to the anterior and posterior leaflets. A posterior papillary muscle, often represented by two or more components, gives rise to chords that attach to the posterior and septal leaflets. Finally, from a variable group of small septal papillary muscles, chords fan out and fasten to the anterior and septal leaflets of the tricuspid valve. A bridge of muscle, the moderator band, stems from the septum, crosses the cavity of the right ventricle to the free wall, and contributes to the origin of the anterior papillary muscle. A tract of specialized tissue associated with the conduction system runs through the moderator band (Fig. 7.2).

Incision

A median sternotomy is the preferred approach for acquired valvular disease because it offers complete exposure for exploration of the mitral, aortic, and tricuspid valves. The tricuspid valve can also be approached through a lower ministernotomy or submammary right thoracotomy (see Chapter 1).

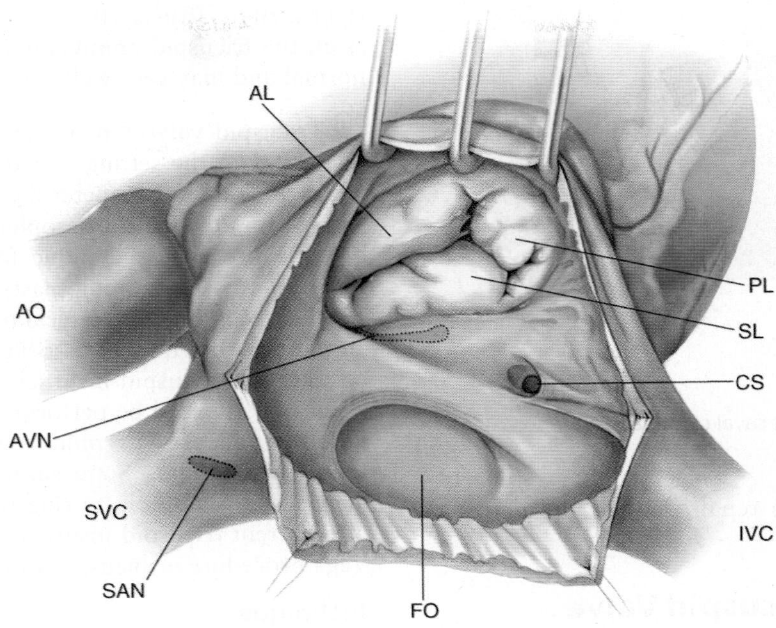

FIG. 7.1 Surgical anatomy of the right atrium and tricuspid valve. AL, anterior leaflet; PL, posterior leaflet; SL, septal leaflet; CS, coronary sinus; IVC, inferior vena cava; FO, fossa ovalis; SAN, sinoatrial node; SVC, superior vena cava; AVN, atrioventricular node; AO, aorta.

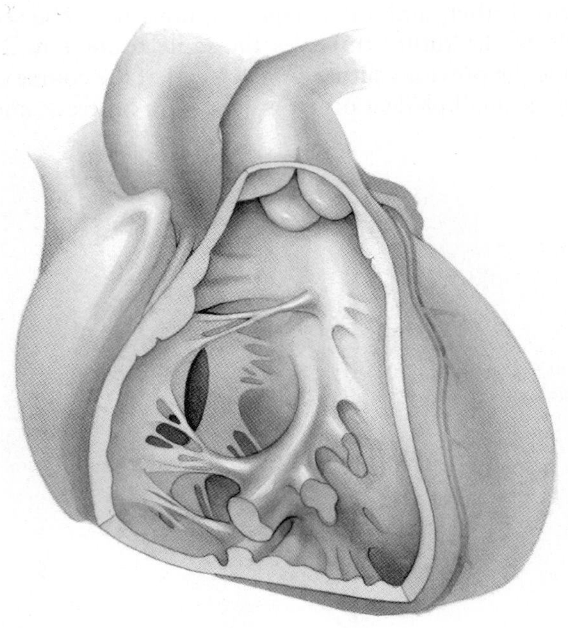

FIG. 7.2 Surgical anatomy of the tricuspid valve as seen from the right ventricle. The free wall of the ventricle has been removed to show the tricuspid subvalvular apparatus and the convex septal wall.

Historically, digital palpation through a purse-string suture on the right atrial appendage was used to assess tricuspid insufficiency before the initiation of cardiopulmonary bypass. Currently, intraoperative transesophageal echocardiography is used to evaluate the tricuspid valve. Because tricuspid insufficiency is load dependent, clinical history, preoperative echocardiography, and/or right heart catheterization data are useful in determining whether the tricuspid valve should be addressed. Some surgeons advocate exploring the tricuspid valve in all patients undergoing mitral valve surgery to directly measure annular size.

Cannulation

When surgery on the tricuspid valve is contemplated, both vena cavae are cannulated directly (Fig. 7.3). A cannula is placed in the ascending aorta, and cardiopulmonary bypass is initiated.

Isolated tricuspid valve surgery can be performed on cardiopulmonary bypass with a warm, beating heart. Most of the time, repair or replacement of the tricuspid valve is performed as part of a combined procedure that includes mitral and/or aortic valve surgery with or without concomitant coronary artery bypass grafting. At the conclusion of these other procedures, the aortic cross-clamp is removed and deairing of the left heart is completed.

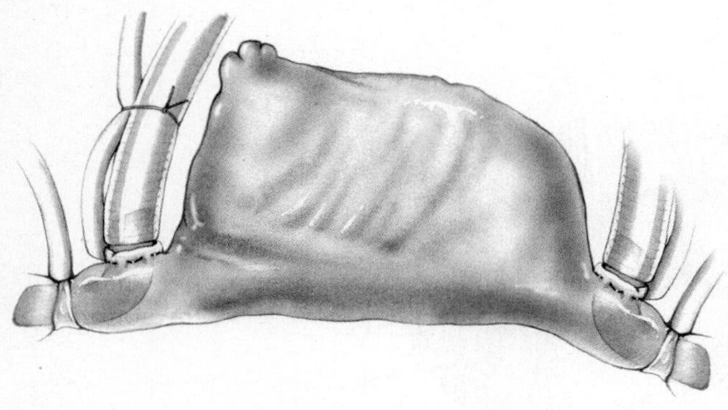

FIG. 7.3 Direct caval cannulation.

The tricuspid valve is then repaired while the patient is being rewarmed.

Exposure of the Tricuspid Valve

A longitudinal or oblique atriotomy is made approximately 1 cm posterior to and parallel to the atrioventricular groove. The atriotomy edges are retracted with sutures, and exposure of the tricuspid valve is further facilitated by means of appropriately sized retractors.

⊘ Injury to the Sinoatrial Node

The sinoatrial node is prone to injury during cannulation and passage of a tape around the superior vena cava. The atriotomy should be well away from the sinoatrial node, and its superior extension should be limited to approximately 1 cm from the superior margin of the right atrium. ⊘

FUNCTIONAL TRICUSPID REGURGITATION

The controversy regarding the management of functional tricuspid insufficiency reflects the difficulty of precisely distinguishing the two stages of the same disease process, that is, irreversible and reversible tricuspid valve insufficiency. Irreversible functional tricuspid insufficiency is the outcome of chronic right ventricular dilation, with a permanent increase in right ventricular volume and tricuspid annular dilation. Certainly, if severe tricuspid regurgitation is present, significant tricuspid pathology must exist, which is most likely irreversible. However, even if the tricuspid insufficiency is only mild or moderate, irreversible tricuspid pathology may still be present. This is because the assessment of the degree of tricuspid regurgitation depends on right ventricular preload and afterload at the time of the study. A better marker of irreversibility may be annular size. The distance from the anteroseptal to the anteroposterior commissure is measured directly through the open right atrium. If it is 70 mm or greater (twice the normal size), the tricuspid annulus will most likely not return to normal and may very well continue to dilate.

NB Tricuspid valve repair is recommended when there is severe TR in the setting of left-sided valvular surgery, or when the annular diameter measures greater than 40 mm (or >21 mm/m^2) on transesophageal echocardiogram. NB

The preferred technique for functional tricuspid regurgitation is ring annuloplasty. De Vega annuloplasty is another technique for surgical management of tricuspid regurgitation, but may be associated with a higher incidence of recurrent tricuspid insufficiency. Bicuspidization of the tricuspid valve can be performed quickly and may be preferred in patients with mild to moderate insufficiency or a less dilated annulus. Some surgeons have found that placement of an annuloplasty ring results in a lower incidence of recurrent tricuspid insufficiency compared with the De Vega procedure or bicuspidization.

Technique

De Vega Annuloplasty

The right atrium is opened obliquely or longitudinally, and the tricuspid valve is inspected. A double-armed suture, usually 2-0 Ticron or Prolene, is started on the annulus at the posteroseptal commissure. It is then extended around the circumference of the valve in a counterclockwise direction, taking deep bites (every 5 to 6 mm) into the endocardium (Fig. 7.4) and into the fibrous ring of the posteroseptal commissure, posterior leaflet, anteroposterior commissure, anterior leaflet, and anteroseptal commissure. The second needle of the suture traverses the same route 1 to 2 mm outside the previous suture. At each end of the course of suturing, a small pledget of felt is used for a buttress, and the

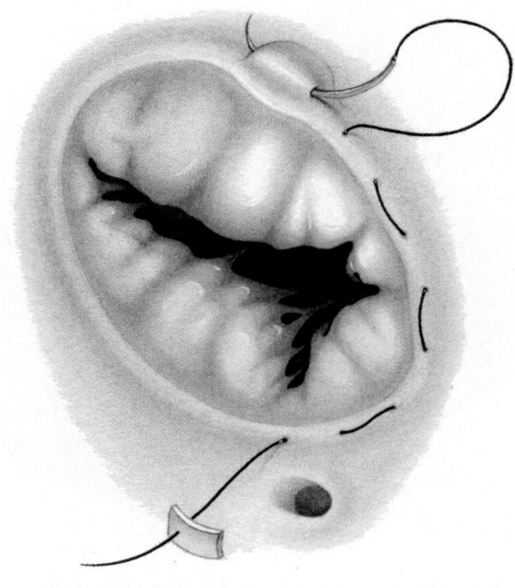

FIG. 7.4 Suturing technique in De Vega annuloplasty.

suture is then tied securely around an appropriately sized mitral valve sizer to ensure a predictable annuloplasty. A strip of autologous pericardium or a C-shaped piece of Teflon felt can be incorporated in the suturing process for additional stability (Fig. 7.5).

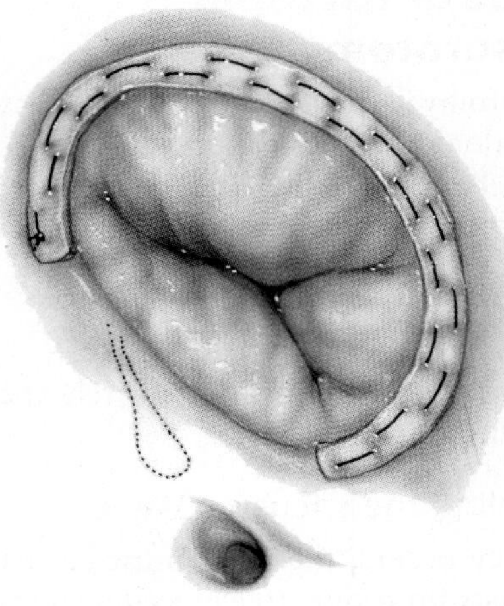

FIG. 7.5 Annuloplasty reinforced with a Teflon felt strip.

Ring Annuloplasty

Several partial rings and flexible annuloplasty bands are available, which conform to the normal shape of the tricuspid valve and do not include the area of the septal annulus. The ring size is determined by the length of fibrous septal annulus, between commissures along the septal leaflet, with a goal of slight undersizing. The ring or band is anchored in position by means of multiple simple or mattress sutures of 3-0 Tevdek incorporating the fibrous annulus of the anterior and posterior leaflets and excluding the septal leaflet (Fig. 7.6A). The sutures are placed closer together on the ring or band to reduce the size of the annulus (Fig. 7.6B). The device is lowered onto the annulus and the sutures tied. The completed annuloplasty using either a band or a ring reduces the size of the tricuspid orifice and attempts to restore the valve to its normal shape (Fig. 7.6C). A potential advantage of a band annuloplasty is that it allows the tricuspid orifice to flex as ventricular contraction occurs.

⊘ Inadequate Suture Depth

The depth of the suture bites at the annulus must be quite substantial; otherwise, the suture will tear through and result in an inadequate annuloplasty. ⊘

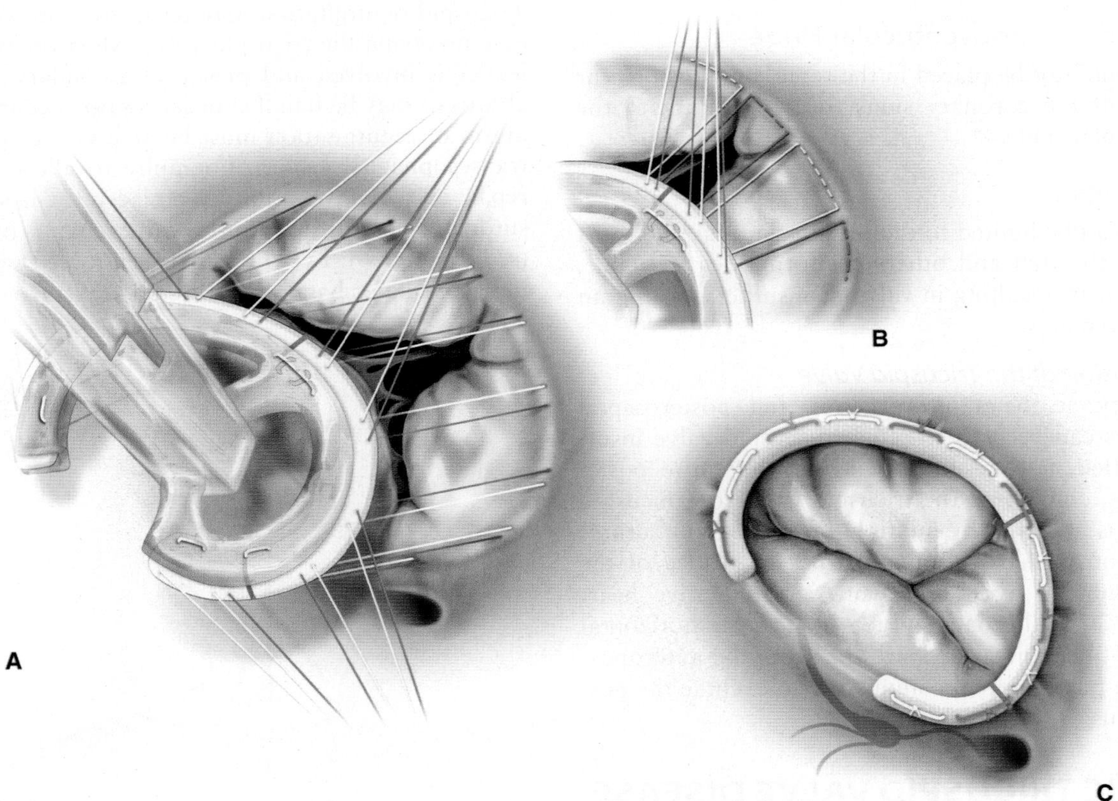

FIG. 7.6 Ring or band annuloplasty. **A:** Anchoring mattress sutures. **B:** Reducing the size of the annulus. **C:** Restoring the valve to its normal configuration.

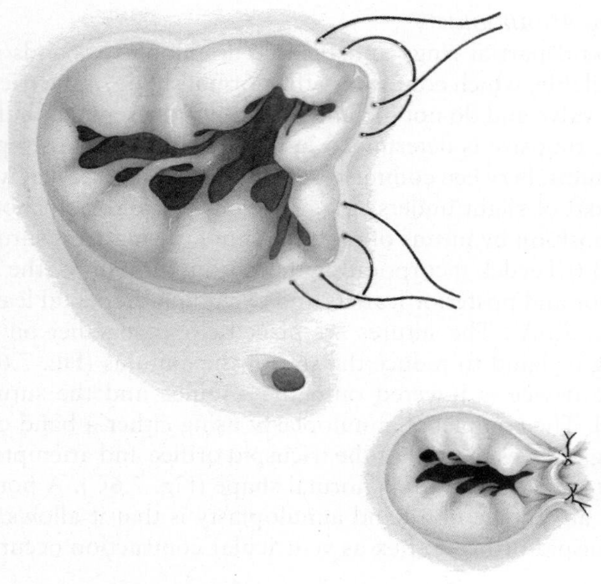

FIG. 7.7 Technique for bicuspidizing the tricuspid valve.

⊘ Injury to the Atrioventricular Node

Sutures should not be placed in the septal annulus or near the orifice of the coronary sinus to avoid injury to the atrioventricular node. ⊘

⊘ Leaflet Tear

Sutures should be limited to the fibrous annulus and must not include the thin and otherwise normal leaflet tissue, which may tear, resulting in valvular insufficiency and an inadequate repair. ⊘

Bicuspidization of the Tricuspid Valve

Annuloplasty at the anteroposterior and posteroseptal commissures can be used to reduce tricuspid valve insufficiency. Often, it is useful to exclude the entire posterior annulus, converting the tricuspid valve to a bicuspid valve. This is achieved by multiple figure-of-eight sutures of 2-0 Ticron placed well away from the orifice of the coronary sinus to avoid producing postoperative heart block (Fig. 7.7). Alternatively, two concentric horizontal pledgeted 2-0 Ticron sutures are run from the anteroposterior to the posteroseptal commissure to exclude the posterior annulus.

ORGANIC TRICUSPID VALVE DISEASE

Rheumatic Tricuspid Disease

Rheumatic involvement of the tricuspid valve generally results in mixed insufficiency and stenosis. Many of these patients require valve replacement (see subsequent text). Occasionally, stenosis is the predominant finding with commissural fusion, thickening of the leaflets, and variable fibrosis and shortening of the chordae tendineae. These patients are candidates for commissurotomy.

Technique of Tricuspid Commissurotomy

Commissurotomy is carried out meticulously with a No. 11 knife blade along the commissures up to 1 to 2 mm from the annulus. Because of the tricuspid nature of the valve, commissurotomy is limited to one or two commissures to avoid producing insufficiency (Fig. 7.8).

⊘ Anterior Septal Commissure

The anterior septal commissure is rarely incised because this often causes insufficiency. ⊘

⊘ Remodeling the Tricuspid Valve

If insufficiency occurs, the valve must be remodeled with an annuloplasty procedure (see preceding text). Frequently, bicuspidization will result in a competent valve. ⊘

Degenerative Tricuspid Disease

Tricuspid regurgitation may result from myxomatous disease involving the tricuspid valve. Most often the anterior leaflet is involved and prolapses secondary to elongated chords or may be flail if chordal rupture occurs. The mechanism of regurgitation must be ascertained in detail from transesophageal echocardiography to allow for accurate repair of the valve. Chordal replacement using Gore-Tex sutures as described for mitral valve repair is often required (see Chapter 6). Every repair is reinforced with an annuloplasty ring or band (see preceding text).

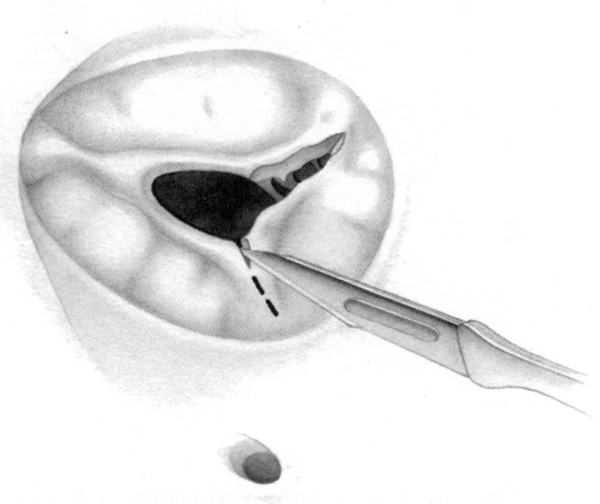

FIG. 7.8 Tricuspid valve commissurotomy.

NB Edge-to-Edge Tricuspid Valve Repair

If severe tricuspid insufficiency persists after all reparative attempts, the addition of an edge-to-edge repair may be considered. This technique may be particularly useful in patients with significant pulmonary hypertension. NB

Technique

The midpoints of the facing edges of the anterior, posterior, and septal leaflets, just at the point of insertion of primary chords, are approximated with multiple U stitches of 4-0 Prolene buttressed with autologous pericardial pledgets. A tri-orifice tricuspid valve is therefore created. The valve is tested with saline for residual leakage or leaflet distorsion. Direct edge-to-edge suturing of adjacent leaflets at the commissures may be added to deal with minor residual insufficiency. The orifices are all measured with Hegar dilators to assure a satisfactory total valve orifice area.

Pacemaker Lead–Induced Tricuspid Regurgitation

The endocardial ventricular lead of a pacemaker may distort and eventually become incorporated into one of the tricuspid leaflets, causing valvular insufficiency. It may be possible to resect the involved portion of the leaflet and reconstruct the valve. The lead is removed and an epicardial ventricular lead is placed. However, if the leaflet involvement is extensive, valve replacement may be required. In this case, the pacemaker lead can be positioned between the sewing ring of the valve and the patient's annulus.

TRICUSPID VALVE REPLACEMENT

Because it is usually possible to repair the tricuspid valve, its replacement is rarely necessary. Nevertheless, when the severity of the valvular distortion prevents a satisfactory reconstructive procedure, valve replacement becomes mandatory. This is occasionally the case with rheumatic involvement of the tricuspid valve. Valve replacement is indicated when patients with carcinoid- or radiation-induced tricuspid disease require surgery. If possible, the subvalvular apparatus is retained and the leaflet tissues are incorporated in suturing the prosthesis to the annulus (see discussion on mitral valve replacement with retaining the subvalvular apparatus in Chapter 6). Often, however, when tricuspid valve replacement becomes necessary, the subvalvular structures and leaflets are diseased to a degree that precludes their use. In these cases, resection of the tricuspid valve is started by incising the anterior and posterior leaflets and dividing the chordal attachments deep in the right ventricle. The mobilized valve may now be inverted up into the right atrium, and with visual control from both the atrial and ventricular sides, the septal leaflet is dissected. A broad zone of the attached margin of the septal leaflet and its chordal attachments is left in place, if possible. Preferably, the septal leaflet or all the leaflets are left intact and used to anchor the appropriate prosthesis. The normal tubular and triangular configuration of the right ventricle is often lost in patients with chronic tricuspid valve disease. The dilated right ventricle can easily accommodate the struts of a tissue prosthesis.

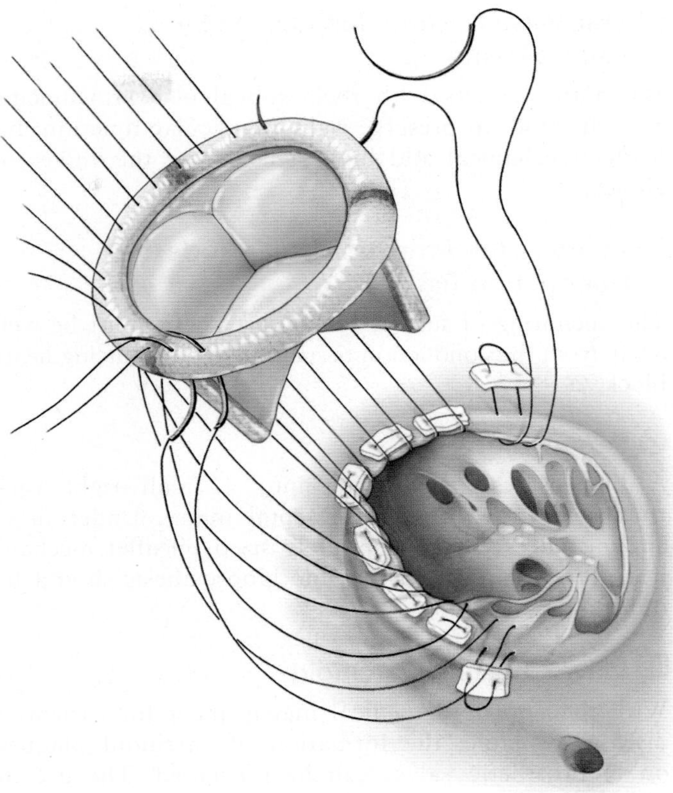

FIG. 7.9 Technique for tricuspid valve replacement.

Size 3-0 Teflon pledgeted sutures are passed through the annulus, except in the region of the septal leaflet. In this area, sutures are placed only through the leaflet tissue and its attached structures to avoid producing heart block. The sutures are then passed through the sewing ring of the prosthesis (Fig. 7.9). The prosthesis is slipped down into its bed, and the sutures are tied and cut. Care is taken to avoid injury to the right ventricular endocardium while introducing the prosthesis into the decompressed ventricle. As in mitral valve replacement, size selection is based not only on the diameter of the atrioventricular ring but also on the size of the ventricular cavity. No problems have been encountered reducing the annulus by placing sutures close together on the sewing ring of the prosthesis. Serious injury to the interventricular septum may occur, however, if too large a prosthesis is placed into the right ventricle.

⊘ Disc Valve Dysfunction Caused by Leaflet Tissue

When the leaflets with their subvalvular attachments are left intact to preserve right ventricular function, bileaflet mechanical and bioprostheses are the valves of choice. ⊘

⊘ Injury to the Atrioventricular Node and Conduction Tissue

The anchoring of sutures for the prosthesis must be well away from the conduction tissue to avoid producing heart block. ⊘

⊘ Septal Injury

A bioprosthesis protruding into a small right ventricular cavity can produce septal injury. Under these circumstances, an appropriately sized bileaflet mechanical prosthesis or a low-profile bioprosthesis should be used. ⊘

NB Valve Choice in Carcinoid

With the improved medical management for carcinoid disease available, the formation of carcinoid plaques on bioprosthetic valves can be prevented. The use of bioprosthetic valves avoids the need for anticoagulation in these patients who have hepatic dysfunction and coagulopathy. NB

NB Consideration should be given to placing permanent epicardial ventricular pacing leads in patients undergoing tricuspid valve replacement. These leads can be buried in a pocket anterior to the posterior rectus sheath in the left upper quadrant for later permanent pacemaker implantation if required. NB

Tricuspid Valve Endocarditis

When tricuspid valve endocarditis does not respond to antibiotic or antifungal therapy, valve excision and replacement may be required. However, attempts should be made to preserve the native valve. Vegetations are usually found to be large and adherent to the leaflet tissue. Often, the infection destroys the leaflet and its attachments. If the posterior leaflet is involved, the necrotic area with a good margin of healthy tissue is removed. Bicuspidization is performed, excluding the posterior annulus, using 2-0 Ticron horizontal mattress sutures with or without autologous pericardial pledgets (Fig. 7.10). When the septal or anterior leaflets are involved, the affected portion is excised in a trapezoidal manner. A limited annuloplasty with horizontal mattress sutures of 2-0 Ticron is then performed, using pericardial pledgets depending on the tissue quality. The resected leaflet edges are reapproximated with interrupted 6-0 or 7-0 Prolene sutures (Fig. 7.11). Because septal leaflet resection and repair may result in complete heart block,

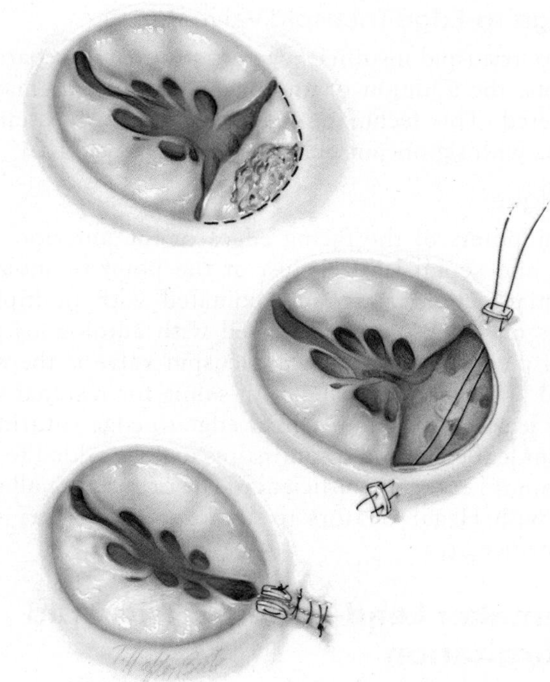

FIG. 7.10 Technique for posterior leaflet resection and bicuspidization of the tricuspid valve.

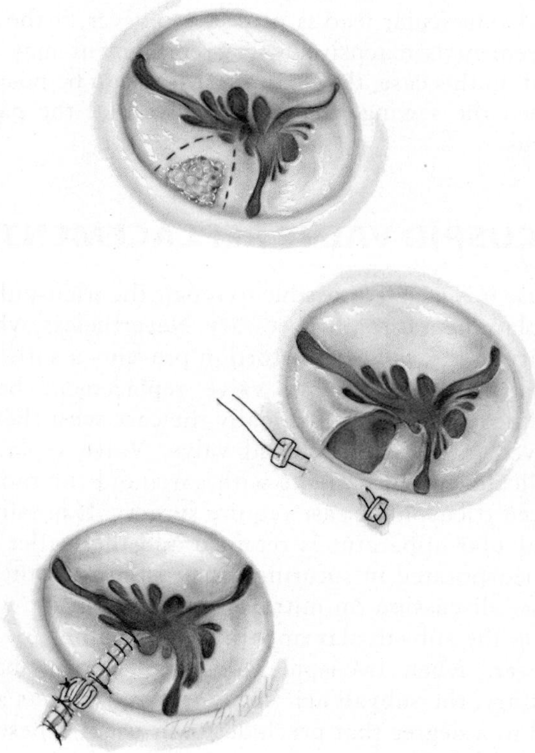

FIG. 7.11 Technique for resection of a portion of tricuspid septal valve leaflet with subsequent annuloplasty and leaflet reapproximation.

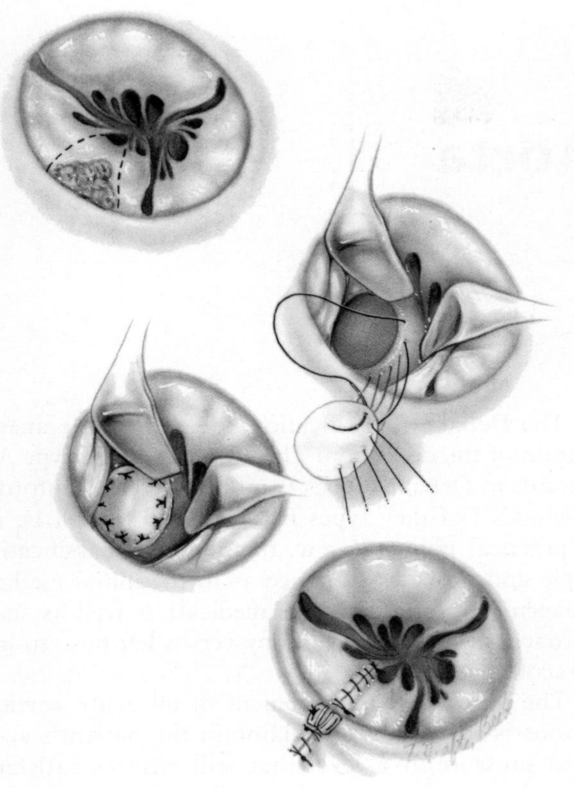

FIG. 7.12 Technique for patch closure of a ventricular septal defect combined with partial septal leaflet resection and reconstruction.

permanent epicardial pacemaker leads should be placed in these patients.

In patients with ventricular septal defects associated with bacterial endocarditis affecting the tricuspid valve, the septal defect is repaired through the tricuspid valve using a pericardial patch (Fig. 7.12). The edges of the ventricular septal defect are first debrided, and the necrotic tissue and vegetations are removed meticulously. A patch of autologous pericardium fixed in glutaraldehyde is then cut to match the size and shape of the resultant defect. This is secured to the edges of the septal defect with running 4-0 Prolene or interrupted horizontal mattress sutures of 4-0 Ticron. At the superior aspect of the ventricular septal defect located under the septal leaflet of the tricuspid valve, the patch is secured to leaflet tissue adjacent to the annulus. If possible, sutures should not be passed through the annulus in this area because the atrioventricular node is likely to be injured. If this portion of the septal leaflet is involved with vegetation and requires excision, an attempt is made to preserve a rim of leaflet tissue next to the annulus. After the ventricular septal defect patch is secured in place, the septal annulus is reapproximated with horizontal mattress sutures of 2-0 Ticron with or without pericardial pledgets, and the leaflet tissue is brought together with interrupted 6-0 Prolene sutures (Fig. 7.12). Results of tricuspid valve repair in patients with endocarditis have been gratifying.

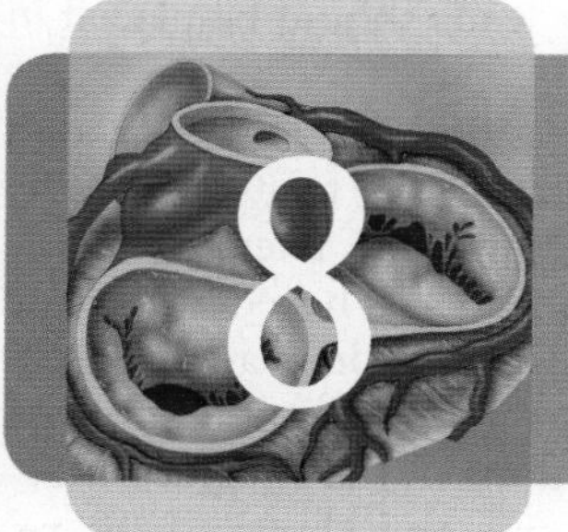

8 Surgery of the Aorta

ACUTE AORTIC DISSECTION

Acute aortic dissection has a sudden onset and is a true surgical emergency. It is usually initiated by a transverse tear in the intima or the intima and media. This disruptive injury gives rise to a hematoma within the media. The pulsatile force of ejection of the left ventricle causes a longitudinal separation of the aortic wall, mainly along and within the media. This dissection can progress both distally and proximally. Distal progression beyond the aortic arch can continue along the course of the descending thoracic and abdominal aorta to a variable extent and can involve its branches. Proximal extension of the dissecting hematoma may infiltrate the aortic root, distorting the aortic valve leaflets or compressing the ostia of the coronary arteries. This can produce aortic valve insufficiency and acute myocardial ischemia, respectively, both of which can cause death. In addition, acute dissection can cause rupture of the aorta into the pericardium, causing tamponade. Therefore, the symptomatology of aortic dissection can be highly variable depending on its effect on the aortic valve, aortic wall, or aortic branches.

The development of acute aortic dissection is thought to involve many factors. Of great significance is medial degeneration or cystic medial necrosis of the aortic wall. Marfan syndrome, an autosomal dominant disorder of vascular collagen, is commonly associated with acute aortic dissection. However, annulo-aortic ectasia can occur in patients without Marfan syndrome and result in acute aortic dissection. Clinically, most cases dissection are associated with hypertension, a bicuspid aortic valve, and coarctation of the aorta.

The current classification (Stanford) distinguishes two types of aortic dissection based on the involvement of the ascending aorta. Type A, or anterior, dissection commonly starts in the ascending aorta, usually 1 to 2 cm above the sinotubular junction, and may progress along the course of the aorta for a variable distance. Type B, or posterior, dissection typically starts in the descending aorta distal to the origin of the subclavian artery. The dissection can progress distally to a variable distance; less commonly, it may extend proximally, thereby resulting in a retrograde type A dissection.

The DeBakey classification is based on the anatomic location of the dissection. Therefore, Stanford type A corresponds to DeBakey types I and II, whereas Stanford type B includes DeBakey types IIIA and IIIB (Fig. 8.1). From the practical point of view, the Stanford classification is simple and provides guidance as to the initial method of management (surgical versus medical) as well as surgical approaches (median sternotomy versus left postero-lateral thoracotomy).

The immediate management of all acute aortic dissections is to reduce and maintain the patient's systolic blood pressure at a level that still ensures satisfactory cerebral and renal perfusion. All patients suspected of acute aortic dissection should immediately undergo computed tomography with contrast. Acute type A aortic dissection is a surgical emergency because conservative therapy is not effective in most instances. On the other hand, patients with acute type B dissection are initially treated medically with antihypertensive therapy. There are occasions when the diagnosis of acute type A aortic dissection cannot be made with computed tomography. In these cases, transesophageal echocardiography should be performed to rule out involvement of the ascending aorta in the dissection process. This can be accomplished in the intensive care unit, the emergency department, or the operating room.

AORTIC ANEURYSMS

Aortic aneurysms are defined as areas of localized aortic dilation and can involve any segment of the aorta. The prevalence of thoracic aortic aneurysms has tripled in the last 20 years. This increase in prevalence may be partly due to the increasingly aging population, better imaging, or a true increase in the incidence. Thoracic aortic aneurysms are now estimated to affect 10 of every 100,000 elderly adults. The ascending aorta is most commonly affected (45%), followed by the descending aorta (35%). The aortic arch (10%) is involved either as an isolated lesion or as an extension of the ascending or, less commonly, descending aortic aneurysms. Progressive enlargement of the aneurysm is an indication for resection and replacement with a

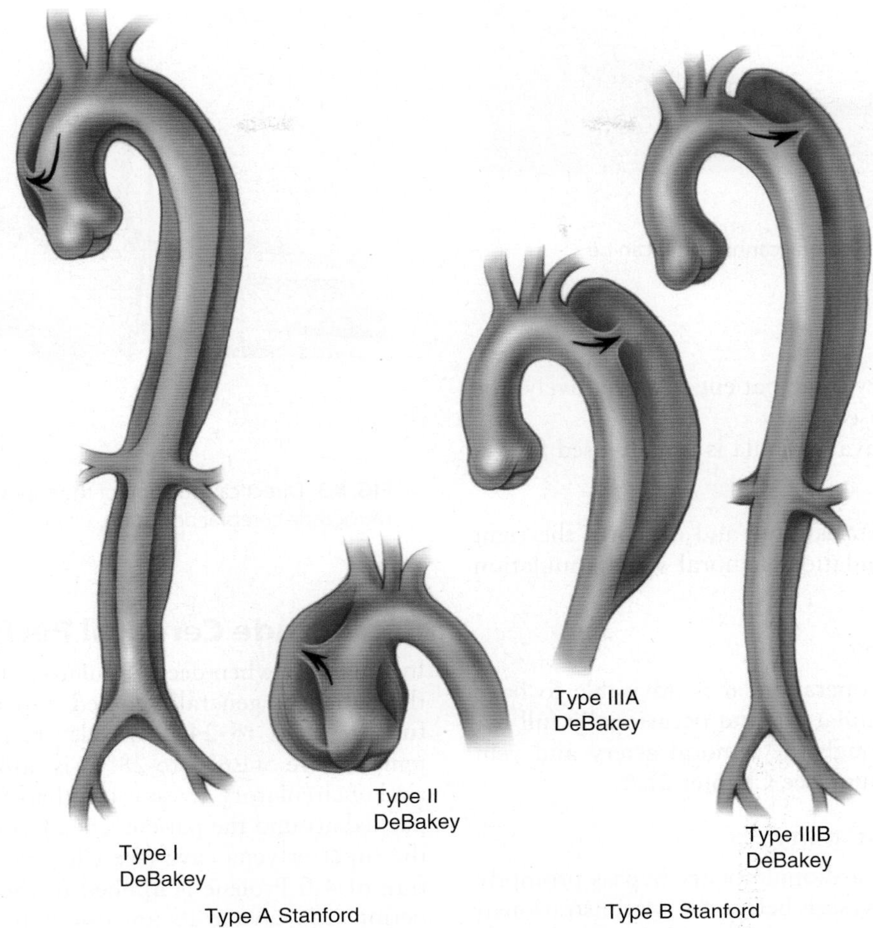

FIG. 8.1 Classification of aortic dissection.

tube graft because it will eventually rupture, culminating in the death of the patient.

The techniques for excision and graft replacement for aneurysms of the ascending and descending thoracic aorta are similar to those described for surgical management of types A and B aortic dissections. In addition, patients with a porcelain or severely atherosclerotic aorta requiring an aortic valve procedure may need replacement of the ascending aorta.

REPLACEMENT OF THE ASCENDING AORTA

The ascending aorta is approached via a median sternotomy. Both groins should be in the operative field and the arterial return is accomplished by cannulating either femoral or external iliac arteries. In patients with ascending aneurysms, direct aortic cannulation in the proximal arch may be feasible. In many centers, the right axillary artery is preferentially used.

NB The right femoral artery is less commonly involved in aortic dissection and therefore should be the second site of choice after the right axillary artery. NB

⊘ Retrograde Perfusion through False Lumen

In patients with aortic dissection, the disease often extends distally, sometimes down to the femoral vessels; therefore, care must be exercised not to cannulate and perfuse through the false lumen of the femoral artery in a retrograde manner. ⊘

⊘ Occlusive Disease of the External Iliac and Femoral Vessels

In elderly patients with severe atherosclerosis, the femoral and iliac arteries are markedly diseased and cannulation may be hazardous. A number of cannulas are available, which can be introduced into these vessels percutaneously or under direct vision using the modified Seldinger technique (Fig. 8.2). The flow through a 20-French cannula is

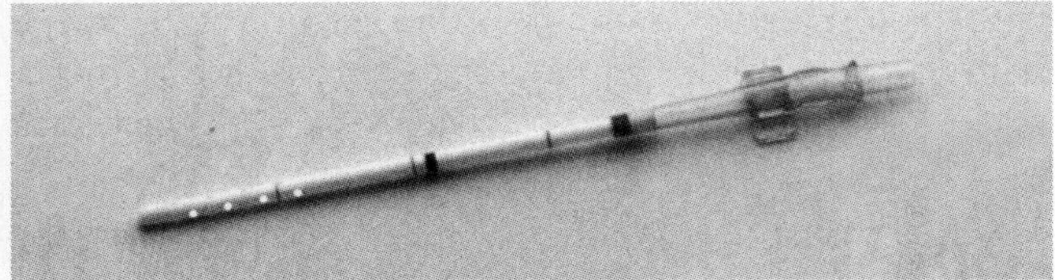

FIG. 8.2 Multiple side hole femoral cannula that can be introduced over a guidewire.

adequate for all but very large patients. Alternatively, the axillary artery may be used.

A dual-stage atriocaval cannula is usually used for venous drainage. ⊘

NB If the ascending aorta is large and obscures the right atrium for venous cannulation, femoral vein cannulation is performed. NB

⊘ Repeat Sternotomy

If the procedure is a reoperation, it is advisable to have arterial and venous cannulation, and occasionally full bypass, accomplished through the femoral artery and vein before opening the sternum (see Chapter 2). ⊘

⊘ Hemodynamic Instability

It is prudent to initiate cardiopulmonary bypass promptly by means of the femoral vessels before the administration of general anesthesia in patients with unstable hemodynamics to prevent circulatory collapse. This is especially important if pericardial tamponade is apparent or suspected. ⊘

Femoral vein cannulation can be achieved by introducing a long cannula with multiple side holes for excellent venous return. The important characteristic of this device is that it comes with a guidewire and contains a tapered, dilated sheath inside the cannula. The guidewire allows easy, comfortable, and safe passage of the cannula over the pelvic brim. The cannula has multiple side holes and may be advanced into the right atrium, providing superior drainage.

⊘ Iliac Vein Injury

Venous cannulas that lack guidewires often hang up at the pelvic rim, resulting in inadequate venous return. If an attempt is made to push the cannula further into the inferior vena cava, perforation of the iliac vein with catastrophic consequences may ensue. It is usually easier to pass the cannula through the right femoral vein because of its straighter course compared to the left side. ⊘

After completion of a median sternotomy, an additional venous cannula is placed in the right atrium if required. A left ventricular vent through the right superior pulmonary vein (see Chapter 4) decompresses the heart and expedites the procedure. Venting is especially important if aortic valve insufficiency is present.

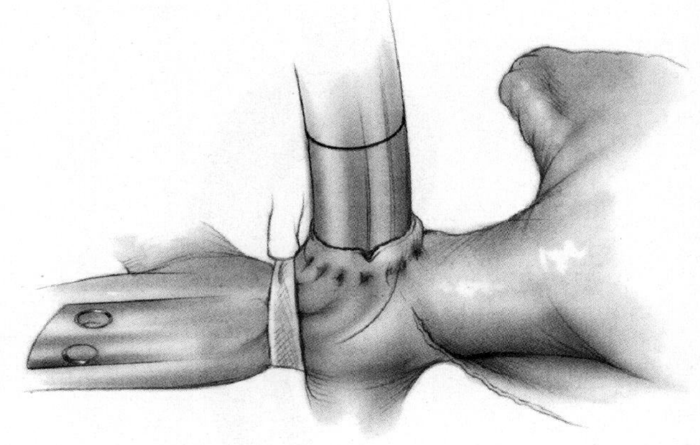

FIG. 8.3 Direct cannulation of the superior vena cava for retrograde cerebral perfusion.

Retrograde Cerebral Perfusion

In situations when deep circulatory arrest is contemplated, the patient is generally cooled down to bladder temperature of 18°C to 24°C. Moderate hypothermia (bladder temperature of 26°C to 28°C) is safe if the anticipated period of circulatory arrest is less than 15 to 20 minutes. Ice is packed around the patient's head. A tape is passed around the superior vena cava (see Chapter 2). A purse-string suture of 4-0 Prolene is applied to the adventitia of the superior vena cava at its junction with the pericardium. The adventitial tissue within the purse-string suture is cleaned off the superior vena cava, and an incision is made on the vein. The opening is enlarged with the tip of a clamp or scissors, and a long right-angled cannula is introduced into the superior vena cava and guided upward past the innominate vein (Fig. 8.3). This cannula is then connected to the side arm of the cardioplegia delivery system or to the arterial line to perfuse cold blood into the superior vena cava whenever circulatory arrest is initiated. The tape around the superior vena cava is snugged down on the cannula to prevent perfusate from flowing back into the right atrium.

⊘ Exclusion of the Azygos Vein

Tape is snugged down on the superior vena cava above the azygos vein to prevent runoff of cold blood into the azygos system (Fig. 8.3). ⊘

NB Some thought has to be given to extending the concept of retrograde cerebral perfusion with cold blood to retrograde perfusion of the gastrointestinal tract and even the rest of the body. Consequently, at times, perfusion of cold blood through the azygos vein may be advantageous. NB

The central venous pressure should not exceed 30 to 40 mm Hg as measured by the side arm of the Swan-Ganz introducer in the internal jugular or subclavian vein. The perfusion flow should be approximately 400 to 800 mL per minute. It is not quite evident if the retrograde cerebral perfusion provides any nutritive support to the brain. However, it is clear that it does provide a uniform cooling of the brain. Its most important benefit is prevention of air or debris from flowing upward into the arch vessels, which would cause cerebral embolization. This can be appreciated when atherosclerotic debris is seen floating in the very dark desaturated blood flowing out of the arch vessels into the operative field.

At the end of circulatory arrest, retrograde cerebral perfusion is discontinued and the cannula is removed. The purse-string suture on the superior vena cava is tied down. If retrograde cerebral perfusion has been accomplished using an arm of the cardioplegia system, retrograde flow is continued for the first 1 to 2 minutes after resuming cardiopulmonary bypass to help prevent air embolism to the arch vessels. It is also important to ensure that the aortic root is filled with blood and devoid of air, before resuming cardiopulmonary bypass.

Selective Antegrade Cerebral Perfusion

A more recent alternative to retrograde cerebral perfusion is selective antegrade cerebral perfusion through the right axillary artery. In conjunction with innominate artery occlusion, this method can provide effective cerebral protection during circulatory arrest by allowing antegrade right carotid artery perfusion. Right axillary perfusion is also used for systemic perfusion during cardiopulmonary bypass.

Before sternotomy, the right axillary artery is exposed through an 5 to 8 cm incision below and parallel to the lateral two-thirds of the clavicle. The pectoralis major muscle is divided in the direction of its fibers. The clavipectoral fascia is incised and the pectoralis minor muscle is retracted laterally. The axillary artery is located superior to the axillary vein. Using sharp dissection, the proximal part of the axillary artery is isolated. After administration of intravenous heparin, a small side-biting vascular clamp is applied to the artery. A longitudinal arteriotomy incision of approximately 1 cm is made and an 8-mm Hemashield Dacron tube graft (Medox Medical, Oakland, NJ) is sewn to the axillary artery in an end-to-side manner using a continuous 5-0 Prolene suture (Fig. 8.4). A 24-French arterial cannula is inserted into the graft, de-aired and secured. Perfusion through a graft is safer than direct cannulation of the axillary artery and allows more accurate cerebral perfusion by monitoring the right radial artery pressure. During hypothermic circulatory arrest, axillary arterial blood flow is adjusted to maintain a right radial artery pressure of 50 to 60 mm Hg.

NB It is important to monitor radial or brachial artery pressures on the side of arterial cannulation in order to prevent hyper-perfusion of the arm, which can lead to adverse outcomes, including limb loss. NB

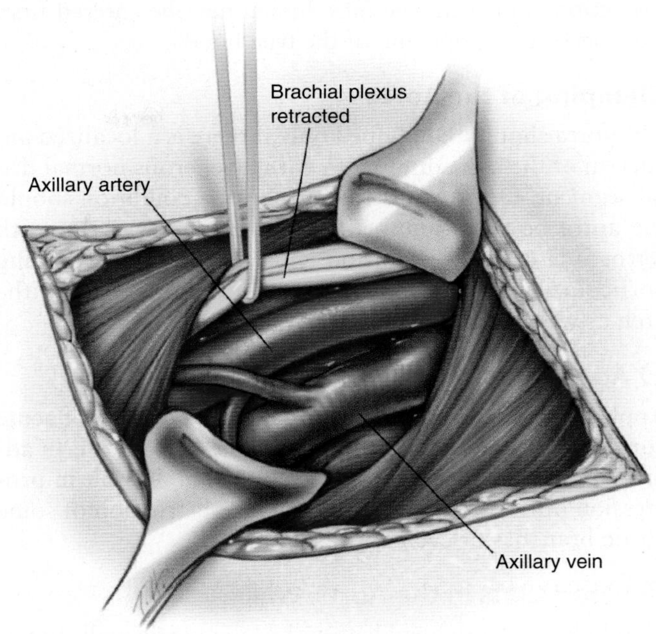

FIG. 8.4 Cannulation of the right axillary artery.

Technique

On cardiopulmonary bypass with the heart decompressed, preliminary evaluation is made. The need for any concomitant additional procedures, such as coronary artery bypass grafting, must be noted. The conduct of the surgery should be choreographed precisely at this time.

When the nasopharyngeal temperature reaches 18°C to 24°C, the patient is placed in the Trendelenburg position. The heart–lung machine is halted, and retrograde cerebral perfusion or selective antegrade axillary perfusion is started. A transverse or longitudinal aortotomy is made on the anterior aspect of the aortic wall (Fig. 8.5). When

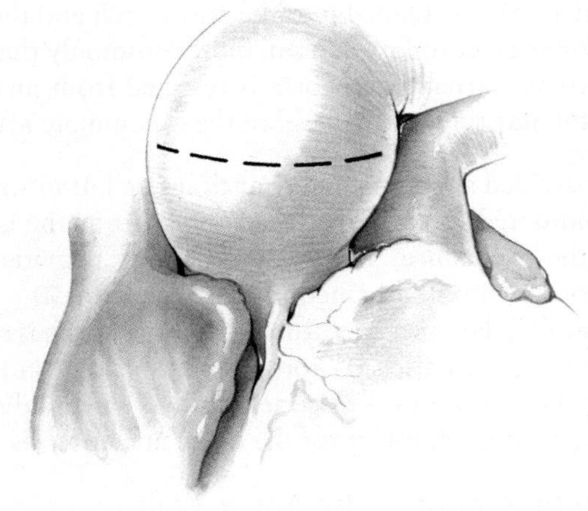

FIG. 8.5 The aortic aneurysm is opened transversely.

dissection is present, the false lumen may be entered first. This necessitates opening of the true lumen.

Clamping of the Aorta

The aorta should be clamped only if there is a localized aneurysm of the ascending aorta with a generous normal distal segment. Only under this very precise condition should the aorta be cross-clamped. Deep circulatory arrest with retrograde cerebral perfusion is used when the ascending aortic aneurysm fades away into the arch or involves the arch as well, as in all patients with aortic dissection.

⊘ Aortic Cross-Clamp Injury

Application of a clamp to the aorta in the presence of acute aortic dissection further traumatizes the aortic wall. In addition, it may pressurize the false lumen and result in progression of the dissection and possible obstruction of some aortic branches or even aortic rupture. ⊘

⊘ Blood Clots in the Aortic Wall

Blood clots are often evident within the aortic wall. In patients with aneurysms, the clots may be old and organized. They must be carefully removed along with atherosclerotic debris to prevent possible subsequent embolization. ⊘

Myocardial Protection

Cold blood cardioplegic solution may be administered antegrade into each coronary artery if deemed necessary. This is especially important if the dissection has involved one of the coronary ostia because the myocardium fed by this vessel may not have cooled sufficiently owing to obstructed flow. Retrograde infusion of cardioplegia into the coronary sinus should also be performed.

NB If the cardioplegic line is used for the retrograde cerebral perfusion with cold blood, this will have to be delayed until the cardioplegic infusion is completed and the line purged of cardioplegic solution. NB

The entry site of the aortic dissection is identified. The dissection may have extended into the aortic arch and the aortic root involving a coronary ostium, most commonly that of the right coronary artery. The aorta is resected from just above the sinotubular ridge to the level of the innominate artery.

NB The divided aortic wall may at times be left *in situ* to be reapproximated loosely over the tube graft at the completion of the procedure. This technique may provide added protection from possible mediastinal infection. NB

Typically, the lesser curvature of the aortic arch is resected to remove as much diseased aorta as possible. A 1-cm cuff of relatively normal aorta is dissected with as much adventitial tissue as possible left intact for the distal anastomosis.

NB Reinforcement of the Aortic Wall

If the distal aortic wall is dissected, BioGlue Surgical Adhesive (CryoLife, Inc., Kennesaw, GA) is injected into the false lumen to bond and strengthen the aortic wall (Fig. 8.6). A sponge is placed in the true lumen to prevent spillage. NB

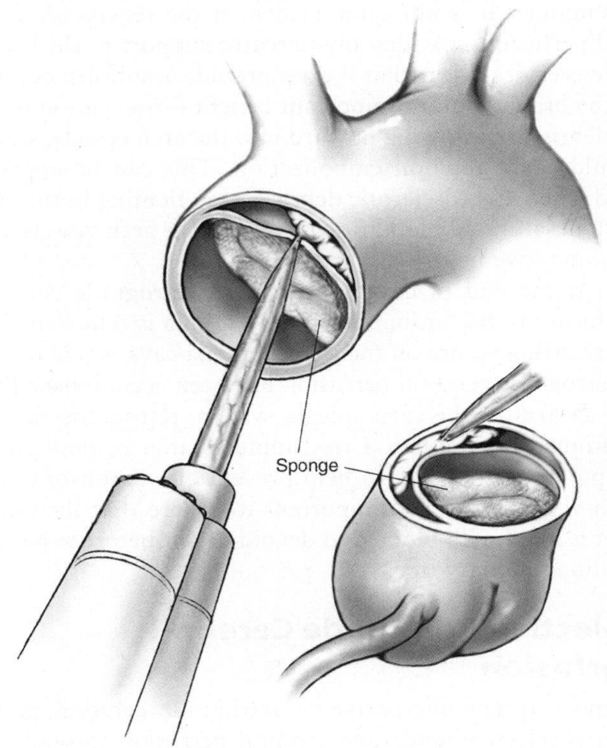

FIG. 8.6 Injection of glue into the false lumen to bond and strengthen the aortic wall.

NB The sponge within the lumen of the aorta is gently pressed against the aortic wall in close proximity to the coronary ostia to prevent the glue material from occluding the coronary arteries. NB

⊘ Glue Embolization

Glue material is not introduced within the dissected distal wall of the aorta if there appears to be reentry sites within the aortic arch. The possibility of glue material becoming detached and embolized through the distal reentry site is a grave complication of this procedure. ⊘

Further reinforcement can be obtained with Teflon felt strips attached to both the inside and/or outside of the aortic wall first with 6 to 10 interrupted mattress sutures or a continuous mattress suture of 3-0 Prolene (Fig. 8.7). Teflon felt strips may not be required if the integrity of the aortic wall appears to be satisfactory with the glue. Alternatively, the outer adventitial layer of the dissected aorta can be cut longer than the inner intimal layer. This layer is then folded into the true lumen and sewn in place with interrupted mattress sutures (Fig. 8.8).

An appropriately sized Hemashield tube graft is cut and tailored obliquely to be attached to the undersurface

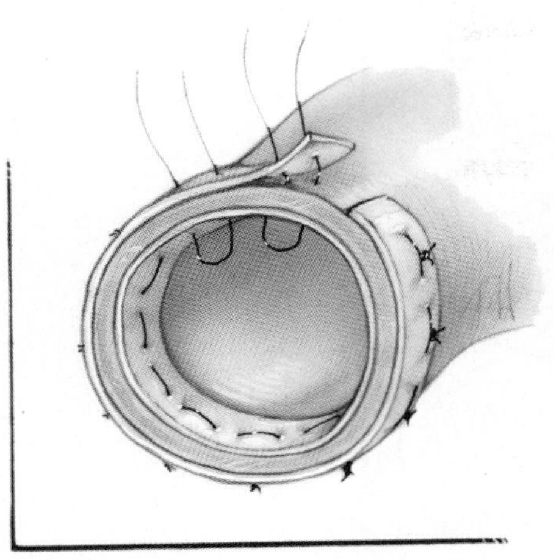

FIG. 8.7 Reinforcement of the distal aorta with double layers of Teflon felt.

of the arch or cut straight to be attached to the aorta at the level of the innominate artery. The tube graft is then anastomosed to the reinforced aortic cuff with a continuous 3-0 Prolene suture.

NB Tension on the Suture Line

It is important for the assistant surgeon to follow the suture meticulously to provide appropriate tension on the suture line. Otherwise, multiple reinforcing interrupted sutures may be required to ensure a watertight anastomosis. NB

With the patient in the Trendelenburg position, the perfusion of retrograde cerebral blood is allowed to accumulate and fill the aortic arch. All air and debris are allowed to flow out through the graft. At this time, another arterial cannula is introduced through the tube graft, and the perfusionist is asked to initiate arterial perfusion through this cannula in an antegrade manner with extremely low flow. A clamp is now applied to the tube graft well away from the anastomosis and proximal to the cannula, and the retrograde cerebral perfusion is gradually discontinued and venous drainage is reinstituted (Fig. 8.9). Normal perfusion flow and pressure are gradually restored, and the patient is rewarmed. The posterior distal suture line is now examined, and additional stitches are placed for control of hemostasis if required.

NB In patients with aortic aneurysm, the femoral arterial cannula may be used to reinstate cardiopulmonary bypass. This retrograde arterial perfusion is gradually increased to normal flow, and rewarming is started. While not essential, antegrade perfusion with a separate cannula through the tube graft allows earlier removal of the femoral arterial cannula and repair of the femoral artery, reducing the risk of limb ischemia. NB

⊘ Retrograde Arterial Perfusion and Aortic Dissection

In patients with aortic dissection, blood gains access through the entry site into the aortic wall. This dissection may result in a reentry site by tearing the intima distally along the course of the aorta. When cardiopulmonary bypass is reinitiated, the retrograde flow may enter the false lumen through this distal intimal tear and reenter the lumen at the entry site. However, when the aorta has been repaired and the entry site is excluded by tube graft interposition, the retrograde flow of blood cannot escape and may cause further dissection of the aorta. Therefore, it is important to establish antegrade flow within the true lumen when resuming cardiopulmonary bypass. ⊘

NB If right axillary artery cannulation has been used, the tube graft can be filled by removing the clamp on the innominate artery. The graft is then cross-clamped, and full flow is resumed. NB

NB After cardiopulmonary bypass is reestablished, additional doses of blood cardioplegic solution are administered by the retrograde technique and antegrade into the

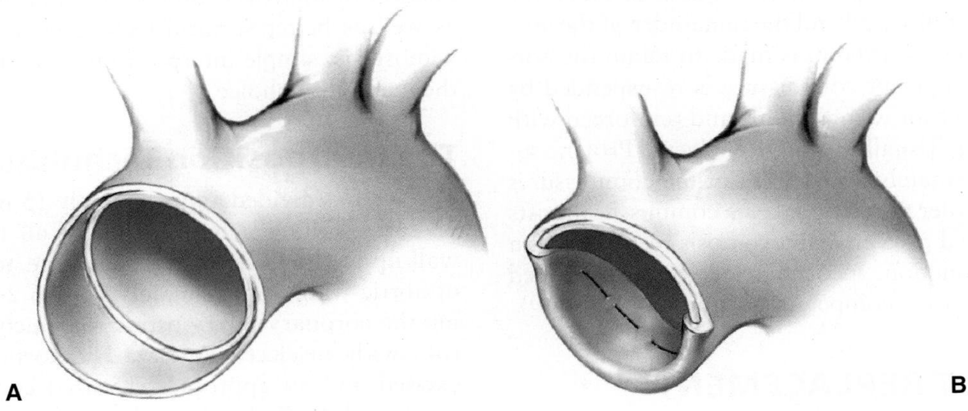

FIG. 8.8 Reinforcing aortic wall with adventitial layer.

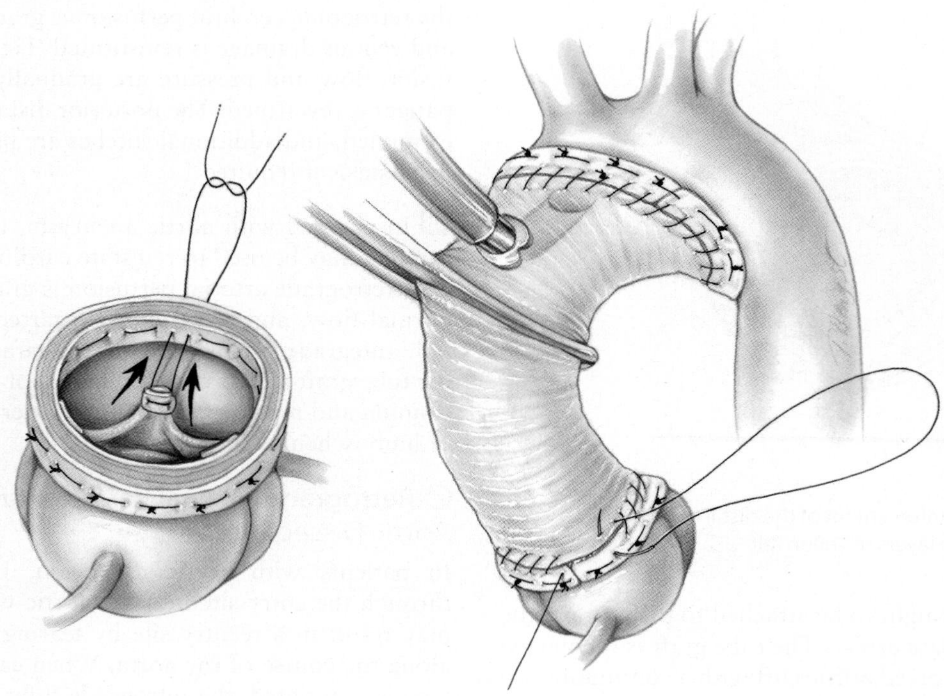

FIG. 8.9 Completion of proximal anastomosis. Inset: Resuspension of an aortic valve commissure.

coronary ostia at 10- to 20-minute intervals (see Chapters 3 and 5). NB

When the aorta is otherwise normal and there is no aortic valve insufficiency, the proximal aorta that has been transected at approximately 1 cm above the level of aortic commissures is reinforced with glue and a single or double layer of Teflon felt, as described for the distal anastomosis. The tube graft is tailored to an appropriate length and anastomosed to the proximal aorta with 4-0 Prolene continuous suture (Fig. 8.9).

Often, however, there may be associated aortic insufficiency due to aortic root dissection or dilation. When the valve leaflets are not diseased and the remainder of the aortic root is normal, every attempt is made to retain the aortic valve. Any incompetent commissure is resuspended by curing the dissected root with BioGlue and reinforced with an external felt strip. Usually, a single pledgeted Prolene suture is placed immediately above each of the commissures and tied down in order to resuspend the commissural posts further. This tailored proximal anastomosis reestablishes a new sinotubular junction, incorporating the resuspended commissures to ensure a competent aortic valve (Fig. 8.9).

AORTIC ROOT REPLACEMENT

When the aortic valve is diseased beyond repair or the dissection extends proximally into the sinuses, complete aortic root replacement with an valved conduit and reimplantation of the coronary arteries become necessary.

Aortic root replacement as originally described by Bentall consisted of replacement of the aortic valve and the ascending aorta including the aortic root, and reimplantation of the coronary arteries into the tube graft all within the native aorta. The tube graft was then wrapped with the redundant aortic wall. There appears to be an increased incidence of pseudoaneurysm formation, probably because of insecure hemostasis at the anastomotic suture lines masked by the wrapping of the aorta. With the introduction of improved tube grafts and aortic root conduits as well as better surgical techniques for anastomosis and hemostasis, simple interposition of a valve conduit is now the method of choice.

The Interposition Technique

The aorta is divided approximately 15 mm above the commissures, followed by excision of all the diseased aortic wall up to the lesser curvature of the aortic arch. Buttons of aortic wall, approximately 1.5- to 2-cm wide, containing the coronary artery ostia are detached from the aortic root with an electrocautery. The aortic valve leaflets are excised and an appropriately sized composite tube graft is selected. St. Jude Medical (Minneapolis, MN) provides a collagen-impregnated tube graft (Hemashield) attached to a bileaflet valve with a tall sewing cuff. Interrupted

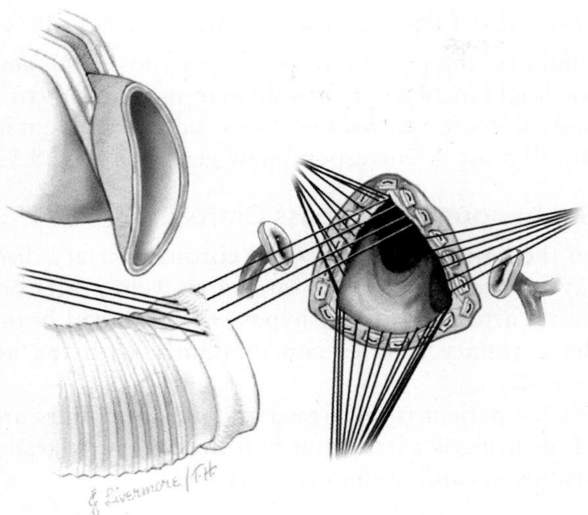

FIG. 8.10 Technique for aortic root replacement: Placement of annular sutures in valve conduit.

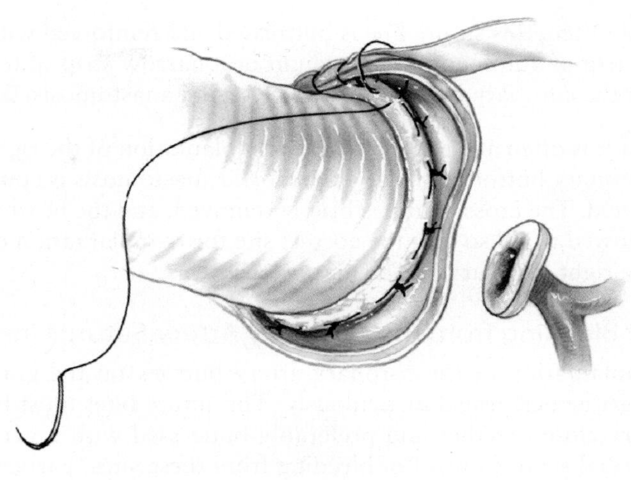

FIG. 8.12 Copeland technique reinforced with a felt strip.

pledgeted sutures of 2-0 Ticron are placed close together in the aortic annulus (Fig. 8.10). Subsequently, they are passed through the lower portion of the sewing ring of the composite valve graft, leaving 2 to 3 mm of the upper sewing cuff free. The prosthesis is lowered into position, and the sutures are tied, taking all the precautions as in aortic valve replacement (see Chapter 5).

NB Six to eight millimeter of the aortic wall should be left attached to the annulus. This remaining aortic wall with its adventitial tissue is now brought forward and sewn to the upper portion of the sewing ring of the prosthesis with a continuous 3-0 Prolene suture (Fig. 8.11). The suture should go through in the order of adventitia, annulus, sewing ring, and then back outside of the folded adventitia. In addition, a Teflon strip can be used to buttress the proximal suture line (Fig. 8.12). This reduces the possibility of leaks at the aortic root. NB

Circular holes are made in the tube graft with an ophthalmologic cautery device for reimplantation of the coronary artery buttons. These openings should preferably be some distance above the sewing ring for ease of suturing. The coronary artery buttons are now attached to these openings with continuous 5-0 Prolene sutures (Fig. 8.13).

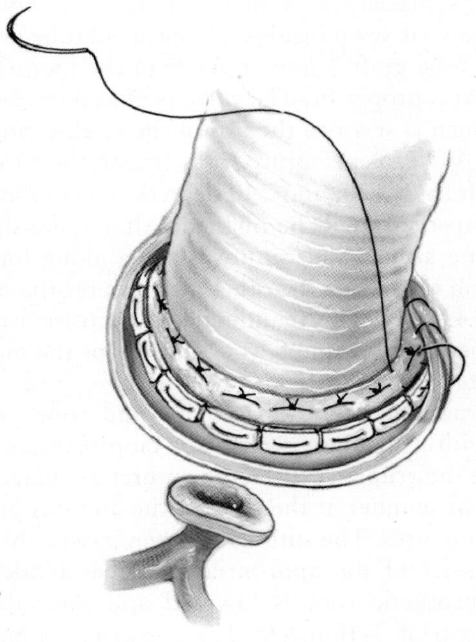

FIG. 8.11 Technique (modified Copeland) for reinforcing the proximal suture line.

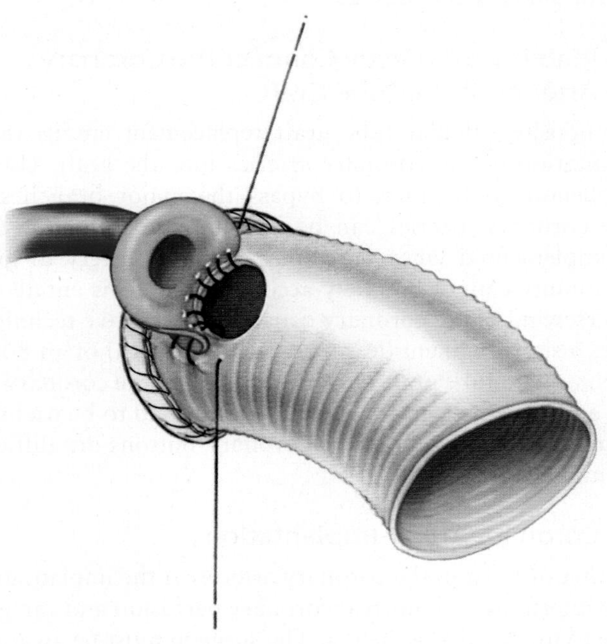

FIG. 8.13 Technique for aortic root replacement: Reimplantation of coronary ostial buttons.

NB Often, this suture line is buttressed and reinforced with a strip of autologous pericardium or a narrow strip of felt on the coronary button for a more secure anastomosis. NB

NB It is often advisable to delay reimplantation of the right coronary button until the distal aortic anastomosis is completed. The cross-clamp is briefly removed, and the heart is allowed to fill so that the correct site for reimplantation of the right coronary can be marked. NB

⊘ Bleeding from the Coronary Artery Suture Line

Implantation of the coronary artery buttons on the graft must be performed meticulously. The suture bites must be very close together and preferably buttressed with a pericardial strip. Control of bleeding from these sites, particularly the left coronary artery anastomosis, at a subsequent stage is challenging. Application of BioGlue to the suture line may assist in hemostasis. ⊘

The tube graft is now cut appropriately and attached to the distal aorta as described earlier. If a tube graft is already attached to the distal aorta, the proximal and distal tube grafts are now tailor cut and anastomosed to each other with a continuous 3-0 or 4-0 Prolene suture.

NB Composite Valve vs. Tube Graft Interposition

Many of these patients have diffuse aortic wall disease. Use of the composite valvular conduit should be preferred to isolated aortic valve replacement followed by tube graft replacement of the aorta above the sinotubular junction. This latter technique may leave behind diseased sinuses of Valsalva and put the patient at risk of later development of aortic sinus aneurysms. NB

⊘ Inability to Directly Connect the Coronary Arteries to the Tube Graft

Composite valvular tube graft replacement entails reimplantation of the coronary arteries into the graft. Use of saphenous vein grafts to bypass the major branches of the coronary arteries can be an alternate technique and is implemented whenever direct coronary artery to graft continuity cannot be safely accomplished. This entails the oversewing of the coronary ostia. An alternative technique uses a short segment (less than 1 cm in length) of an 8-mm Hemashield tube graft interposed between the coronary ostia and the aortic graft. This has been found to be useful in some patients in whom the coronary buttons are difficult to mobilize. ⊘

⊘ Coronary Artery Implantation

A kink or twist of the coronary arteries at the implantation site interferes with normal coronary perfusion and can give rise to myocardial ischemia. The surgeon must be aware of this possibility during anastomosis of the coronary ostia to the graft to prevent misalignment. ⊘

⊘ Stenosis of the Coronary Artery Ostia

To minimize the possibility of ostial stenosis, the anastomosis should incorporate a wide margin of the aortic wall around each coronary ostium. The window that is cut in the graft wall must be correspondingly generous (Fig. 8.13). ⊘

NB Saphenous Vein Bypass Grafts

When the patient has associated coronary artery disease, it may be necessary to use saphenous vein grafts or appropriate arterial grafts to bypass the occluded branches of the coronary arteries concomitantly with the aortic surgery. NB

As the patient is rewarmed and all suture lines are secured, deairing is carried out and the patient is gradually weaned from cardiopulmonary bypass.

NB Aortic root venting is performed with an air vent needle through the graft before removing the clamp across the tube graft. The clamp is then reapplied partially across the anterior portion of the graft distal to the needle vent (see Venting and Deairing of the Heart section in Chapter 4). NB

⊘ Air Removal

The vent needle for air removal should not be inserted in the aorta distal to the graft to avoid starting a new site of dissection. ⊘

Techniques for Aortic Root Replacement with a Bioprosthesis

When a tissue valve is preferred during concomitant valve and root replacement, a stented porcine or bovine pericardial valve is sewn inside a Hemashield tube graft. Generally, a tube graft 3 mm larger than the bioprosthesis is chosen for a proper fit. The valve is placed inside the tube graft, which is sewn to the top of the sewing ring using a running 4-0 Prolene suture. It is important to mark the tube graft at 0, 120, and 240 degrees, where the struts of the bioprosthesis will be aligned. After tying down two knots, one arm of one suture is sewn along one half of the sewing ring while the other arm secures the other side (Fig. 8.14A, B). This handmade composite valve graft conduit is then implanted as described for the mechanical composite valve graft.

Alternatively, the aortic valve and root can be replaced with a stentless aortic root bioprosthesis. A series of simple interrupted 4-0 Ticron sutures are placed closely in a planar manner at the level of the annulus and below the commissures. The sutures are then passed through the Dacron skirt of the appropriately sized stentless valve. The bioprothetic root is lowered and the sutures tied over a strip of Teflon felt. The coronary stumps of the bioprosthesis are removed and the coronary buttons are reimplanted into their respective openings using 5-0 Prolene sutures. The bioprosthesis can be extended with a

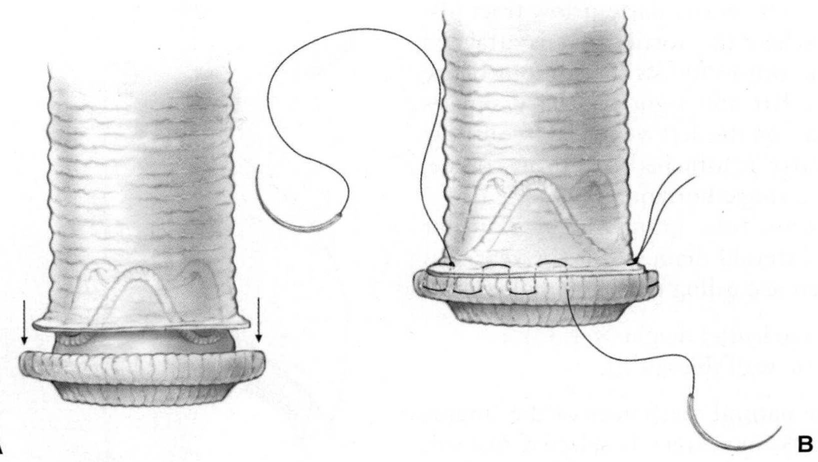

FIG. 8.14 Constructing a bioprosthetic valve conduit.

Hemashield Dacron tube graft, if necessary, to replace the ascending aorta.

NB The Freestyle bioprosthesis can usually be oriented in its anatomic position without tension on the coronary button anastomoses. In fact, the outpouching nature of bioprosthetic coronary stumps reduces the need for extensive mobilization of the coronary artery buttons. However, when the native coronary buttons are more than 120 degrees apart as in a congenitally bicuspid valve, the stentless valve should be rotated 120 degrees. For reattachment of the coronary artery buttons, only one of the coronary stumps is removed and a second opening is made in the noncoronary sinus of the bioprosthesis using a 4-mm aortic punch. The remaining coronary stump is reinforced with a 5-0 Prolene suture. NB

Aortic Valve-Sparing Root Replacement

Patients with aortic root disease, such as those with Marfan syndrome, have progressive dilation of the aortic sinuses and aortic annulus, which can lead to aortic valve insufficiency despite normal aortic valve leaflets. In these patients, it is possible to replace the diseased aortic root and preserve the aortic valve by reimplanting it inside a Dacron tube graft.

The aorta is transected just beyond the aneurysmal dilation. Both coronary arteries are mobilized as individual buttons, as described previously. The root is dissected circumferentially down to a level just below the nadir of the aortic annulus. All three sinuses of Valsalva are excised, leaving approximately 5 mm of arterial wall attached to the aortic annulus (Fig. 8.15A). A series of 12 to 14 interrupted horizontal mattress sutures of 2-0 Ticron are passed

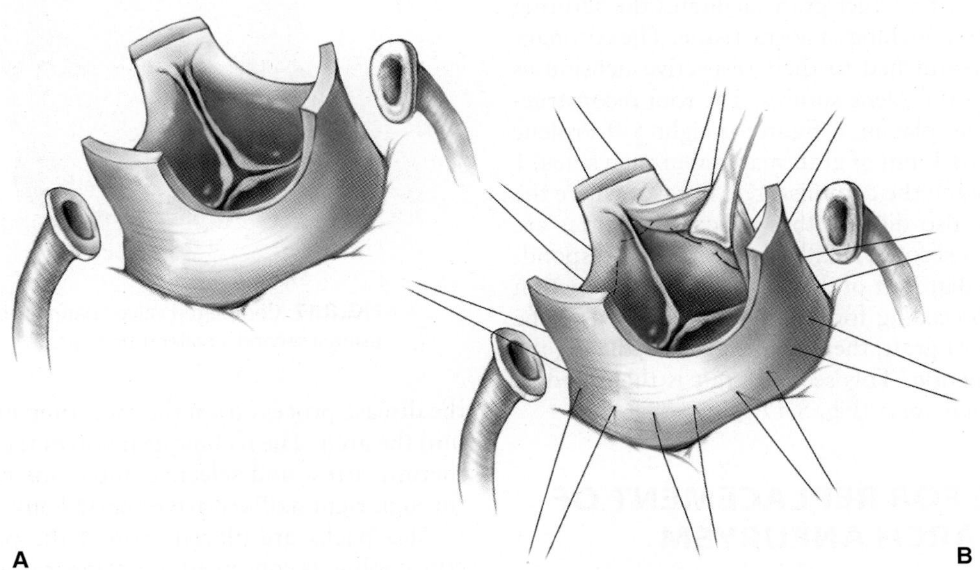

FIG. 8.15 Valve-sparing root replacement: **A:** Excising coronary arteries as buttons. **B:** Interrupted proximal sutures.

from inside to outside the left ventricular outflow tract just below the aortic valve. Where the aortic valve is attached to ventricular muscle, the sutures follow the contour of the commissure between the left and right coronary sinuses (Fig. 8.15B). On the side of the left ventricular outflow tract where the aortic valve is attached to fibrous tissue, the sutures are placed in a single horizontal plane.

Traditionally, a Dacron tube graft with a diameter matching the calculated external diameter of the ventriculoaortic junction is chosen according to the formula:

$$\text{Diameter} = (\text{Average leaflet height} \times 1.33) + (2 \times \text{Aortic wall thickness}).$$

However, to simulate the natural mechanics of the sinuses of Valsalva, a graft 4 to 6 mm larger is selected instead. Theoretically, the creation of these pseudosinuses minimizes systolic contact between the valve cusps and the Dacron graft and reduces diastolic closing leaflet stresses, both of which may enhance valve durability. Three equidistant marks are made at one end of the tube graft. The previously placed horizontal mattress sutures are then passed through the Dacron graft, taking care to match the commissures to the markings on the graft. Because there are more sutures in the fibrous portion of the left ventricular outflow tract in patients with annuloaortic ectasia, they are placed correspondingly closer in the Dacron graft, thereby correcting the dilation. The tube is lowered over the scalloped aortic valve and the sutures are tied on the outside with a narrow strip of felt sandwiched into the suture line. The graft is cut 2 to 3 cm above the commissures, which are suspended to the graft with mattress 4-0 Prolene sutures reinforced with pledgets. The graft is filled with saline solution to confirm the correct orientation of the commissures and the competence of the valve. The valve is reimplanted inside the graft using the 4-0 or 5-0 Prolene sutures in a running manner (Fig. 8.16). The use of a larger graft facilitates the suturing of the valve without bunching of aortic tissue. The coronary buttons are then reattached to their respective neosinuses on the graft using 5-0 Prolene sutures. The root reconstruction is completed by placing a figure of eight 5-0 Prolene suture to plicate 2 to 3 mm of graft material in each sinus, 1 cm above and between the commissures. In cases where the ascending aorta is also dilated, these plicating sutures are not used. Instead, a second, smaller tube graft corresponding to the external diameter of the ventriculoaortic junction according to the preceding formula is anastomosed to the top of the aortic root graft, thereby effectively reducing the neosinotubular junction. This second graft is then used to replace the ascending aorta (Fig. 8.17).

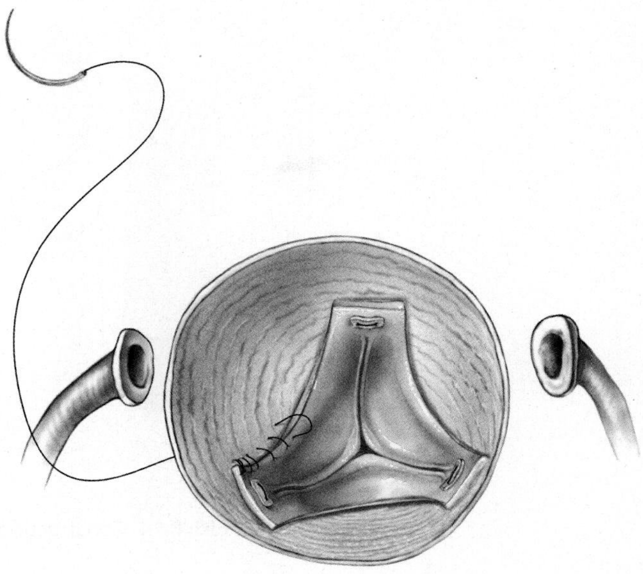

FIG. 8.16 Valve-sparing root replacement: Distal suture line.

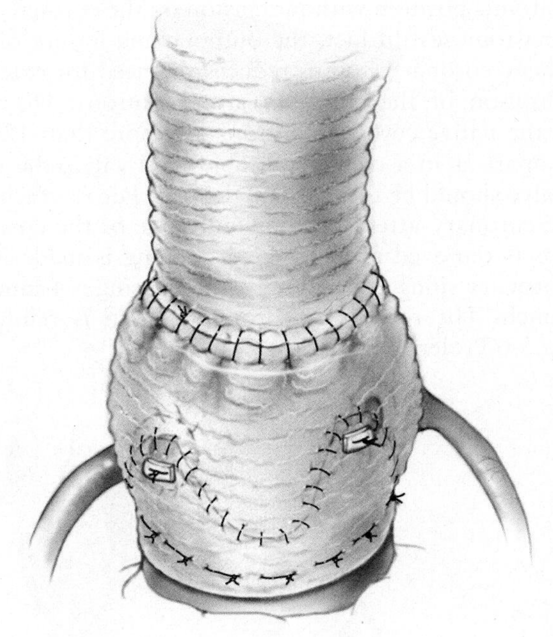

FIG. 8.17 Completed valve-sparing root replacement using a second smaller tube graft.

TECHNIQUE FOR REPLACEMENT OF AN AORTIC ARCH ANEURYSM

The aortic arch may have to be replaced if there is an enlarging aneurysm affecting the arch or there is extension of the disease process from the ascending or descending aorta into the arch. The technique involves the use of deep hypothermic arrest and selective antegrade cerebral protection through right axillary artery perfusion.

Ice packs are placed around the patient's head, and core cooling is continued to a temperature of 18°C. During core cooling, the aortic arch and brachiocephalic vessels are dissected and mobilized. A trifurcation graft is constructed

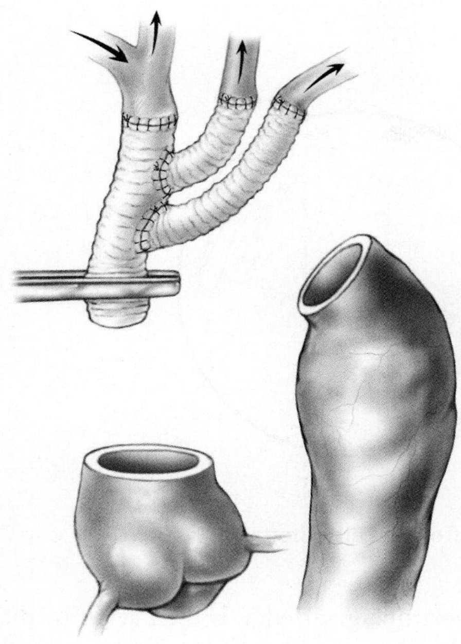

FIG. 8.18 Arch replacement: Completed trifurcation graft to left subclavian, left carotid, and innominate arteries.

by sewing two 8-mm branch Hemashield Dacron grafts to a 12-mm graft or two 10-mm side-branch grafts to a 14-mm graft in an end-to-side manner. After circulatory arrest is achieved, the arch vessels are clamped and divided 0.5 cm beyond their origins. Selective antegrade cerebral perfusion is begun and the flow adjusted to maintain a perfusion pressure of 50 to 60 mm Hg. The limbs of the trifurcation graft are trimmed to appropriate lengths and sutured sequentially to the arch vessels with 5-0 Prolene beginning with the left subclavian artery, then the left carotid artery, and finally the innominate artery (Fig. 8.18). The clamps on the left subclavian and left carotid arteries are released. With an intact Circle of Willis, there is usually back bleeding to allow flushing of air and debris through these side branches into the main graft. The innominate artery is then unclamped for final deairing. The main graft is clamped proximal to the side branches to allow antegrade perfusion to the head and upper extremities.

Attention is now directed to the arch reconstruction. An aortotomy is made across the arch, the redundant arch tissue with debris and blood clots is removed, and ascending and descending aortic segments are completely divided. A Hemashield tube graft of appropriate size is introduced into the lumen of the descending aorta (Fig. 8.19). It is sewn to the normal aortic wall with a continuous suture of 3-0 Prolene. Sometimes, it is buttressed with a Teflon felt strip on the outside of the descending aorta (Fig. 8.20). The suture line may be further secured with BioGlue. The tube graft is then pulled out of the descending aorta (Fig. 8.21). An arterial cannula is inserted into the arch graft, which

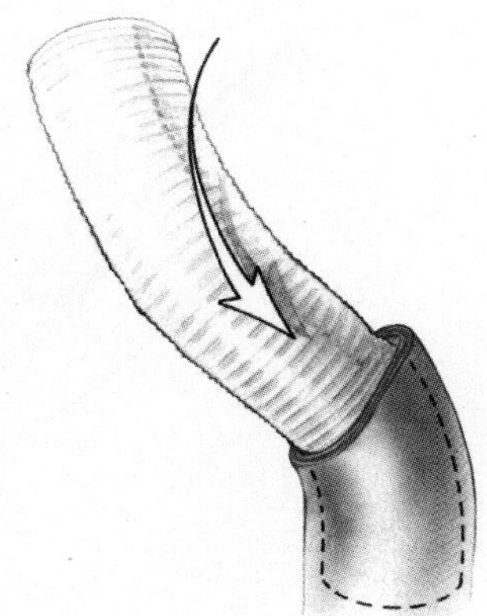

FIG. 8.19 Arch replacement: Insertion of a tube graft into the descending aorta and performance of distal suture line.

is then clamped. Perfusion to the lower body is gradually instituted while the arch graft is aspirated to evacuate air. The arch graft is then sutured to the transected end of the ascending aorta using 4-0 Prolene. At this time, an opening in the arch graft is made and the beveled end of the trifurcation graft is sewn to the arch graft with 5-0 Prolene suture (Fig. 8.22) without interrupting perfusion. During this anastomosis, the heart is perfused with warm blood through the retrograde cardioplegia cannula. After deairing maneuvers, all clamps are released.

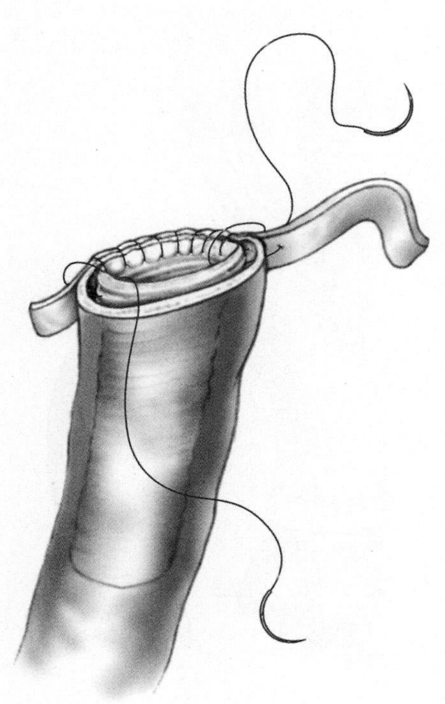

FIG. 8.20 Arch replacement: Sewing a graft to the aortic wall.

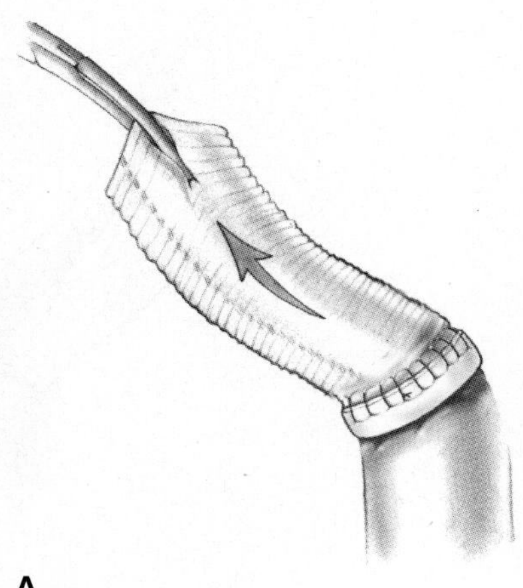

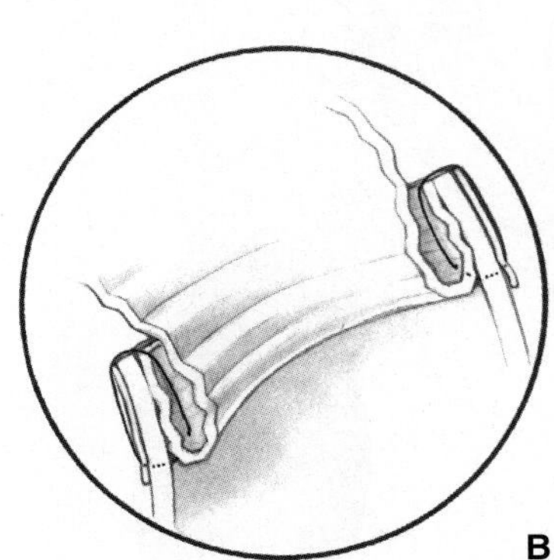

FIG. 8.21 Arch replacement. **A:** Tube graft is withdrawn from the distal aorta. **B:** Close-up of an inverted distal suture line.

Elephant-Trunk Technique

When the descending aorta is also diseased and requires subsequent excision and replacement, an elephant-trunk technique is used. This entails inverting approximately 3 cm of Hemashield tube graft on itself.

NB Tube Graft Inversion

The short segment is on the outside of the larger segment of the tube graft. NB

The double-layer tube graft is introduced into the lumen of the descending aorta as before (Fig. 8.23). The double-layer tube graft edge is then sewn to the descending aorta, buttressed with a Teflon felt strip on the outside with a continuous suture of 3-0 Prolene. Again, the use of BioGlue may reinforce the anastomosis.

NB The needle bite includes the two layers of tube graft, aortic wall, and a Teflon felt strip. NB

At the completion of the anastomosis, the longer segment of the graft is pulled out of the lumen of the tube graft, leaving a "trunk" of approximately 3 cm behind within the lumen of the descending aorta.

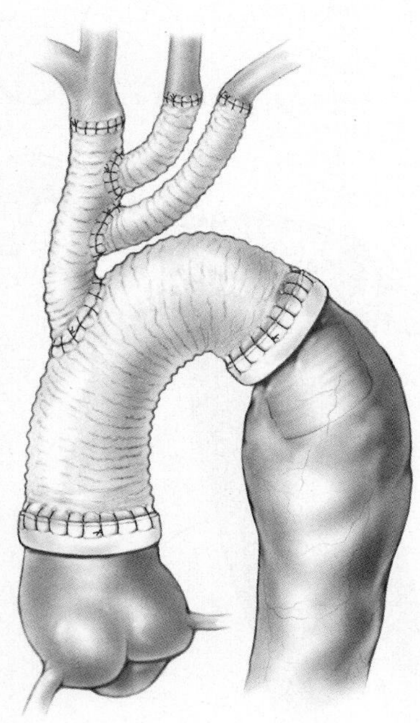

FIG. 8.22 Completed arch replacement with elephant-trunk extension into descending aorta.

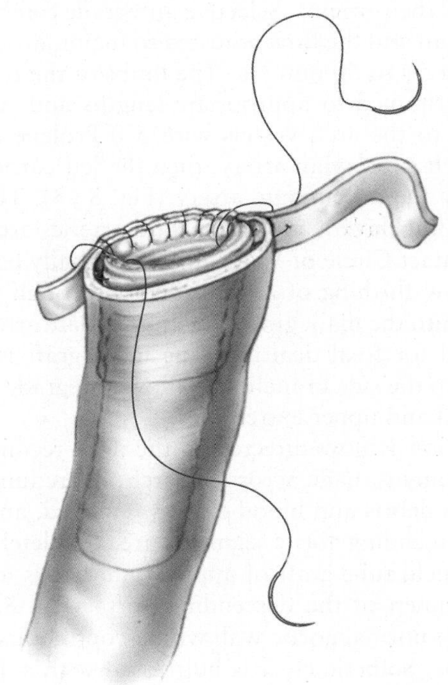

FIG. 8.23 Elephant-trunk technique: A double-layer graft is sewn to the aortic wall.

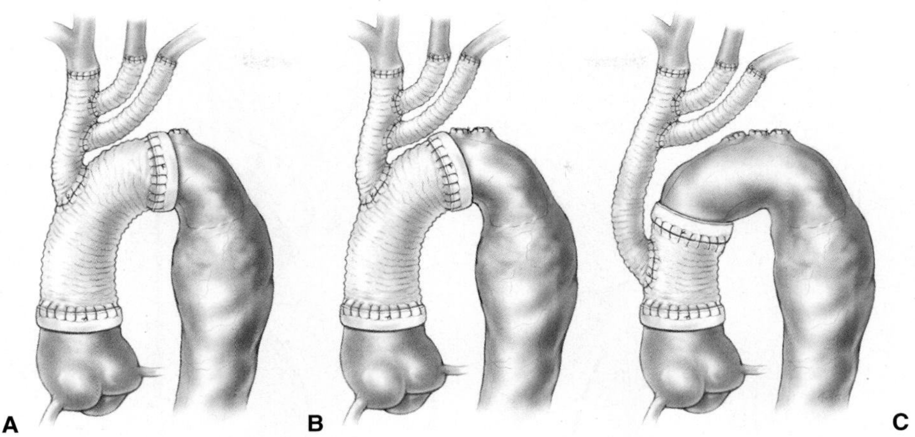

FIG. 8.24 Performing elephant-trunk anastomosis more proximally on aortic arch or distal ascending aorta.

NB The trunk is anastomosed to another tube graft when excision of the descending thoracic aorta is undertaken weeks to months subsequently. NB

NB If a neck for the elephant-trunk anastomosis is not present distal to the left subclavian artery, the site of the distal suture line can be as far proximally as the ascending aorta depending on the narrowest part of the aortic arch (Fig. 8.24). In these cases, the arch vessel stumps are oversewn with 4-0 Prolene sutures. NB

MANAGEMENT OF TYPE B AORTIC DISSECTION

Initial management of patients with type B dissection affecting the descending aorta is to control the high blood pressure with medical therapy. In contradistinction to type A aortic dissection, which requires urgent surgical intervention, patients with type B dissection have a relatively good prognosis with medical therapy. However, elective surgical intervention remains the best form of management and provides superior long-term results in patients who are young and free of other concomitant diseases. Therefore, replacement or stenting of the descending thoracic aorta is the treatment of choice in young, otherwise healthy patients with chronic type B dissection and in older patients with expanding descending aortic aneurysms. Nevertheless, patients who continue to have pain despite maximal medical management, have evidence of contained rupture, or have ischemia of a limb or major organ owing to involvement of an arterial branch by the dissection process should undergo urgent surgical intervention.

NB Interventional radiologists have been important participants in the care of patients with aortic dissections. They are often able to reestablish flow to compromised or occluded aortic branches by fenestrating the intimal flap or stenting the true or false lumen. This may allow a patient with a type B dissection to be stabilized and have surgery on an elective basis. More recently, segments of contained rupture in the acutely dissected descending aorta have been stent grafted (see subsequent text). Some patients with type A dissections continue to demonstrate clinically significant obstruction to flow in one or more aortic branches after ascending aortic replacement. These patients may also be successfully treated by the interventional radiologist. NB

Technique for Replacement of the Descending Thoracic Aorta

A postero-lateral thoracotomy through the fifth intercostal space provides adequate exposure of the descending thoracic aorta. At times, a second lower incision may facilitate the distal anastomosis. Adhesions must be taken down with utmost care to prevent injury to the lung or the diseased aorta. A plane of dissection is identified, and vascular loops or umbilical tapes are passed around the transverse arch between the left carotid and the left subclavian arteries, the left subclavian artery, and the descending aorta distally. The left groin area is always prepared and should be within the operative field in all cases.

We routinely use partial left-sided heart bypass for nearly all surgeries on the descending thoracic aorta. The femoral artery is cannulated for arterial return, and either the femoral vein, pulmonary artery, or pulmonary vein is selected for venous drainage (see Replacement of the Ascending Aorta section). The use of partial bypass allows control of the patient's blood pressure. It also provides perfusion of the lower body and may protect the spinal cord.

Initially, the transverse arch and the left subclavian artery are clamped. The distal aorta is clamped a short distance below the proximal clamp, although the distal extent of aortic dissection may have progressed well below the

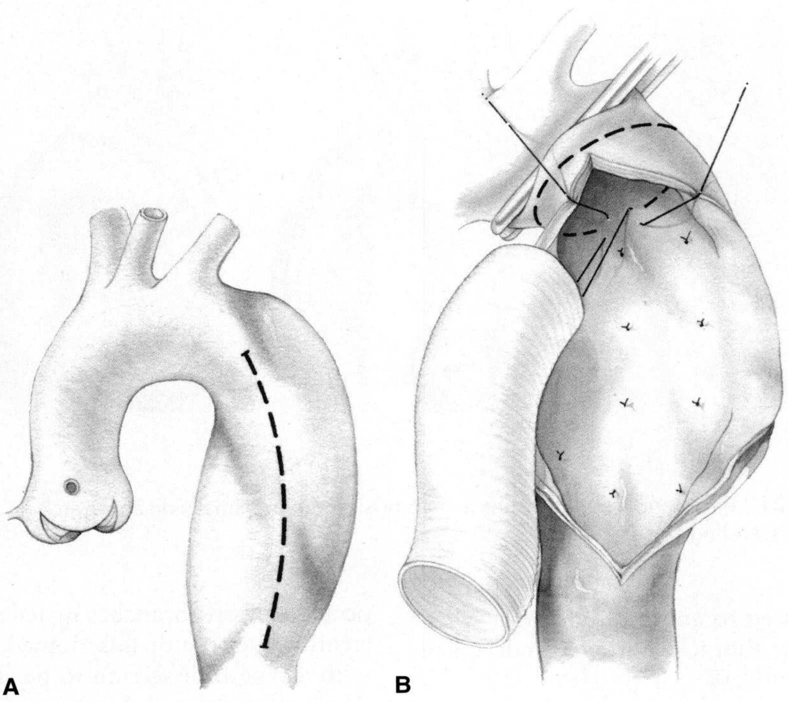

FIG. 8.25 Stepwise technique for the replacement of the descending aorta. A: An aortotomy. B: The proximal suture line.

diaphragm. A short aortotomy is made; it is then extended to provide adequate exposure (Fig. 8.25A). When the aorta is opened and decompressed, it is often possible and preferable to reapply a single clamp below the origin of the subclavian artery above the site of dissection to ensure perfusion through the left subclavian artery because this may decrease the incidence of paraplegia. The ostia of the intercostal arteries are oversewn with 3-0 Prolene sutures.

An appropriately sized Hemashield tube graft is sewn into the proximal aortic lumen with continuous sutures of 3-0 Prolene (Fig. 8.25B). The suture line is always buttressed and reinforced with strips of Teflon felt, which may be outside and around the aorta or within its lumen or both. A clamp is then applied to the tube graft, and the proximal clamp placed on the aorta is removed. The suture line is checked for bleeding, and additional sutures are placed if deemed necessary. Use of BioGlue on the outside of the anastomosis will provide additional reinforcement of the suture line. The tube graft is cut to the precise length and sewn to the distal aortic wall with continuous 3-0 Prolene suture incorporating a strip of Teflon felt in the suturing to reinforce the anastomotic line (Fig. 8.26A). The remaining aortic wall is then reapproximated over the graft (Fig. 8.26B). Alternatively, the aorta may be transected at the proposed site of anastomosis. A generous cuff of aortic wall is dissected free and reinforced with a strip of Teflon felt. The tube graft is then interposed, and both proximal and distal anastomoses are completed with continuous suture of 3-0 Prolene.

NB Reimplantation of the intercostal arteries

The lower thoracic intercostal arteries may on occasion be quite large in patients with chronic dissection or aneurysm. Although oversewing them has been the accepted technique, consideration should be given to their reimplantation to reduce the incidence of paralysis. NB

Technique

A small, elliptic segment of the tube graft overlying the intercostal arteries is removed. The island of intercostal arteries is then sewn to the tube graft with deep bites of continuous suture of 3-0 Prolene (Fig. 8.27). Use of BioGlue may additionally secure the suture line.

In patients who have previously undergone ascending aorta and arch replacements with the so-called elephant-trunk technique, the proximal anastomosis is simplified. After the initiation of cardiopulmonary bypass, the blood pressure is temporarily lowered to 60 mm Hg. The distal aorta is opened, the graft extension is identified, and the clamp is placed on this graft (Fig. 8.28). The proximal descending graft is then anastomosed to the trunk extension with running 3-0 or 4-0 Prolene sutures. The distal anastomosis is completed as described previously.

The surgery can also be performed without the use of left-sided cardiopulmonary bypass. Often the aorta is clamped only proximally. Blood from the distal aorta is removed through a cell saver sucker for reinfusion. The distal anastomosis is carried out by this open technique unimpeded by the distal clamp.

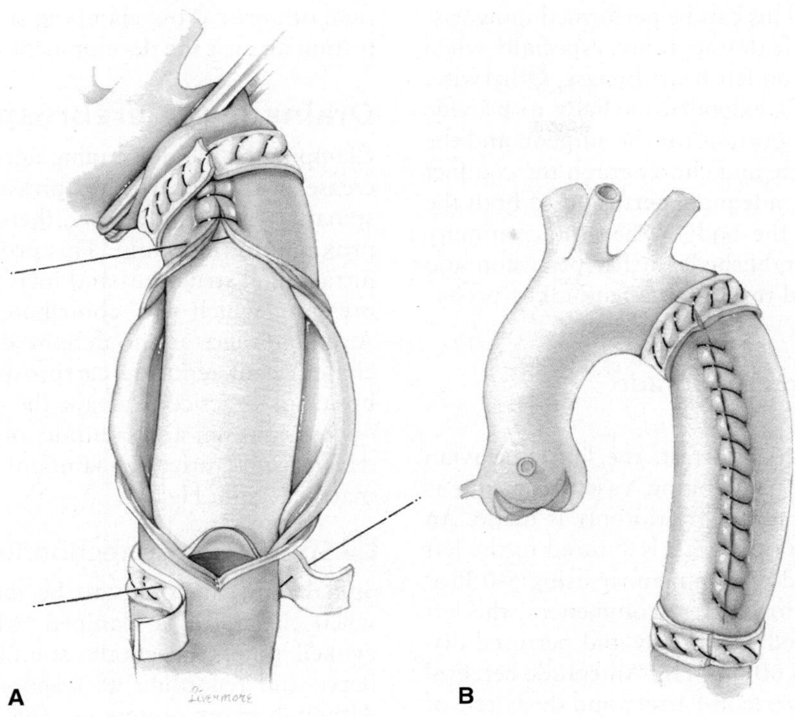

FIG. 8.26 Stepwise technique for the replacement of the descending aorta. A: The distal suture line. B: Wrapping the graft.

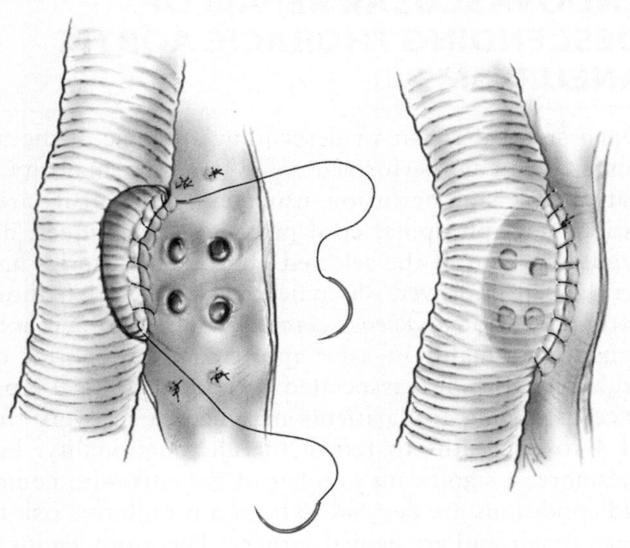

FIG. 8.27 Stepwise technique for the replacement of the descending aorta: Reimplantation of the intercostal arteries into the tube graft.

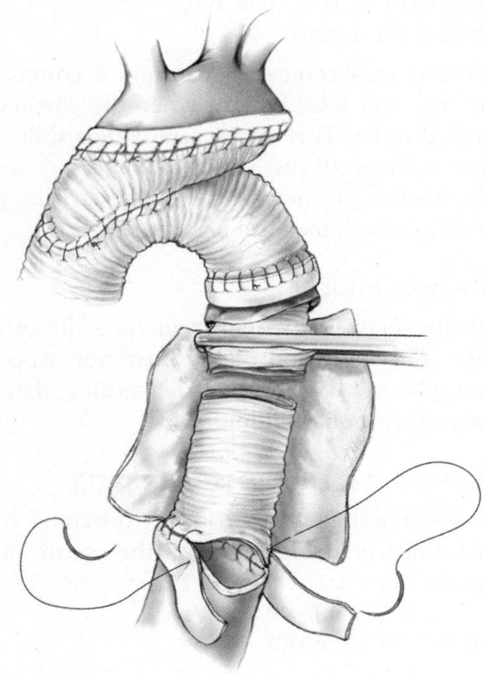

FIG. 8.28 Completing the descending aortic replacement after an elephant-trunk procedure.

NB Perfusion of Upper Body

Rarely, one may encounter a situation while on left heart bypass in which the descending aortic aneurysm has been opened, only to note that the appropriate proximal margin of resection is indeed beyond the proximal clamp within the arch of the aorta. This necessitates total circulatory arrest. As retrograde perfusion through the femoral artery cannot perfuse the head and the upper part of the body with the thoracic aorta cross-clamped, the ascending aorta needs to be cannulated separately. This can be performed quite easily through the standard left thoracotomy, especially when the heart is decompressed on left heart bypass. Otherwise, the thoracotomy incision is extended medially to provide adequate exposure. It is important for the surgeon and the perfusionist to communicate and choreograph the conduct of the procedure to ensure adequate perfusion of both the lower and upper parts of the body. When the continuity of the aorta has been reestablished, further perfusion and rewarming can be achieved through the femoral or preferably the aortic cannula. NB

NB Circulatory Arrest and Antegrade Cerebral Protection

During cooling for circulatory arrest, the left subclavian artery is isolated. A small side-biting vascular clamp is applied and a 1 cm longitudinal arteriotomy is made. An 8-mm Hemashield Dacron tube graft is sutured to the left subclavian artery in an end-to-side manner using 5-0 Prolene suture. When circulatory arrest commences, the left subclavian artery is clamped proximally and perfused distally at a pressure of 50 to 60 mm Hg. Antegrade cerebral perfusion through the left vertebral artery and the Circle of Willis is confirmed by the backflow coming out of the left carotid and innominate arteries. NB

NB Connection of the True with the False Distal Lumen

It is of utmost importance to maintain a connection between the true and false lumens when the chronic dissection extends distally. This entails removing a short segment of the intima flap wall just distal to the distal anastomosis. In this manner, all the aortic branches arising from the false as well as true lumen are perfused. NB

⊘ Esophageal Injury

Deep suturing may inadvertently include the esophagus. Transection and dissection of the posterior aspect of the aorta allow precise placement of the sutures, thereby preventing possible esophageal injury. ⊘

⊘ Hypertension from Cross-Clamping

Aortic cross-clamping often produces proximal hypertension, which must be controlled with the use of antihypertensive agents. ⊘

⊘ Spinal Cord Ischemia

A significant decrease in distal perfusion pressure can occasionally result in paraplegia. This is a grave complication that should be prevented using all available means. Many techniques, including partial bypass from the left atrium or pulmonary artery to the femoral artery, or the femoral vein to the femoral artery have been employed with some success. Heparin-bonded tubes for left-sided heart bypass have also been used. However, it appears that keeping the time of aortic cross-clamping short provides the best protection against the development of paralysis. ⊘

Drainage of Cerebrospinal Fluid

Clamping of the descending aorta causes a significant decrease in distal perfusion pressure, including that to the spinal arteries. Conversely, there is resultant hypertension proximal to the clamp. This produces engorgement of the intracranial structures and increases in cerebrospinal fluid pressure, which may contribute to spinal cord ischemia. Although there are no definite data to support the beneficial effect of reducing cerebrospinal fluid pressure, it has been our practice to drain the cerebrospinal fluid in the operating room and continue drainage for the first 1 or 2 days postoperatively, maintaining a pressure of approximately 10 mm Hg.

NB Spinal Cord Protection Techniques

Spinal cord function can be monitored during the time when the aorta is clamped. Monitoring somatosensory evoked potentials entails stimulating the posterior tibial nerve and recording its response in the cerebral cortex. Although many centers use this monitoring technique, its clinical pertinence has not been fully established. NB

ENDOVASCULAR REPAIR OF DESCENDING THORACIC AORTIC ANEURYSMS

Open surgical repair of descending thoracic aortic aneurysms can be performed safely in great majority of patients. Distal perfusion using extracorporeal circulation, multiple spinal cord protection techniques, and reimplantation of the selected intercostals arteries have resulted in improved outcomes. However, a left thoracotomy incision and cross-clamping of the thoracic aorta constitute a highly invasive approach. The reported cumulative morbidity associated with open surgical repair exceeds 50%. Most patients may need a recovery time of 4 to 6 months to return to full functionality. Furthermore, a significant number of patients with comorbid conditions are deemed to be at a prohibitive risk for open repair and are denied surgery. Therefore, endovascular repair of descending thoracic aortic aneurysms is an attractive approach.

Candidates for endovascular repair should have an inner aortic diameter of 23 to 37 mm adjacent to the aneurysm without significant thrombus or calcification in these so-called landing zones. They should have at least 2 cm of normal aorta both proximal and distal to the aneurysm to ensure adequate fixation of the device (Fig. 8.29). A number of endografts are now commercially available and able to accommodate various neck geometries and angulation.

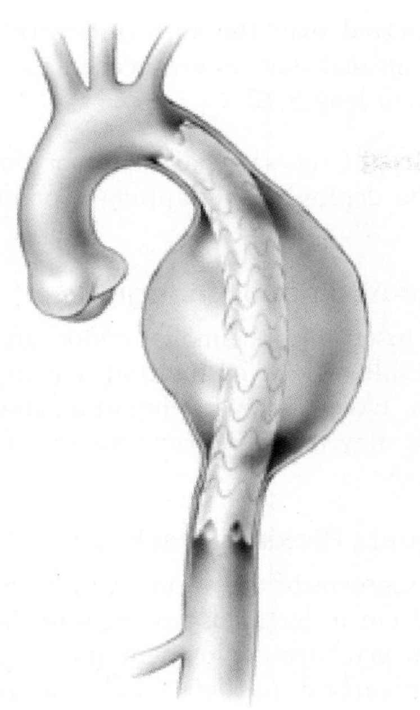

FIG. 8.29 Endograft with adequate distal and proximal fixation.

⊘ Type I Endoleak

With poor fixation, a type I endoleak of the aneurysm may be encountered. An aneurysm with the type I endoleak is considered untreated. Type I endoleaks may occasionally be treated with balloon dilation of the fixation segments. But more frequently, deployment of proximal or distal extension cuffs is required to exclude the aneurysm completely. ⊘

NB Correct Sizing of the Endograft

Endografting of the descending thoracic aorta requires preoperative measurements of the diameter of the proximal and distal necks of the aneurysm, treatment length, and proximal and distal angulation. This information can be obtained from computed tomographic angiography using three-dimensional reconstruction (Fig. 8.30). Center-line distances should be used to estimate the length of prosthesis that is required. Undersizing of the endograft will result in poor fixation, endoleak, or migration of the device. Excessive oversizing of the graft may cause crimping and occlusion of the graft or aortic injury and rupture. NB

Technique

The procedure is performed in a surgical or angiography suite equipped with a fluoroscopy machine. Most patients are placed under general endotracheal anesthesia. Most endovascular devices can be inserted through a 20, 22, or 24 French sheath. The size of the sheath is determined on the basis of the device size. The preoperative computed tomography images with contrast should include the abdomen and pelvis to assess the femoral and iliac arteries for size, tortuosity, and calcification. A 24 French sheath has an outer diameter of approximately 9 mm. If the femoral arteries cannot accommodate the intended sheath, a Dacron

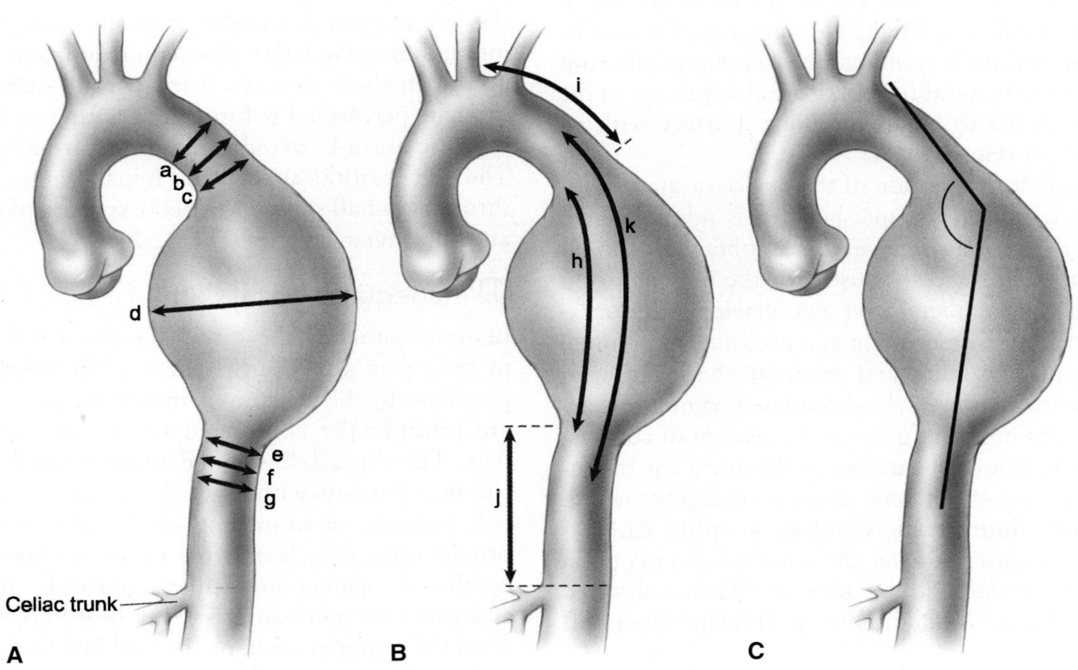

FIG. 8.30 Required preoperative measurements of the diameters, lengths, and angulation of the descending thoracic aorta. (From the GORE TAG training manual.)

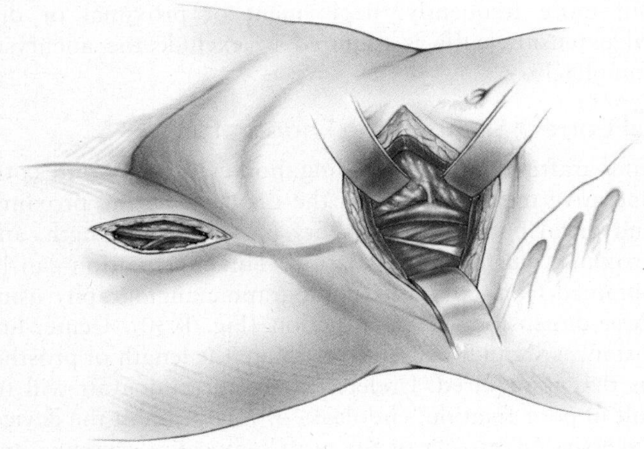

FIG. 8.31 Surgical exposure of the terminal aorta, common, internal, and external iliac arteries through a flank incision.

conduit should be anastomosed to the iliac artery for the insertion of sheath. This anastomosis can be performed through a small flank incision (Fig. 8.31).

⊘ Iliac Artery Injury

If a sheath larger than the external iliac artery diameter is inserted, iliac artery injury can occur. This injury is usually manifested upon withdrawal of the sheath after deployment of the device. The iliac artery injury and massive retroperitoneal bleeding will present as severe hypotension. If guidewire access is maintained, a balloon occlusion catheter (CODA balloon, Cook, Bloomington, IN) can be quickly passed into the terminal aorta to temporarily stop the bleeding. An ipsilateral retroperitoneal approach to the iliac artery is needed to repair the injured artery with an interposition graft (Fig. 8.31). ⊘

In general, before insertion of the device or anastomosis of an iliac conduit, systemic heparin is administered. A contralateral femoral artery access is obtained using a 5 French sheath. This access is used for the insertion of a pigtail arteriography catheter over a guidewire. Arteriography of the aortic arch, descending and proximal abdominal aorta is performed to mark and roadmap the location of the arch and mesenteric vessels. Adequate imaging and arteriography of the aorta require rapid injection of contrast using a power injector. The access to the aorta for the insertion of the device is obtained using an exchange length guidewire under fluoroscopic control. A utility catheter (Glide catheter) is inserted over the guidewire to maintain access. The large sheath with the tapered dilator is inserted over a stiff guidewire (Lunderquist or Amplatz super stiff guidewire).

NB All guidewire, catheter, and sheath insertions must be performed under fluoroscopic control to avoid false passages and intimal injury. Under fluoroscopic control, the device is inserted over the stiff guidewire and deployed. Usually, additional devices are needed to achieve the desired treatment length. NB

NB Endografts of the same diameter or one to two sizes larger can be deployed overlapping a previously inserted graft. NB

⊘ Sizing of Additional Endografts

Inadvertent insertion of a smaller endograft inside a larger graft will result in lack of fixation and migration of the smaller graft. Excessive oversizing of an endograft inside a smaller graft may result in crimping and occlusion of the larger graft. ⊘

NB Inadequate Proximal Neck

If a normal segment of the aorta 23 to 37 mm in diameter of at least 2 cm in length is not present distal to the left subclavian artery, then deployment in the arch between the left common carotid and left subclavian arteries may be considered. NB

⊘ Occlusion of Subclavian Artery

In general, occlusion of the left subclavian artery with the endovascular graft may be well tolerated without adjunctive procedures. However, there are patients who are dependent on antegrade subclavian blood flow. These include patients with a diminutive right vertebral artery and a dominant left vertebral artery who would be at risk for a posterior cerebral vascular accident. Patients who have previously undergone coronary artery bypass grafting of the left anterior descending coronary artery using the left internal thoracic artery also require a patent left subclavian artery. In these patients, a left carotid–subclavian bypass must be performed before endografting of the descending thoracic aorta to avoid cerebral or cardiac complications. The left carotid–subclavian bypass may be performed through a small supraclavicular exposure of the left carotid and subclavian arteries (Fig. 8.32). ⊘

NB Inadequate Distal Cuff

In some patients, the distal aneurysm extension is close to the celiac artery such that a 2 cm length of the aorta proximal to the celiac axis in not present. These patients are traditionally considered for a thoracoabdominal repair. The thoracoabdominal repair should be considered for most patients with low risk for open surgery. In higher risk patients, de-branching of the abdominal aorta may provide adequate length for endovascular repair. In this combined open-endovascular approach, the celiac and superior mesenteric arteries may be bypassed using grafts from the terminal aorta or the iliac arteries. These patients still require a transperitoneal abdominal or retroperitoneal approach to the abdominal aorta. After rerouting of the mesenteric vessels, the thoracic portion of the aorta can be repaired using an endograft. This approach obviates the

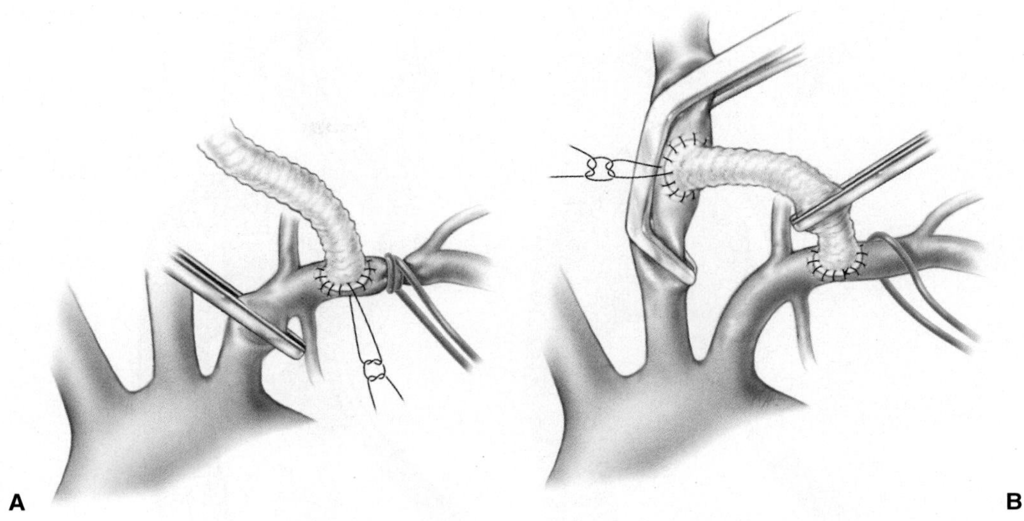

FIG. 8.32 Supraclavicular exposure and completion of a left carotid–subclavian artery bypass.

need for a combined thoracic and abdominal incision and cross-clamping of the aorta. NB

NB Patients at High Risk for Spinal Ischemia

Some patients may have previously undergone repair of abdominal aortic aneurysms or may have occlusion of the internal iliac arteries. Other patients may have extensive aneurysms from the proximal arch to the level of the diaphragm requiring multiple overlapping endografts. These patients have been found to be at increased risk for spinal cord ischemia after endovascular repair of thoracic aortic aneurysms. Occlusion of the left subclavian artery with the endovascular graft may exacerbate this risk due to compromise of the vertebral artery as a collateral to the anterior spinal artery. In these patients, insertion of a lumbar drain preoperatively may reduce the risk. In addition to the lumbar drain, avoiding intraoperative and postoperative hypotension is an important consideration to maintain spinal perfusion. NB

NB Endoleaks

Some aneurysms maintain continuity with the circulation after placement of endovascular grafts. These endoleaks may be recognized at the time of treatment on the completion angiogram of the aorta. Frequently, the endoleaks are recognized on follow-up imaging such as computed tomography with contrast. Depending on the type and location of the endoleaks, various therapeutic options may be available. NB

Type I leak is the most commonly encountered type, and involves a leak from the proximal or distal fixation site. Treatment is usually successful with the placement of a graft extension cuff.

Type II leaks occur from side-branch vessels such as intercostal or lumbar arteries that continue to remain patent in the aneurysm sac. They are generally treated with catheter-based coil embolization.

Type III leaks result from a tear in the graft, attachment of the modular grafts, graft disconnection, or graft disintegration. These should be treated routinely, usually with additional endografts within the old graft.

Type IV occurs when blood leaks through the suture holes between the graft material and the metal stent. If persistent, treatment involves the insertion of a covered stent-graft (endograft) inside the original graft.

Type V or endotension refers to the expansion of the aneurysm despite treatment without any documented leak into the aneurysm sac, potentially through the graft fabric. If the aneurysm continues to expand, redo endografting may be performed.

The patients who have undergone endovascular repair of thoracic aortic aneurysms are followed up closely with serial computed tomography of the chest, abdomen, and pelvis. Routinely, after an uneventful repair, the first postoperative scan is obtained 2 to 4 weeks after surgery and annually thereafter. The follow-up computed tomographic scans with contrast are carefully examined. All postoperative type I and type III endoleaks should be treated. Type II endoleaks (patent intercostal arteries) in general may be observed if there is no expansion of the aneurysm. Persistent type II endoleaks may be treated with embolization of the culprit patent intercostal artery.

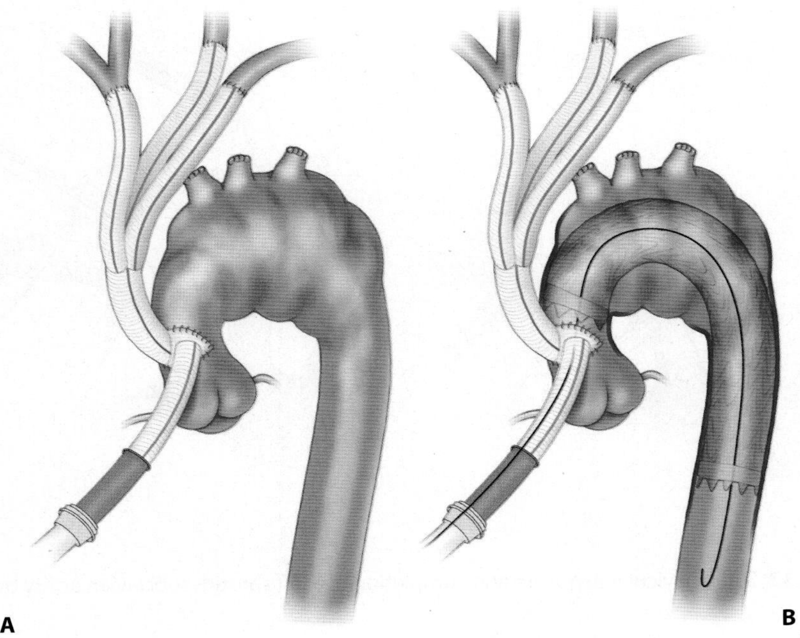

FIG. 8.33 Debranching of the aortic arch. **A:** The distal ends of graft limbs are anastomosed to the left subclavian, the common carotid, and the innominate arteries. **B:** The stent-graft is deployed.

ENDOVASCULAR REPAIR OF AORTIC ARCH ANEURYSM

In patients who are at high operative risk with open surgical repair of aortic arch and circulatory arrest, an endovascular approach (debranching procedure) may be considered. In this combined open-endovascular procedure, the innominate, left carotid and left subclavian arteries are bypassed using a graft(s) from the ascending aorta. The aneurysmal aortic arch is then stented with occlusion of the origin of the head vessels.

Technique

A number of debranching techniques and modifications are now available depending on the aortic pathology. All include diversion of blood flow to the head vessels followed by endovascular coverage of the diseased aorta and coverage of the origin of the head vessels. The operation can be performed without the use of cardiopulmonary bypass through a median sternotomy. In cases when the ascending aorta is not diseased, a side-biting clamp is placed on the mid-ascending aorta. An anastomosis is performed to the main body of a bifurcated or trifurcated graft. The distal anastomoses are performed to the left subclavian, the common carotid and the innominate arteries individually (Fig. 8.33A). These can be performed in an end-to-end or end-to-side fashion. Finally, a stent-graft is deployed either antegrade through the branched graft or retrograde through the femoral vessels as described previously (Fig. 8.33B).

NB Inaccessible Left Subclavian Artery

In cases when the left subclavian artery is difficult to mobilize, a left carotid–subclavian bypass is performed through a separate supraclavicular approach (Fig. 8.32). NB

NB Inadequate Length of Ascending Aorta

If a limited amount of aorta is available between the sinotubular junction and the take-off of head vessels, cardiopulmonary bypass with aortic cross clamping should be utilized. NB

If the ascending aorta is diseased and needs to be replaced (porcelain arota or severe atherosclerotic disease), a hybrid approach to the aorta may reduce the period of circulatory arrest and the complexity of the operation. In these operations, cardiopulmonary bypass is initiated in a standard manner using axillary or distal arch aortic cannulation. After cooling and application of the cross clamp, the ascending aorta is reconstructed using a 4-branched graft (Fig. 8.34A). After adequate cooling, a period of circulatory arrest is initiated, usually with the use of antegrade or retrograde cerebral perfusion. The head vessels are dissected and the distal end of the dacron graft is attached to

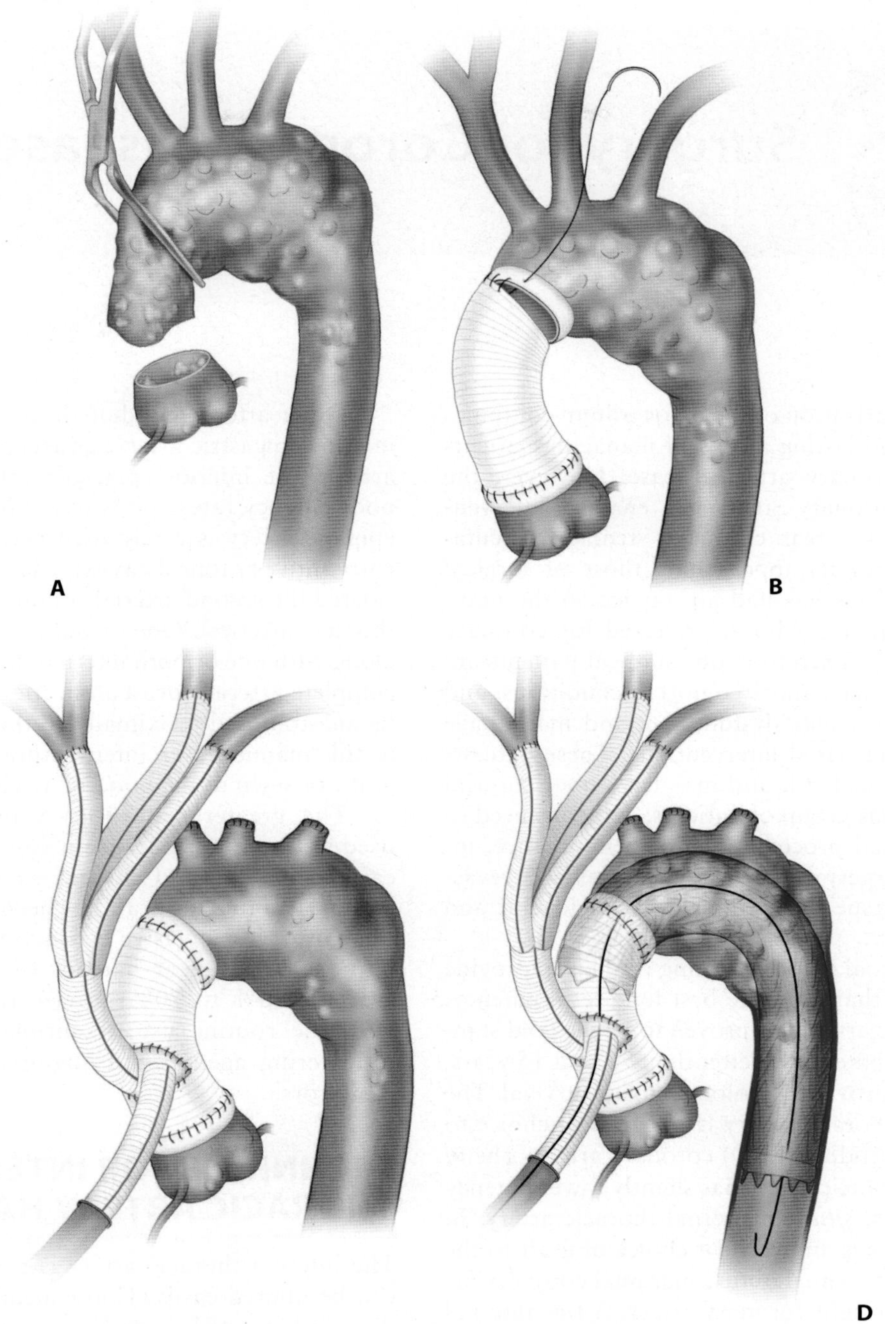

FIG. 8.34 Replacement of ascending aorta and debranching of aortic arch. **A:** Proximal anastomosis of the aortic graft. **B:** Distal anastomosis of the aortic graft, under circulatory arrest. **C:** Head vessels are attached to the limbs. **D:** Deployment of the stent-graft.

the aortic arch (Fig. 8.34B). Now circulation is established through the 4th limb of the graft and the individual head vessels are attached to the graft branches (Fig. 8.34C). Each branch is de-aired and unclamped before the next head vessel anastomosis. The origins of the head vessels can now be stapled. This is then followed by warming, separation from bypass, and finally stent-graft deployment through the 4th limb of the graft (Fig. 8.34D).

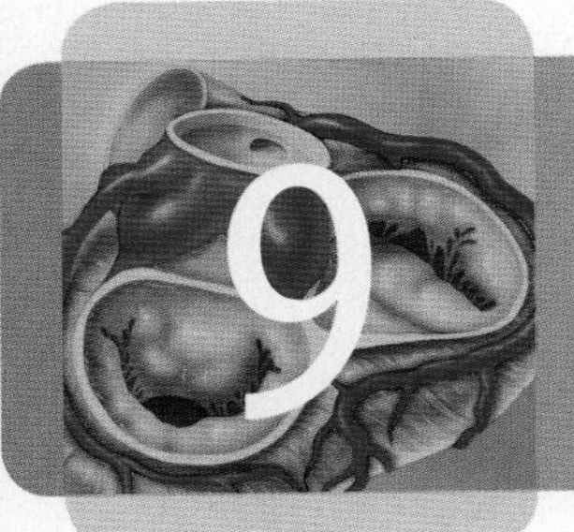

9 Surgery for Coronary Disease

Surgery for revascularization of the myocardium continues to be an effective and lasting means of managing patients with multivessel coronary artery disease. However, the evolution of intracoronary stents has enabled interventional cardiologists to treat coronary stenoses percutaneously with early results approaching those of surgical bypass procedures. This has had an impact on the number and types of patients who are referred for coronary artery bypass surgery. Therefore, our surgical patients are now generally older, have more comorbid conditions, and more severe left ventricular dysfunction, and many have had previous catheter-based interventions. These patients are at increased surgical risk and may have poor surgical targets. To handle this group of patients, surgeons need to incorporate additional procedures into their practice, including off-pump surgery and transmyocardial laser revascularization, and pursue such strategies as angiogenic and cell-based technology.

Ultimately, the goal in the operating room is to provide patients with grafts that have the best long-term patency. The internal thoracic artery has proven to be the gold standard of conduits. Its patency is better than 90% at 15 years, and its use has been proven to prolong patient survival. The *in situ* left internal thoracic artery is the graft of choice to the left anterior descending (LAD) coronary artery. The *in situ* right internal thoracic artery has slightly lower patency compared with the *in situ* left internal thoracic artery. In younger patients, this is an excellent choice of graft to the ramus intermedius, proximal obtuse marginal coronary artery, or mid to distal right coronary artery. A free internal thoracic artery graft has a lower patency rate than an *in situ* graft.

⊘ Right Coronary Artery Ischemia

If the right coronary artery is dominant and of good size, the right internal thoracic artery flow may be inadequate. ⊘

⊘ Sternal Complications

Bilateral internal thoracic arteries should be avoided in patients with insulin-dependent diabetes because of increased sternal complications. ⊘

Other arterial conduits have been used, including the inferior epigastric artery, gastroepiploic artery, and radial artery. The inferior epigastric artery was found to have poor patency rates and is used rarely if at all. The gastroepiploic artery is rarely used because its harvest requires entry into peritoneal cavity. The radial artery is now considered the second arterial conduit of choice (after internal thoracic arteries). One or both radial arteries can be used along with one or both internal thoracic arteries to provide complete arterial revascularization. The radial artery may be anastomosed proximally to the aorta, sewn in an end-to-side manner to an internal thoracic artery to create a Y graft, or sewn to the hood of a vein graft.

The greater saphenous vein has been extensively used as a conduit because it can be quickly procured, is easy to handle, and ensures excellent inflow. Renewed enthusiasm for this graft has been generated by the development of less invasive endoscopic vein-harvesting techniques. The 10-year patency of greater saphenous vein grafts is 60% to 70%; however, this may be improved with the routine use of antiplatelet agents, cholesterol-lowering agents, and angiotensin-converting enzyme inhibitors.

TECHNIQUE FOR INTERNAL THORACIC ARTERY HARVEST

The internal thoracic artery is a very delicate vessel that can be injured easily. Consequently, the artery should be dissected as a pedicle with great care.

A median sternotomy is made in the usual manner. The parietal pleura and pericardium are depressed gently, and the course of the internal thoracic artery is identified from its origin near the first rib to its termination beyond its bifurcation in the rectus sheath. A Favaloro retractor provides excellent exposure. The Rultract System retractor also provides superb exposure and is probably less traumatic. The posterior rectus sheath is freed from the undersurface of the sternum and costal cartilages, allowing more extensive retraction with improved exposure of the internal thoracic artery.

⊘ Injury to the Ribs and Costochondral Junction

Overzealous elevation of the hemisternum by retractors may result in rib fractures or even costochondral disruption. This is more apt to occur in patients with pectus deformities or morbid obesity and in elderly patients with osteoporosis. ⊘

Although it is possible to dissect the internal thoracic artery without entering the pleural cavity, we prefer to routinely open the left pleura widely to provide excellent exposure and greatly facilitate harvesting of the internal thoracic artery.

NB Opening the pleura allows the left internal thoracic artery pedicle to fall away from midline. This decreases the risk of injury at reoperation. NB

Alternatively, the left internal thoracic artery can be harvested through a lower ministernotomy, dividing the left half of the sternum (see Chapter 1). A Favaloro retractor allows the left hemisternum to be elevated to provide adequate exposure for mobilizing the internal thoracic artery. This approach allows off-pump bypass grafting of the left internal thoracic artery to the LAD coronary artery (see subsequent text).

The internal thoracic artery is usually harvested as a pedicle with extensive use of electrocautery for chest wall hemostasis but not pedicle hemostasis. The parietal pleura on the internal intercostal musculofascial layer of the chest wall is incised approximately 7 to 10 mm medial to the internal thoracic artery along its entire course (Fig. 9.1). The blade of the electrocautery is then used to depress and dissect the pedicle from the chest wall. The lowest current is used to coagulate the internal thoracic artery and vein branches, well away from the parent trunks. The side branches on the artery are then occluded with fine metal clips. The pedicle is dissected from the level of the rectus sheath to the level of the subclavian vein where the artery passes beneath this vessel. Care is taken to identify and divide two intercostal branches, one passing anterior to the subclavian vein and a high first intercostal branch coursing laterally above the subclavian vein.

⊘ Unstable Hemodynamics

When the patient's condition is unstable, it may be preferable to harvest the internal thoracic artery while the patient is on cardiopulmonary bypass. ⊘

⊘ Injury to the Internal Thoracic Artery

Because the internal thoracic artery is a delicate structure, any undue stretching, clamping, or misplaced metal clips results in permanent vascular injury and therefore unsatisfactory short- and long-term results. Excessive traction during mobilization should be avoided as it can lead to dissection of the vessel wall. ⊘

⊘ Heat Injury

When an electrocautery is used to divide the internal thoracic artery branches after application of metal clips, the heat and the electric current may conduct through the metal clip adjacent to the parent trunk and cause a burn injury. Therefore, branches must be divided with scissors or coagulated well away from the metal clip adjacent to the internal thoracic artery. ⊘

⊘ Maximal Length of the Internal Thoracic Artery

The internal thoracic artery pedicle must be dissected free from the chest wall along its entire course, from near its origin in the first intercostal space to well past its bifurcation into the rectus sheath to provide maximal length. ⊘

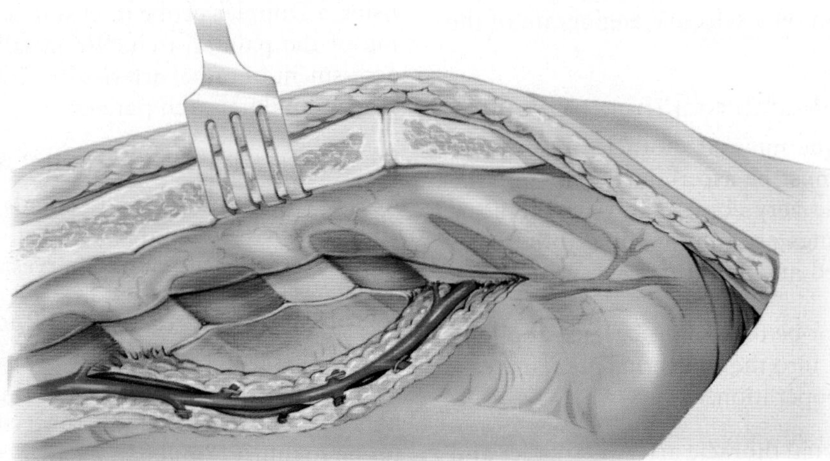

FIG. 9.1 Harvesting an internal thoracic artery.

⊘ Internal Thoracic Steal Syndrome

The first intercostal branch of the internal thoracic artery must be identified and divided to avoid any possible steal phenomenon from the internal thoracic flow. ⊘

Before commencing cardiopulmonary bypass, papaverine is sprayed gently over the pedicle and the adequacy of flow is determined. If there is no flow, a 1-mm vascular probe (Parsonnet) is cautiously introduced into the lumen of the vessel for a varying distance. This should be done with extreme care to avoid intimal injury. Usually, very good flow is noted. Unless traumatized during harvesting, the internal thoracic artery usually provides adequate flow and should not be discarded.

NB In elderly patients, it may be preferable to skeletonize the internal thoracic artery rather than harvesting it as a pedicle. This may decrease the incidence of avascular necrosis and infection affecting the sternum. NB

The pedicle is laid on the heart to judge the appropriate length. The end of the pedicle is then grasped and occluded with forceps, allowing the internal thoracic artery to distend with blood. The artery is then cleaned free of the surrounding tissues, using sharp dissection. The artery is transected obliquely with the heel on the fascial side of the pedicle and prepared as a large-hood orifice.

NB The internal thoracic artery can be lengthened considerably with multiple pedicle fasciotomies. Maximal length can be obtained by skeletonizing the vessel along its course. Division of the internal thoracic veins should be avoided when performing the fasciotomies. If the pedicle remains too short, the artery may be divided proximally and used as a free graft. NB

⊘ String Sign

Excessive stretch and tension on the internal thoracic artery result in narrowing of the lumen and graft failure. This is seen as a string sign on a selective angiogram of the artery. ⊘

⊘ Optimal Length of the Internal Thoracic Pedicle

Before the distal end of the internal thoracic artery is divided, its correct length must be ascertained. The internal thoracic pedicle should lie very comfortably on the heart when it is full and the lungs are fully inflated; otherwise, the artery will be stretched and could become detached at the anastomotic site. ⊘

Similarly, it should not be redundant because too long a pedicle may curl or kink into the substernal area, increasing the risk of injury at reoperation.

NB The caliber of the internal thoracic artery is smaller and resistance to flow is higher the longer the pedicle is. A tortuous internal thoracic artery course makes later catheter intervention difficult. NB

⊘ Clot Formation within the Internal Thoracic Artery

The internal thoracic artery, when fully mobilized and divided, is occluded with an atraumatic bulldog clamp after the patient has been fully heparinized to prevent any clotting within the lumen of the vessel. ⊘

NB Incising the Pericardium for Bypass Grafting to the Circumflex Coronary Artery

The pericardium is divided with electrocautery where the internal thoracic artery pedicle crosses it down to 1 cm above the left phrenic nerve. This allows the pedicle to assume a more lateral position and lie against the medial surface of the lung instead of coursing over the apex of the lung. This is especially important when the left internal thoracic artery is grafted to an obtuse marginal branch of the circumflex coronary artery. NB

NB Course of the Right Internal Thoracic Artery

An *in situ* right internal thoracic artery can easily reach the diagonal, ramus intermedius or a proximal obtuse marginal branch of the circumflex coronary artery. The pedicle should cross the distal ascending aorta near the innominate vein. Thymic tissue and fat can be used to cover the pedicle. If the right internal thoracic artery is grafted to the LAD coronary artery, its course will be across the more proximal aspect of the ascending aorta, which puts it at high risk of injury during reoperative procedures. NB

TECHNIQUE FOR RADIAL ARTERY HARVEST

Usually, the nondominant arm is identified preoperatively for radial artery harvest. Intravenous catheters and venipunctures are avoided in this arm. Allen test is performed using a Doppler probe to ensure adequate ulnar artery filling of the palmar arch. We usually perform preoperative assessment of radial arteries by ultrasound and Doppler for size and palmar arch patency.

⊘ Calcification of the Radial Artery

The distal portion of the radial artery tends to calcify. Unless the extra length is needed, the most distal segment of the artery should not be harvested and left *in situ.* ⊘

⊘ Injury to the Superficial Radial Nerve

The superficial radial nerve provides cutaneous innervation to the radial aspect of the thumb and dorsum of the hand. It follows the middle third of the radial artery and is prone to injury. Similarly, excessive lateral retraction of the brachioradialis muscle may lead to injury to this nerve and resultant numbness of the thumb. This may occur in 5% to 10% of the patients undergoing radial artery harvest. ⊘

NB Preventing Radial Artery Spasm

The graft is gently flushed with heparinized blood and papaverine after harvesting. In addition, we routinely use intravenous nitrates or calcium channel blockers intraoperatively as well as postoperatively until the patient can tolerate oral medications. Most patients with free arterial grafts will be discharged with oral isosorbide dinitrates. NB

Endoscopic Radial Artery Harvest

In the operating room, the arm is abducted to 90 degrees. Under sterile conditions, the arm is prepared and draped on an armboard. A sterile blood pressure cuff is placed around the upper arm and connected to a sphygmomanometer. In addition, a small roll is placed under the wrist to hyperextend the hand. A 1-in. longitudinal incision is made over the radial artery distally, such that it will be covered with the sleeve of a shirt (Fig. 9.2A). Under direct vision, the radial artery is dissected for a short distance proximally and distally. The blood pressure cuff is inflated to 20 mm above the patient's systolic blood pressure. The endoscope is inserted through the incision while the tunnel is being insufflated. The tissue plane under the radial artery is dissected first, followed by circumferential mobilization. The branches are freed gently for a sufficient length so that cautery can be applied without injury to the radial artery wall. The dissector is then replaced with scissors equipped with cautery to divide all side branches (Fig. 9.2B). A counter incision at the elbow is made, and the proximal end of the radial artery is divided and controlled. Alternatively, an endoloop can be advanced through the tunnel and proximal control can be obtained. The latter technique avoids the counter incision. After removal of the radial artery from the tunnel, metal clips are applied to the branches (Fig. 9.2C). The distal radial artery is ligated and divided. Under endoscopic visualization, the blood pressure cuff is deflated and optimal hemostasis is ensured. The wrist incision is closed in two layers and a sterile pressure dressing is applied. The radial artery is irrigated with heparinized saline. Papaverine may be sprayed on the pedicle to prevent spasm.

Open Radial Artery Harvest

The arm is abducted to 90 degrees and under sterile conditions prepared and draped on an armboard. An incision is made in the midportion of the forearm over the belly of the brachioradialis muscle. The opening is then extended for a variable distance proximally toward the groove between the brachioradialis and biceps tendon (Fig. 9.3). Distally, the incision is extended toward the wrist crease. With experience, the opening in the forearm can be fairly limited in length and still allow adequate exposure to harvest the radial artery.

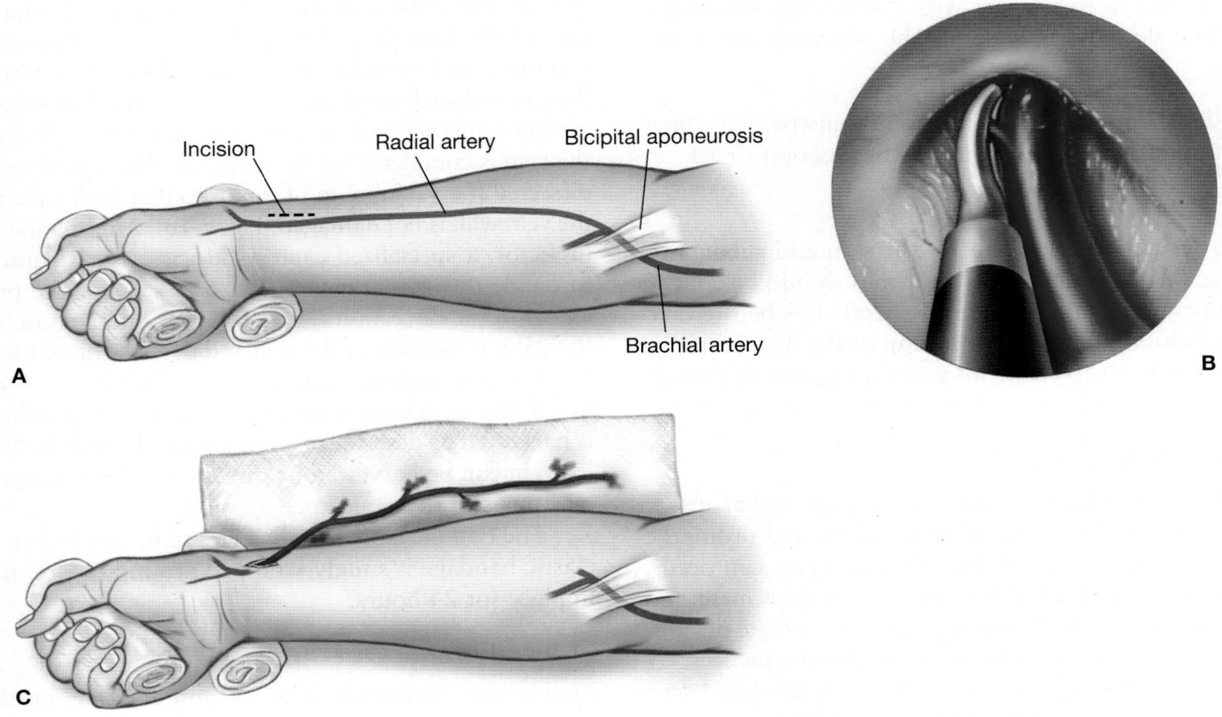

FIG. 9.2 A–C: Endoscopic harvesting of radial artery.

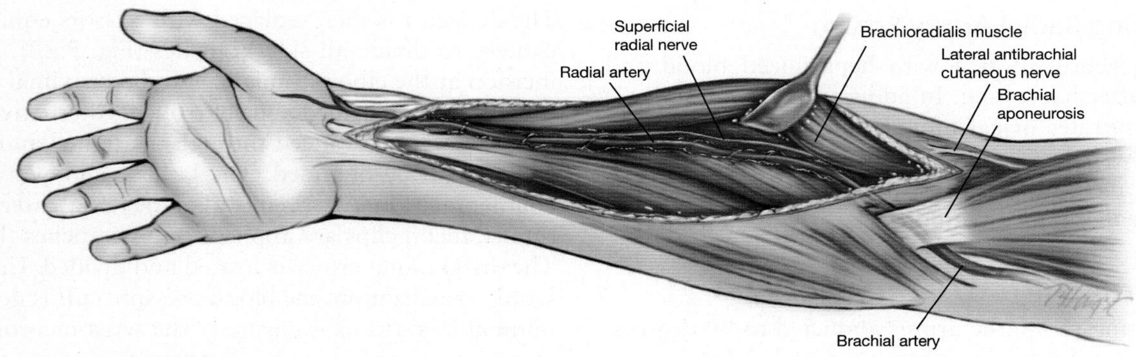

FIG. 9.3 Open harvesting of radial artery.

The dissection of the radial artery begins distally by dividing the fascia and then proceeding proximally between the belly of the brachioradialis and flexor carpi-radialis muscles. A vessel loop is then passed around the radial artery to facilitate exposure. The artery is dissected along with the two venae comitantes, double clipping and sharply dividing all the branches. When the radial artery is completely mobilized, the radial recurrent artery is identified proximally and the superficial palmar artery is seen distally. These two large branches define the limits of the dissection and should be preserved (Fig. 9.3). The radial artery is divided distally and proximally and placed in a solution of heparinized blood and papaverine. The arm incision is closed in two layers with continuous absorbable suture. The deep layer includes the subcutaneous tissue distally.

NB The distal limit of the skin incision should be 3 cm above the wrist joint to decrease postoperative discomfort. NB

⊘ Hematoma Formation

An electrocautery is used only on the skin and subcutaneous tissue. All the radial artery branches should be clipped proximally and distally with small metal clips before division. In addition, the proximal stump of the divided radial artery should be oversewn with a suture ligature to prevent late bleeding and hematoma formation. ⊘

⊘ Compartment Syndrome

Compartment syndrome occurs rarely after radial artery harvest. However, if not recognized and treated promptly, extensive muscle loss and distal ischemic injury can occur. The hand must be checked for unrestricted movement and intact sensation at routine intervals in the immediate postoperative period to prevent such devastating consequences. ⊘

The distal end of the radial artery is dissected free of the accompanying veins and surrounding tissue. An oblique opening is created, which can be enlarged to match the coronary artery opening by making a short longitudinal incision at the heel.

TECHNIQUES FOR GREATER SAPHENOUS VEIN HARVEST

Traditional open vein harvesting through one long incision or multiple interrupted incisions can result in significant wound morbidity, including infection and chronic leg edema. The endoscopic approach avoids the healing problems associated with a long leg incision and may, in particular, benefit patients with diabetes, obesity, or peripheral vascular disease.

Endoscopic Saphenous Vein Harvest

A 2-cm transverse incision is made just above the medial aspect of the knee (Fig. 9.4A). The greater saphenous vein is identified and encircled with a vessel loop. An endoscope is then introduced using carbon dioxide insufflation to dissect a plane superficial to the vein. Circumferential dissection of the vein is completed by the dissector. The side branches are dissected for a minimum of 5 mm so that with cauterization the vein wall is not damaged (Fig. 9.4B). After removal of the dissector, a specialized cautery device/scissors is introduced to divide the side branches (Fig. 9.4C). Once the proximal extent of the dissection is reached, a counterincision is made to facilitate division of the vein and oversewing of the stump. The vein is then gently withdrawn through the knee incision.

If two vein graft segments are required, the thigh vein is harvested as described. For additional conduit, the lower leg vein can be harvested by directing the endoscope inferiorly through the same knee incision.

The two incisions are then closed in two layers, and an elastic bandage is snugly wrapped around the leg and kept in place for 24 hours.

⊘ Intraluminal Clot

Endoscopic dissection with carbon dioxide insufflation causes vein compression and can lead to stasis of blood flow. Heparin should be administered intravenously before endoscopic vein harvest to prevent intraluminal thrombus formation. ⊘

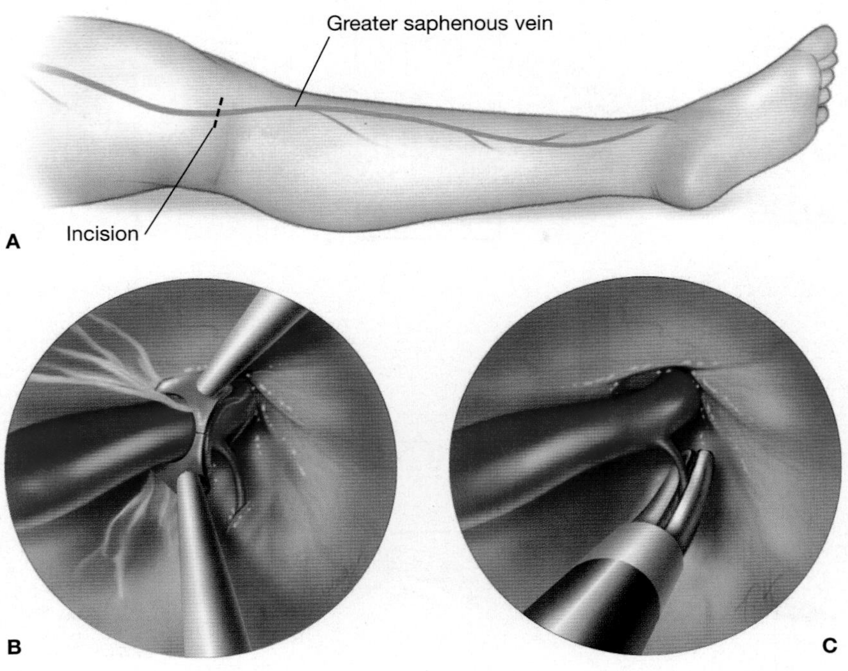

FIG. 9.4 **A–C:** Endoscopic harvesting of greater saphenous vein.

⊘ Hematoma Formation

Hemostasis must be meticulously achieved using an electrocautery to avoid the development of a hematoma. If a large area of dead space has been created by the dissection, a soft drain connected to a closed drainage system should be placed along the endoscopic tract and left in place for at least 24 hours. ⊘

⊘ Traction Injury to the Vein

Excessive traction on the vein to mobilize it and withdraw it from the endoscopic tract can lead to intimal injury and avulsed branches. This must be avoided by extensive dissection with the cautery device and endoscopic scissors. ⊘

The learning curve for using endoscopic equipment is significant. With experience, it adds little time to the overall operation. Endoscopic vein harvesting is our procedure of choice when two or more vein conduits are required.

Open Greater Saphenous Vein Harvest

An incision is made in the groin, one fingerbreadth medial to the femoral artery pulse. The subcutaneous tissue is dissected to expose the greater saphenous vein as it curves to pierce the cribriform fascia of the femoral sheath and join the femoral vein. The skin incision is then extended downward along the course of the vein. The incision can alternatively be started at the ankle, anterior to the medial malleolus, and extended upward. Many surgeons consider this approach convenient and elect to use it routinely.

The vein is harvested using the "no touch" technique. This entails handling of the vein only by its adventitia with an atraumatic vascular forceps. The vein is then gently removed from its bed by careful dissection and division of its branches.

⊘ Skin Infection or Ulceration

Harvesting veins from limbs with evidence of infection or ulceration should be avoided if possible. ⊘

⊘ Accidental Division of the Vein

With the aid of a pair of sharp scissors, the skin incision is extended over the surgeon's index finger, which has tunneled above and parallel to the saphenous vein. This technique prevents accidental division of a more superficially placed saphenous vein and eliminates the development of unnecessary dead spaces or redundant skin flaps. ⊘

⊘ Nerve Injury

The saphenous nerve runs a course along the greater saphenous vein. Special care should be taken not to divide it to avoid postoperative paresthesia. ⊘

⊘ Skin Incision along the Knee

The incision alongside the knee joint is subjected to much strain and stretch in several directions as the joint moves. This may give the patient significant discomfort and interferes with satisfactory healing. Therefore, the skin in this location is usually left intact (Fig. 9.5). ⊘

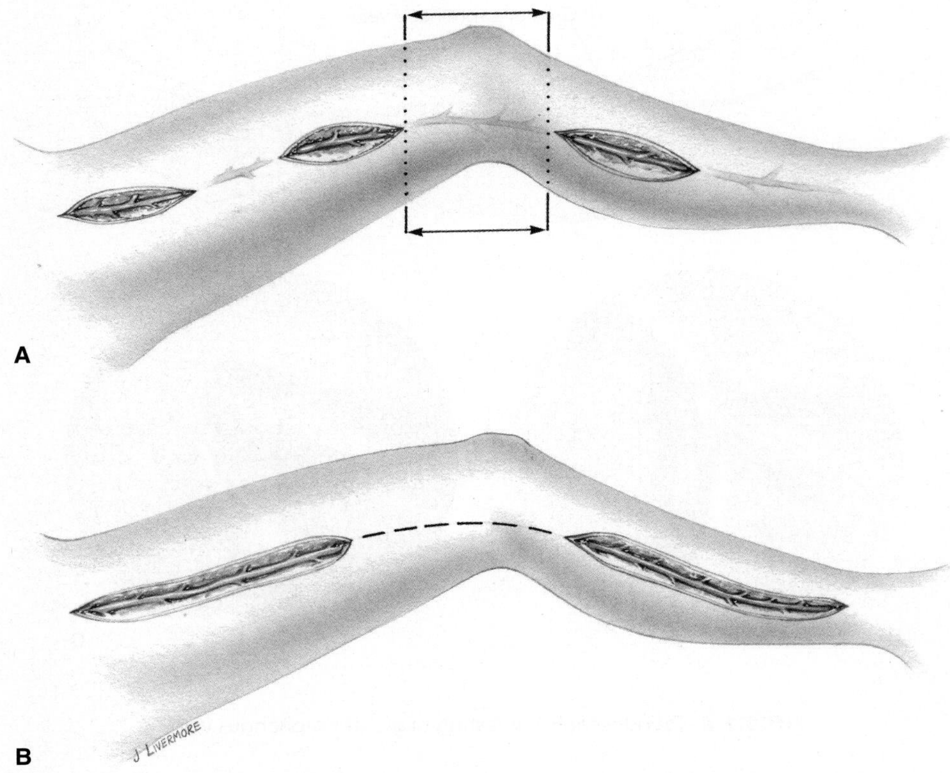

FIG. 9.5 Open harvest of a greater saphenous vein. **A:** Multiple skin incisions. **B:** Long incisions leaving a skin bridge alongside the knee joint.

NB Interrupted Skin Incisions

In patients who are diabetic or have peripheral vascular disease and are prone to poor wound healing, multiple skin incisions are made, leaving intervening bridges of skin intact. This allows better closure of the wound and minimizes ischemic changes along the skin edges (Fig. 9.5A). NB

⊘ Wound Healing

A wound in the lower leg tends to heal slowly; this is of particular significance in the elderly diabetic patient with peripheral vascular disease. Meticulous handling of tissues and careful wound closure are mandatory. ⊘

NB It is perhaps preferable not to harvest veins from the lower legs of elderly patients with diabetes or peripheral vascular disease. NB

When both greater saphenous veins have been stripped for varicosities or removed for previous bypass procedures, a search should be made for one or both lesser saphenous systems. Often, an adequate segment of vein can be procured. In these cases, the patient should be prepared and draped in such a manner that the back of the legs can be exposed.

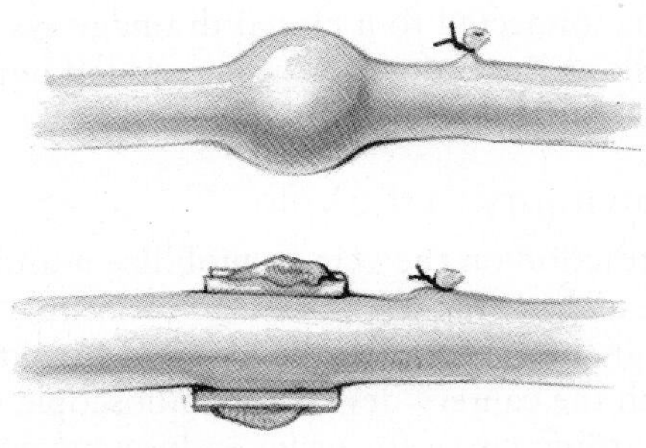

FIG. 9.6 Excluding a localized varicosity.

⊘ Varicosities

Saphenous veins with varicosities should be avoided. The walls of these vessels are dilated and abnormal, and the large caliber predisposes to lower flow velocity and possibly early graft thrombosis and occlusion. ⊘

⊘ Localized Varicosities

Localized varicosities can be detected along the vein wall when it is being gently distended. They may be partially excluded by the application of metal clips on the redundant tissue parallel to the vein wall (Fig. 9.6). ⊘

⊘ Intimal Injury

The vein must never be pulled or stretched to facilitate dissection. The intimal layer is very delicate and may tear, giving rise to the formation of a nidus for platelet aggregation and possible subsequent early occlusion of the graft (Fig. 9.7A). This is more likely to occur when multiple skin incisions are made and the vein has to be harvested from beneath the skin bridges. ⊘

⊘ Overdistention of the Vein

The vein graft should be gently distended; any excessive pressure can result in intimal tear and disruption. Devices are commercially available to prevent the intraluminal pressure from exceeding 150 mm Hg. ⊘

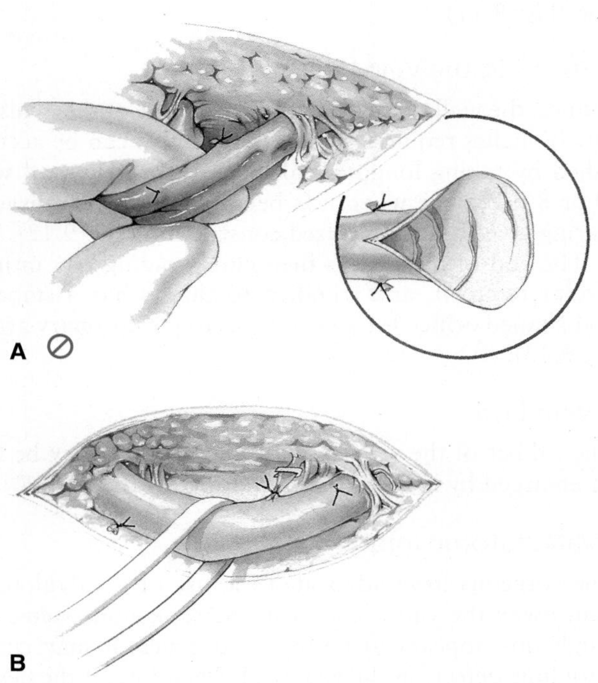

FIG. 9.7 A: Pulling or stretching vein injures the intima. **B:** Gentle retraction with an elastic band.

⊘ Avulsion Injury

Stretching of the vein may also result in avulsion injury owing to tension on small side branches. These tears on the vein wall can be oversewn with 7-0 or 8-0 Prolene sutures to ensure adequate hemostasis; however, the vein integrity remains disrupted. ⊘

The vein can be gently retracted by means of elastic vessel bands whenever necessary (Fig. 9.7B).

The side branches are identified and ligated; alternatively, they can be occluded with metal clips and then divided (Fig. 9.8).

⊘ Branch Stump

The branches should be ligated or clamped approximately 1 mm from the vein wall to minimize the presence of a stump, which may predispose to thrombus formation and early graft occlusion (Fig. 9.9A). Any stump can easily be eliminated by application of a fine metal clip behind the tie, parallel with the vein wall (Fig. 9.9B). ⊘

⊘ Graft Narrowing

Conversely, the tie or metal clip should never occlude part of the vein wall itself. This gives rise to localized constriction (Fig. 9.9C). The tie or clip should be gently removed. Applying pressure with a heavy needle driver on the closed loop of the metal clip will separate the two ends and facilitate its removal. The tie or metal clip is replaced or reapplied appropriately. ⊘

⊘ Adventitial Constriction

The adventitial tissue may at times be caught in the tie around one of the branches, creating a localized constriction. The adventitial band should be carefully divided with Potts scissors (Fig. 9.10). ⊘

When an adequate segment of vein is dissected free, it is divided at each end and removed. The vein stumps in the groin and the ankle are securely ligated.

Skin Closure

The leg wound is closed in layers with absorbable sutures. In the groin region or where the wound is deep, an

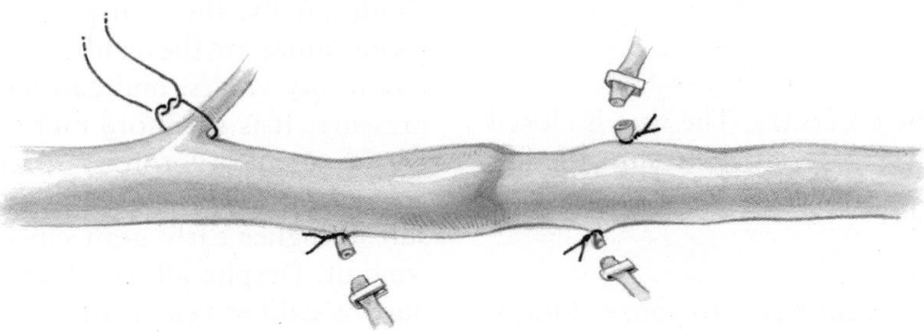

FIG. 9.8 Ligating or clipping vein branches.

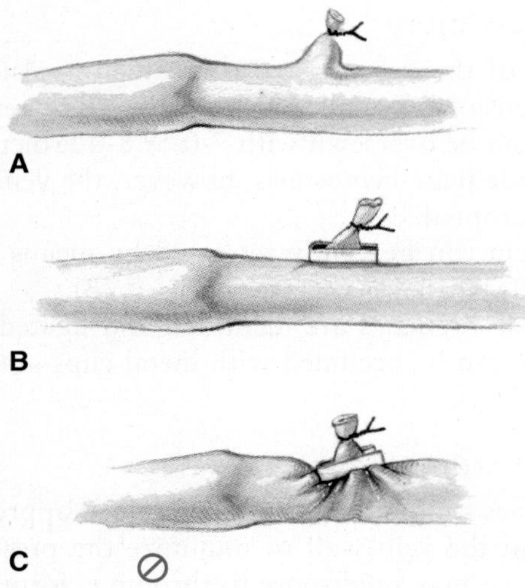

FIG. 9.9 **A:** Leaving excess stump on a vein branch. **B:** A metal clip eliminates stump. **C:** A clip constricting vein.

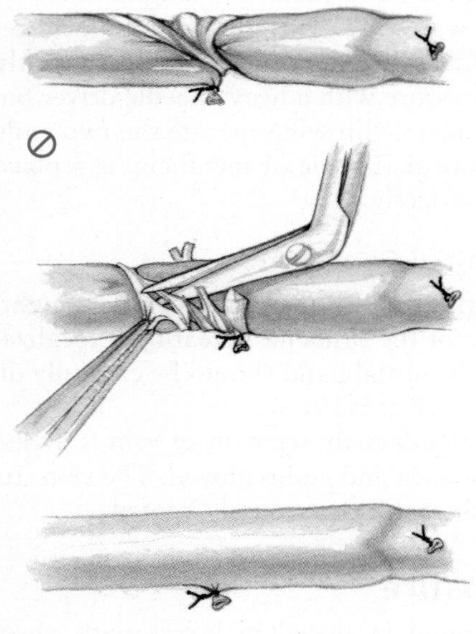

FIG. 9.10 Dividing the adventitial band to relieve constriction.

extra layer of closure may be necessary. The skin is closed with fine absorbable suture material in a subcuticular manner.

⊘ Wound Drainage

If the wound is deep or continues to ooze blood, closed-system drainage for 24 hours should be used. This prevents hematoma formation and possible infection. ⊘

⊘ Wound Infection

Patients with diabetes and patients with peripheral vascular disease are at increased risk of this complication. Therefore, the wound must be closed atraumatically and without leaving any dead space. Absolute hemostasis must be achieved before closure is begun. The subcuticular skin closure may be reinforced with deeply placed, interrupted horizontal mattress monofilament sutures that are left in place until satisfactory healing has been completed, usually for at least 2 to 3 weeks. ⊘

Regardless of harvest technique, an olive-tipped cannula is introduced into the distal end of the vein. The vein is gently distended with autologous heparinized blood. Any avulsed branches are identified and securely ligated with 4-0 silk or oversewn with 7-0 or 8-0 Prolene sutures, taking all the aforementioned precautions into consideration (Fig. 9.11).

⊘ Suturing the Vein Wall

At times, the wall of the vein itself at the site of the avulsion of its branches requires suture closure; this can be accomplished by taking longitudinal bites of the vein wall with 7-0 or 8-0 Prolene when it is being distended. Transverse suturing gives rise to localized constriction (Fig. 9.12). ⊘

The end of the vein is then cut, avoiding any intimal valvular remnant, and trimmed so that is has a smooth, hood-shaped orifice for anastomosis to the coronary artery (Fig. 9.13).

NB Vein End

If the caliber of the vein is small, the opening may be further enlarged by incising the vein orifice at the heel. NB

⊘ Valvulotome Injury

Some surgeons have advocated the use of a valvulotome to cut away the valve leaflets in the saphenous veins. Although this appears to be useful at times, it may create buttonhole defects in the vein wall. Therefore, if the device is used, great caution must be exercised. We do not routinely remove the valve leaflets unless they are located at the anastomotic sites. ⊘

NB Lower Versus Upper Leg Veins

Traditionally, the vein procured from the lower leg conforms more to the caliber of the coronary arteries, has few if any valves, and can withstand higher intraluminal pressure. It is therefore more suitable for bypass grafting of the smaller coronary arteries. However, the normal arterialization process and intimal hyperplasia may result in higher early graft closure of small saphenous vein conduit. Despite all its advantages, the proximal end of a narrow-caliber vein graft may be too small for a standard aortic anastomosis. The proximal anastomosis will have to be carried out to a smaller aortic opening rather than a regular punched-out hole. NB

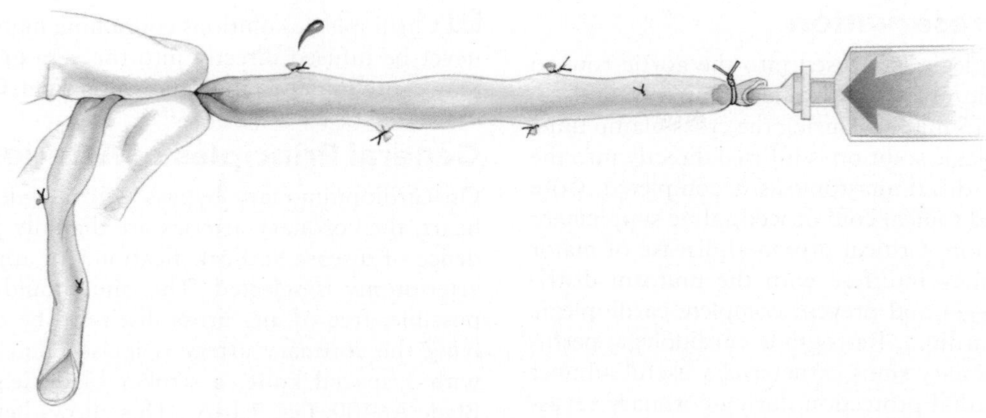

FIG. 9.11 Gently distending a vein.

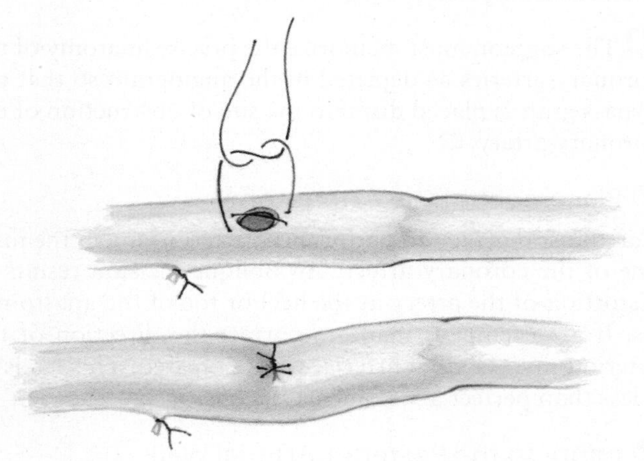

FIG. 9.12 Transverse closure of an avulsed branch leads to constriction of a vein.

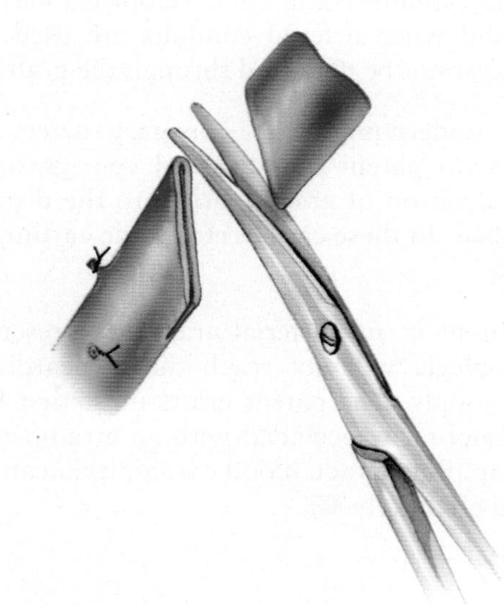

FIG. 9.13 Trimming the end of a vein to create a hood.

CORONARY ARTERY BYPASS GRAFTING WITH CARDIOPULMONARY BYPASS

Although many approaches have been used in the last decade for coronary artery bypass surgery, including limited thoracotomy incisions and techniques, a median sternotomy is considered the incision of choice in most cases today. Although off-pump coronary artery bypass grafting is a valuable technique in selected cases, cardiopulmonary bypass is used in majority of coronary revascularization cases.

Venous drainage is accomplished through a single atriocaval cannula in most patients undergoing coronary artery bypass surgery. Bicaval cannulation is used when concomitant procedures necessitating an opening into the right side of the heart are indicated. Oxygenated blood is returned to the patient by direct cannulation of the ascending aorta. In rare instances when aortic cannulation is not feasible because of an ascending aortic aneurysm or extensive aortic wall calcification, the femoral or axillary arterial route is chosen instead (see Chapter 2).

Venting of the left side of the heart through the right superior pulmonary vein or through the pulmonary artery has been used, but it is unnecessary in most instances (see Chapter 4). In rare instances, when reoperative surgery for a single bypass to the circumflex coronary artery is needed, a left thoracotomy is an alternate approach. In such cases, cardiopulmonary bypass is achieved by both femoral artery and femoral vein cannulation (see technique described in Chapter 2).

Myocardial Preservation

Cold blood cardioplegia is infused into the aortic root to achieve cardioplegic arrest of the heart initially and repeated every 10 to 15 minutes during the cross-clamp time. Additional cardioplegic solution is infused directly into the vein graft after the distal anastomosis is completed. Core cooling to 34°C and topical cold or iced saline supplement myocardial protection. Critical proximal disease of major coronary arteries may interfere with the uniform distribution of cardioplegia and prevent complete cardioplegic arrest of the myocardium. Retrograde cardioplegic perfusion through a coronary sinus catheter is a useful adjunct for optimal myocardial protection during coronary revascularization (see Chapter 3).

In patients with acute coronary occlusion and impending infarction, the culprit vessel is grafted first to allow cardioplegic solution to be delivered through the vein graft to the involved myocardial territory.

NB Retrograde administration of cardioplegia may be particularly useful when arterial conduits are used because cardioplegia cannot be delivered through the graft. NB

NB Patients undergoing redo coronary artery bypass procedures with patent but diseased vein grafts are at risk of embolization of graft debris into the distal coronary artery bed. In these cases, retrograde cardioplegia is indicated. NB

NB When patent *in situ* arterial grafts are present, antegrade cardioplegia will not reach the myocardium that these grafts supply. The patent grafts must first be identified and temporarily occluded with an atraumatic small bulldog clamp. Retrograde blood cardioplegia can then be administered effectively. NB

NB Cardioplegic solutions containing high potassium must never be infused directly into the vein grafts because this may cause injury to the vein wall intima. NB

General Principles of Arteriotomy

On cardiopulmonary bypass with a quiet, decompressed heart, the coronary arteries are digitally palpated for evidence of disease and calcification. An appropriate site for arteriotomy is selected. This site should be, as much as possible, free of any gross disease. The epicardium overlying the coronary artery is incised and spread sideways with a special knife, a stroker blade (e.g., Beaver Mini-Blade A6400, Fig. 9.14A). This allows better inspection of the coronary artery wall. After the exact site of arteriotomy has been established, a poker blade (e.g., Beaver Micro-Sharp Blade A7513) is used to incise the anterior wall of the coronary artery (Fig. 9.14B).

NB The surgeon must memorize the precise anatomy of the coronary arteries as depicted in the angiogram so that the bypass graft is placed distal to the site of obstruction of the coronary artery. NB

⊘ Placement of the Arteriotomy

Care must be taken to perform the arteriotomy in the midline of the coronary artery. An oblique incision results in distortion of the artery at the heel or toe of the anastomosis. If an attempt is made to correct the direction of the arteriotomy, a flap of arterial wall is created. This leads to a less than perfect anastomosis (Fig. 9.15). ⊘

⊘ Injury to the Posterior Arterial Wall

Special precautions must be taken not to damage the posterior wall of the coronary artery. This can happen if the

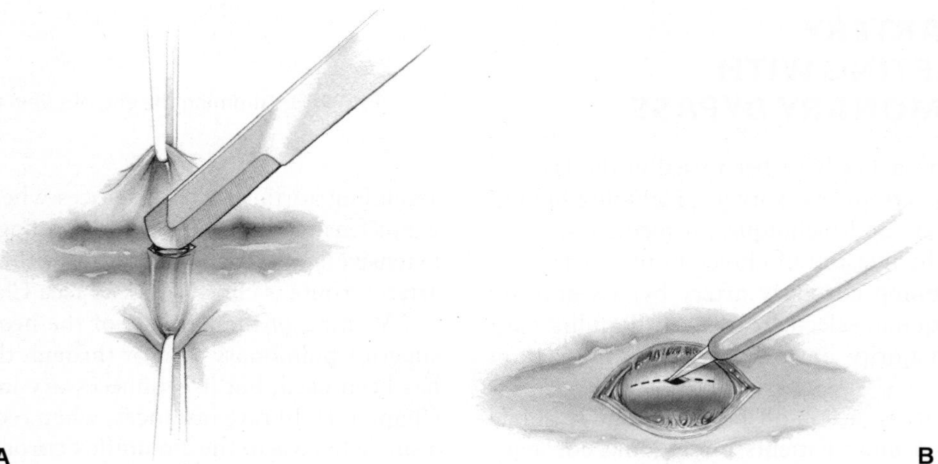

FIG. 9.14 A: A stroker blade is used to expose coronary artery. **B:** A poker blade is used to incise the anterior wall of a coronary artery.

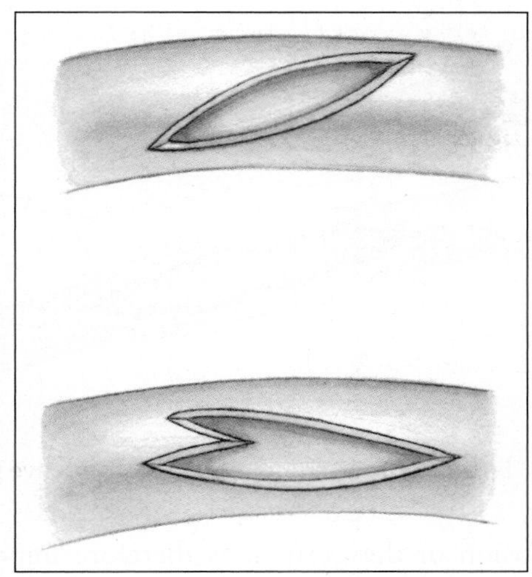

⊘ FIG. 9.15 Oblique arteriotomy and attempted correction create a flap of arterial wall.

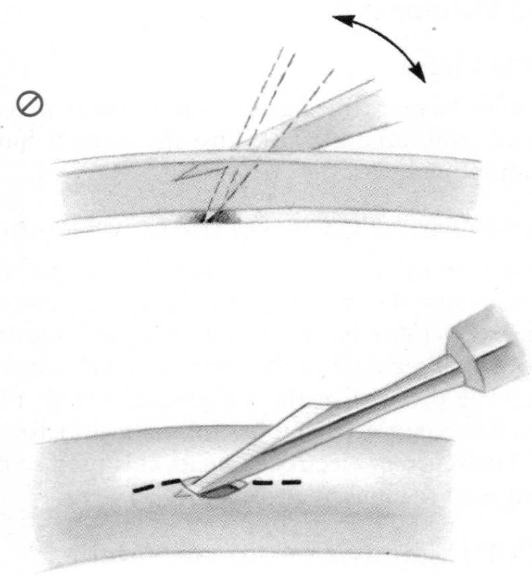

⊘ FIG. 9.16 Perpendicular angle of a blade damages the posterior wall of a coronary artery.

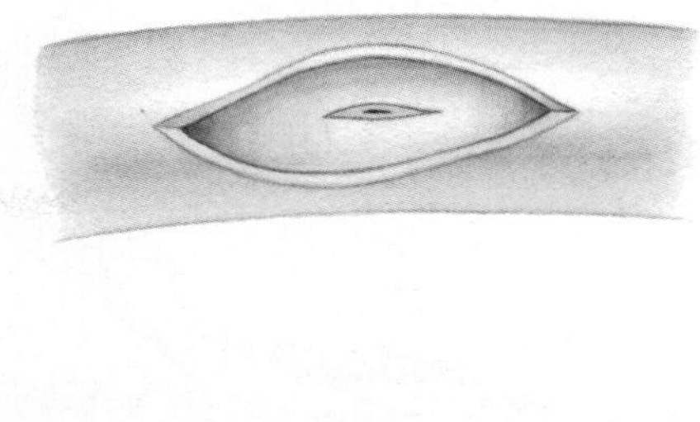

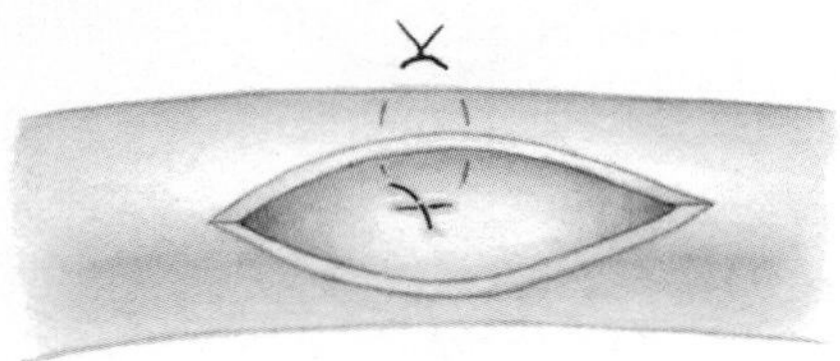

FIG. 9.17 Incision through the posterior wall of a coronary is repaired with a suture tied outside the vessel.

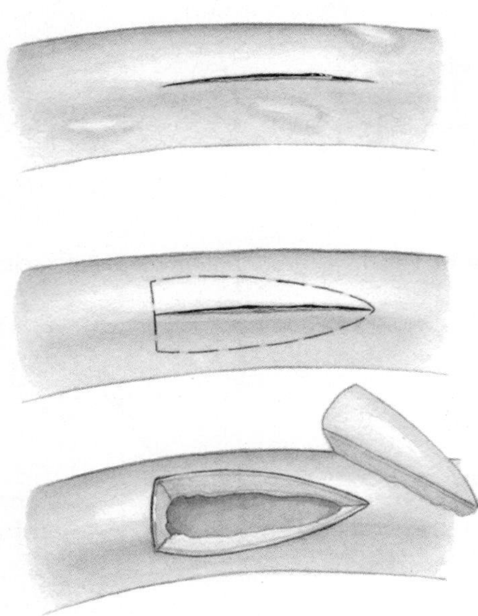

FIG. 9.18 Removing a triangular segment from a calcified coronary artery.

angle of the blade is perpendicular to the vessel. The angle should always be approximately 45 degrees with respect to the coronary artery (Fig. 9.16). If the posterior wall has been incised through the adventitia by the blade, it should be approximated with a fine suture of 8-0 Prolene tied on the outside of the vessel (Fig. 9.17). ⊘

⊘ Calcified, Nonpliable Arterial Wall

Sometimes the arterial wall is inflexible and heavily calcified, making it impossible to tailor a satisfactory arteriotomy to perform a functioning anastomosis. A button of anterior wall is removed at the arteriotomy site. The technique essentially entails the removal of a triangular segment of anterior arterial wall from the site of the anastomosis. The calcified arterial wall would otherwise restrict the lumen of the graft anastomosis (Fig. 9.18). ⊘

The arteriotomy is then enlarged both proximally and distally (Fig. 9.19). A special modification of Potts scissors is available to enlarge a coronary artery in particularly difficult locations. The diameter of the coronary artery lumen as well as the presence of distal obstructive plaques may be

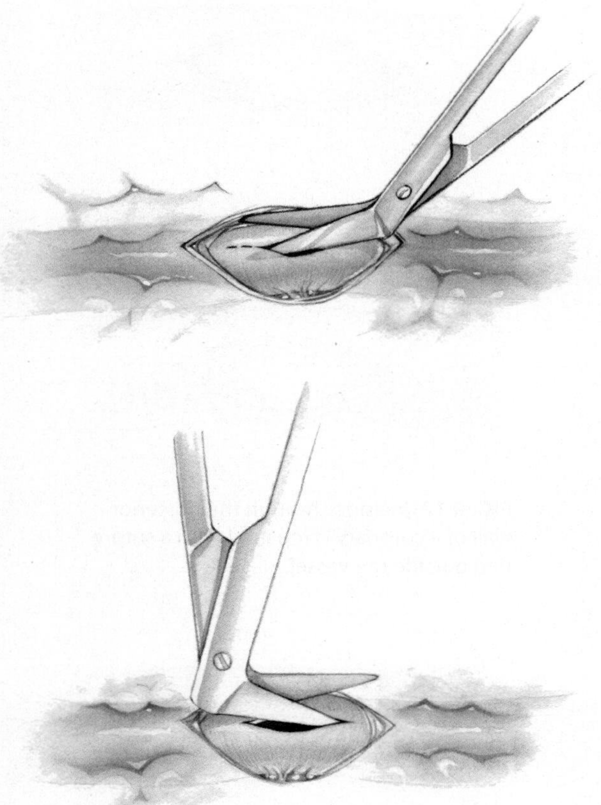

FIG. 9.19 Enlarging an arteriotomy with Potts scissors.

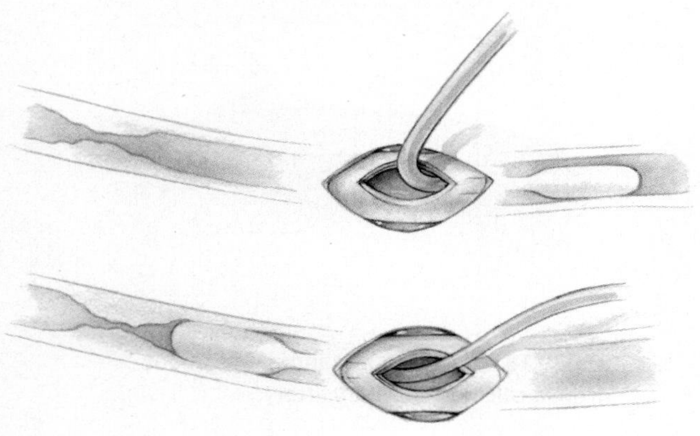

FIG. 9.20 Calibrating the lumen of a coronary artery with a probe.

evaluated by gently inserting calibrated probes through the arteriotomy site (Fig. 9.20).

⊘ Distal Obstructive Plaque

Although every attempt is made to identify a relatively normal site for the anastomosis, at times localized plaques at the toe of the anastomosis may limit the flow and cause

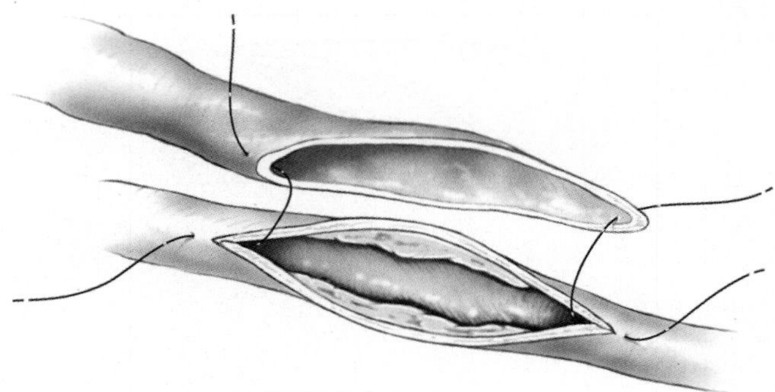

FIG. 9.21 Enlarging an arteriotomy across obstructive plaque.

early occlusion of the graft. It is therefore important to enlarge the arteriotomy by cutting across the obstructive plaque (Fig. 9.21). Similarly, the distal opening of the conduit is enlarged and an anastomosis is then carried out. If the obstructing segment is too long and this procedure is not feasible, a second bypass graft must be placed distal to the site of obstruction. ⊘

⊘ Intimal Injury

Probing must be performed gently, taking every precaution not to force too large a probe into the arterial lumen to prevent an intimal tear. ⊘

⊘ Intramyocardial Course of the Coronary Artery

The artery may follow an intramyocardial course. It must be followed into the muscle, and the myocardial bridge over the artery must be divided with great caution. The intramyocardial segment of the artery is nearly always disease free. The division of the myocardial bridge must be limited to the extent needed to perform a satisfactory anastomosis. Low-current electrocoagulation is used to cauterize the edges of the muscular bridge. ⊘

⊘ Difficulty Identifying Coronary Arteries

In some patients, epicardial fat along the course of the coronary artery prevents the precise identification of the vessel. Under such circumstances, the side branches of the artery are identified first and then followed toward the parent trunk. The artery is then dissected clear of the fatty tissue. When the LAD coronary artery cannot be identified, it may be useful to locate the posterior descending artery and follow it to the apex of the heart. The distal anterior descending coronary artery should be near this site. ⊘

Positioning the Heart to Expose Coronary Arteries

Exposure of the Anterior Surface of the Heart

A laparotomy pad soaked in ice-cold saline solution is placed into the pericardium behind the empty and flaccid heart. This maneuver usually exposes the anterior surface

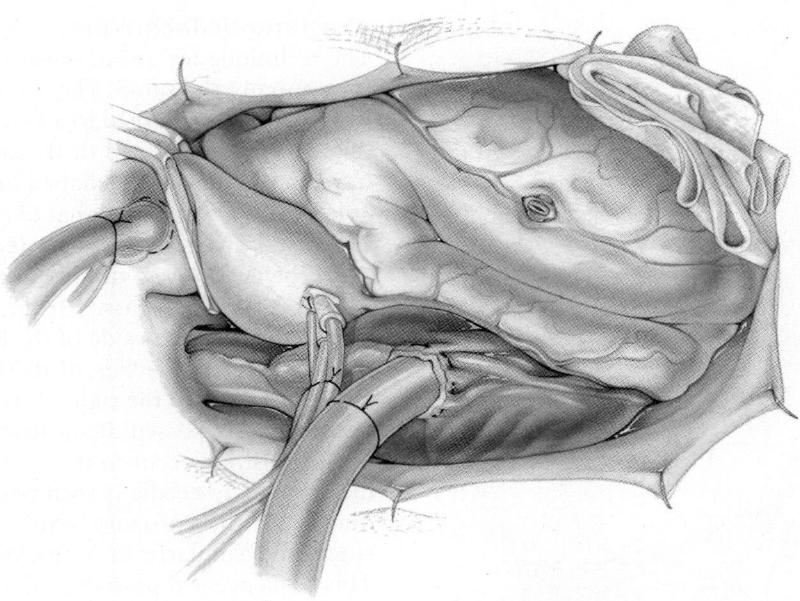

FIG. 9.22 Positioning the heart to expose anterior coronary artery branches.

of the heart quite well. The LAD, diagonal, and, with some minor adjustments, ramus intermedius coronary arteries can be viewed with ease (Fig. 9.22).

Exposure of the Right Coronary Artery and Branches

The right coronary artery is usually a large vessel and is covered by epicardial fat in the right atrioventricular groove. Its distal branches, the posterolateral and right posterior descending arteries, tend to be more superficial as they course toward the apex of the heart.

The operating table is elevated, and the patient is placed in a slight Trendelenburg position. The acute margin of the right ventricle is gently elevated and held in position by the assistant surgeon's hand. The distal right coronary artery and the proximal segment of its branches are brought into view (Fig. 9.23). Distal right coronary artery is usually palpable. The epicardium over the atrioventricular groove is incised. The distal right coronary is identified and dissected for a short distance. To provide exposure for the posterior descending or posterolateral arteries, the apex of the heart is elevated toward the patient's right shoulder (Fig. 9.24).

Exposure of the Circumflex Coronary Artery and Branches

The operating table is lowered slightly and its left side raised. Cold lap pads are placed behind the heart, near left atrium. The empty, flaccid heart is gently elevated and held by the assistant surgeon's right hand. This maneuver, with some minor adjustments, brings all the obtuse marginal and posterior lateral branches of both the circumflex and right coronary arteries into view (Fig. 9.25).

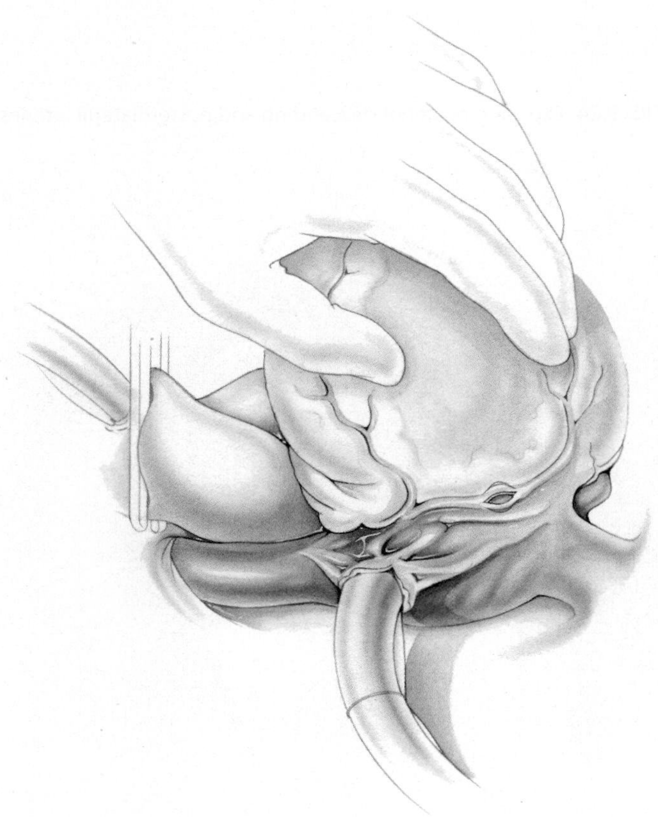

FIG. 9.23 Positioning the heart to expose the right coronary artery and branches.

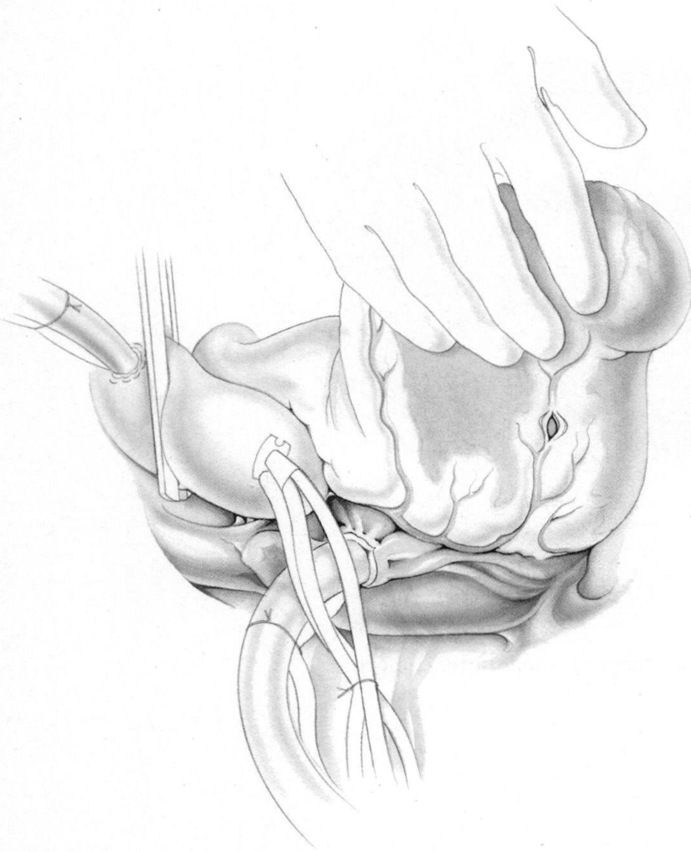

FIG. 9.24 Exposing posterior descending and posterolateral arteries.

Anastomotic Techniques

The technique for anastomosis to all the coronary arteries is essentially the same. The arteriotomy is made at the selected site. It is enlarged to a length of 5 to 7 mm with Potts scissors. The distal end of the conduit must be tailored to have an oblique, hood-shaped lumen with a circumference at least 25% larger than that of the arteriotomy (Fig. 9.13). The distal anastomosis is started with 30-in. long, 7-0 or 8-0 Prolene sutures, double armed with tapered needles. The first needle is passed from the outside of the graft 2 mm to the surgeon's side of the heel. It is then passed from the inside to the outside of the lumen of the coronary artery, 2 to 3 mm to the right of its heel (Fig. 9.26). The same needle is now passed again from the outside to the inside of the graft, adjacent to the previous suture in a clockwise direction. The needle is then passed from the inside to the outside of the coronary artery, adjacent to the previous stitch and similarly in a clockwise direction (Fig. 9.27). This sequence is repeated until four rounds of sutures have been placed in the internal thoracic artery graft or the vein graft. By gently pulling on both ends of the suture in a see-saw manner, the graft is lowered into position (Fig. 9.28).

Traditionally, the vein or the thoracic artery is held by the assistant surgeon with two atraumatic forceps (Fig. 9.26). The forceps ideally should hold the adventitial tissue of the conduit. This may be difficult, and the whole wall thickness including the intima is often grasped by the forceps. This damages the wall of the conduit and may lead to early graft closure.

The conduit can be held between the surgeon's left thumb and index finger; the anastomosis is carried out with the right hand (Fig. 9.29). This technique eliminates any

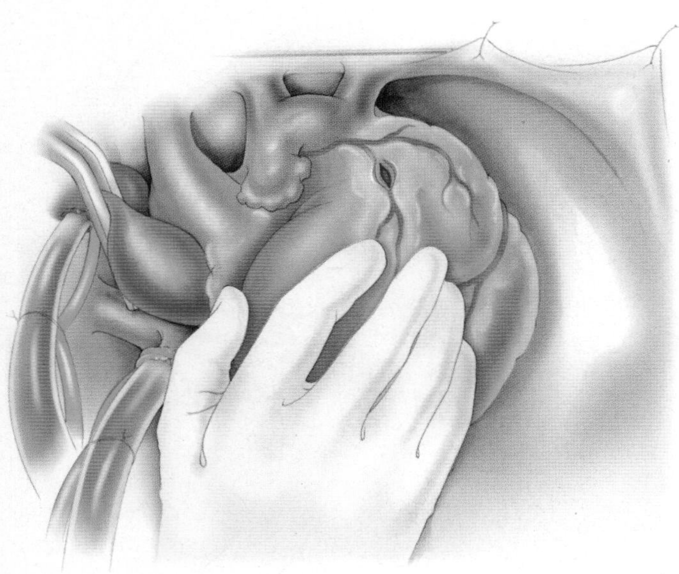

FIG. 9.25 Positioning the heart to expose the circumflex coronary artery and branches.

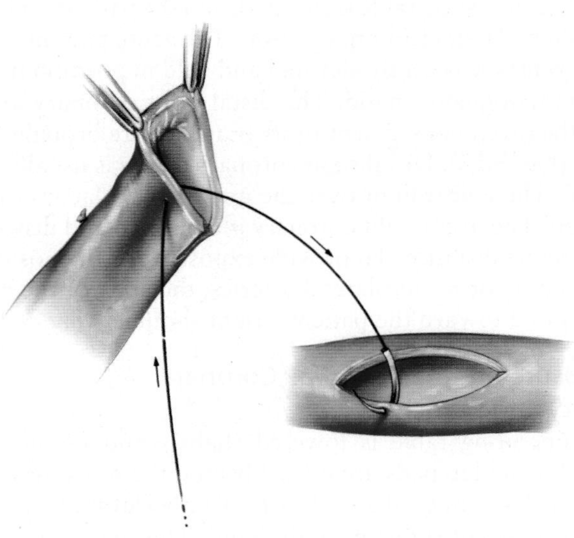

FIG. 9.26 Stepwise technique for a distal anastomosis.

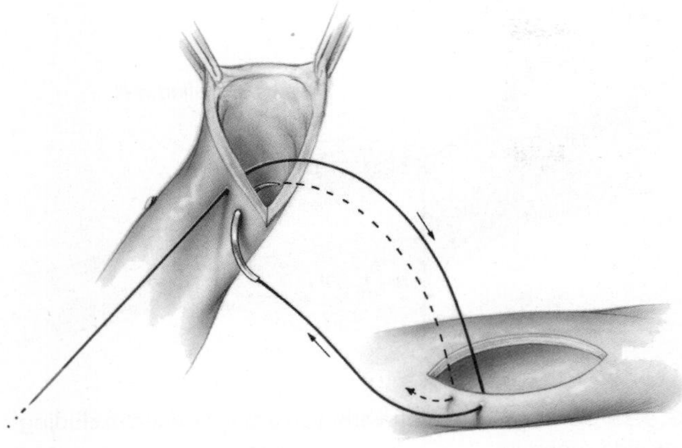

FIG. 9.27 Stepwise technique for a distal anastomosis.

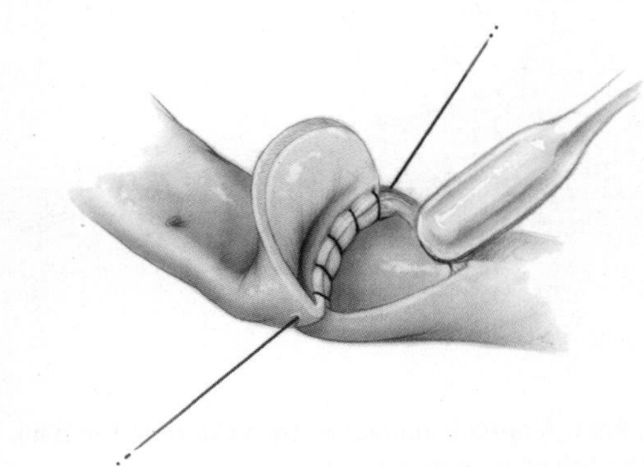

FIG. 9.28 Stepwise technique for a distal anastomosis.

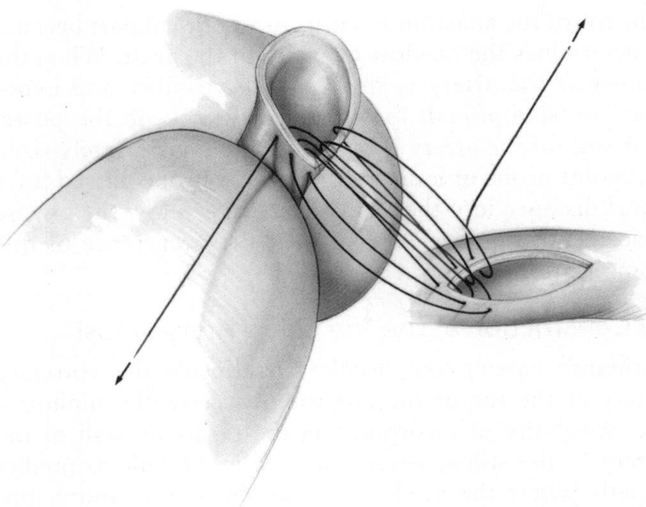

FIG. 9.29 Holding a vein graft between the left thumb and index finger.

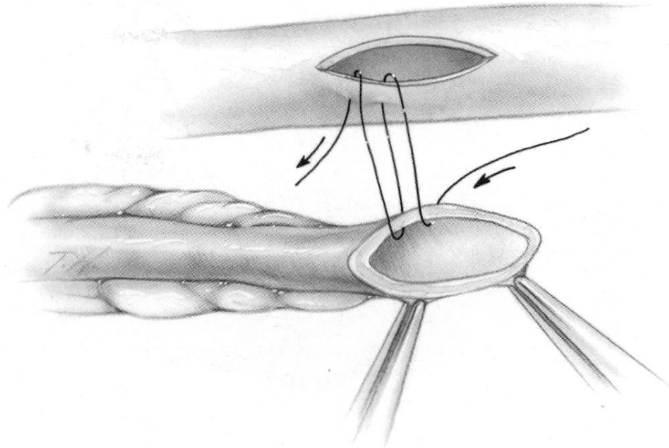

FIG. 9.30 Placing conduit on the heart next to the anastomotic site on a coronary artery.

possible forceps injury to the conduit and does not require the expertise of an assistant surgeon. Moreover, although initially it may appear to be somewhat clumsy and difficult, with a little experience, this technique becomes easy and actually expedites the anastomosis. Alternatively, the conduit is placed on the heart adjacent and parallel to the anastomotic site on the coronary artery (Fig. 9.30). Some surgeons prefer to suspend the conduit from the drape with a fine adventitial traction suture. The sequence of suturing remains the same for all the techniques described.

⊘ Anastomotic Leak at the Heel

The sutures at the heel must be extremely close to each other to minimize the possibility of leaks. Subsequent placement of reinforcing sutures in this area is difficult and may compromise the lumen of the anastomosis. ⊘

⊘ Patency of the Lumen at the Heel of the Anastomosis

An appropriately sized ballpoint probe is now introduced into the lumen of the coronary artery, the internal thoracic artery, or the vein conduit for a short distance to ensure a satisfactory anastomosis at the heel (Fig. 9.28). ⊘

NB This probe can be left in the lumen of the coronary artery to stop the flow of blood and allow accurate placement of stitches. NB

The left arm of the suture is tagged with a rubber-shod clamp to provide gentle traction. The needle at the other end of the suture is now continued as an over-and-over stitch, outside in on the conduit and inside out on the coronary artery (Fig. 9.31). This is continued forward, passing well around the toe of the anastomosis (Fig. 9.32).

The needle should take small and superficial bites very close to each other on the coronary artery at the toe.

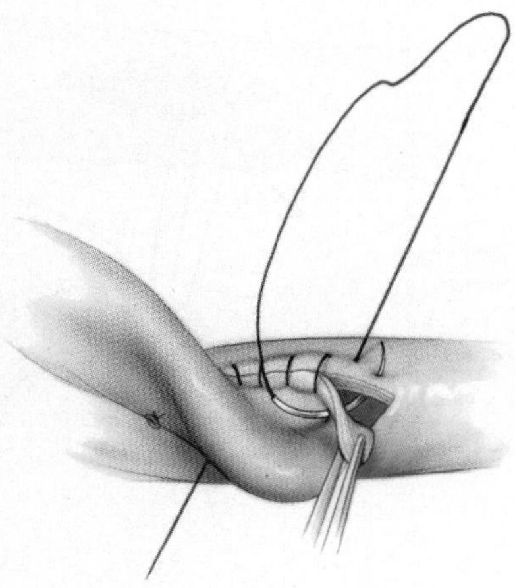

FIG. 9.31 Completing a distal anastomosis.

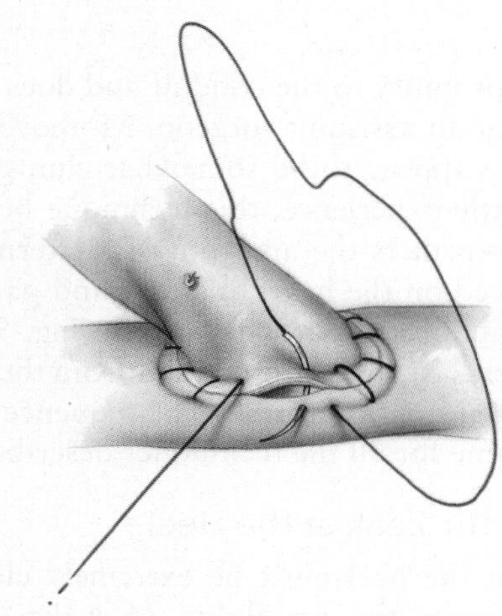

FIG. 9.32 Completing distal anastomosis.

NB The needle may include a very thin segment of the surrounding epicardium to minimize anastomotic leaks. NB

At this time, an appropriately sized probe is passed through the toe of the anastomosis to ensure its patency. The suturing is continued until the other suture end is reached.

⊘ Calcified Arterial Wall

When the wall of the coronary artery is heavily calcified, a diamond-tipped needle swaged on a 7-0 Prolene suture is used to perform the anastomosis. These needles are much stronger and can pierce the calcified plaques with minimal difficulty. Alternatively, when the edge of the coronary arterial wall is calcified, the vein graft can be sewn in place within the arterial lumen, excluding the calcified segment. Because the diameter of the vein is larger than that of the artery, the lumen of the anastomosis will be adequate (Fig. 9.33). ⊘

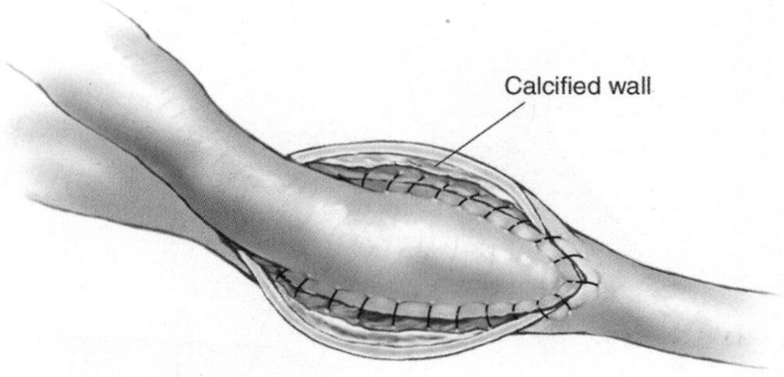

FIG. 9.33 Sewing a vein graft within an arterial lumen excluding a calcified segment.

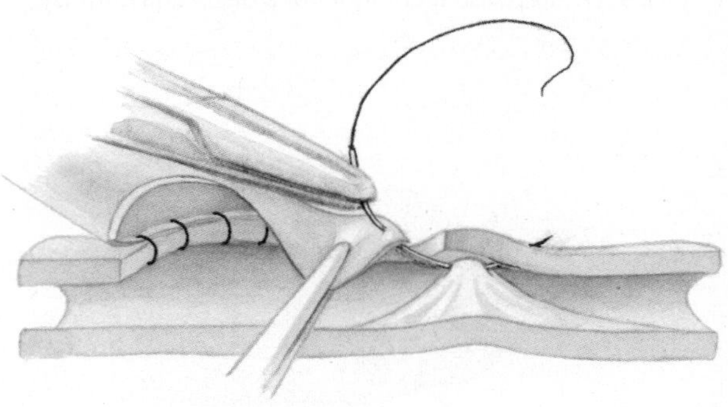

⊘ FIG. 9.34 A needle inadvertently picking up the back wall at the toe of an anastomosis.

⊘ Inadvertent Suturing of the Posterior Wall

The toe of the anastomosis is its most critical part because it determines the outflow capacity of the graft. When the lumen of the artery is small or the visibility and exposure are suboptimal, the needle may pick up the posterior wall of the artery (Fig. 9.34). An appropriately sized ballpoint probe or a disposable plastic probe passed for a short distance into the distal artery may allow the precise placement of sutures and prevent the occurrence of this complication. ⊘

⊘ Constriction at the Toe of the Anastomosis

Although passing the needle from inside the coronary artery at the toe of the anastomosis certainly minimizes the possibility of incorporating the posterior wall of the artery in the stitch, nevertheless, it is difficult to predict exactly where the needle will exit the artery, and a longer and larger segment of arterial wall may become included in the stitch. When tightened, the stitch produces some dimpling and stenosis of the anastomosis at the toe. Every precaution must be taken to avoid this complication (Fig. 9.35). ⊘

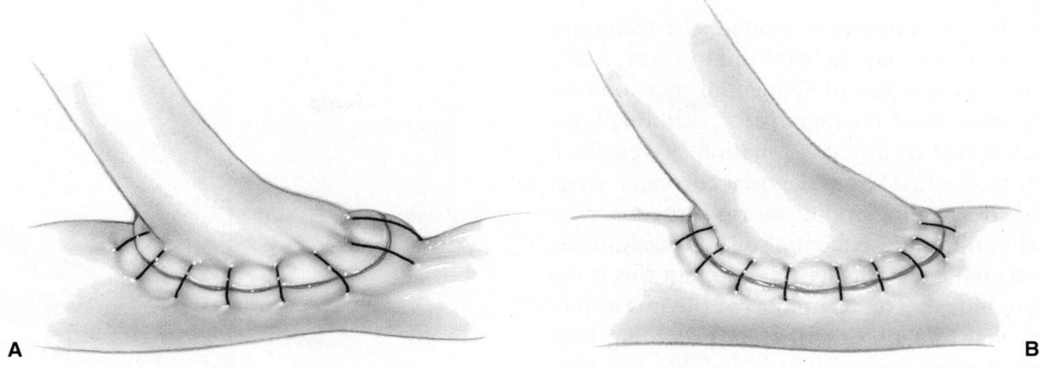

FIG. 9.35 **A:** Dimpling and narrowing at the toe of the anastomosis. **B:** Small, close-together suturing at the toe prevents narrowing of the anastomosis.

NB Appearance of the Anastomosis at the Toe

Sutures should be placed further apart on the graft than the coronary artery at the toe of the anastomosis. When blood flow is established, the graft will bulge and provide a "hood" over the anastomosis. NB

Blood cardioplegic solution is gently infused through the graft before tightening the suture line to allow air to escape and prevent any air embolization to the coronary arteries. The sutures are tightened with care and securely tied (Fig. 9.36). Similarly, in the case of the internal thoracic artery, the bulldog clamp is removed. It is reapplied after the sutures have been tied if other coronary anastomoses are still to be done.

NB Often this step of the procedure is preceded by retrograde infusion of blood cardioplegia to wash out any debris and air from within the distal coronary artery. NB

NB Incorporation of the Epicardium into the Anastomosis

The epicardial tissue on each side of the coronary arteriotomy is very often incorporated into the suturing process to ensure a more secure anastomosis. NB

The pedicle of the internal thoracic artery is tacked to the epicardium on each side of the anastomotic site with simple 6-0 Prolene sutures. This prevents the pedicle from twisting on itself and therefore obstructing flow through the vessel.

⊘ Flattening of the Thoracic Pedicle

If the tacking sutures are placed too far from the coronary artery, the pedicle may be stretched when the heart fills. This lateral traction may compress the internal thoracic artery and compromise the graft flow. ⊘

⊘ Anastomotic Leak

Infusion of blood cardioplegic solution through the vein graft reveals any anastomotic leaks. These are best controlled at this time with a separate suture, taking care not to impinge on the lumen of the anastomosis. The surrounding epicardial tissue can be incorporated in the suture over the leak site. ⊘

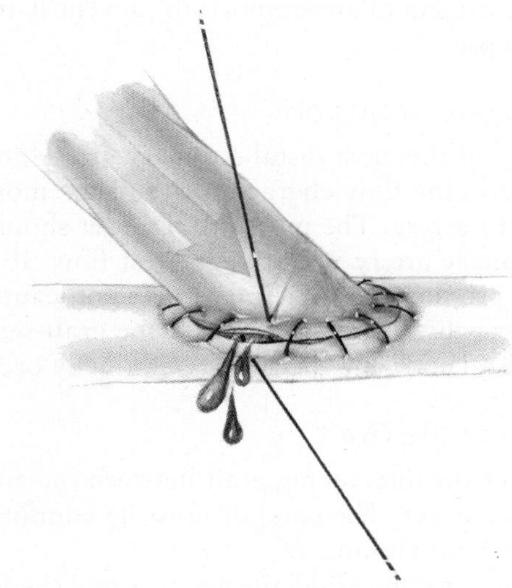

FIG. 9.36 Infusing cardioplegia down a graft before tying the suture.

Alternate Distal Anastomotic Techniques

Interrupted Suture Technique

The anastomosis can also be accomplished with interrupted sutures; this is considered a superior technique, at least on theoretic grounds. Many surgeons combine both continuous and interrupted techniques, reserving the latter for the toe of the anastomosis. The general principles are the same as described previously for the continuous suture technique, but the incidence of anastomotic leaks is considerably higher, requiring additional reinforcing sutures.

Sequential Anastomosis

When the availability of conduits is limited, the technique for sequential anastomosis may be helpful. However, many surgeons prefer the routine use of sequential anastomoses for possible improved flow characteristics. Although the technique can be applied to any combination of vessels, it is most applicable to the LAD and diagonal coronary arteries or the posterior descending and distal right coronary arteries. Occasionally, multiple sequential distal anastomoses with only one proximal anastomosis are used, but this is not generally considered ideal. The technique of the anastomosis is the same as that already described in preceding text. However, the alignment of the incisions is variable, resulting in side-to-side, T-, Y-, or diamond-shaped configurations.

⊘ Large Arteriotomy

The surgeon should always avoid large arteriotomies when performing sequential anastomosis to prevent flattening of the anastomosis. ⊘

⊘ Distal Graft Occlusion

The patency of the most distal coronary artery anastomosis depends on the flow characteristics of the more proximal coronary artery. The most distal target should be the largest coronary artery with the greatest flow. If the flow in the most proximal coronary artery is significantly higher than the most distal coronary artery, the graft segment to the more distal coronary artery may gradually occlude. ⊘

⊘ Kinking of the Graft

The length of the intervening graft between the anastomoses must be correct. The conduit must lie comfortably on the heart without kinking. ⊘

If all these technical details are accomplished and adhered to, excellent long-term results can be achieved with the technique for sequential anastomosis.

Toe-First Anastomosis

Occasionally, the course of the coronary artery, particularly the branches of the right coronary artery are such that this technique may facilitate the anastomosis. The first suture needle is passed from the outside into the lumen of the artery at the toe of the anastomosis (Fig. 9.37). It is then passed from the inside to the outside of the conduit. The same needle is now passed again from the outside into the arterial lumen adjacent to, but to the surgeon's right of, the previous suture (Fig. 9.38) and through the conduit from the inside to the outside (Fig. 9.39). This arm of the suture is clamped. The graft is now lowered into position. At this point, an appropriately sized probe is introduced into the lumen of the coronary artery to ensure a patent anastomosis at the toe.

The needle at the other end of the suture is passed through the graft wall and then through the arterial wall from the inside to the outside (Fig. 9.40). The suturing is thus continued as an over-and-over stitch to a point well around the heel of the anastomosis (Figs. 9.41 through 9.44). The needle is then

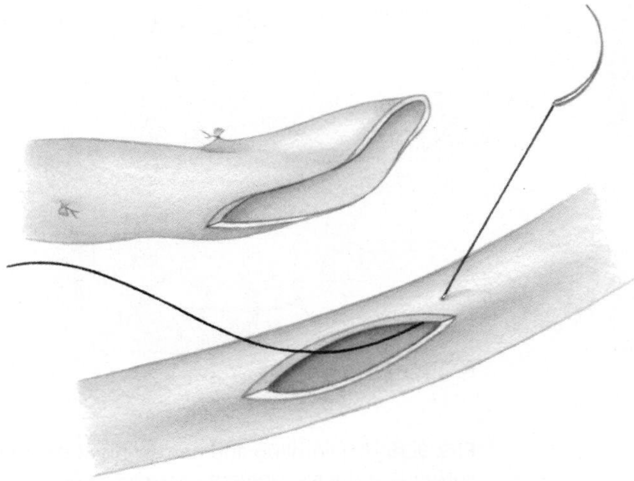

FIG. 9.37 Stepwise technique for a toe-first distal anastomosis.

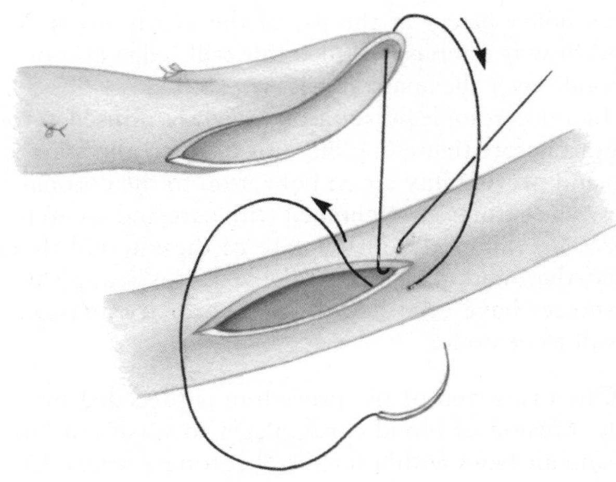

FIG. 9.38 Stepwise technique for a toe-first distal anastomosis.

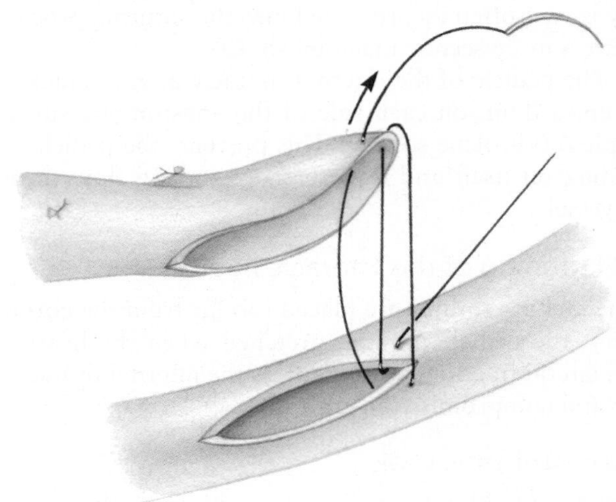

FIG. 9.39 Stepwise technique for a toe-first distal anastomosis.

clamped. The other needle is passed through the arterial wall from the outside to the inside and then from the inside to the outside of the graft (Fig. 9.45). The anastomosis is then completed and the suture ends tied after deairing by infusion of cardioplegic solution into the graft (Fig. 9.46).

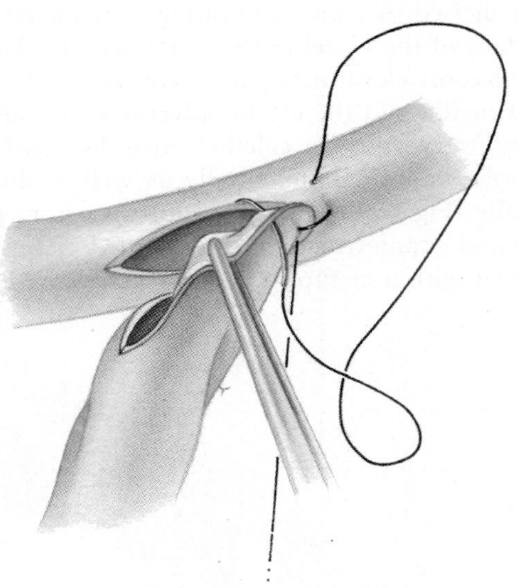

FIG. 9.40 Stepwise technique for a toe-first distal anastomosis.

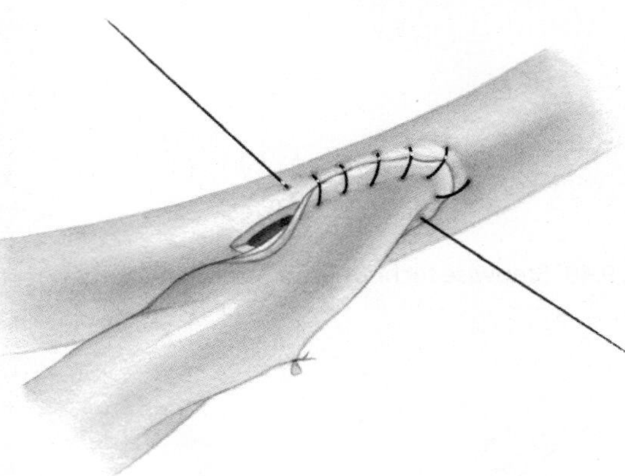

FIG. 9.41 Stepwise technique for a toe-first distal anastomosis.

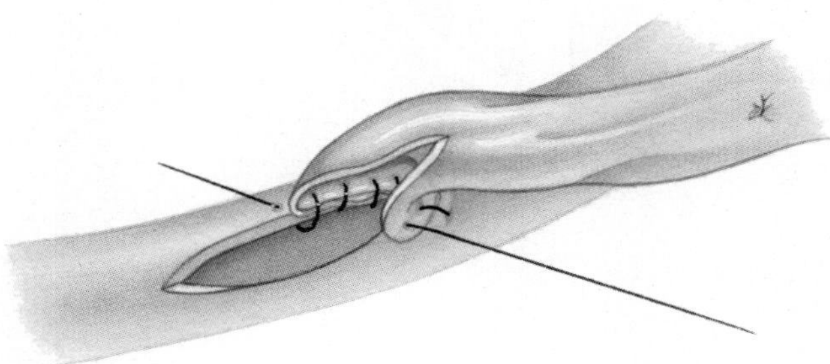

FIG. 9.42

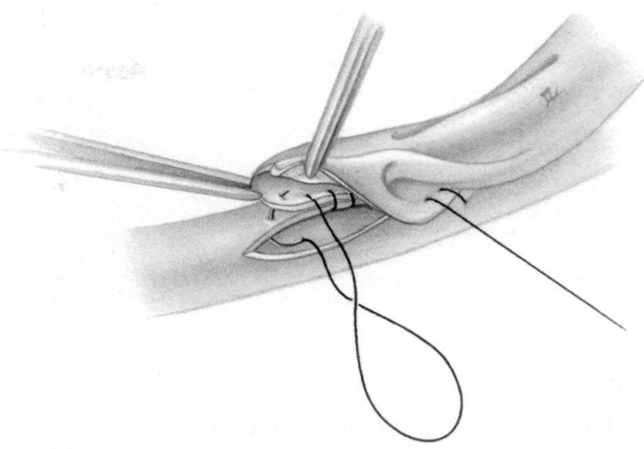

FIG. 9.43

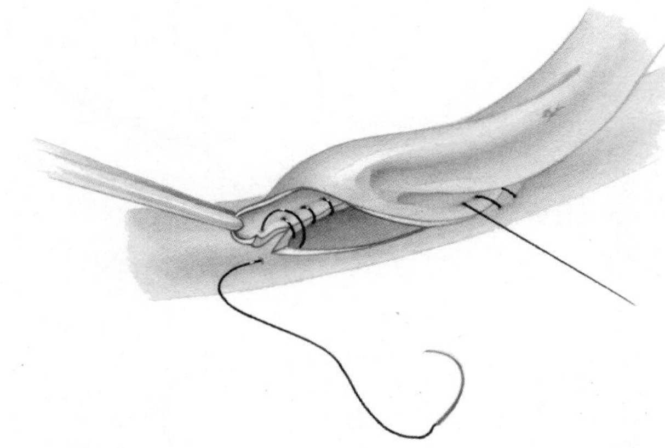

FIG. 9.44

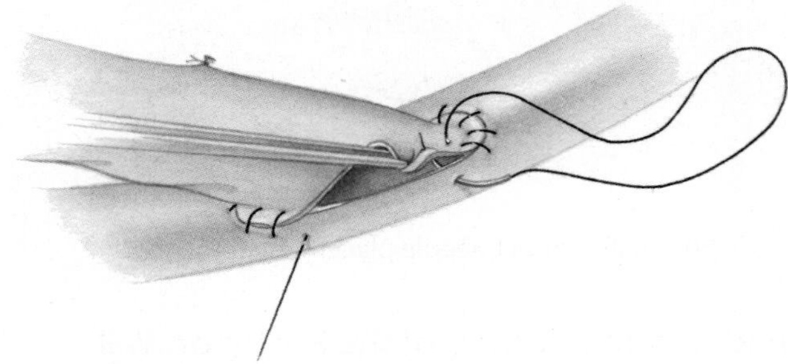

FIG. 9.45

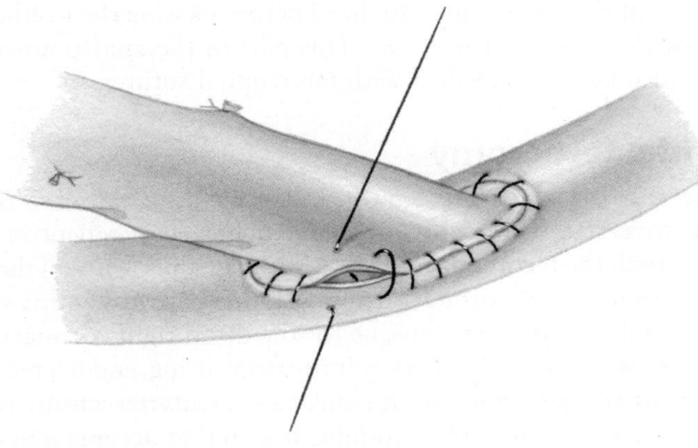

FIG. 9.46

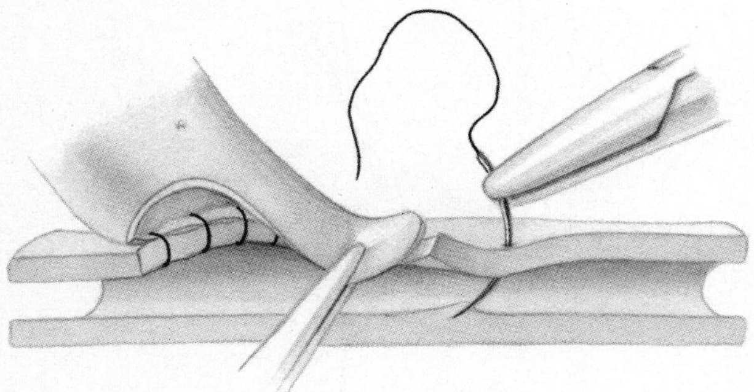

⊘ FIG. 9.47 A needle picking up the back wall of a coronary artery at the toe.

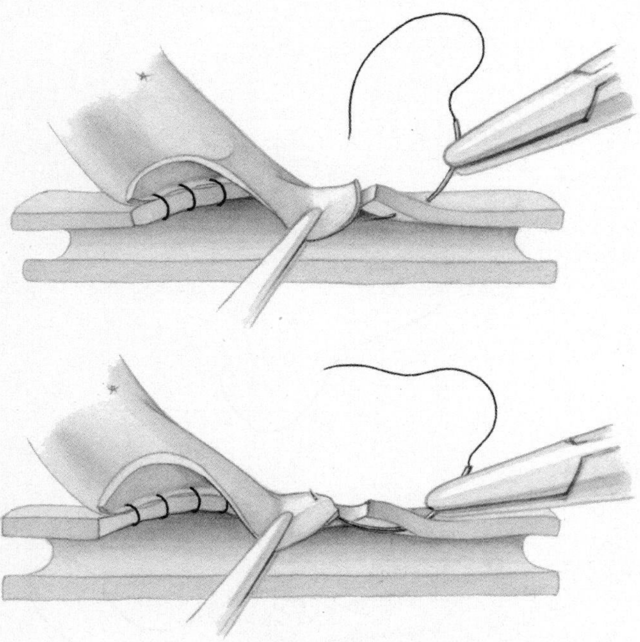

FIG. 9.48 Correct needle placement at the toe.

⊘ Inadvertent Suturing of the Posterior Wall

The needle may pick up the posterior wall of the coronary artery (Fig. 9.47). This complication can be prevented if the lumen at the toe is fully visualized before passing the needle through the graft (Fig. 9.48). This part of the anastomosis can also be accomplished with interrupted sutures. ⊘

Endarterectomy

The role of endarterectomy in coronary artery disease is controversial. Many surgeons have achieved excellent results with the technique and use it when dealing with all the main branches of coronary arteries. Others are less enthusiastic and reserve the technique for the distal right coronary artery, whereas still others refrain from using endarterectomy at all. Nevertheless, in many cases, endarterectomy is the only way to provide a suitable lumen that accepts a bypass graft. It may well be that endarterectomized coronary arteries have decreased late patency and that the technique leads to increased perioperative myocardial infarction. It is nonetheless a useful technique and, when used appropriately, does provide excellent results.

Technique

The epicardium over the diseased segment of the coronary artery is incised. A 1-cm arteriotomy is made on the anterior surface of the vessel in the usual manner. With a fine endarterectomy elevator, a plane is developed between the calcified media and the elastic adventitial segment of the coronary artery wall. The calcific core is dissected free from the arterial wall circumferentially as well as distally and proximally (Fig. 9.49). With peanut dissectors providing traction and countertraction, the calcified plaque is gently withdrawn with a clamp or a pair of forceps (Fig. 9.50).

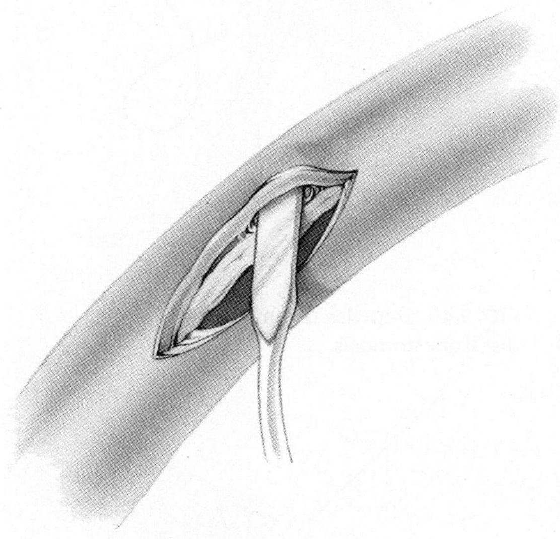

FIG. 9.49 Stepwise technique for a coronary endarterectomy.

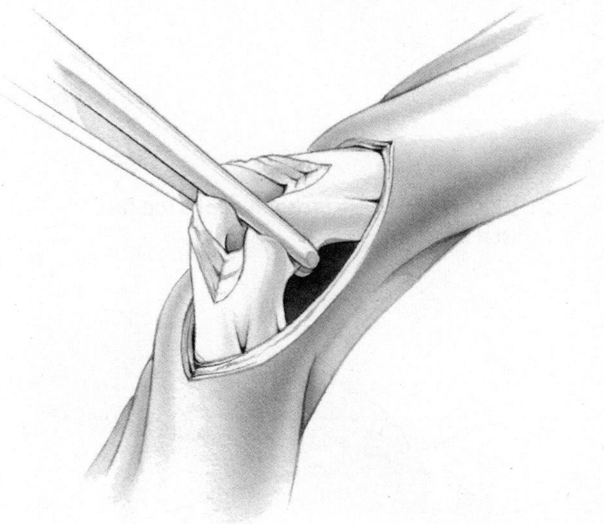

FIG. 9.50 Stepwise technique for a coronary endarterectomy.

The calcific core is withdrawn proximally and then divided with scissors. The distal segment is gently pulled and withdrawn until it becomes detached.

⊘ Tear of the Coronary Arterial Wall

Often the calcific core is adherent to the arterial wall to such an extent that its removal may create a tear in the arterial wall. Dissection must therefore be carried out with great caution. If a tear occurs, it should be directly sutured, provided that the lumen is adequate. Alternatively, the injured site is incorporated into the arteriotomy and the vein graft anastomosis. ⊘

The lumen of the endarterectomized coronary artery is irrigated profusely to remove any debris, and the vein graft is anastomosed to it in the usual manner.

⊘ Constriction of the Anastomotic Site

Often the length of the anastomosis may be quite extensive. Care should be taken to prevent the purse-string constrictive effect of the continuous suture technique. ⊘

⊘ Septal Branch Occlusion

Detachment of calcific plaque may occlude some of the arterial branches. This is particularly important whenever the LAD coronary artery is endarterectomized because total occlusion of the septal branches may result in perioperative myocardial infarction. ⊘

NB The internal thoracic artery should preferably not be used as a conduit when endarterectomy is performed because the internal thoracic artery is prone to distortion at the heel and compromised inflow when a long arteriotomy is required. NB

Proximal Anastomoses

Increasingly, all proximal anastomoses are being performed with the aortic cross-clamp in place. This technique appears to be associated with a reduced incidence of intraoperative stroke owing to detachment of calcific plaques caused by clamp injury to the aorta. It is important for a surgeon to commit to memory the size of the heart before the initiation of cardiopulmonary bypass and to envision how the vein grafts are to lie. With the heart empty and flaccid, estimation of the correct length of the vein graft may be difficult. A good rule is to estimate the length of the vein graft by the contour of the parietal pericardium. Alternatively, the heart can be filled and the correct length of the conduit ascertained.

Another technique is to remove the aortic cross-clamp and allow the heart to beat normally. The vein grafts are

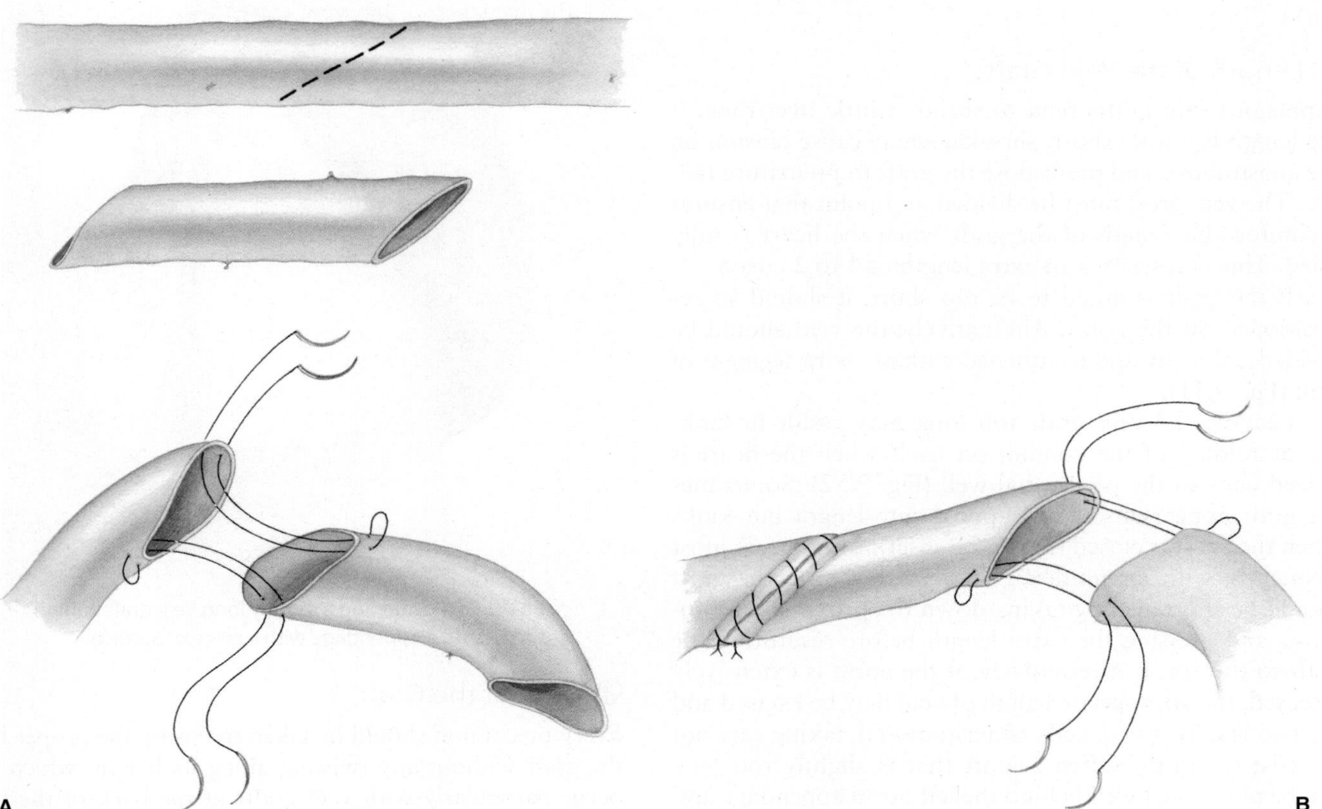

FIG. 9.51 Lengthening a vein graft with an extra vein segment.

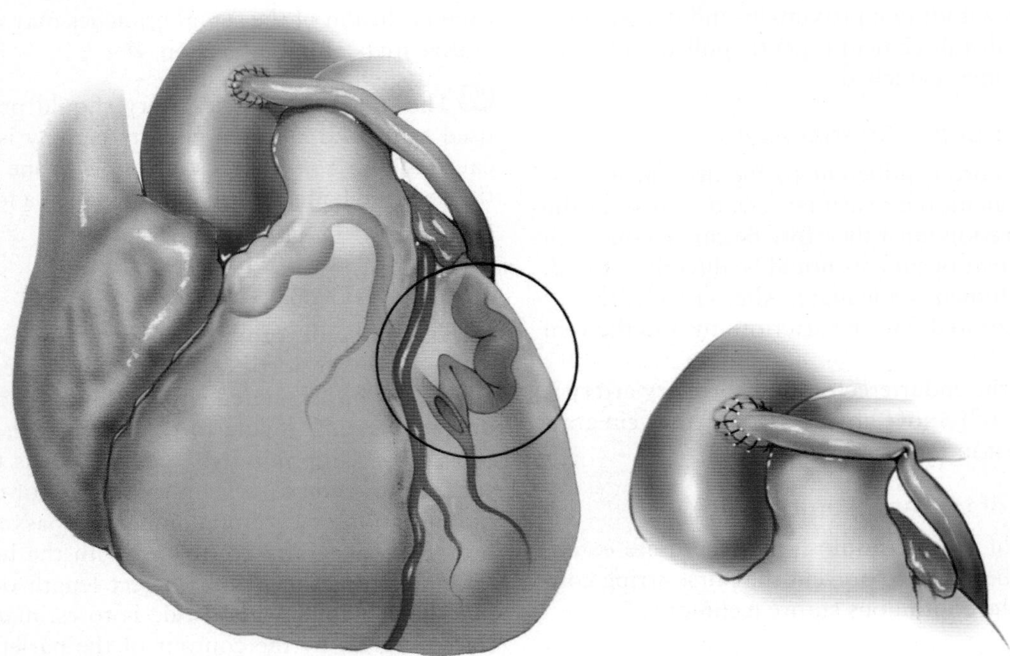

⊘ **FIG. 9.52** A vein graft that is too long kinks or folds on itself behind the heart. **Inset:** Graft kinking when the chest is closed.

cut to the optimal length, and the proximal anastomoses are performed with a side-biting clamp applied to the aorta.

⊘ Length of the Vein Graft

Saphenous vein grafts tend to shrink a little over time. If the length is a little short, shrinkage may cause tension on the anastomosis and predispose the graft to premature failure. The vein graft must be divided at a point that ensures a comfortable length of the graft when the heart is fully filled. This necessitates an extra length of 1 to 2 cm. ⊘

If the graft is noted to be too short, it should be repositioned on the aorta. Alternatively, the vein should be divided obliquely and lengthened with an extra segment of vein (Fig. 9.51).

Leaving the vein graft too long may result in kinking or folding of the conduit on itself when the heart is placed back in the pericardial well (Fig. 9.52). Sometimes the graft appears to be the appropriate length but kinks when the chest is closed (Fig. 9.52, inset). This occurs most frequently with circumflex grafts. In this case, the graft should be shortened by taking down the proximal anastomosis and excising the extra length before resuturing the graft to the aorta. Alternatively, if the aorta is extensively diseased, the appropriate length of vein may be excised and the two resulting vein ends reanastomosed, taking care not to twist the graft. Often a graft that is slightly too long can be positioned well behind the left atrial appendage and kept in place with a piece of Surgicel (Fig. 9.53).

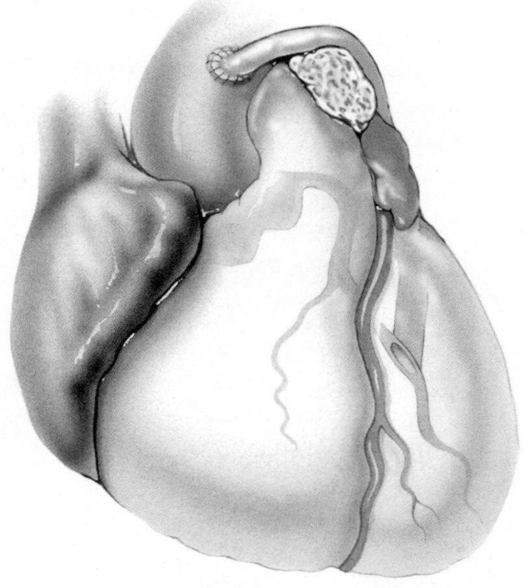

FIG. 9.53 Positioning a slightly long vein graft behind the left atrial appendage with a piece of Surgicel.

⊘ Twist of the Graft

Every precaution should be taken to ensure the proper lie of the graft without any twisting along its length, which may occur particularly with vein grafts at the back of the heart (Fig. 9.54). In rare cases, when this occurs, the proximal

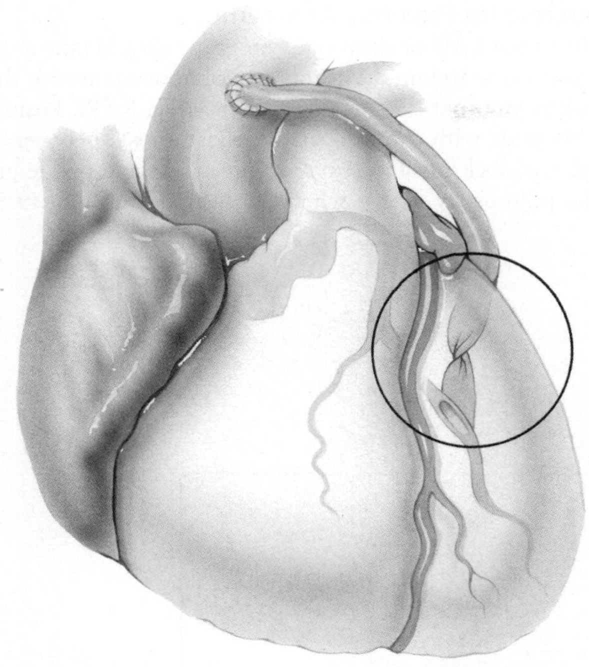

⊘ **FIG. 9.54** Twisting of a vein graft.

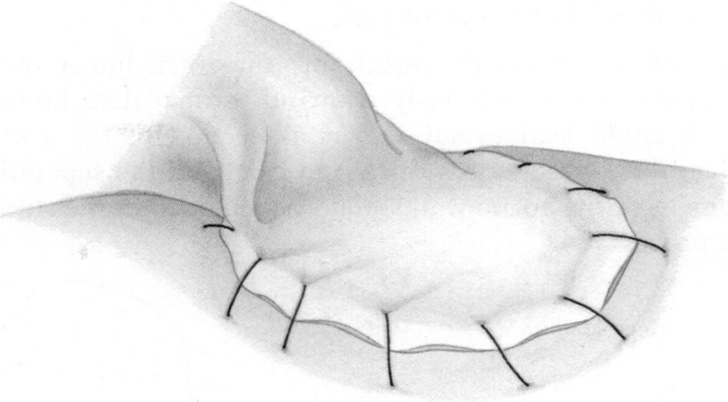

⊘ **FIG. 9.55** The hood of a vein graft is flattened owing to too large an aortic opening.

anastomosis must be redone. If for any reason this is not feasible, the vein graft may be divided and reanastomosed after being untwisted. Some surgeons prefer to mark the vein graft with a methylene blue stripe to prevent this complication. ⊘

The vein end is tailored to have a large, wide, hood-shaped opening (Fig. 9.13). This can be accomplished by dividing the vein approximately 30 degrees obliquely with respect to its length and then extending the incision generously downward at the heel to create a vein graft opening that is at least 20% larger than the aortic opening.

⊘ Mismatch between the Vein Graft and Aortic Opening

The circumference of the vein graft must be at least 20% larger than the aortic opening; otherwise, the vein stretches out flat and compromises the lumen (Fig. 9.55). ⊘

NB If the vein caliber is small, the aortic opening should be limited to a narrow slit corresponding to the incision at the heel of the graft. NB

NB If the aortic opening is inadvertently made too large, the opening can be narrowed to the appropriate diameter with a purse-string 4-0 Prolene suture (Fig. 9.56). NB

With a no. 11 blade, a 3- to 4-mm slit-like incision is made at a precise site for each proximal anastomosis. The opening is dilated slightly with the tip of a fine forceps. A disposable punch is introduced into the slit-like opening, and a circular part of the aortic wall, 4.0 to 4.8 mm in diameter, is removed (Fig. 9.57).

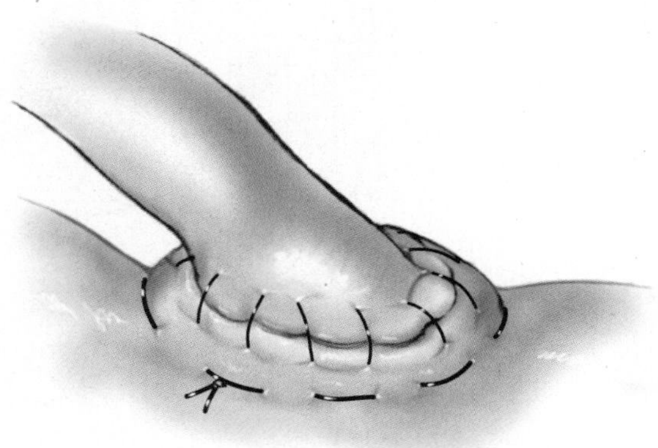

FIG. 9.56 Narrowing too large an aortic opening with a purse-string suture.

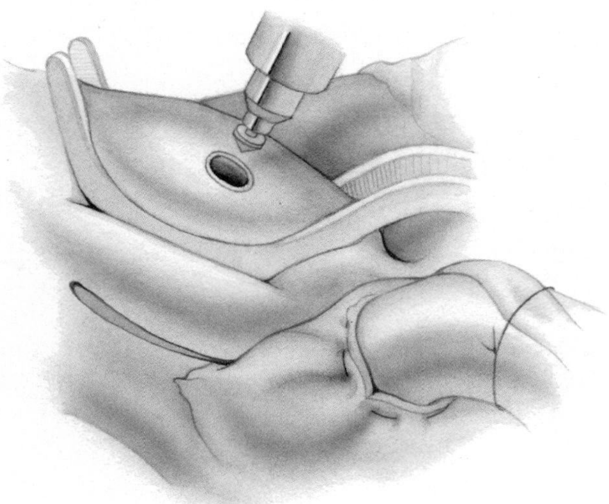

FIG. 9.57 Creating aortic opening with a disposable punch.

⊘ Intimal Wall Detachment

The introduction of the punch into the aortic lumen must be performed meticulously to avoid intimal detachment, which could lead to subsequent dissection of the aorta. When the aortic wall is thick and calcified, the separated segment of the aortic wall should be included in the suturing process. ⊘

Technique for Proximal Anastomosis

The lie of the LAD or diagonal vein grafts should take a deep concave course to join the aorta in an oblique manner at the 2 o'clock position at the anastomotic site (Fig. 9.58). Positioning this graft with the heel of the anastomosis between the 3 and 5 o'clock positions may result in kinking of the graft by the pulmonary artery when the heart is full (Fig. 9.59).

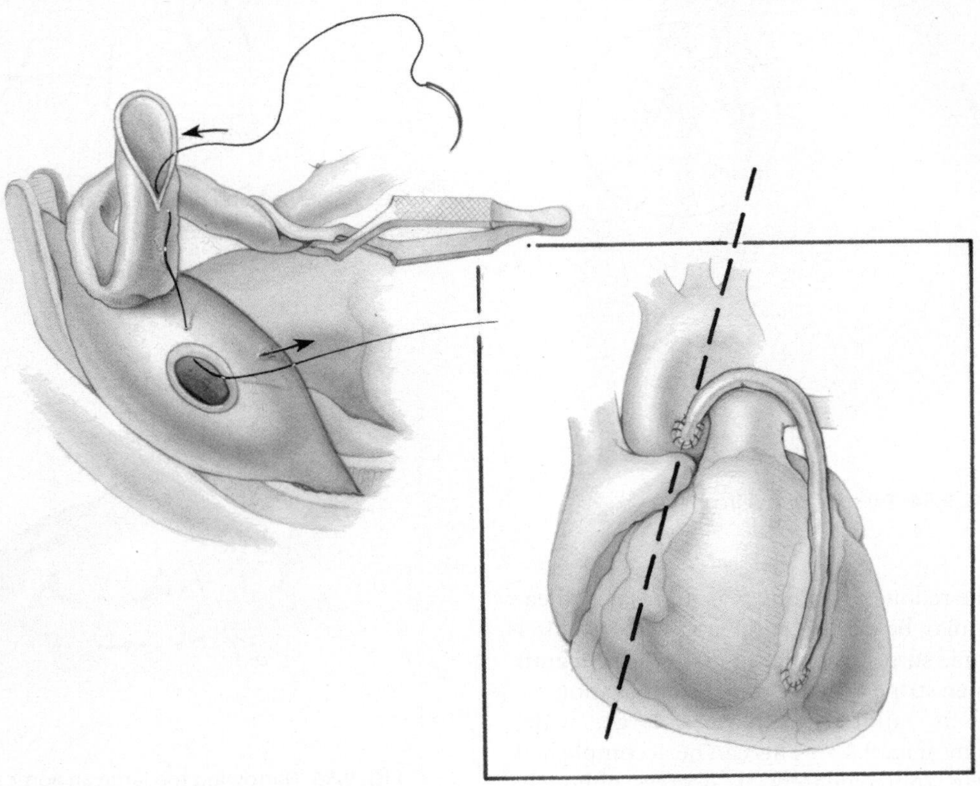

FIG. 9.58 Correct orientation of a proximal vein graft to the left anterior descending or diagonal coronary artery.

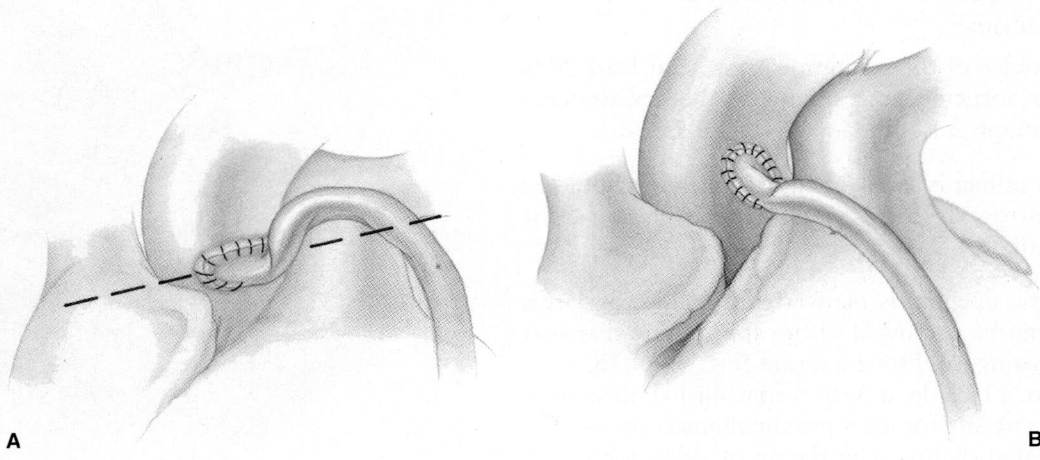

FIG. 9.59 Incorrect orientation of a proximal vein graft leading to kinking by the pulmonary artery. A: A graft to the left anterior descending artery. B: A graft to the right coronary artery.

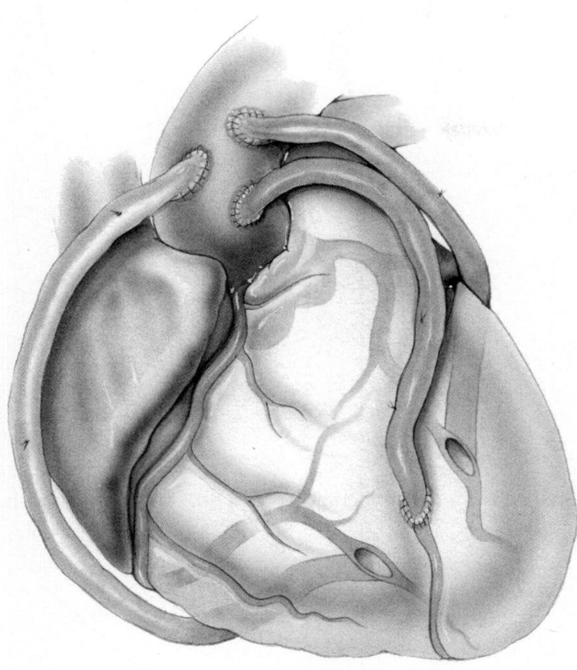

FIG. 9.60 Correct placement and orientation of the proximal vein grafts.

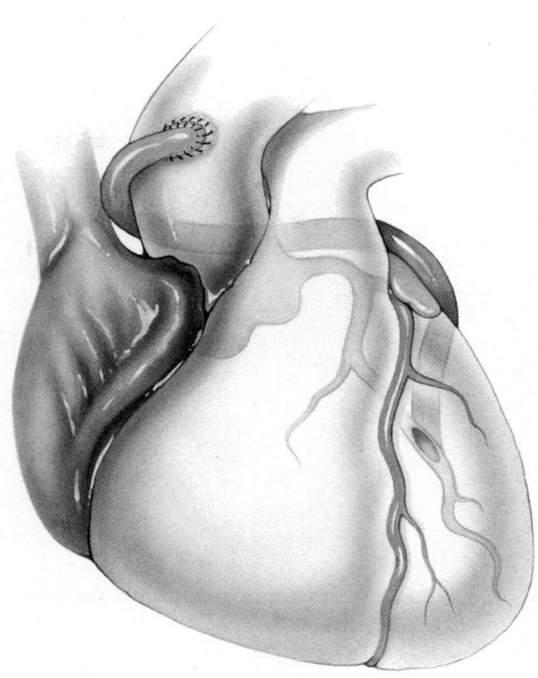

FIG. 9.61 Routing a graft through the transverse sinus.

The ramus and obtuse marginal grafts join the aorta horizontally at the 3 o'clock position. The distal right vein graft takes a course along the atrioventricular groove and joins the ascending aorta at the 6 to 7 o'clock position, and the posterior descending artery grafts take a course lateral to the atrium and join the aorta at approximately the 8 o'clock position. The right-sided grafts are anastomosed to the anterior right lateral aspect of the aorta relatively high on the aorta (Fig. 9.60). This prevents the graft from being kinked by the superior vena cava or the right ventricular outflow tract (Fig. 9.59B). Under special circumstances, the left-sided grafts can be passed behind the aorta through the transverse sinus and be anastomosed to the right side of the aorta (Fig. 9.61). The latter technique is particularly useful when there is calcification of the left side of the ascending aorta or when the vein is short. Nevertheless, this technique predisposes the vein graft to possible twisting behind the aorta and makes control of any bleeding from a side branch difficult.

NB The surgeon must always anticipate the possibility that the patient may require aortic valve replacement at some time in the future. Therefore, the proximal anastomoses should be placed high on the aorta to allow a subsequent aortotomy to be made without interfering with the proximal graft sites. NB

The proximal anastomosis is started with a 30-in. long 5-0 or 6-0 Prolene double-armed suture. The precise lie and course of direction of the vein graft are envisioned.

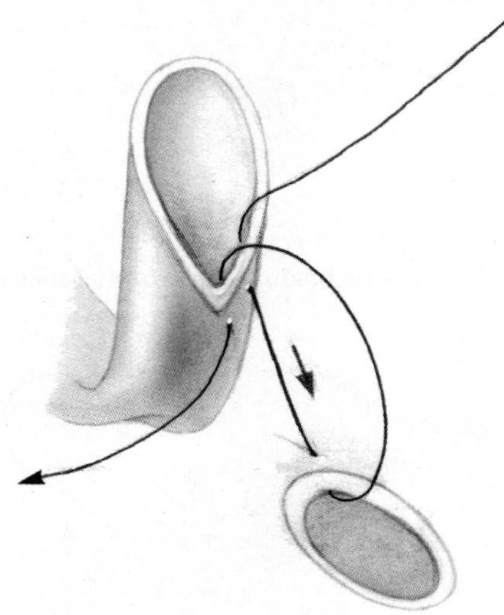

FIG. 9.62 Stepwise technique for a proximal anastomosis.

The first stitch is passed from the inside of the graft to the outside and then passed from the outside to the inside of the aorta in a counterclockwise direction (Fig. 9.62). After three to five rounds of suturing, the graft is lowered into position, and the needle is clamped (Fig. 9.63). The needle at the other end of the suture is now passed in a backhand manner, from the inside to the outside of the aorta (Fig. 9.64), followed by outside to inside of the vein graft in a clockwise direction (Fig. 9.65). This over-and-over

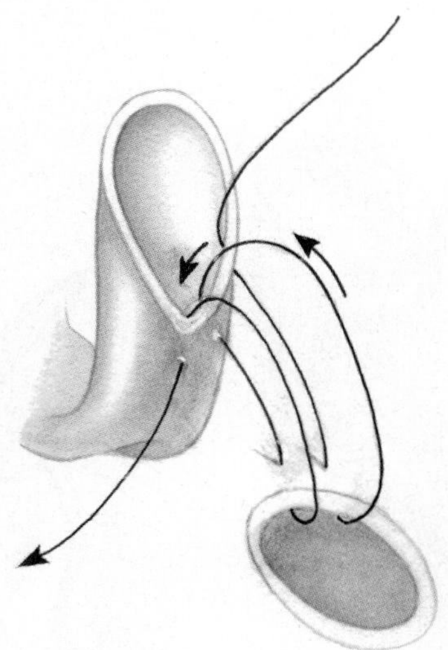

FIG. 9.63 Stepwise technique for a proximal anastomosis.

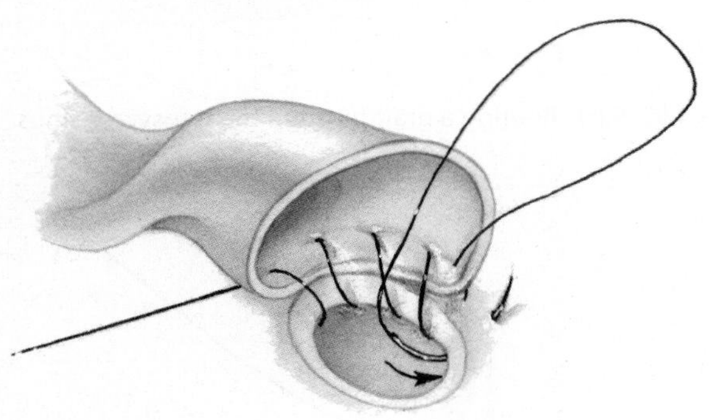

FIG. 9.64 Stepwise technique for a proximal anastomosis.

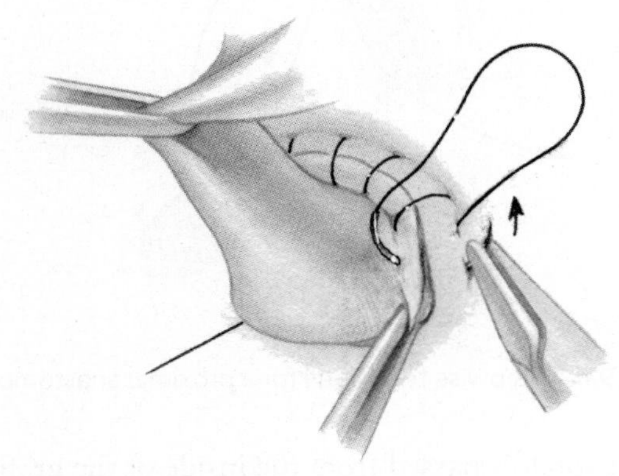

FIG. 9.65 Stepwise technique for a proximal anastomosis.

suturing is continued to meet the other arm of the suture (Fig. 9.66). When all the proximal anastomoses are completed, the vein grafts are each occluded with atraumatic bulldog clamps. The perfusion pressure is temporarily reduced, and the aortic clamp is removed. Blood is allowed to

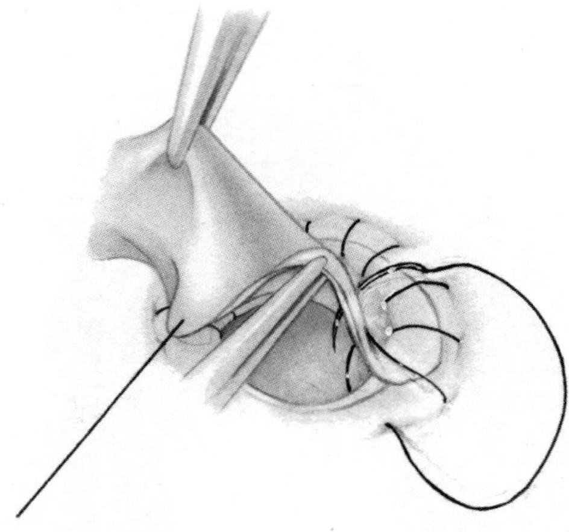

FIG. 9.66 Stepwise technique for a proximal anastomosis.

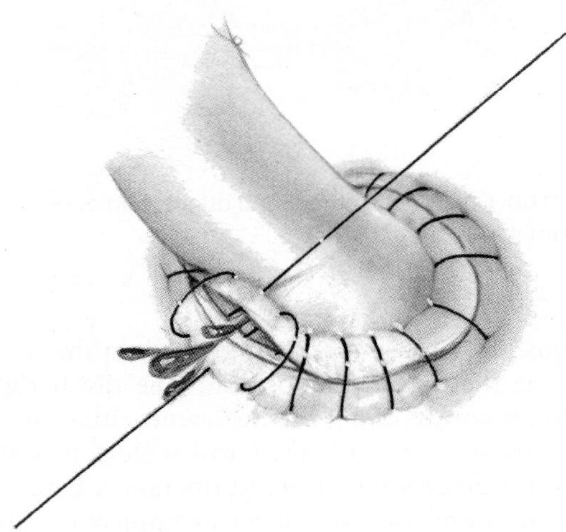

FIG. 9.67 Stepwise technique for a proximal anastomosis.

distend the vein grafts and to leak through the anastomoses (Fig. 9.67). This maneuver displaces air, allows the vein graft to assume its hood shape, and prevents purse-string constriction of the anastomosis. The suture ends are now tied securely. Normal perfusion pressure is resumed when all sutures have been tied.

NB Calcified Aorta

Placement of proximal anastomoses should be on the normal aortic wall. Calcific sites should be avoided. However, aortic walls are sometimes very diseased and at times calcified. Often, "toothpaste" material is squeezed out of the aortotomy site; at other times, there are calcific plaques within the aortotomy. The edges of the aortotomy should be free of any debris. It is cleaned with a dry gauze, and the aortic clamp is loosened slightly to allow blood to gush out of the aortotomy and wash away any debris or particles. NB

Technical points to ensure good proximal anastomoses include tailoring a generous opening in the proximal vein because the aortic wall is not pliable. In addition, deep bites of all the layers of the aortic wall must be taken.

NB Epiaortic Ultrasonographic Scan

Atherosclerotic changes of the aorta are very common in elderly patients. Epiaortic ultrasonographic scanning can be used to detect localized atheromatous areas that may not be detectable by digital palpation. At times, the aorta may be so diseased that proximal vein grafts may have to be placed on the innominate artery. A totally calcified lead pipe aorta may have to be replaced (see Chapter 8). NB

NB Free Internal Thoracic and Radial Arterial Grafts

If a free internal thoracic or radial arterial graft is used, a small aortic opening must be made. Unless the aortic wall is fairly thin, it may be preferable to anastomose the proximal arterial conduit to a vein graft hood or to a patch of vein or pericardium that has already been sewn to an aortic opening. NB

NB Marking of Proximal Anastomoses

To facilitate angiographic location of the proximal anastomoses in the future, some surgeons incorporate a radiopaque ring into the proximal suture line. NB

NB Aortic Wall Adventitial Tissue

In preparing the site for proximal anastomosis, adventitial tissue on the aortic wall should be incorporated in the suturing process. This is particularly important in elderly patients with delicate aortic walls. The adventitial tissue acts as "natural" pledgets, providing a secure anastomosis and adding strength to the aortic wall. NB

OFF-PUMP CORONARY ARTERY BYPASS GRAFTING

Traditionally, coronary artery bypass grafting has relied on the aid of cardiopulmonary bypass to obtain a bloodless and stationary operating field. However, despite the many advances made, blood contact with the artificial surfaces of the cardiopulmonary bypass circuit continues to produce a well-documented diffuse inflammatory response that affects multiple organ systems and is responsible for much of the noncardiac morbidity after open-heart surgery. Off-pump coronary bypass grafting has been associated with decreased transfusion requirements, and may be a preferred strategy in high-risk patients with cerebrovascular disease or aortic calcific disease.

NB Relative Contraindication to Off-Pump Surgery

Patients who have had recent myocardial infarction with impaired left ventricles and patients with dilated ventricles are not ideal candidates for off-pump bypass procedures. Similarly, in patients with more than mild mitral insufficiency, grafting the branches of the circumflex coronary artery may cause hemodynamic instability. These patients may be best managed by performing the revascularization procedure on the beating heart with cardiopulmonary support. The aorta is not clamped and cardioplegia is not administered. The heart is kept empty, providing optimum myocardial protection and hemodynamic stability. NB

Anesthetic Considerations

The main goal of anesthesia management is to maintain hemodynamic stability during the various manipulations of the heart during off-pump coronary surgery. Ideally, an oximetric pulmonary artery catheter is used to continuously measure mixed venous oxygen saturation and cardiac output. Transesophageal echocardiography may have limited value when the heart is displaced to a vertical position. The key to avoiding emergent conversion to cardiopulmonary bypass is to be proactive, rather than reactive, in optimizing surgical conditions to prevent hypotension and low cardiac output. Intravascular volume should be replenished because the most common cause of low blood pressure is decreased venous return with positioning of the heart. Hemoglobin level, electrolytes, acid–base status, and arterial blood gases should be maintained within a normal range. Although inotropic support may be necessary, it is kept to a minimum to prevent tachycardia, which can interfere with optimal suture placement and increase myocardial oxygen consumption. Most important, continuous communication is needed between the operating surgeon and the anesthesiologist.

NB Positioning the Heart

The most critical aspect of off-pump coronary bypass surgery is the positioning of the heart to expose the target vessel adequately without hemodynamic compromise. This can be accomplished through strategic placement of four deep pericardial sutures (Fig. 9.68) and appropriately placing the patient in various positions. The first pericardial suture is placed above the left inferior pulmonary vein well below the phrenic nerve, the second near the inferior vena cava, and the last two equidistant in a line drawn between the first two sutures. Rommel tourniquets are used to avoid abrasions on the epicardium by the pericardial sutures. By sequentially increasing the tension on each suture from the pulmonary vein to the inferior vena cava, coupled with steep Trendelenburg positioning of the

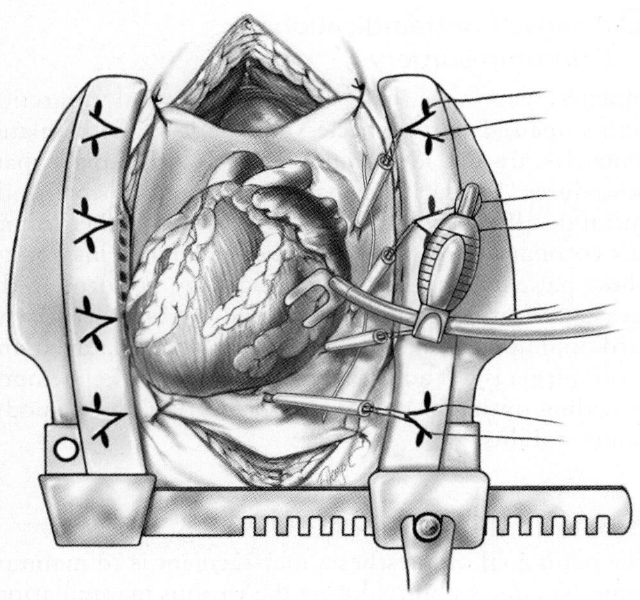

FIG. 9.68 Strategic placement of deep pericardial sutures.

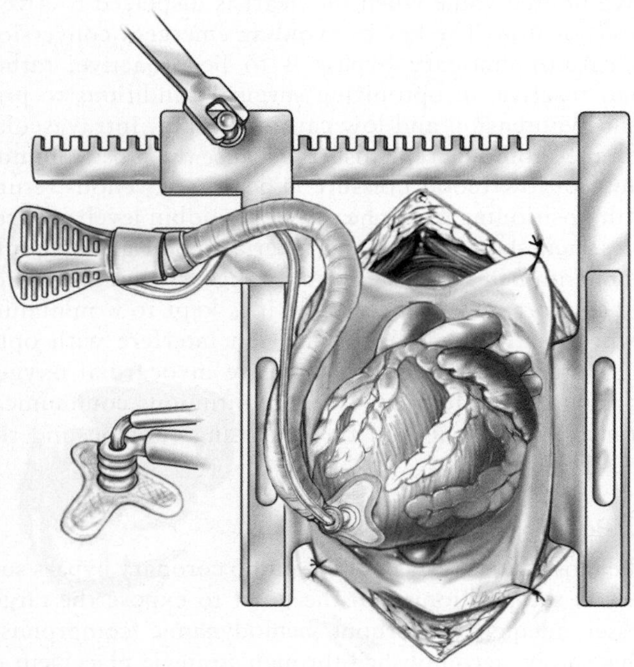

FIG. 9.69 An apical suction device for exposing lateral and posterior vessels.

operating table rotated toward the surgeon, the heart can be lifted out of the pericardial sac to expose the LAD and diagonal target vessels. Generally, lifting the heart to a vertical position is relatively well tolerated. Commercially available apical suction devices (Fig. 9.69) can be used to lift the heart vertically so that the lateral and posterior targets can be visualized. The flexible joint at the hinge point of the apex device allows the heart to freely twist about its long axis. NB

NB Mechanical stabilization

There are several devices that can locally immobilize the target coronary artery during off-pump surgery. The Acrobat System (Maquet Cardiovascular, Wayne, NJ) utilizes both suction and compression (Fig. 9.70) to stabilize the target vessel. The Octopus System (Medtronic, Inc. Minneapolis, MN) obtains stabilization by applying high-pressure suction to the surrounding tissue through multiple suction cups (Fig. 9.71). NB

⊘ Stabilizer Myocardial Injury

It is important that the stabilizer is used for local immobilization of the myocardium only. It should not be used as a retraction device, which may cause hemodynamic compromise. ⊘

Anterior Vessels

Left Anterior Descending and Diagonal Branch

Generally, the anterior vessels are grafted first. Revascularization of the LAD artery with the internal thoracic artery allows immediate perfusion of a sizable portion of the myocardium.

NB Sometimes the diagonal artery may need to be grafted before the LAD artery because the internal thoracic pedicle

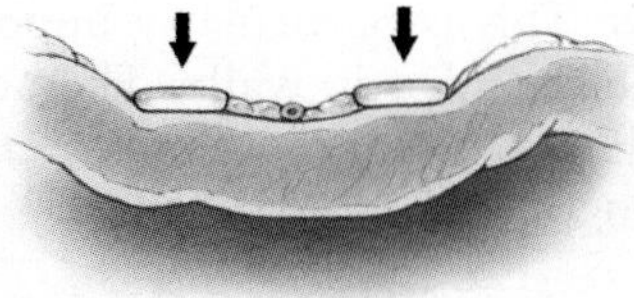

FIG. 9.70 Target stabilization using compressive forces.

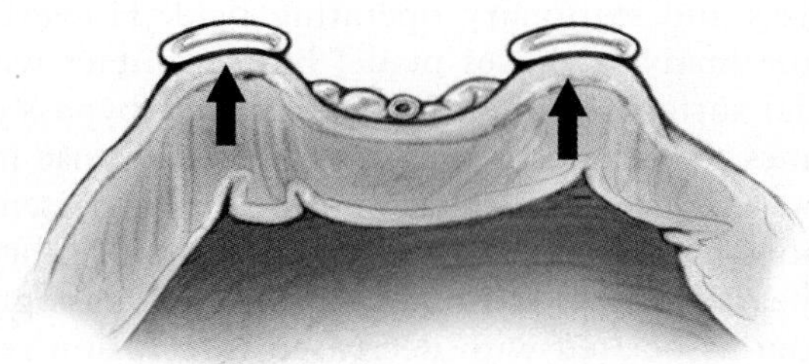

FIG. 9.71 Target stabilization using high-pressure suction.

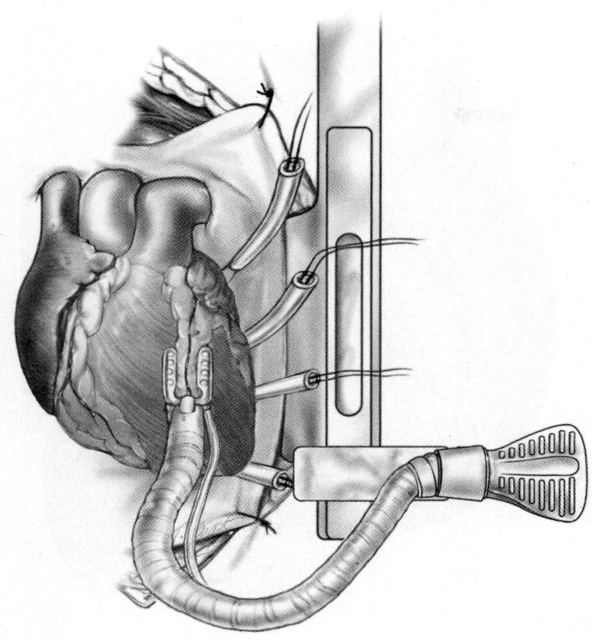

FIG. 9.72 Exposure and stabilization of the left anterior descending artery.

can make placement of the stabilizer for immobilization of the diagonal branch difficult. NB

These anterior branches are exposed by gentle traction on the deep pericardial sutures to rotate the apex of the heart into the surgical field. The stabilizer is placed on the target site with the tips toward the base of the heart (Fig. 9.72).

NB The LAD artery is usually grafted at the distal one-third to one-half where the vessel normally emerges from its intramyocardial location. Occasionally, grafting of the artery is required more proximally. Proximal occlusion with a soft silastic tape (see subsequent text) is performed before arteriotomy as significant coronary bleeding may occur. Many surgeons routinely use intraluminal shunts to minimize distal bed ischemia. NB

Ramus Intermedius and High Obtuse Marginal Branches

These are often intramyocardial and require grafting near the base of the heart that cannot be mobilized into the field. However, displacement of the heart into a vertical position allows easier access for arteriotomy and suturing. The stabilizer is placed with the tips toward the base of the heart (Fig. 9.73). Placing the patient in Trendelenburg position and rotating the table toward the surgeon may facilitate exposure.

⊘ Injury to the Left Atrial Appendage

Although the stabilizer can be positioned with the heel toward the base of the heart, bleeding from the left atrial appendage can occur if it is allowed to rub against the stabilizer arm (Fig. 9.74). ⊘

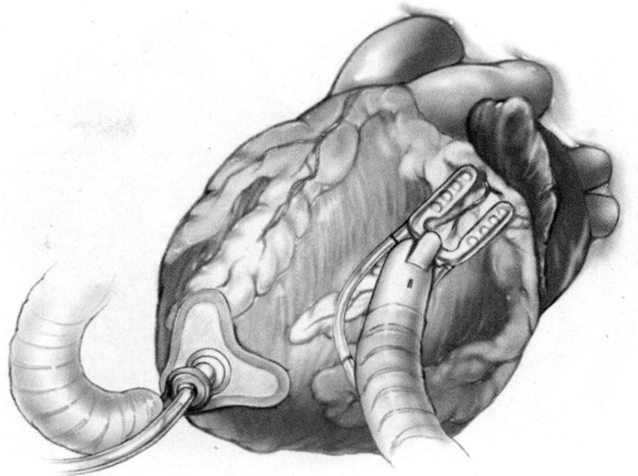

FIG. 9.73 Exposure and stabilization of the ramus intermedius and high obtuse marginal branches.

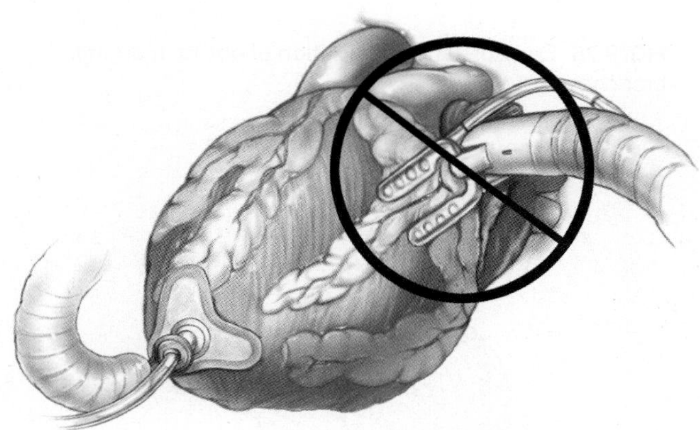

⊘ FIG. 9.74 Injury to the left atrial appendage from inappropriate placement of a stabilizer.

Posterior Vessels: Obtuse Marginal Branches

Other lower obtuse marginal branches can be best accessed with the heart in the vertical position and slightly rotated to the right. The stabilizer is attached on either the crossbar or the right side of the retractor and placed with the tips toward the base of the heart (Fig. 9.75).

NB Exposure of the circumflex coronary artery and some of the obtuse marginal branches may be difficult at times, particularly when the left ventricle is dilated. Opening of the right pleura will provide better access. NB

⊘ Obstruction of Venous Return

The heart should not be rotated excessively in an attempt to provide better target exposure because this may cause obstruction of venous return. ⊘

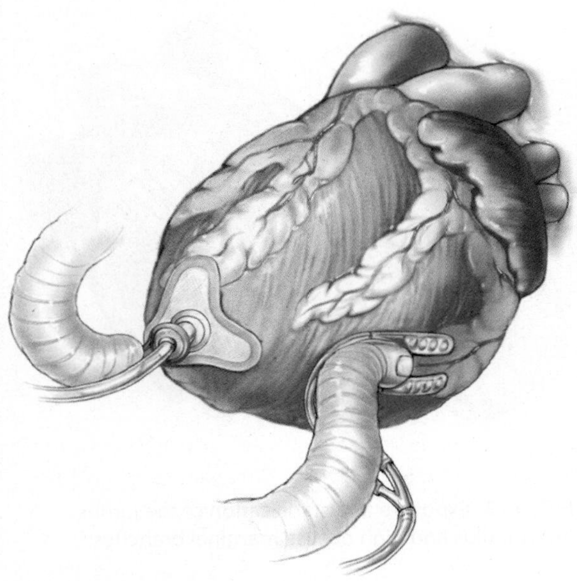

FIG. 9.75 Exposure and stabilization of obtuse marginal branches.

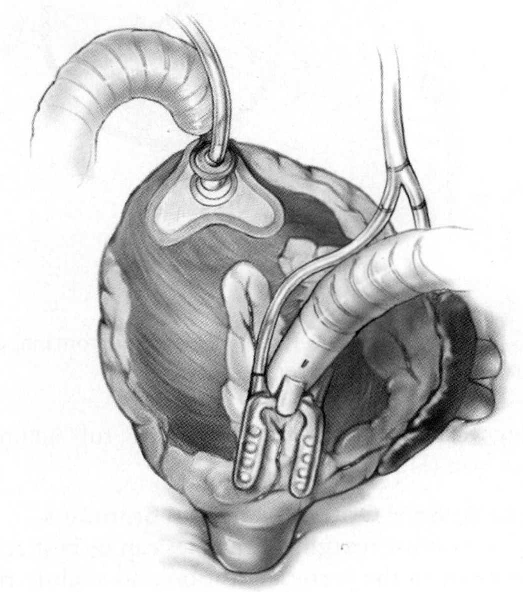

FIG. 9.76 Exposure and stabilization of the posterior vessels.

Posterior Vessels

Posterior Descending Artery

Exposure of this vessel is usually very well tolerated without hemodynamic instability. The heart is displaced vertically without any rotation. The stabilizer is attached to the left side of the retractor and placed toward the base of the heart (Fig. 9.76).

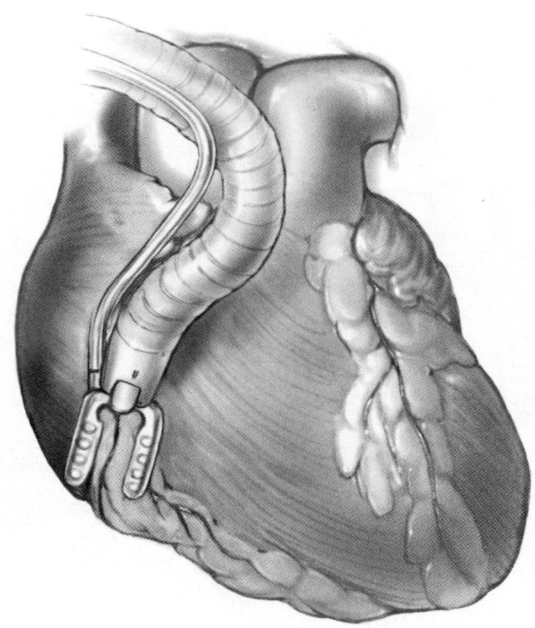

FIG. 9.77 Exposure and stabilization of the distal right coronary artery.

Distal Right Coronary Artery

Adequate exposure can usually be accomplished without lifting the heart out of the chest. The stabilizer is attached to the right side of the retractor with the tip directed downward along the course of the artery (Fig. 9.77).

NB It is preferable to graft the right posterior descending artery rather than the distal main right coronary artery. Occlusion of posterior descending artery rarely causes hemodynamic problems. If the right coronary artery itself must be grafted, a shunt may be required to avoid ischemia and hemodynamic instability. NB

⊘ Right Ventricular Distention and Bradycardia

It is not uncommon for bradycardia and right ventricular distension to occur with proximal occlusion of the right coronary artery. Therefore, alligator clips should be applied to the epicardium and attached to a pacemaker before coronary occlusion. Alternatively, an intraluminal shunt can be used. ⊘

Conduct of the Surgery

As in on-pump coronary artery surgery, the heart is exposed through a median sternotomy and all conduits are harvested in the usual manner. The operative technique for grafting vessels during an off-pump case is similar to that used with on-pump surgery. After an arteriotomy is made, an intravascular shunt is inserted and the proximal silastic tape is released. In vessels too small for shunting, the silastic tape is placed under traction to control bleeding.

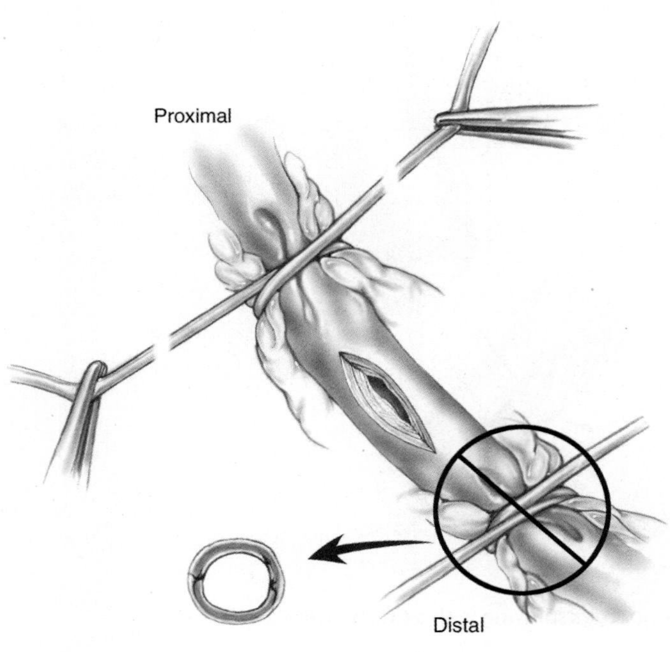

FIG. 9.78 Avoid the use of distal occlusion.

⊘ Injury to the Artery Distal to the Anastomosis

Distal vessel occlusion should be avoided because it may cause intimal injury and subsequent stenosis (Fig. 9.78). ⊘

A bloodless field is obtained with a CO_2 mist blower.

⊘ Lifting an Intimal Plaque

Vigorous spraying with the CO_2 blower can either lift an intimal plaque or separate the intimal layer to cause a localized dissection (Fig. 9.79). Use of the CO_2 blower should be limited to the time that the needle passes through the target vessel and only when sufficient blood is present to obscure the field. Focus should be on the site of each needle passage with attention to the back wall and edges. A completely bloodless field is not necessary. ⊘

NB After each distal anastomosis, the graft is deaired by gently flushing with warm blood (or removing the internal thoracic artery occluder) before tightening and securely tying the suture. NB

With a relatively disease-free aorta, proximal vein graft anastomoses are performed using a partial occlusion clamp. The systemic arterial blood pressure is lowered to a systolic level of approximately 100 mm Hg before the clamp is applied. The clamp should be tightened just enough for hemostasis but securely enough to not slip off.

⊘ Aortic Dissection

Applying the clamp too tightly or during hypertension can cause aortic dissection, especially in the elderly with a fragile aorta. ⊘

NB In patients with atherosclerotic or calcific aortic disease in whom the side-biting clamp cannot be placed safely, alternative sites for proximal anastomoses such as the innominate artery may be considered. Another strategy in this clinical situation is the use of the Heartstring System if a soft spot on the ascending aorta can be identified. The Heartstring III Proximal Seal System (Maquet Cardiovascular, Wayne, NJ) allows creation of a proximal handsewn anastomosis without clamping the ascending aorta (Fig. 9.80). NB

Transmyocardial Revascularization

Transmyocardial revascularization (TMR) is an adjunct to the surgical management of coronary artery disease. Carbon dioxide laser, holmium:YAG laser, and xenon chloride eximer laser have all been used to create channels into the left ventricular cavity. TMR with laser is used in patients with stable angina despite optimal medical therapy and with a region of myocardium that cannot be directly vascularized. In this patient population, TMR has been shown to improve anginal symptoms and is associated with improved left ventricula perfusion. Although the mechanism of the beneficial effects of TMR is unknown, it is believed that local intramyocardial delivery of blood and/or angiogenesis play a role in this process.

NB Patients with ejection fractions less than 30% or acute ischemia are generally not candidates for TMR. NB

NB Although TMR is usually applied only to areas of myocardium that cannot be directly revascularized, patients with diffusely diseased coronary arteries may benefit from combined treatment. NB

Technique

TMR can be performed as an isolated procedure through an anterior thoracotomy or thoracoscopic approach. However, it is typically performed after bypass grafting is completed, while the patient is still on cardiopulmonary bypass. The viable ischemic area is exposed. The laser is fired to create between 15 and 20 channels 1 cm apart, covering the ischemic but not directly the revascularized area. Bubbles are seen by transesophageal echocardiography when the laser beam reaches the ventricular cavity, confirming a completed channel. The carbon dioxide laser should be synchronized to the patient's electrocardiogram so that the pulse is delivered on the R wave, to minimize the likelihood of arrhythmia. After cardiopulmonary bypass is discontinued and protamine is administered, most channels readily seal at the epicardial surface with gentle digital pressure. Occasionally, a figure-of-eight 6-0 Prolene suture may be required for hemostasis. NB

NB Many surgeons combine laser with therapeutic angiogenesis.

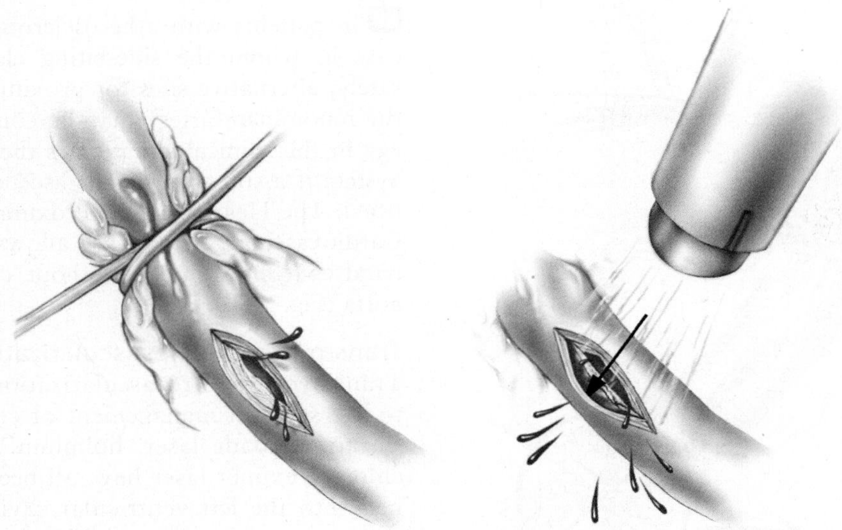

FIG. 9.79 Separation of intimal plaque from vigorous spraying with a CO_2 blower.

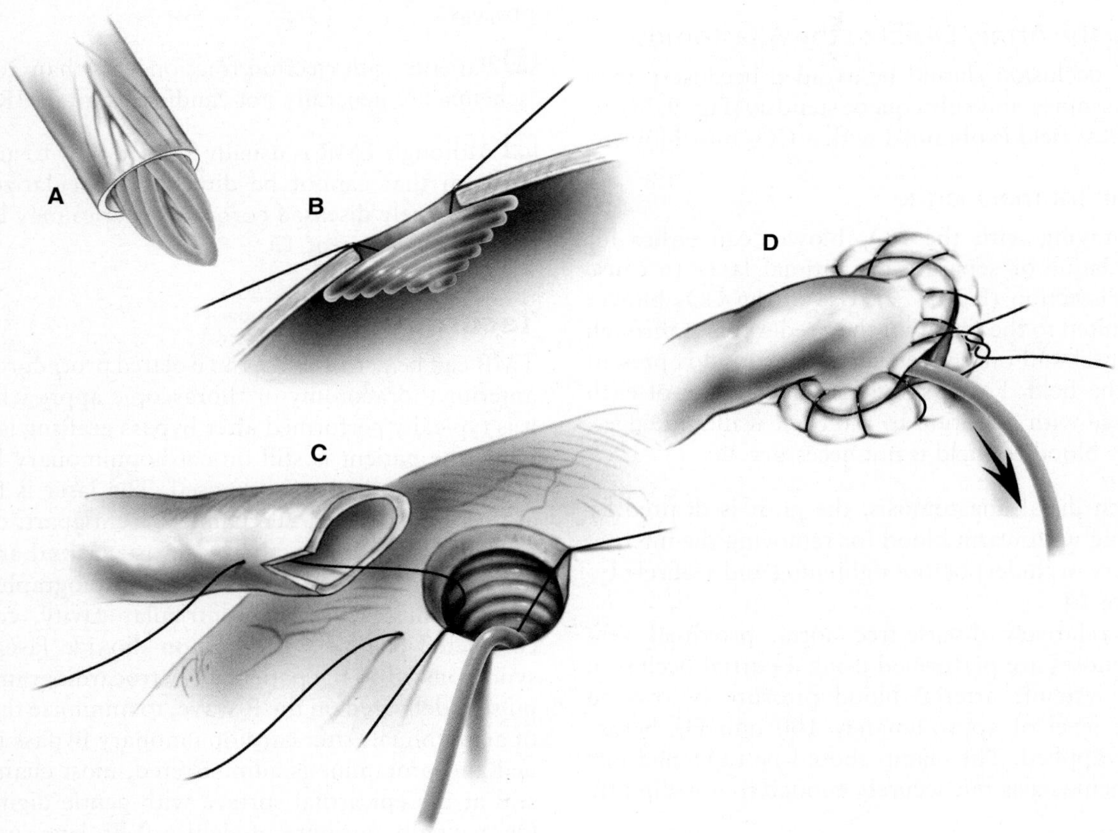

FIG. 9.80 Heartstring II proximal seal system for proximal aortic anastomosis.

CONSIDERATIONS IN REOPERATIVE CORONARY ARTERY BYPASS SURGERY

The operative strategy for performing redo coronary surgery is similar to the primary procedure. Some important points need to be considered. General precautions for repeat sternotomy need to be followed (see Chapter 1). If a patent *in situ* right internal thoracic graft is present and crossing the midline, or if a redundant left internal thoracic pedicle lies directly beneath the sternum, great care must be exercised to prevent injury to these grafts.

If a patent *in situ* internal thoracic graft is present, the pedicle must be identified and mobilized if the redo procedure is to be done on cardiopulmonary bypass with cardioplegic arrest of the heart. The pedicle must be occluded with an atraumatic bulldog clamp during the cross-clamp interval. The safest technique for identifying the left internal thoracic pedicle is to begin the dissection from the diaphragm and proceed superiorly. The anastomotic site is therefore encountered first, and the pedicle can then be gently encircled for later clamping.

NB If a thoracic pedicle is injured, it may be primarily repaired using surrounding adventitial tissue. If repair and reestablishment of flow is not feasible, urgent initiation of cardiopulmonary bypass is advisable. Replacement of injured graft is then undertaken. Alternatively, the injured graft may be cannulated with an olive-tipped catheter and perfused with a line connected to an aortic or femoral artery catheter. NB

NB There is always concern regarding having adequate conduits for a coronary reoperation. It is important to evaluate the patient preoperatively for the availability and quality of remaining conduits. This may entail Doppler studies to identify residual greater saphenous vein segments or usable lesser saphenous vein. At the time of angiography, it is useful to inject any internal thoracic vessel not previously used to demonstrate its patency. Occasionally, the internal thoracic vessels are injured or occluded during chest closure, and therefore would not be available as conduits for the reoperation. NB

NB If conduits are limited, sequential anastomoses should be considered. This strategy also reduces the number of proximal anastomotic sites on an already overcrowded and scarred ascending aorta. NB

The ascending aorta is often quite thickened and diseased in patients undergoing redo coronary artery procedures. Therefore, it is generally safer to perform all distal and proximal anastomoses under a single aortic cross-clamp period. The hood of the old vein graft is usually free of disease and provides a good location for a proximal anastomosis.

NB The patent arterial grafts often provide satisfactory sites for the proximal anastomosis of short arterial grafts. This can be performed without clamping the aorta. NB

Patent but diseased saphenous vein grafts should not be manipulated to prevent embolization of debris into the distal coronary artery bed. Some controversy exists as to whether antegrade cardioplegia should be administered down diseased vein grafts. Some surgeons divide all old, patent vein grafts once on cardiopulmonary bypass and flush debris out of them with retrograde cardioplegia. The two ends are oversewn after the distal anastomosis of the new graft is completed.

⊘ Inadequate Flow through Internal Thoracic Artery

An internal thoracic artery may not provide sufficient flow to a previously grafted coronary artery with a diseased but patent vein graft. This is especially true if the surgeon elects to divide and oversew the old graft to prevent embolization of debris. In this case, another vein graft is preferred. ⊘

NB How to deal with a patent or stenotic vein graft when an internal thoracic artery is to be used is somewhat controversial. In our practice, we tend to leave the old vein graft intact and anastomose the internal thoracic artery to the coronary just distal to the old graft. If the vein graft has been injured, then it is replaced with another vein graft. If there is not an anastomotic stenosis, a 1-mm rim of the old vein graft is left at the distal anastomotic site and the new vein graft is sewn to it. Alternatively, another vein graft and the internal thoracic artery may be connected to this coronary artery, with the risk of competitive flow causing a string sign of the arterial conduit. NB

NB Often the coronary artery disease has progressed and given rise to new stenotic lesions distal to the occluded graft. In such situations, the occluded graft must be replaced to provide perfusion to the proximal coronary bed. In addition, a second graft is required to provide flow beyond the new stenotic lesion. NB

⊘ Injury to the Lung

The internal thoracic pedicle often lies between the lung and the heart. If dissection is carried out superiorly to locate the pedicle, the lung tissue is frequently injured in multiple locations. This results in air leaks that may persist for several days postoperatively. ⊘

NB If the internal thoracic pedicle cannot be safely found, the surgery may be performed as an off-pump procedure or on cardiopulmonary bypass with deep hypothermic arrest. NB

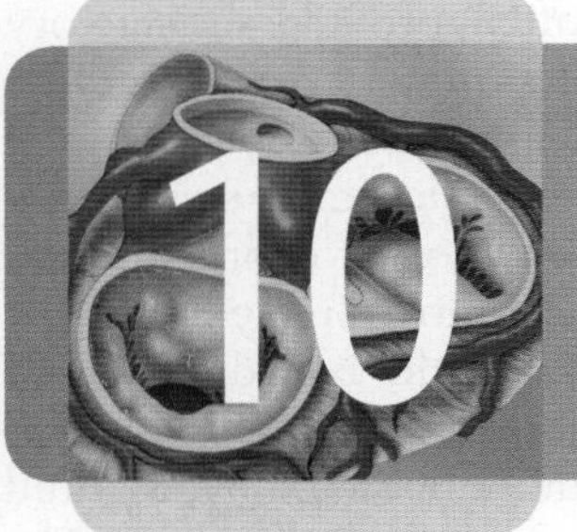

10 Surgery for Mechanical Complications of Myocardial Infarction

The mechanical complications of acute myocardial infarction have serious clinical implications and are generally associated with a poor prognosis. The onset of ischemia is usually heralded by pain that may be followed by shock and ventricular failure owing to significant myocardial injury. The severity of symptoms and clinical manifestations are intimately related to the magnitude of myocardial necrosis and loss of contractile strength.

Necrosis of the free ventricular wall may cause acute myocardial rupture. Necrosis of the ventricular septum may result in an acute septal defect and sudden left-to-right shunt, leading to hemodynamic instability. Necrosis of papillary muscles will result in papillary muscle dysfunction or rupture, causing severe mitral valve insufficiency.

Patients are initially stabilized with medical management and intraaortic balloon counterpulsation before undergoing cardiac catheterization and coronary angiography. Most of them will require emergent surgery because of intractable and progressive cardiogenic shock. Concomitant coronary artery bypass grafting should always be contemplated, whenever possible, to achieve complete myocardial revascularization. A small subgroup of these patients may compensate and present late with a pseudoaneurysm, left ventricular aneurysm, ventricular septal defect, or ischemic mitral valve insufficiency.

EXPOSURE AND CANNULATION OF THE HEART

The heart is exposed through a median sternotomy. Venous drainage is accomplished through bicaval cannulation, although a single large atrial cannula is adequate whenever the right heart remains a closed system during the procedure. Arterial blood is returned by direct aortic cannulation.

NB Contained Bleeding within the Pericardium

When there is evidence of contained bleeding within the pericardium due to a pseudoaneurysm or rupture of the heart, it is prudent to cannulate the aorta through a small enough opening in the pericardium overlying the aorta to allow volume replacement during venous cannulation and initiation of cardiopulmonary bypass. Alternatively, femoral cannulation should be contemplated. NB

NB Cardiogenic Shock

Most patients requiring surgical intervention for management of acute mechanical complications of myocardial infarction are in cardiogenic shock. Many may be on intraaortic balloon pump support. Cardiopulmonary bypass is initiated, and the heart is decompressed by a vent catheter introduced into the main pulmonary artery or through the right superior pulmonary vein into the left ventricle. Core cooling to 30°C to 32°C is carried out, and the aorta is clamped. Cold blood cardioplegic solution is then administered through the aortic root followed by retrograde delivery into the coronary sinus (see Chapter 3). NB

ACUTE MYOCARDIAL RUPTURE

Cardiorrhexis is a dramatic and lethal event. It is virtually always associated with a transmural infarction. Through a rent in the ventricular endocardium, blood gradually leaks into the area of infarction and distends the necrotic tissue. This hematoma continues to expand and finally ruptures the myocardium. The incidence of myocardial rupture after myocardial infarction has decreased with the introduction of modern management strategies for acute coronary events.

The sudden onset of cardiogenic shock 3 to 4 days after acute myocardial infarction may herald the development of cardiac tamponade due to myocardial rupture. Equalization of pressures in the right atrium, right ventricle in diastole, and pulmonary artery wedge, as measured with a Swan-Ganz catheter and aspiration of blood from the pericardial cavity are significant clues to the accurate diagnosis.

Immediate surgical exploration through a standard median sternotomy should be undertaken. If the heart has actually overtly ruptured, only a salvage operation may be successful. This entails prompt initiation of cardiopulmonary bypass. The infarcted necrotic tissue is removed. An appropriate patch of Hemasheild or bovine pericardium is sewn to the healthy normal myocardium with a continuous suture of 3-0 Prolene buttressed with a strip of felt to cover the defect. The suture line may have to be reinforced with additional sutures.

More commonly, the rupture consists of a small rent in the myocardium. The infarcted segment becomes spongy, oozing with blood. At times there may be a small hole through which blood spurts out. This may be amenable to suturing a large patch to the surrounding normal myocardium without resecting any muscle. Surgical management of this type of myocardial injury has been simplified with the use of biocompatible glues, such as cyanoacrylate or histoacryl. The technique entails applying the glue to the relatively dried surface of the infarcted myocardium, and covering the area with an appropriately sized patch of Teflon felt or bovine pericardium. The procedure does not require cardiopulmonary bypass support, and can be performed expeditiously with improved patient survival.

NB The sutureless technique for left ventricular rupture is a lifesaving procedure. Coronary artery bypass grafts are not performed, and generally these patients are taken directly to the operating room without undergoing coronary angiography. NB

VENTRICULAR SEPTAL RUPTURE

The ventricular septum receives blood from perforating branches of the left anterior descending artery as well as perforating branches of the posterior descending artery. Despite this dual blood supply, there is frequently no septal collateral flow. Consequently, the interventricular septum remains quite vulnerable to ischemia and occasionally ruptures after myocardial infarction. This is seen notably in patients whose infarction is the result of single-vessel disease. As with ventricular aneurysm, the anteroapical area is the most common site; it is involved in 65% of patients with ventricular septal rupture. The posterior segment of the septum is involved in 17% of the cases, and the middle segment in 13% of the cases; only 4% of the ruptures involve the inferior segment of the septum.

There is frequently a rapid progressive hemodynamic deterioration with myocardial failure following the rupture of the ventricular septum. The initial diagnosis is confirmed by echocardiography and is later followed by cardiac catheterization and coronary angiography. The goal of preoperative management is to decrease the left-to-right shunt by reducing systemic vascular resistance but at the same time ensuring adequate systemic blood pressure and cardiac output. Because these patients tend to die of end-organ failure rather than heart failure, prompt temporary stabilization is achieved with the support of an intraaortic balloon pump, ionotropic agents, and diuretics to maintain optimal tissue perfusion.

The operative mortality in this subgroup of patients is relatively high, but without urgent surgery, most of them would not survive.

Technique for the Surgical Treatment of a Ventricular Septal Defect

The septal defect is approached through an incision parallel to the course of the left anterior descending coronary artery in the center of the left ventricular infarct (Fig. 10.1). The septal defect and the extent of surrounding friable necrotic tissue are identified. With a continuous 3-0 Prolene suture, a generous patch of bovine pericardium is sewn to the left ventricular side of the septum, taking deep bites of normal, healthy muscular tissue as far away from the necrotic rim of the defect as possible. At times, this may necessitate sutures being placed close to the mitral valve annulus. The septal necrosis often extends to the ventriculotomy. The pericardial patch is then allowed to protrude outside the heart and be incorporated in the ventriculotomy closure (Fig. 10.2).

This technique essentially excludes the infarcted area. The suture line on the septum is inspected and checked for any residual defects. It is reinforced with multiple interrupted sutures buttressed with felt pledgets. The patch is anchored to the anterior edge of the left ventricular wall with a felted suture. This technique is based on the concept that the higher left ventricular pressure will force the pericardial patch against the entire septum, thereby obliterating the septal defect. Because sutures are placed on the

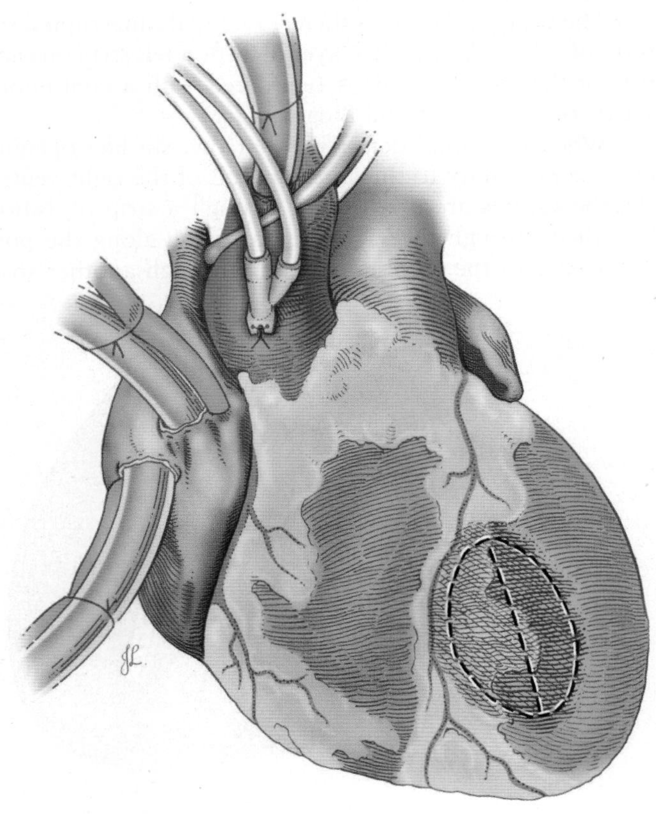

FIG. 10.1 Technique for surgical treatment of a ventricular septal defect.

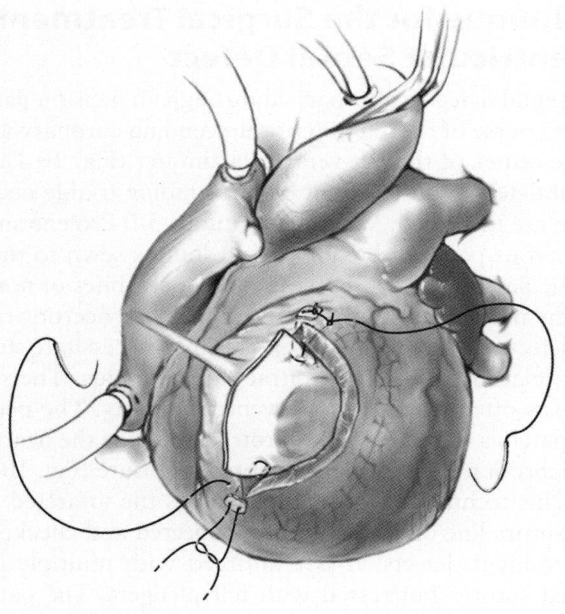

FIG. 10.2 A generous patch of bovine pericardium is sewn to the normal septal wall away from the defect.

normal healthy tissue, well away from the necrotic edges, the repair should be secure.

The ventriculotomy is then closed with interrupted sutures of 3-0 Prolene with a layer of Teflon felt strip on each side of the incision. This is reinforced with a continuous suture of 3-0 Prolene and Bioglue.

When the septal defect is a narrow, slit-like opening in close proximity to the anterior wall of the right ventricle, the sutures are first passed through a strip of Teflon felt, then through the viable septal tissue along the posterior edge of the defect, and again through another strip of Teflon felt on the right ventricular side of the septum (Fig. 10.3A). The sutures are brought out through the anterior wall of the right ventricle before they are passed through another strip of Teflon felt. Finally, the sutures are tied down, and the ventriculotomy is closed as described previously (Fig. 10.3B). Alternatively, the single pericardial patch technique could be used.

If the apex of the heart has infarcted and is necrotic, it is amputated. The viable tissue is then reapproximated in a sandwich manner by means of four strips of Teflon felt, one on each side of the septum and one each on the right and left exterior ventricular walls, with a series of interrupted horizontal mattress sutures (Fig. 10.4).

The approach to a rupture of the posteroinferior aspect of the septum through the infarcted inferior left ventricular wall is more challenging. Often the posteromedial papillary muscle is also involved in the necrotic process, and concomitant mitral valve replacement may become necessary. Closure of the ventricular septal defect is performed using the patch technique as described in preceding text. Most often, the inferior wall of the ventricle is closed using an appropriately sized Hemashield patch so as not to interfere with the normal geometry of the left ventricle. Coronary bypass grafting is performed judiciously on all bypassable vessels to ensure full revascularization of the remaining myocardium.

NB The liberal application of biological glue (i.e., Bioglue Surgical Adhesive, Cryolife Inc., Kennesaw, GA) on all suture lines has been a satisfactory hemostatic tool. NB

NB Percutaneous closure of postinfarction ventricular septal defects has become an alternative strategy in many critically ill patients. This can be done in conjunction with coronary angiography and possible percutaneous coronary revascularization. NB

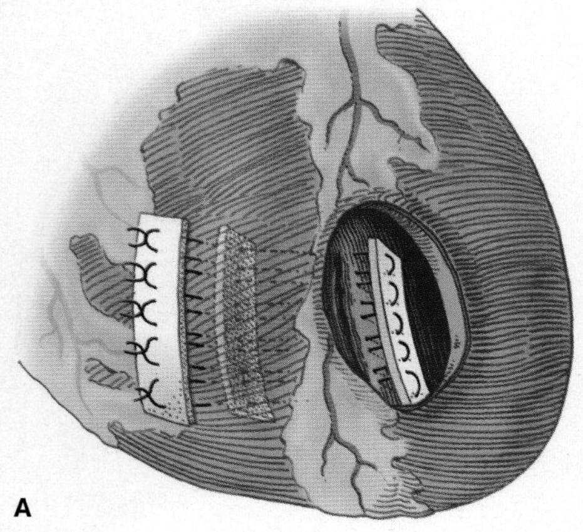

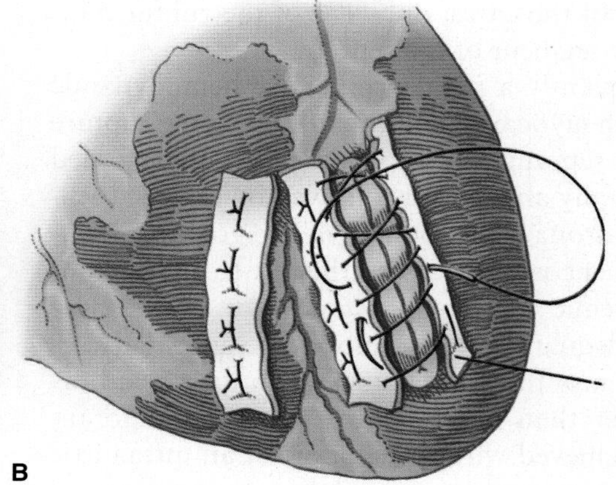

FIG. 10.3 **A:** The slit-like ventricular septal defect is closed with interrupted sutures incorporating strips of Teflon felt on both sides of the septum and anterior wall of the right ventricle. **B:** The knots are then tied, and the ventriculotomy is closed.

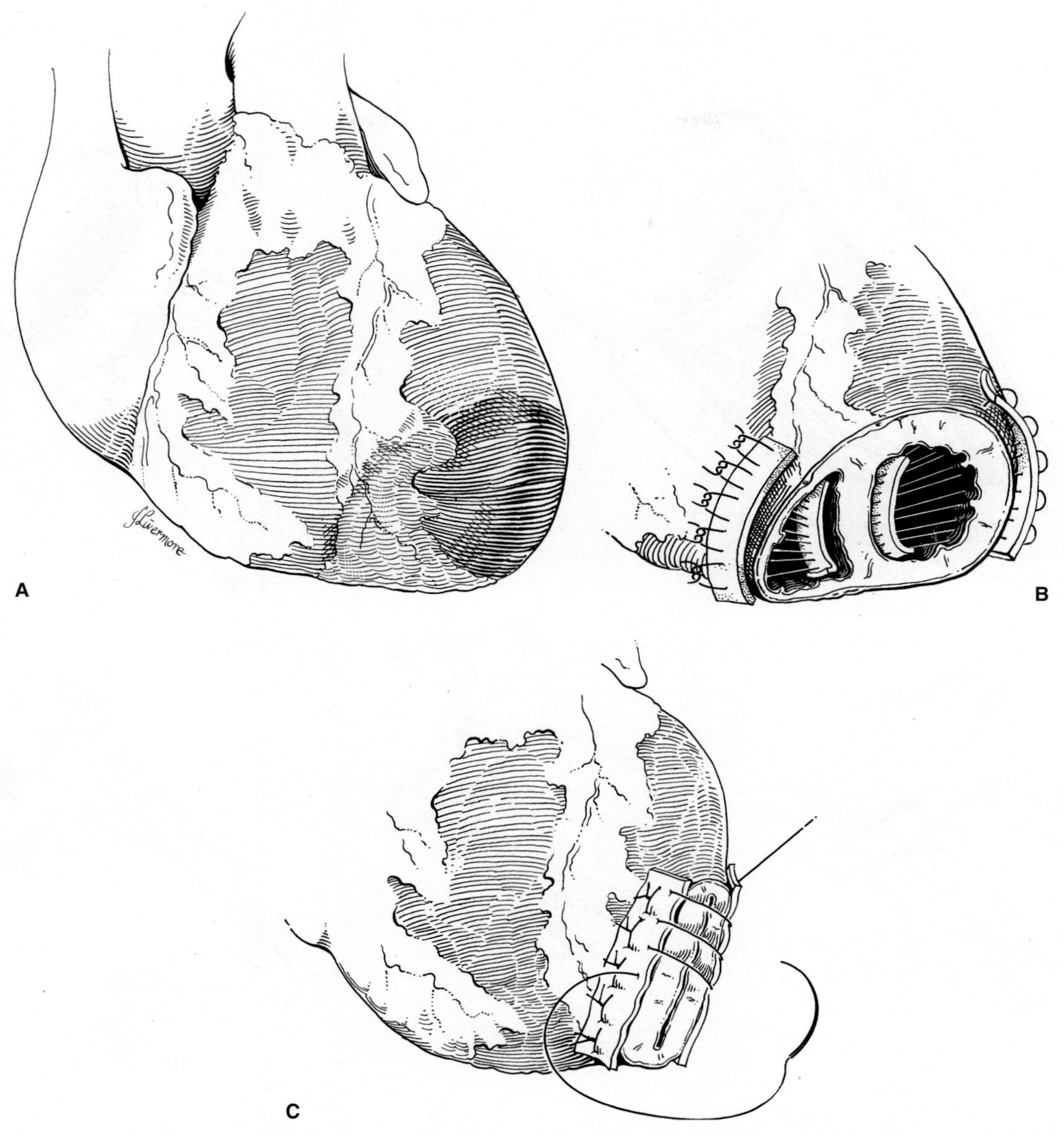

FIG. 10.4 **A:** Ventricular septal defect as the result of apical infarction. **B:** The necrotic apex of the left ventricle is amputated. **C:** The septal defect and ventricular walls are reconstructed with interrupted sutures incorporating strips of Teflon felt.

NB The very few patients who survive the acute phase may present in congestive heart failure at a later date. By 3 to 4 weeks after acute myocardial infarction, some fibrosis occurs in the necrotic areas so that the tissues are strong enough to hold sutures safely and surgical repair can be performed more easily. NB

PAPILLARY MUSCLE RUPTURE

The anterolateral papillary muscle has a rich blood supply from both the left anterior descending and left circumflex coronary arteries. In 90% of hearts, the right coronary artery is dominant and supplies the posteromedial papillary muscle. In the remaining 10%, its blood supply is provided by branches of the left coronary artery system. Therefore, infarction of the posterior wall of the left ventricle frequently results in necrosis of the posteromedial papillary muscle. A papillary muscle rupture usually occurs during the first week after infarction or later with reinfarction. Because both leaflets of the mitral valve are attached to each papillary muscle by chordae tendineae, complete disruption of either one, usually the posteromedial papillary muscle, results in gross mitral insufficiency, acute pulmonary edema, and death unless surgical intervention is

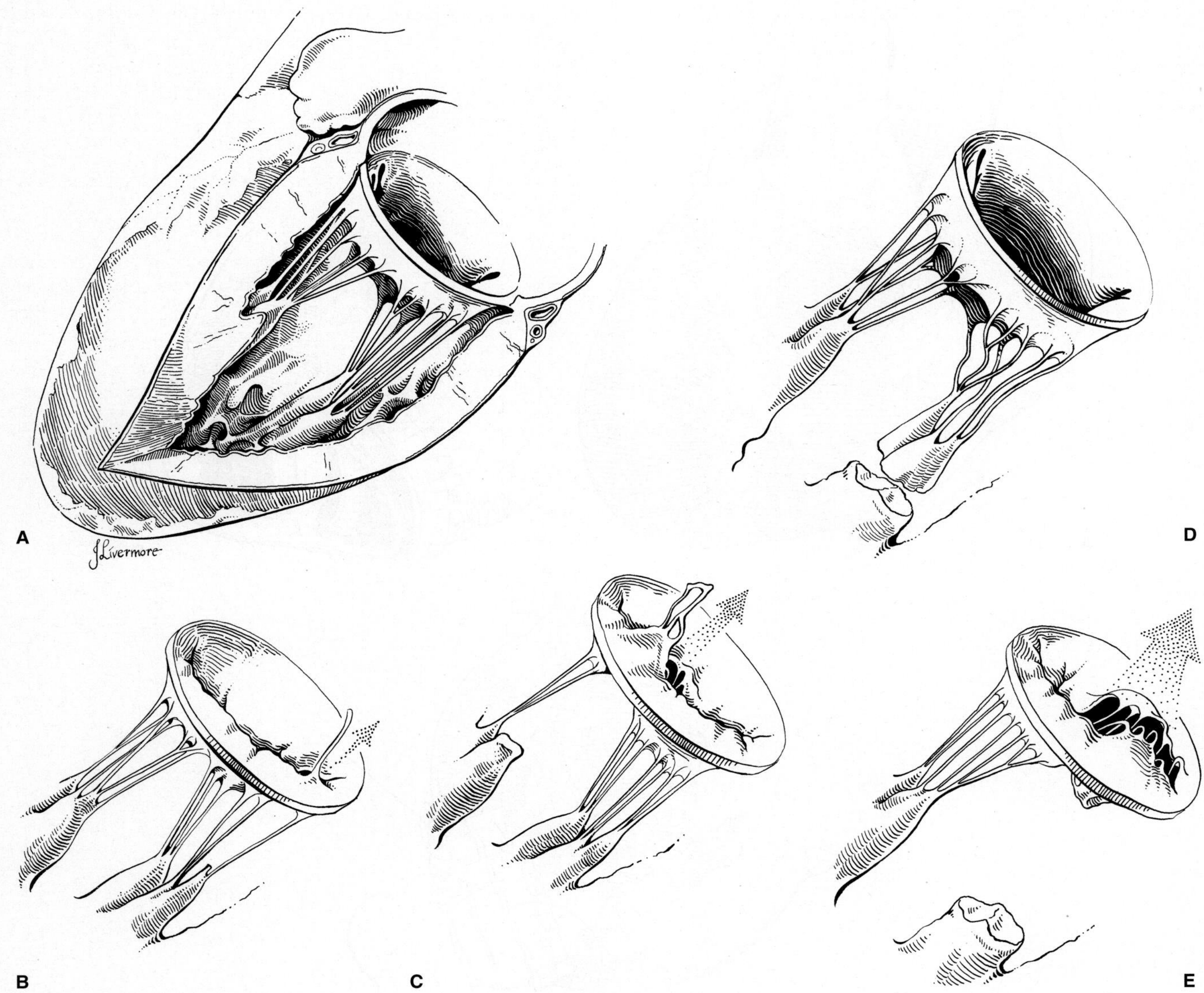

FIG. 10.5 A: Spatial relationships of the anatomic components of the mitral valve apparatus. **B:** Rupture of chordae tendineae. **C:** Partial rupture of the head of the papillary muscle. **D:** Complete tear of the papillary muscle giving rise to gross valvular insufficiency **(E).**

prompt. A tear of the apical head of a papillary muscle that supports a small segment of only one of the mitral leaflets may result in a milder degree of mitral regurgitation (Fig. 10.5). Dysfunction of the papillary muscle is probably more common. If myocardial infarction is not massive and left ventricular function is not severely impaired, these patients can compensate long enough to undergo coronary angiography before semiurgent surgical treatment.

Most commonly, conservative surgery will not be adequate because the infarcted papillary muscle is friable and necrotic. Occasionally, a ruptured papillary muscle can be reimplanted, but it may be hazardous if the reimplantation site is necrotic. Mitral valve replacement is the procedure of choice in most patients and can be performed expeditiously with relative safety (see Chapter 6). Coronary artery bypass grafting to bypassable vessels is highly desirable to revascularize the viable myocardium as completely as possible.

Significant mechanical complications occurring during the acute phase of myocardial infarction are quite rare. Most patients following myocardial infarction will continue on a medical regimen and live a symptom-free productive life. There is, however, a subgroup of patients who develop symptoms reflecting the effects of chronic changes secondary to an old myocardial infarction. Diagnostic evaluation of these patients with ischemic cardiomyopathy may reveal the presence of a large dyskinetic (aneurysmal) or akinetic segment of left ventricle, a pseudoaneurysm, and/or ischemic mitral valve disease, all of which may require surgical intervention.

SURGICAL VENTRICULAR RESTORATION

Following myocardial infarction, a discrete scar develops, resulting in an akinetic or dyskinetic segment. Traditionally, surgical ventricular restoration for ischemic cardiomyopathy has focused on recognizing the borders of the scar tissue and excluding the scar by excision and primary closure or placement of a patch at the junction between scar and normal muscle. More recently, the importance of ventricular chamber size and shape has been appreciated. The goal of surgery to reconstruct the left ventricle is to achieve a normal-sized cavity and to convert the more spherical shape to a more conical pattern.

Technique

Cardiopulmonary bypass is initiated in the standard manner. Usually, a single atriocaval cannula is adequate for venous return. Cardioplegic arrest of the heart is accomplished by infusion of cold blood cardioplegic solution through the aortic root after clamping the aorta. This is complemented by infusion of cold blood cardioplegia into the coronary sinus by the retrograde technique (see Chapter 3). Venting of the left ventricle through the right superior pulmonary vein helps to keep the field dry. When the heart is still and vented empty, the extent of the old infarct is evaluated. The scar segment of the left ventricular wall, devoid of myocardium, tends to be sucked in by the vent suction. The heart is carefully dissected free from the pericardium. Traction sutures are placed in the scar tissue, and an incision is made through it (Fig. 10.6). The opening is then enlarged, and some excess scar tissue may be excised to provide easy access for removal of blood clots from within the left ventricle and/or aneurysm wall (Fig. 10.7).

⊘ Adherent Calcified Aneurysm Wall

Occasionally, there may be marked fibrous reaction or even calcification of the aneurysm wall, making its mobilization tedious and time-consuming. The involved segment of the aneurysm can be amputated free from the heart and left adherent to the pericardium and pleura (Fig. 10.8). ⊘

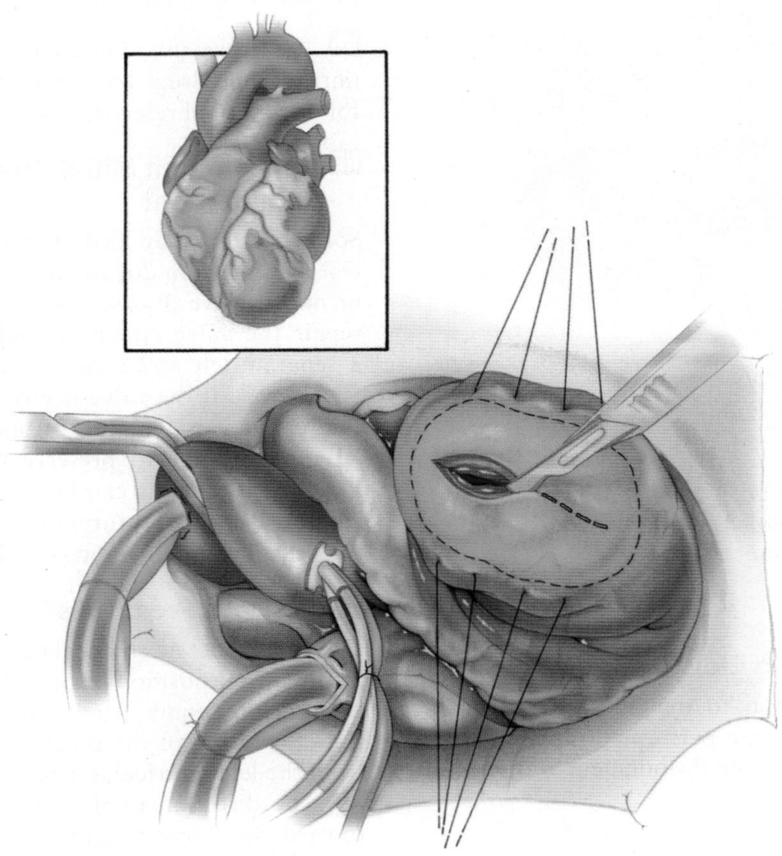

FIG. 10.6 Ventriculotomy through scar tissue.

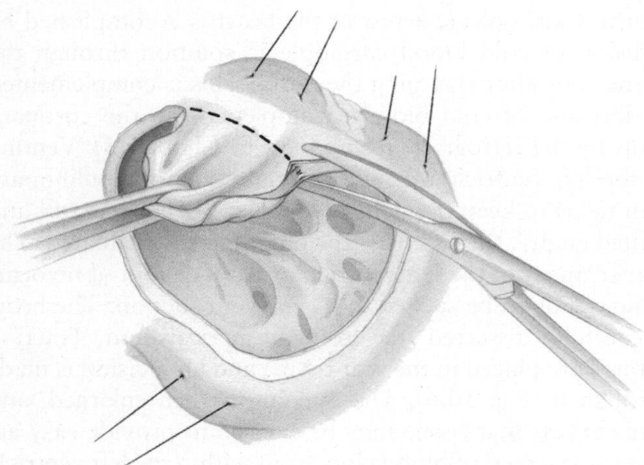

FIG. 10.7 Excision of a scarred ventricular wall.

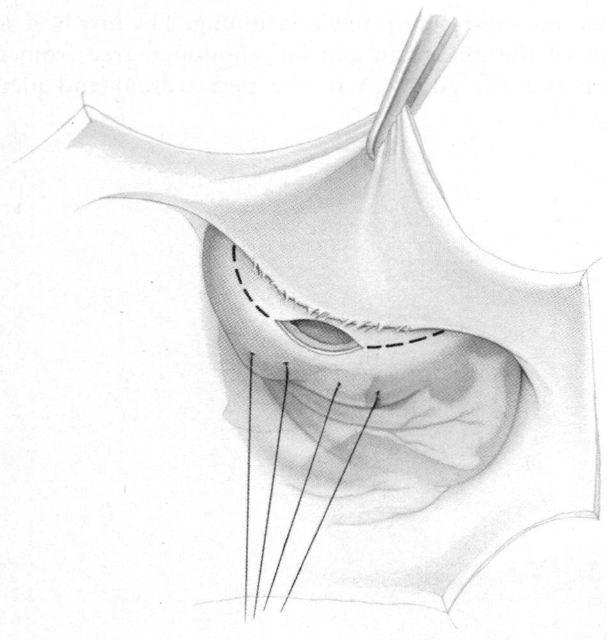

FIG. 10.8 Technique for leaving a scarred ventricular wall adherent to the pericardium.

⊘ Dislodgment of Blood Clots

Manipulation and dissection to free the left ventricular wall from the pericardium are performed after the aorta has been cross-clamped to avoid dislodgment and systemic embolization of blood clots. ⊘

⊘ Loose Blood Clots

There are often loose blood clots in the ventricular cavity. A sponge should be placed in the outflow tract of the left ventricle near the aortic valve before attempting to remove blood clots and debris from the ventricular cavity. The sponge will prevent the escape of blood clots into the aortic root and possible embolization into the coronary arteries. The interior of the left ventricle is then thoroughly irrigated with cold saline solution to wash away any debris. ⊘

With sharp scissor dissection, a 3-mm thick layer of the endocardial fibrous lining of the left ventricular cavity is stripped *en masse* for approximately 1 to 2 cm from the edge of the infarcted area. This theoretically removes any abnormal foci of electrical activity.

NB Radical Endocardial Dissection

If a patient has a history of ventricular arrhythmia, it is advisable to carry out a radical endocardial resection while performing the left ventricular remodeling. The procedure entails the dissection of a 2- to 3-mm thickness of the endocardium of the left ventricle. The resection should be extensive, reaching to the base of the papillary muscle and the aortic root, to ensure complete removal of any scattered arrhythmogenic foci. Cryoablation of the transitional zone between the scar tissue and myocardium in patients with a ventricular aneurysm may be helpful. Care must be taken not to damage the papillary muscle to avoid causing mitral insufficiency. Most of these patients are candidates for implantation of an internal cardioverter-defibrillator device. NB

NB The liberal use of internal cardiac defibrillators and antiarrhythmic drugs has markedly decreased the indication for endocardial resection. NB

NB Concomitant Mitral Valve Repair or Replacement

Some patients may have hemodynamically significant mitral regurgitation due to papillary muscle dysfunction and/or mitral valve disease. Every attempt should be made to repair the valve either through the ventricle or through a separate left atrial incision in the traditional way (see Chapter 6). If the valve is grossly diseased and unsuitable for repair, it is replaced through the ventriculotomy. An attempt is made to preserve the subvalvular apparatus. Excess leaflet tissue can be excised or incorporated in the sutures. Pledgeted sutures of 2-0 Ticron are used to anchor the prosthesis in position (Fig. 10.9). NB

⊘ Choice of Prosthesis

Only a bileaflet mechanical or bioprosthesis should be used in the mitral position, especially if implanted through the left ventriculotomy. Particular attention should be given to the orientation of the prosthesis, which is not as familiar from the left ventricular aspect. ⊘

The direction of the sutures is from the left atrium toward the left ventricular cavity. The sutures are then passed from the superior aspect of the prosthetic sewing ring to its inferior aspect so that when the sutures are tied, the knots are on the left ventricular side (Fig. 10.9). Care

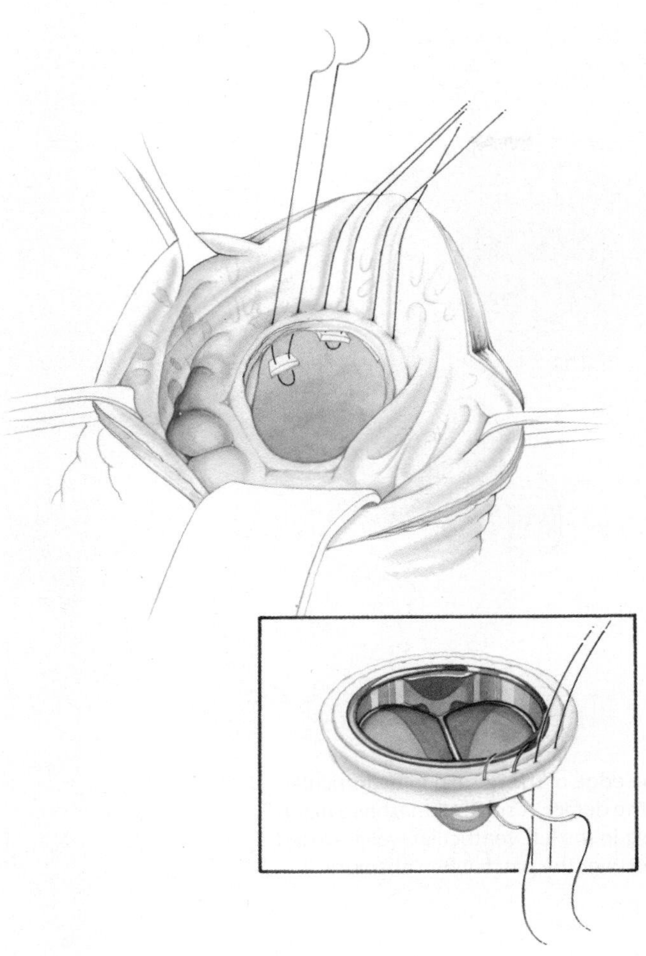

FIG. 10.9 Technique for mitral valve replacement through a left ventriculotomy.

must be taken to ensure that the knots of the sutures do not interfere with the occlusive mechanism of the prosthesis.

The ventricle should be closed in such a manner as to restore its normal geometry. This entails excluding the akinetic and dyskinetic segment of the infarcted ventricular wall and thereby reducing the left ventricular volume. A continuous 2-0 monofilament suture is placed deep into the scar along the edge of the normal left ventricular wall and tied to create a purse-string effect (Fig. 10.10A).

NB The infarction frequently affects both the anterior wall of the left ventricle as well as a segment of the septum. It is therefore important to include the edge of the scar on the septum in the purse-string suture. This reduces the size of the defect in the left ventricular wall to a great extent and gives the left ventricular cavity a relatively normal shape and geometry (Fig. 10.10B). NB

NB The "ideal" size of the left ventricular cavity can be approximated with commercially available sizers. The recommended cavity size is 60 mL per square meter of body surface area of the patient. The appropriately sized balloon is placed in the left ventricular cavity and a 2-0 Prolene suture is placed in the scar tissue along the border of normal tissue. This is accomplished in a purse-string manner over the sizer, which is removed before the suture is tied. NB

A Hemashield patch is cut into the appropriate size and shape of the defect and sewn into place with a continuous suture of 3-0 Prolene, taking deep bites of the surrounding scar tissue. The suture line may have to be tightened with a nerve hook and reinforced with a few interrupted sutures buttressed with felt pledgets. BioGlue can be applied to the suture line for added security. Only when the patient has been weaned off cardiopulmonary bypass and there is no bleeding from the patch site should the excess left ventricular wall be approximated over the patch to prevent the accumulation of blood and clot between the patch and ventricular wall (Fig. 10.10C).

NB Tissue Covering the Left Ventricular Patch

Covering the left ventricular patch with infarcted wall minimizes the possibility of graft infection should mediastinitis occur. NB

Coronary artery bypass grafting to diseased vessels is performed when possible to achieve maximal revascularization of the heart. Special care is taken to deair the heart before removing the patient from cardiopulmonary bypass (see Chapter 4).

NB A multicenter clinical trial did not demonstrate that addition of surgical ventricular restoration to coronary bypass surgery in suitable patients with ischemic cardiomyopathy reduces mortality. However, this procedure can restore ventricular geometry and volume in properly selected patients. NB

PSEUDOANEURYSM

Postinfarction false aneurysm is a rare phenomenon. It occurs when blood leaking from a myocardial rupture slowly accumulates in the pericardial cavity. Reactionary adhesions limit the size of the pseudoaneurysm. Two-dimensional echocardiography and ventricular angiography delineate the lesion quite vividly. Unlike left ventricular aneurysms, eventual rupture of the pseudoaneurysm is virtually certain. Therefore, surgical management must always be carried out on a semiurgent basis.

The surgical technique is similar to that described for true aneurysms. However, false aneurysms are often very thin walled and may rupture easily during dissection and manipulation of the heart. Therefore, it is prudent to initiate cardiopulmonary bypass by cannulating the femoral artery and vein (see Chapter 2). A median sternotomy is then performed; the aorta is cross-clamped and cardioplegic arrest of the heart achieved before addressing the pseudoaneurysm. If the pseudoaneurysm ruptures before aortic clamping, blood is removed from the field and returned to

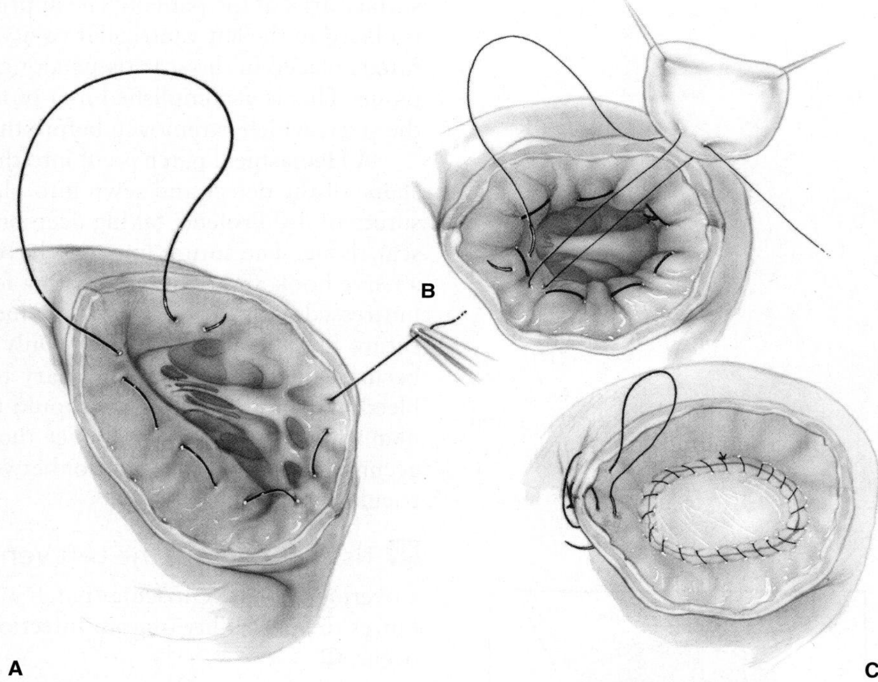

FIG. 10.10 **A:** Suture placed in the scar along the edge of the normal left ventricular wall. **B:** Purse-string suture reducing the size of the defect. A small Hemashield patch is sutured in place to cover the defect. **C:** The defect in the left ventricular wall is closed, and the scarred aneurysmal wall is approximated over the patch when absolute hemostasis is achieved.

the pump by suckers. The aorta is quickly clamped, bleeding is brought under control, and cardioplegic arrest of the heart is then accomplished.

Pseudoaneurysms usually have small openings. The defect is closed with a patch of Hemashield using interrupted 3-0 Ticron sutures buttressed with felt pledgets. The suture line is reinforced with a continuous suture of 3-0 Prolene. Absolute hemostasis is obtained, and the heart is deaired (see Chapter 4).

ISCHEMIC MITRAL REGURGITATION

Besides complete or partial papillary muscle rupture, ischemic mitral valve prolapse may be caused by elongation of a papillary muscle following infarction. Occasionally, necrosis of a separate commissural head of papillary muscle gives rise to rupture of the commissural chord (Fig. 10.5B). However, ischemic mitral regurgitation encountered following the acute postinfarction period is predominately functional. It is due to annular dilation secondary to left ventricular enlargement and/or local left ventricular remodeling of the inferior wall causing papillary muscle displacement with restricted motion of the mitral leaflets. The surgical approach to chronic ischemic mitral regurgitation requires a precise understanding of the mechanisms involved (see Chapter 6).

INTRAAORTIC BALLOON PUMP

Occasionally, patients may require intraaortic balloon pump support after a cardiac surgical procedure. Depressed left ventricular function, ongoing myocardial ischemia, and ventricular arrhythmias are all indications for placement of an intraaortic balloon pump.

Technique for Placement of Intraaortic Balloon Pump

If the patient has a palpable femoral pulse, the intraaortic balloon pump can be placed percutaneously using the Seldinger technique. After the common femoral artery is entered, the guidewire is passed through the needle, which is then removed. The dilator is introduced over the wire. The sheath is then passed over the wire into the artery. The deflated prewrapped balloon catheter is then introduced through the sheath and positioned in the descending thoracic aorta with the tip just distal to the takeoff of the left subclavian artery. Use of transesophageal echocardiography aids in proper positioning of the intraaortic balloon.

⊘ Bleeding in Heparinized Patients

During or immediately after cardiopulmonary bypass, the patient is fully heparinized. Use of the percutaneous technique may lead to hematoma formation, retroperitoneal hemorrhage, or bleeding around the balloon sheath. This is especially likely to occur if it is difficult to palpate the femoral pulse, leading to inadvertent punctures of the femoral vein or back wall of the femoral artery. ⊘

⊘ Improper Placement of the Balloon Catheter

The balloon catheter should be placed through the common femoral artery. If it is inserted through the superficial femoral artery, lower extremity ischemia may result. The entry site of the balloon should be caudad to the inguinal ligament. Placement above this level may lead to bleeding, which is difficult to control by external pressure when the balloon catheter is removed. ⊘

NB Management of Lower Extremity Ischemia

If a patient develops evidence of leg ischemia after balloon pump placement, removing the sheath may allow improved distal blood flow. Alternatively, smaller diameter balloon catheters are available and should be used in patients with small femoral arteries. NB

In the operating room, when difficulties are encountered during weaning from cardiopulmonary bypass, placement of an intraaortic balloon may be helpful. In these patients, often no femoral pulse can be palpated. Limited exposure of the common femoral artery is achieved through a small longitudinal incision with minimal dissection. A purse-string suture of 4-0 Prolene incorporating only adventitial tissue is placed on the anterior surface of the common femoral artery. The needle, wire, dilator, and balloon catheter are sequentially passed through this purse-string site. The suture is left long with the ends secured together by a metal clip and buried in the wound. The incision is closed in layers around the balloon catheter. Subsequently, the balloon may be removed under local anesthesia at the patient's bedside. The femoral arteriotomy is closed by simply tying the previously placed Prolene suture (Fig. 10.11).

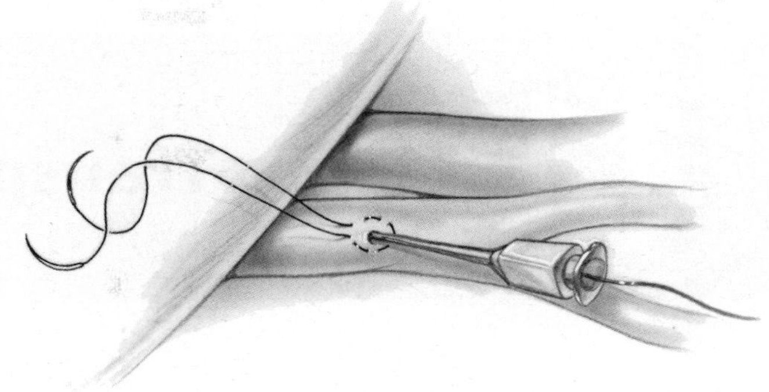

FIG. 10.11 Technique for placement of intraaortic balloon catheter.

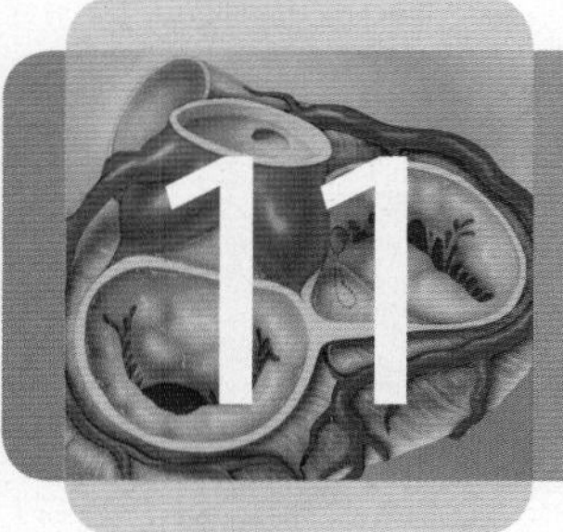

11 Heart Transplantation

Heart transplantation has emerged as an effective therapy for patients with end-stage heart diseases. In 2005, a total of 2,125 heart transplants were performed in the United States. The major obstacle to more widespread application of heart transplantation is donor shortage.

DONOR SELECTION

Matching of a donor heart to a specific recipient requires consideration of many donor and recipient factors, several of which have changed over time. Although there is no absolute maximum age for cardiac donors, many centers use an upper age limit of 55 to 65 years.

A history of diabetes mellitus in the donor with microvascular disease, long-standing donor hypertension with left ventricular hypertrophy (by electrocardiogram or echocardiogram), or prolonged high-dose donor heart inotropic requirement may be associated with an increased risk of early graft failure. Segmental or global wall motion abnormality of the donor heart can be associated with brain death and should not be considered a contraindication to transplantation. Resuscitation with thyroid hormone or the addition of inotropes and/or vasoconstrictors may lead to improvement in left ventricular function. The donor can then be reassessed with a repeat echocardiogram or a pulmonary artery catheter.

It is generally recommended that male donors older than 40 years and female donors older than 45 years undergo a coronary angiogram if available. Presence of significant coronary artery disease (>50% lesions) in two or more major coronary arteries is usually a contraindication to utilization of a donor heart. However, for critically ill recipients, donor hearts with discrete coronary stenoses can undergo bypass grafting using recipient conduits *ex vivo*, and be transplanted with acceptable short-term outcomes.

Aside from the considerations mentioned earlier, other contraindications to the use of a donor heart include positive human immunodeficiency virus (HIV) serology, positive hepatitis C serology, donor malignancies other than primary brain tumor, and systemic bacterial infection (especially with gram-negative organisms).

NB It is important to match the donor heart to the clinical situation of the recipient. For a critically ill recipient, the donor criteria may be relaxed, as the alternatives of either continued waiting on the list or a ventricular assist device may carry a higher mortality risk. NB

Size matching of the donor and recipient is important. Severe undersizing can lead to the inability of the donor heart to support the recipient's circulation, especially if there is evidence of primary graft dysfunction. Most programs require a donor-to-recipient weight ratio of at least 0.7. Oversizing can lead to restrictive physiology due to limited recipient mediastinal space. This issue is especially relevant in patients whose native heart disease is not dilated. Donor–recipient size matching has to be considered in association with other donor and recipient variables (i.e., an undersized female donor heart may not be suitable for a male recipient with pulmonary hypertension, especially in a setting of mild donor left ventricular hypertrophy and/or long ischemic time). Caution needs to be exercised when using a donor with multiple risk factors: older age, left ventricular hypertrophy, long ischemia time, and others.

PRESERVATION SOLUTION

The ideal preservation solution will ensure microvascular, cellular, and functional integrity of the donor heart during the ischemic phase. Experience with the currently used preservations solutions (University of Wisconsin and Celsior solution) have shown excellent myocardial functional recovery, especially when the ischemic time is less than 6 hours.

University of Wisconsin solution is an "intracellular" based solution (low sodium, high potassium) and contains several classes of impermeable molecules to minimize cellular swelling. Because of the concern about the deleterious effects of high potassium concentrations on microvasculature, Celsior solution, which is an "extracellular" solution, was developed. In addition to many impermeable molecules, Celsior also has glutamate that serves as a substrate for energy production. Several studies have shown that both solutions afford similar protection to the donor heart during preservation. We currently use University of Wisconsin solution as our preservation solution of choice.

DONOR OPERATION

Upon arrival at the donor hospital, the procurement surgeon will review the donor's medical records to ensure the accuracy and completeness of all data. The donor is placed in supine position with arms extended by the side. Because most donors are multiorgan donors, the donor is prepped from neck to midthigh. Midline sternotomy incision is performed as previously described. In smaller community hospitals, a sternal saw may not be available and a Lebsche knife may be used. The pericardium is opened and pericardial sutures are placed. The right pleural space is opened widely. The heart is systematically examined for size, evidence of right ventricular dysfunction, contusion, aneurysm, segmental wall motion abnormality, or a thrill suggestive of valvular heart disease. The course of the coronary arteries is palpated for evidence of calcification or plaques. If the quality of the donor heart is acceptable, this information is communicated to the recipient hospital.

The dissection of the donor heart is started by freeing the superior vena cava from pericardial reflection to the innominate vein. The azygous vein is usually tied and divided to ensure sufficient length of the superior vena cava.

NB For recipients with congenital heart disease who have previously undergone a classic or bidirectional Glenn procedure, a longer segment of innominate vein may be required. **NB**

The aorta is dissected distally beyond the innominate artery take-off. The needle for administration of preservation solution is inserted into the ascending aorta and secured (Fig. 11.1). When the other procurement teams have completed their respective organ dissections, heparin at a dose of 300 units per kilogram of body weight is administered.

The most important step in heart procurement is to ensure that the donor heart is emptied. The pericardium on the right side is incised at the level of the hemidiaphragm down to the inferior vena cava. The superior vena cava is clamped and the inferior vena cava is transected so that the blood from the heart empties into the right chest cavity.

NB If the lungs are being harvested, exsanguination has to be done into the abdomen by the abdominal team. **NB**

When the heart is empty (usually after 5 to 10 beats), the aortic cross-clamp is applied and the preservation solution is administered into the aortic root. We measure pressure in the ascending aorta and maintain it between 50 and 70 mm Hg. The apex of the heart is elevated toward the right side, and the left inferior pulmonary vein is incised where it joins the left atrium (Fig. 11.2). The pericardium is filled with ice slush to ensure topical cooling. A total

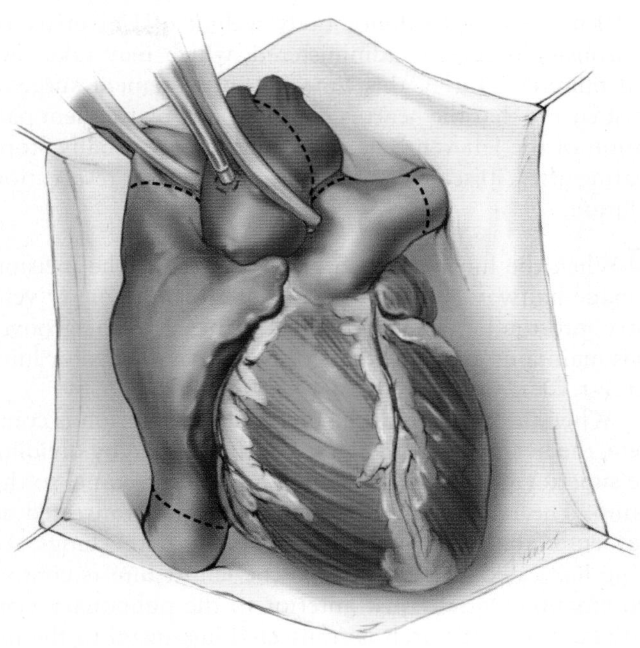

FIG. 11.1 The donor heart is prepared. Antegrade cardioplegia needle has been placed, and the aortic cross-clamp is applied.

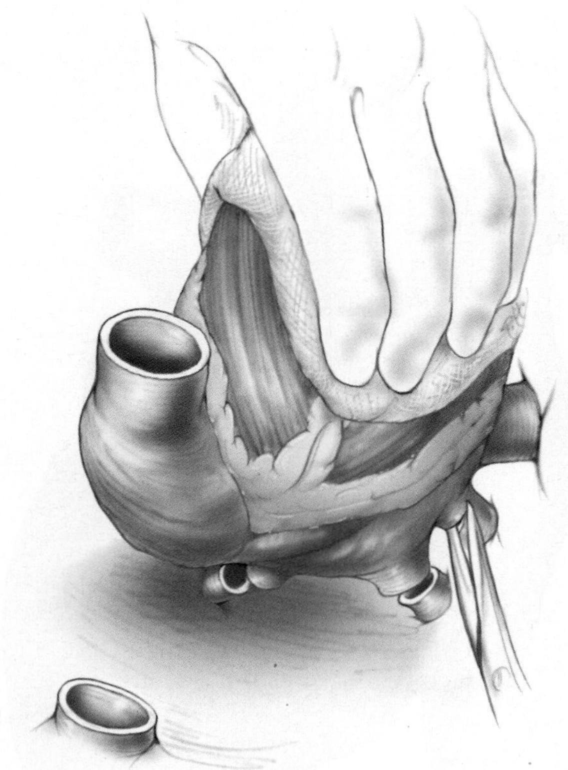

FIG. 11.2 After dividing the inferior vena cava, the left inferior pulmonary vein is transected at its point of entry into the left atrium (when lungs are not being harvested).

of 10 mL per kg of donor body weight of University of Wisconsin solution is administered, which may take several minutes. During this time, the procurement surgeon must ensure that the heart is not distended by frequent palpation of the left ventricle. The donor heart usually stops beating after 30 seconds of perfusion with the preservation solution.

NB When the lungs are also being harvested, the incision is made halfway between the left inferior pulmonary vein entry into the left atrium and the atrioventricular groove. This maintains adequate cuffs of pulmonary veins for lung harvest. NB

When the infusion of the preservation solution is complete, the heart is excised. This is accomplished by dividing the superior vena cava or innominate vein proximal to the clamp. The remaining pulmonary veins are transected as they enter the left atrium. Alternatively, if the lungs are being harvested, the incision on the left atrium is continued circumferentially just anterior to the pulmonary vein orifices. The aortic arch is transected just distal to the innominate artery and the main pulmonary artery is divided. If the lungs are not being harvested, the proximal right and left pulmonary arteries can be divided to provide extra pulmonary artery length (Fig. 11.3).

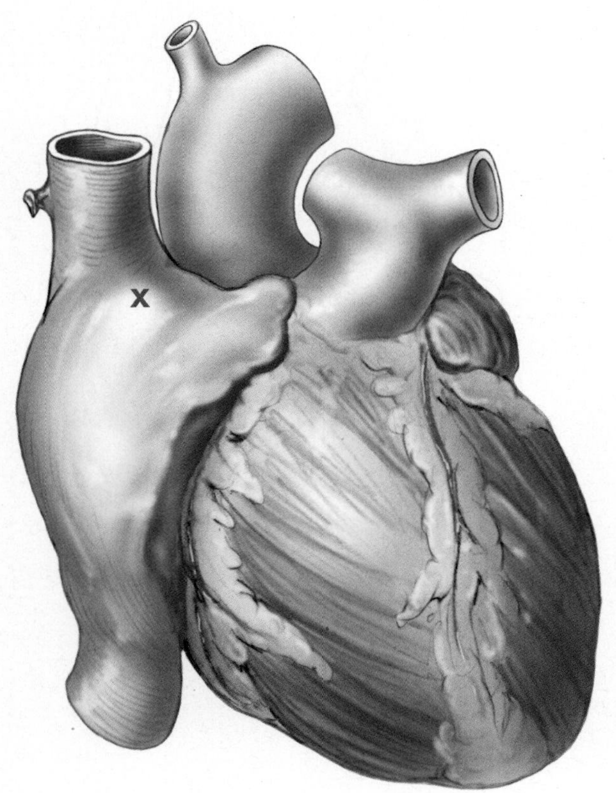

FIG. 11.3 Excised donor heart. The sinoatrial node is marked with an X.

The heart is removed from the donor and taken to the back table. It is inspected for the presence of a patent foramen ovale or valvular abnormalities. If a patent foramen ovale is found, it is closed with a figure-of-eight or continuous Prolene suture through the inferior vena caval opening, using forceps to expose the interatrial septum. The valves are visualized to rule out vegetations, small perforations, or clots that may have been missed by the preoperative echocardiogram. A piece of donor pericardium is also harvested and packed with the donor heart.

NB Strips or pledgets of donor pericardium are very useful in reinforcing aortic and pulmonary artery suture lines. NB

The donor heart is packed in a minimum of three sterile plastic bags and then placed in a plastic container full of ice for transport. Several donor lymph nodes are also taken for prospective cross-matches.

RECIPIENT SURGERY

A pulmonary artery catheter and an arterial line are placed in the recipient. The recipient does not undergo general anesthesia until the donor heart has been examined and found to be satisfactory. We usually allow 1 hour from skin incision to the arrival of the donor heart for recipients who have not undergone a previous sternotomy. In patients with a prior sternotomy, this period is extended to 2 hours to allow adequate time to complete the dissection of the native heart.

NB Right Ventricular Wall Injury

In patients with a prior sternotomy and biventricular failure with a distended right ventricle, the surgeon may expose the femoral artery and vein before opening the chest. If the right ventricle is injured during sternal opening, expeditious femoral cannulation and cardiopulmonary bypass can be achieved. NB

⊘ Recipient Coagulopathy

Excellent hemostasis is critical during the dissection of the recipient's native heart. Recipients with right heart failure usually have liver congestion and coagulopathy, which may lead to excessive blood loss. ⊘

In redo surgeries, the native heart is dissected so that the superior vena cava, inferior vena cava, and the ascending aorta are accessible for cannulation and cross-clamping. The remainder of the dissection can be completed once the heart is arrested.

⊘ Clot Embolization

Patients with end-stage heart disease and global hypokinesis are at high risk of developing left ventricular thrombus. It is important to minimize the manipulation of the native heart before aortic cross-clamping in order to reduce the risk of clot dislodgment and possible embolization. ⊘

⊘ Injury to Bypass Grafts

In patients who have undergone previous coronary artery bypass grafting, it is important to identify the left internal thoracic artery and other conduits and to protect them during dissection of the heart. Any graft injury or manipulation leading to spasm or distal embolization of debris may result in hemodynamic instability. ⊘

Aortic and bicaval venous cannulation are performed (see Chapter 2). The superior and inferior venae cavae are cannulated as distant from the heart as possible. This will allow adequate vena caval cuffs for tension-free anastomoses to the donor heart. Cardiopulmonary bypass is initiated once the donor heart is in the operating room and the patient is cooled to 28°C. The aortic cross-clamp is applied, and cardioplegia is administered into the aortic root until the native heart is arrested. The snares around the superior and inferior venae cavae are tightened and the native heart is excised.

BICAVAL TECHNIQUE

The excision of the recipient's native heart is begun with an incision in the right atrial appendage, 1 cm from and parallel to the atrioventricular groove. The incision is extended inferiorly toward the inferior vena cava. Superiorly, the incision is extended onto the roof of the left atrium, between the superior vena cava and aorta. The aorta is then transected circumferentially approximately 1 cm distal to the sinotubular junction. The pulmonary artery is divided approximately 2 cm distal to the pulmonic valve. The atrial septum, which is now exposed, is incised through the fossa ovalis. The incision is extended superiorly to the dome of the left atrium to meet the superior extension of the right atrial incision. It is then directed toward the base of the left atrial appendage. Inferiorly, the incision extends across the posterior left atrial wall parallel to the coronary sinus. The inferior aspect of the right atrial incision is extended onto the medial aspect of the inferior vena cava and posterior to the coronary sinus to meet the left atrial incision. With the apex of the heart elevated out of the pericardium, this incision is extended to the base of the left atrial appendage, completing the left atrial excision. The recipient's native heart is delivered off the field. A portion of the remaining wall of the right atrium is removed, leaving cuffs of superior and inferior venae cavae. The cuffs of recipient left atrium, inferior vena cava, superior vena cava, aorta, and main pulmonary artery are prepared for anastomosis to the donor heart (Fig. 11.4). Optimal hemostasis of exposed muscle in the left atrial wall is accomplished with electrocautery before bringing the donor heart onto the operative field. A vent is placed through the recipient's right superior pulmonary vein into the left atrium with the tip in the left inferior pulmonary vein. The vent is inserted through a purse-string suture and connected to an active suction to remove the pulmonary venous return that can warm the donor heart.

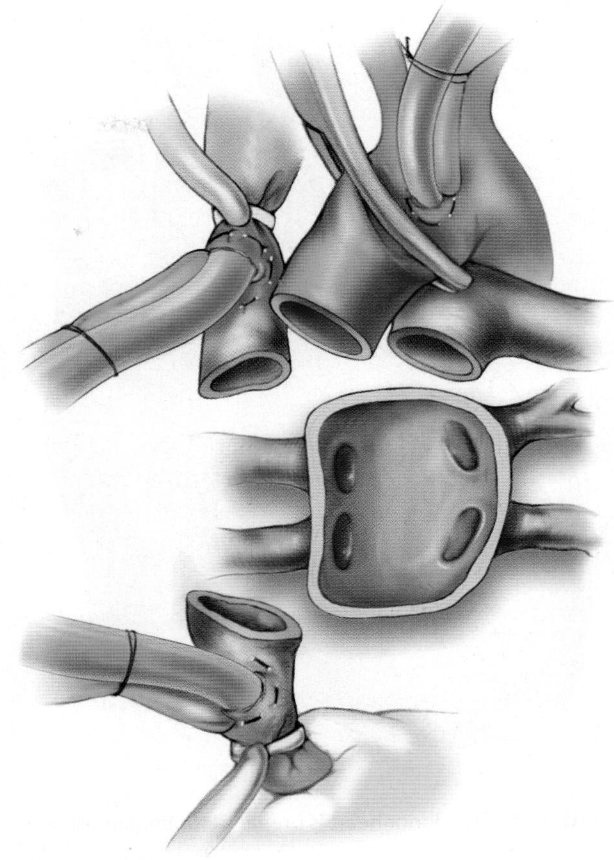

FIG. 11.4 The recipient's native heart has been removed, leaving a cuff of left atrium. The transected pulmonary artery, aorta, inferior and superior venae cavae are shown.

⊘ Warm Ischemia of Donor Heart

If a vent is not used, the accumulation of venous return from the lungs can lead to warming of the donor heart which may negatively impact the function of the allograft. ⊘

The donor heart is inspected again for a patent foramen ovale and valvular lesions by the implanting surgeon.

NB Any clots noted on the valves are removed by cold saline irrigation. NB

Incisions are made connecting the two right and two left pulmonary vein orifices of the donor heart. A third incision then connects these two openings to create one large left atrial cuff (Fig. 11.5). The aorta and the pulmonary artery are dissected free from one another. If the donor heart has been harvested with attached branch pulmonary arteries, these are incised posteriorly to create a confluence, which is then trimmed to the appropriate length (Fig. 11.5). The implantation of the donor heart is begun with the left atrial anastomosis, which is started at the level of the left atrial appendage (Fig. 11.6). This suture line is performed with 3-0 Prolene using an everting-edge technique,

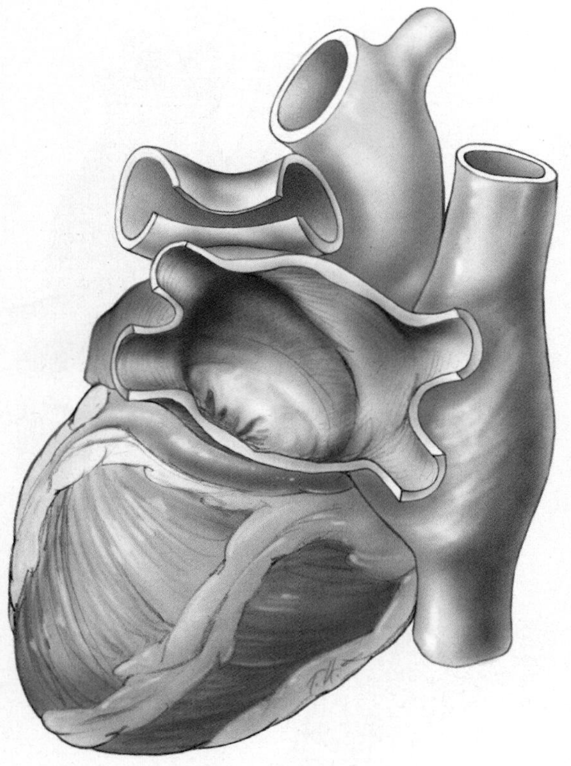

FIG. 11.5 The donor heart is prepared for implantation.

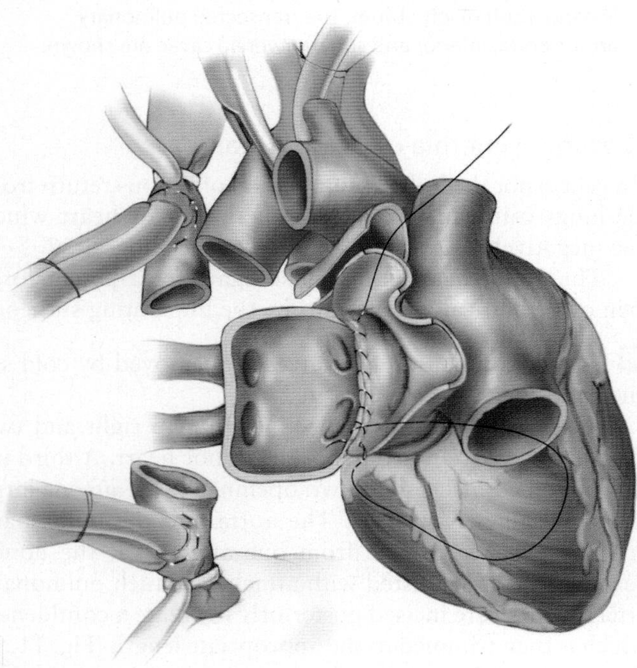

FIG. 11.6 The implantation of the donor heart begins with the left atrial anastomosis.

approximating intima to intima, which minimizes the risk of suture line clot formation.

NB The use of a large noncutting circular needle allows adequate bites of both the donor and recipient left atrial walls to be taken. By incorporating 8 to 10 mm of donor and recipient tissue in this everting manner, hemostasis is better ensured. This is especially important for the left atrial suture line, which is difficult to expose after the transplant is completed. NB

The left atrial suture line is continued inferiorly and then anterior to the recipient's right inferior pulmonary vein. The suture is tagged when the suture line reaches the level of the right superior pulmonary vein. The second needle is used to complete the left atrial suture line superiorly. Before securing the suture line, a 12-French chest tube flushed with cold plasmalyte is placed under direct vision into the left ventricle and the suture is snared around the chest tube. The flow of plasmalyte is begun and adjusted to 300 to 500 mL per hour for optimal cooling of left ventricular cavity.

⊘ Malalignment of the Venae Cavae

The surgeon must be sensitive to the respective positions of the recipient and donor inferior and superior venae cavae while constructing the left atrial suture line. If the inferior and superior venae cavae are not lined up appropriately, these anastomoses may be compromised. ⊘

The pulmonary artery of the donor heart is anastomosed to the recipient's pulmonary artery using 4-0 Prolene suture. In patients with preexisting pulmonary hypertension, this suture line may be reinforced with a strip of donor pericardium.

⊘ Pulmonary Artery Kinking

Kinking of the pulmonary artery may occur when the heart is filled. This may be caused by leaving the donor pulmonary artery too long. It also may occur if the donor ascending aorta and pulmonary artery are not adequately dissected free of one another. In either case, a gradient is created across the pulmonary artery anastomosis, which results in right ventricular hypertension and dysfunction. ⊘

While the patient is being rewarmed, the aortic anastomosis is performed using 5-0 Prolene continuous suture (Fig. 11.7). This suture line is always reinforced with a strip of donor pericardium. After the completion of this anastomosis, the left ventricle is deaired before reperfusion of the heart begins. The chest tube that was used for cooling the inside of the left ventricle is removed, and the left atrial suture line is secured.

Modified reperfusion solution is administered into the aortic root at a pressure of 40 mm Hg for 3 to 5 minutes. After this period, the modified reperfusion is switched to leukocyte-depleted blood until the aortic cross-clamp is removed (for a minimum total of 10 minutes).

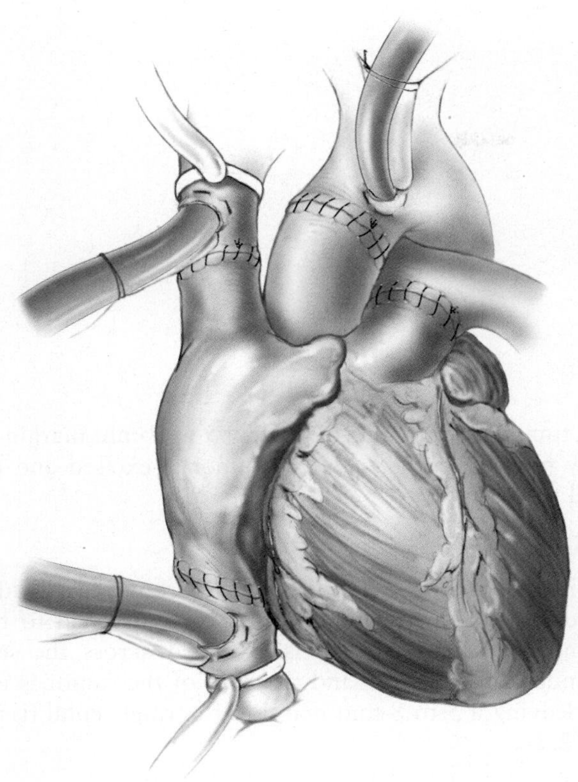

FIG. 11.7 Completed bicaval heart transplant.

NB There is ample experimental data suggesting that modification of the initial reperfusate improves myocardial functional recovery after regional or global ischemia. The modification of the initial reperfusate involves leukofiltration, addition of substrates such as aspartate, glutamate, and glucose for metabolism, addition of magnesium to minimize calcium influx, supplementation with dextran to reduce cellular swelling, and addition of nitroglycerin to ensure homogeneous distribution of reperfusate. NB

During this period of reperfusion, the inferior vena caval anastomosis followed by superior vena cava anastomosis is performed using 4-0 Prolene continuous sutures. These anastomoses are performed in such a way that endocardium is attached to endocardium in an everting manner. This technique minimizes the risk of clot formation.

⊘ Narrowing of Caval Anastomosis

Suturing of the cavae should be done carefully to avoid narrowing or purse-stinging of the anastomosis, which could complicate future endomyocardial biopsies. ⊘

This allows for direct measurement of left ventricular filling pressures during the immediate postoperative period. A left atrial line is placed through the right superior pulmonary vein and secured in place with two pledgeted Prolene sutures. The patient is then gradually weaned off cardiopulmonary bypass. Transesophageal echocardiography is always used to assess both right ventricular and left ventricular function during the weaning process.

⊘ Trapped Left Atrial Line

After securing the left atrial line, it is important to pull on the catheter to ensure that it can be removed easily in the postoperative period. ⊘

NB Training the Right Ventricle

Preexisting pulmonary hypertension and the effects of cardiopulmonary bypass on pulmonary vascular resistance may give rise to perioperative right ventricular dysfunction, following heart transplantation. To minimize the risk of right ventricular dysfunction and to "train" the right ventricle of the donor heart, we use a segmental strategy in weaning cardiopulmonary bypass. This entails maintaining the systemic perfusion pressure while at the same time reducing the right ventricular afterload. The technique involves leaving the pulmonary artery anastomosis suture line untied and snared. A sucker with 3/4 in. tubing (to minimize the risk of hemolysis) is inserted into the pulmonary artery and placed on suction at approximately 1 L per minute. The systemic perfusion pressure is maintained at 60 mm Hg or above by the perfusionist. If the donor right ventricular function remains stable with acceptable central venous pressure, the venting of the pulmonary artery is slowly decreased and the suction tubing is removed. The pulmonary artery suture line is tied. This "segmental weaning protocol" has been associated with a low incidence of postoperative right ventricular dysfunction. NB

⊘ Postoperative Hypoxemia

Persistence of a patent foramen ovale postoperatively can lead to right-to-left shunting and hypoxemia, especially if the pulmonary vascular resistance is high. ⊘

⊘ Sinoatrial Node Injury

The sinoatrial node of the donor heart should not be manipulated during harvest or implantation to minimize the risk of sinoatrial node injury. ⊘

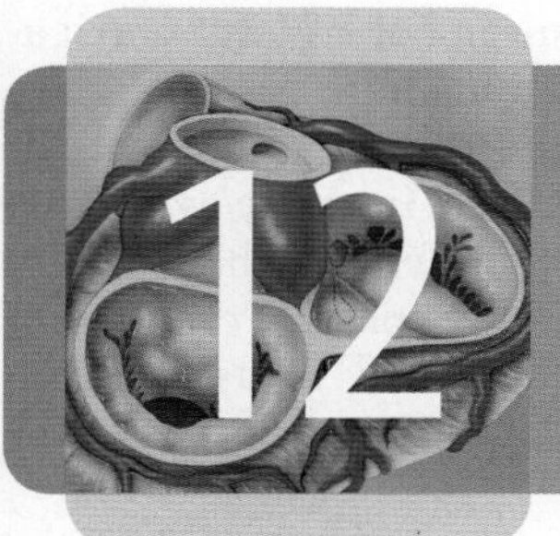

12 Cardiac Tumors

BENIGN TUMORS

Myxoma

Primary tumors of the heart are very rare. More than half of the benign tumors are myxomas. Although they can occur in any chamber of the heart, most myxomas arise from the interatrial septum and are seen most commonly in the left atrium. In approximately 15% of patients, the tumor is located within the right atrium.

The diagnosis may be suggested by the patient's symptoms, often related to obstruction of flow through the mitral orifice or systemic embolization. Echocardiography confirms the diagnosis.

Technique

The heart is exposed through a median sternotomy. The aorta is cannulated in the usual manner. The superior and inferior venae cavae are both directly cannulated (see Chapter 2). This is accomplished with great care to avoid manipulation of the atria.

⊘ Venous Cannulation through the Right Atrium

The introduction of large cannulas into the superior and inferior venae cavae through the right atrium may dislodge tumor fragments as well as clutter the operative field during tumor resection. Therefore, direct cannulation of both cavae is always preferred. ⊘

The aorta is clamped, and the heart is arrested with cold blood cardioplegia administered into the aortic root (see Chapter 3). Previously placed snares around both venae cavae are snugged down on the venous cannulas. An oblique incision is begun on the right superior pulmonary vein with a long-handled no. 15 blade. The opening is extended obliquely across the right atrial wall. Two small retractors are placed on the atriotomy edges to expose the right atrial cavity, interatrial septum, and any right atrial tumor that may exist (Fig. 12.1).

Right Atrial Myxoma

Myxomas occurring in the right atrium are usually bulky and may have a relatively wide base. The incision is now extended across the interatrial septum, encircling the base of the tumor with an approximately 5-to-8-mm margin of grossly normal septal wall. The tumor is excised and removed (Fig. 12.1).

Left Atrial Myxoma

Myxomas occurring in the left atrium are usually pedunculated and have a relatively small base attached to the septum. The septal incision is extended across the septum under direct vision, and the base of the tumor is excised, leaving a 5-to-8-mm margin of normal septal tissue (Fig. 12.2).

⊘ Artery to the Sinoatrial Node

The artery to the sinoatrial node traverses the atrial septum superiorly. Injury to this vessel may result in sick sinus syndrome. The base of a myxoma in this vicinity should be shaved off. ⊘

⊘ Injury to the Atrioventricular Node

Dissection near the anterior aspect of the coronary sinus orifice may cause atrioventricular node injury with resultant heart block. ⊘

NB Myxomas can occasionally arise from the atrial wall. The base of the tumor is removed with a margin of normal atrial wall. The resection need not be full thickness. The defect, if any, is approximated with fine Prolene sutures or patched with a piece of autologous pericardium. To minimize the risk of local recurrence, we usually apply a cryoprobe to the edges of the defect, especially when transmural resection cannot be done. NB

The septal defect is closed with a patch of autologous pericardium treated with glutaraldehyde or bovine pericardium using a continuous suture of 4-0 Prolene. The opening on the superior pulmonary vein and the right atriotomy are closed with a running 4-0 Prolene suture (Fig. 12.3). Dearing is carried out, and the aortic clamp is removed.

NB Thick Atrial Septum

Occasionally, the atrial septum is thickened with hypertrophied muscle and fatty tissue. It is important to position the pericardial patch on the endothelial surface of the left

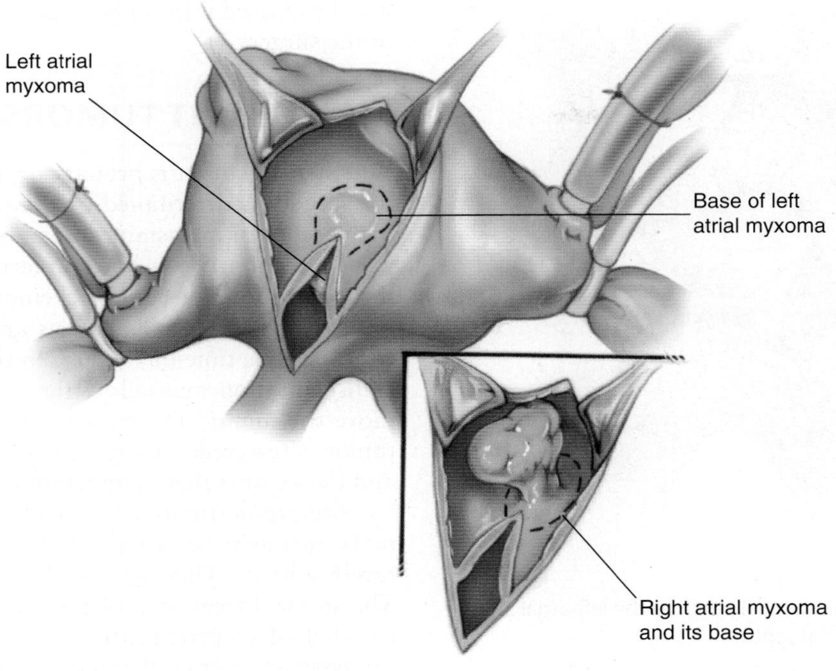

FIG. 12.1 Exposure of a left atrial myxoma and its base. Inset: Exposure of a right atrial myxoma and its base.

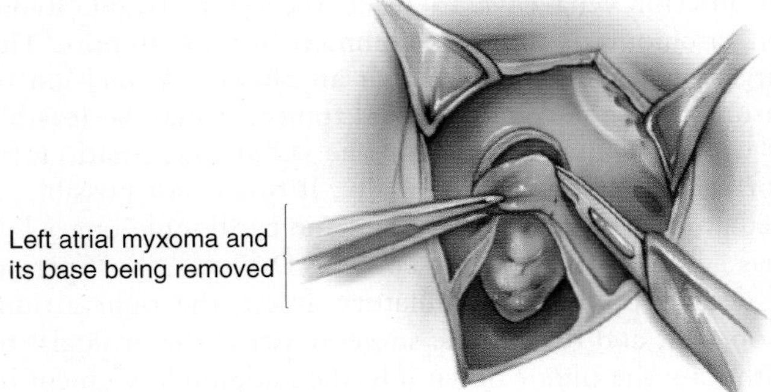

FIG. 12.2 Excision of a left atrial myxoma and its base with a generous margin of septal wall.

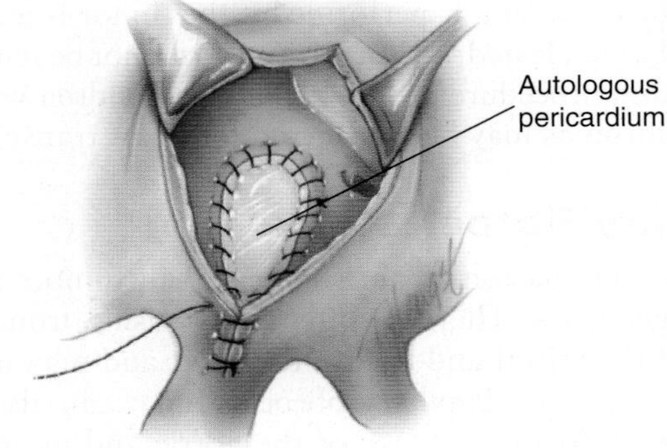

FIG. 12.3 Closure of a septal defect with autologous pericardium.

atrial side of the septum to prevent possible embolism of fatty tissue or thrombus formation (Fig. 12.4). NB

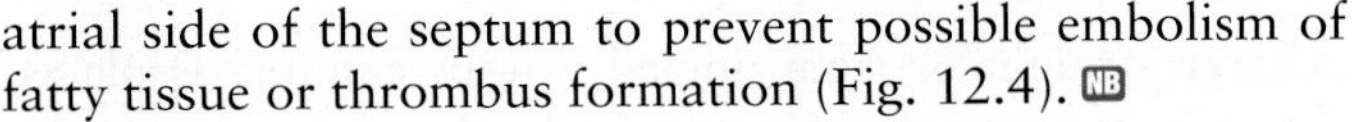

Rhabdomyoma

Rhabdomyomas arise from cardiac myocytes and are most commonly seen in infants and children. It is usually part of the disease complex tuberous sclerosis. The gray-white tumor mass often may disappear totally with time. Rhabdomyomas tend to grow as multiple tumors from the ventricular septum and cause obstruction of the inflow and outflow tracts of both sides of the heart. The most common symptom is heart failure caused by obstruction of a cardiac chamber or valve orifice.

Surgery is indicated before 1 year of age in patients without tuberous sclerosis when it may be possible to enucleate the tumor. Unfortunately, symptomatic patients with tuberous sclerosis often have extensive, multiple tumors and surgery has little to offer.

Fibroma

A fibroma arises from fibrous tissue cells as a single mass and is the second most common benign cardiac tumor. The majority of fibromas occur in children. Classically, it presents as a solitary white whorley mass in either ventricle, and frequently undergoes calcification. The symptoms are secondary to the obstruction of blood flow through the

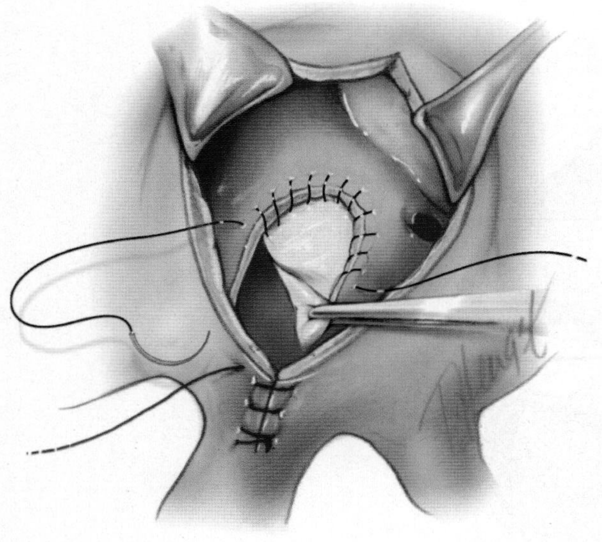

FIG. 12.4 Attaching a pericardial patch to the left atrial aspect of a thickened atrial septum.

affected segment of the heart. If calcified, it may be appreciated on a chest x-ray. Echocardiography confirms the presence and location of the mass.

Surgical excision is performed if the tumor is localized and can be enucleated. If the entire mass cannot be removed, a debulking procedure can be palliative. Children with extensive fibromas may be considered for heart transplant.

Papillary Fibroelastoma

Papillary fibroelastomas are solitary small tumors resembling vegetations. They are often seen arising from atrial aspect of the mitral and tricuspid valves, and may involve chordal structures. Papillary fibroelastomas can also arise from the ventricular surface of the aortic and pulmonary valves. These tumors are generally asymptomatic, but they can obstruct flow and embolize. They may be found incidentally at the time of surgery or seen on echocardiogram mimicking vegetations on the valves.

Because they can cause devastating complications, papillary fibroelastomas should be removed when diagnosed. A conservative resection, allowing for a valve repair rather than replacement, should be performed.

Lipoma

Lipomas are generally localized discrete tumors. They can occur anywhere in the heart or on the pericardium. Lipomas are generally asymptomatic. Large tumors causing significant symptoms should be resected. If a smaller lipoma is noted incidentally during a cardiac procedure, it may be excised if it can be done without increasing the risk of the surgery.

MALIGNANT TUMORS

Whether the tumor is primary or metastatic, the indication for surgery is determined by the tumor size, location, and the absence of metastatic spread beyond the heart. If complete resection is possible, surgery results in better palliation than radiation and/or chemotherapy alone. Complex left-sided cardiac malignancies are difficult to adequately expose at the time of surgery. In these cases, cardiac autotransplantation may allow the surgeon to completely remove the tumor. The patient's heart is explanted and the tumor is resected. Any resulting defects are reconstructed, and the heart is then reimplanted.

Metastatic tumors are much more common than primary malignancies of the heart. Cardiac metastases are rarely solitary. They commonly cause pericardial effusion. The surgical treatment of these patients is usually limited to relief of recurrent effusions by subxiphoid pericardial drainage or a pericardial window procedure.

Right Atrial Extension of Tumors below the Diaphragm

Abdominal and pelvic tumors may invade and grow up the inferior vena cava to reach the right atrium. Renal cell carcinoma is the most common of these tumors. The surgery is approached through an abdominal incision to ensure resectability of the renal tumor. It may be feasible to withdraw the tumor from the subdiaphragmatic inferior vena cava transabdominally. If this is not possible, a median sternotomy is performed and cardiopulmonary bypass achieved for systemic cooling. During a short period of deep hypothermic circulatory arrest, the right atrium is opened, and the cardiac surgeon assists the urologist to withdraw the tumor down into the abdominal segment of inferior vena cava and remove it. Cardiopulmonary bypass is reinstituted, the patient is rewarmed, and weaned from bypass in the usual manner.

⊘ Cannulation of Right Atrium

A large straight or right angled venous cannula is placed through a purse-string suture into the right atrium for a limited distance to avoid contact with the tumor. A dual-staged cannula should not be used. ⊘

⊘ Coagulopathy

These patients have significant problems with coagulopathy following cardiopulmonary bypass with profound hypothermia. This technique should be reserved for patients in whom the tumor cannot be removed through the inferior vena cava just below the diaphragm. ⊘

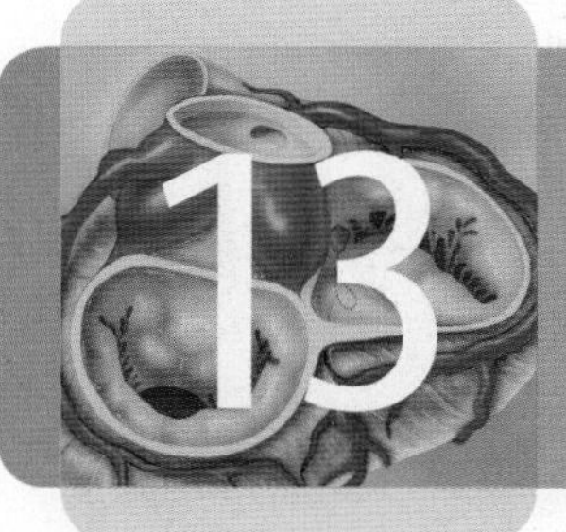

13 Surgery for Atrial Fibrillation

The Maze procedure was developed and modified by Dr. James Cox and has proved to be effective for treating atrial fibrillation associated with valvular and ischemic heart disease and isolated atrial fibrillation refractory to medical therapy. The Cox-Maze III cut and sew technique is the gold standard against which modifications should be measured because of its greater than 95% cure of atrial fibrillation. However, this procedure adds significantly to the aortic clamp time and incurs the risk of serious bleeding from the back of the heart. Several different energy sources have been used to ablate atrial tissue, creating the same lesion pattern as the Maze III operation in less time and with less bleeding potential. The ideal energy source for performing a full or partial Maze procedure should be fast and produce a transmural lesion without causing damage to surrounding structures. It would be advantageous if it could be applied through a minimally invasive approach without the use of cardiopulmonary bypass. Radiofrequency systems heat tissue, causing thermal injury and conduction block. Unipolar systems have been modified by adding irrigation to minimize the surface charring, which can lead to thrombus formation, and to prevent injury to adjacent structures, particularly the esophagus. Bipolar radiofrequency clamps can be used epicardially, assure transmural lesions, and avoid damage to surrounding tissue. However, not all of the Maze lesions can be performed with the bipolar device. Cryoablation is performed with a nitrous oxide–cooled probe. Its advantage is the lack of tissue vaporization, resulting in a smooth tissue surface. It takes 2 to 3 minutes to produce each transmural lesion. Microwave produces conduction block by thermal injury, but unlike radiofrequency, it does not cause surface charring. It is also more likely to produce a transmural lesion because of greater tissue penetration. Focused ultrasonography results in deep heating and coagulation necrosis, and can be delivered through tubular or planar transducers. Both the Nd:YAG laser and infrared coagulator produce transmural photocoagulation necrosis at relatively low tissue temperatures with no tissue vaporization. We have used a combination of bipolar radiofrequency clamp and a cryoprobe to recreate the lesions of Cox-Maze III procedure (which is called Cox-Maze IV procedure). This procedure can also be performed using a combination of other energy sources. Patients with chronic atrial fibrillation undergoing mitral valve surgery are candidates for this procedure, which adds approximately 20 minutes to the cross-clamp time.

TECHNIQUE

A median sternotomy is used, and standard bicaval cannulation is performed. The initial right atrial incisions and lesions are accomplished on cardiopulmonary bypass with a beating heart.

We first encircle right and left pulmonary veins. Using the radiofrequency clamp, we create transmural lesions around the pulmonary veins (Fig. 13.1). After tightening the caval tourniquets, the right atrial appendage is excised. Using the radiofrequency clamp passed through the right atrial appendage opening, a linear lesion is created toward SVC, on the aortic side of the appendage (Fig. 13.2). We then perform a vertical incision on the right atrial free wall. Using the bipolar clamp, linear lesions are created up to SVC and down to IVC (Fig. 13.3).

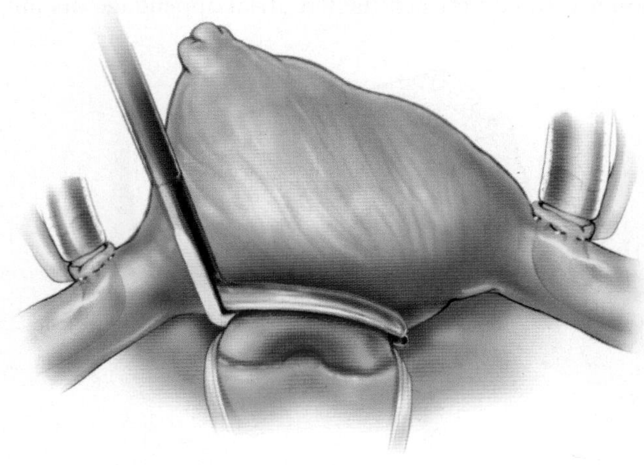

FIG. 13.1 The bipolar clamp is used to create lesions around the right and left pulmonary veins.

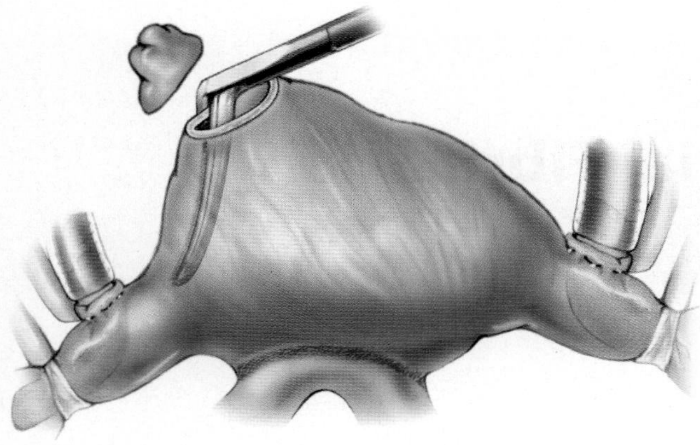

FIG. 13.2 Excision of the right atrial appendage and lesion line on the aortic side of SVC.

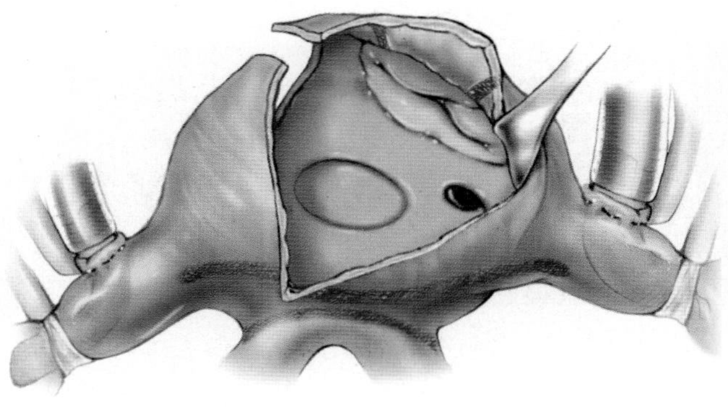

FIG. 13.4 Radiofrequency lesions from the amputated appendage to the tricuspid valve annulus and from the atriotomy free wall to the tricuspid annulus.

With the atrial free wall retracted, linear endocardial lesions are created from the superior aspect of atriotomy to 2 o'clock and 10 o'clock positions of the tricuspid vale annulus (Fig. 13.4). These two lesion sets are usually performed with bipolar radiofrequency clamp on the free wall to save time. The segment near AV groove needs to be performed endocardially with cryoprobe.

Omitting Right Atrial Ablation Lines

It is generally agreed that most of the right-sided lesions are not required in most patients. However, the ablation line from the coronary sinus inferiorly into the inferior vena cava should probably be included to prevent right atrial flutter (Fig. 13.5).

After placing a retrograde cardioplegia catheter, we then close the right atriotomy and start the left-sided lesion set. Aorta is cross-clamped and heart is arrested. Left atrial appendage is amputated and through the opening, a lesion is created between the left atrial appendage opening and left superior pulmonary vein (Fig. 13.6). Left atrial appendage base closed. We then mark the coronary sinus with a marking pen between the right and left coronary artery circulations. A standard left atriotomy is performed, with extension superiorly into the dome of left atrium or inferiorly around the right inferior pulmonary vein. Using the bipolar clamp, a lesion is created from the inferior aspect of the atriotomy to the inferior left pulmonary vein. Similarly, another lesion is created toward the mitral valve annulus and across the coronary sinus (Fig. 13.7). We then use the cryoprobe to create endocardial lesions connecting the PV lesions and to connect the left PV lesion set to the annulus of the mitral valve (Fig. 13.8). Lastly, the epicardial cryoablation of the coronary sinus is performed to complete the mitral isthmus ablation.

⊘ Patent Foramen Ovale

If a patent foramen ovale or small atrial septal defect is present, the right atrial lesions must be performed after the aorta is cross-clamped or with induced ventricular

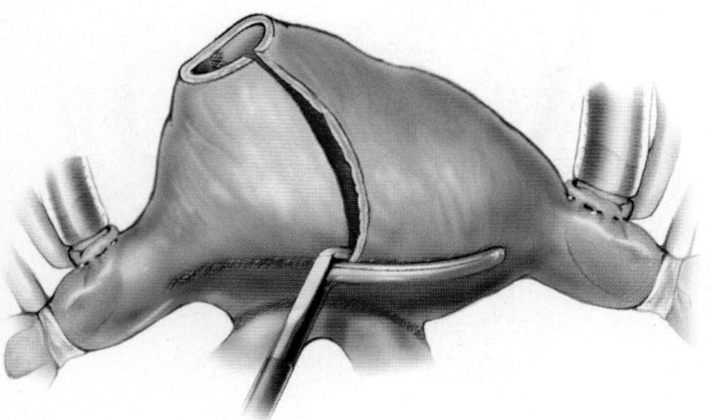

FIG. 13.3 Linear lesions are created through the atriotomy up the SVC and down to IVC.

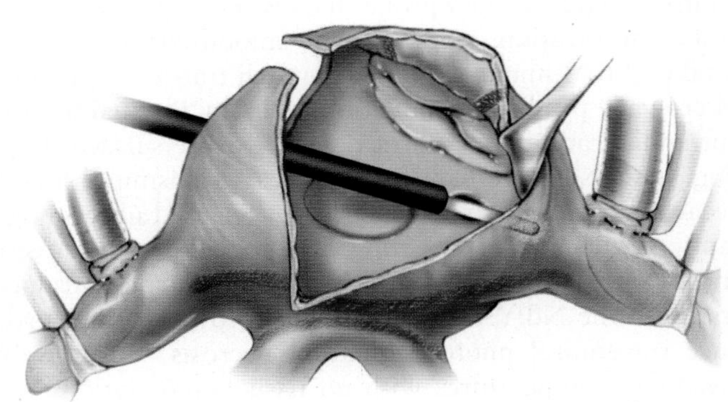

FIG. 13.5 Ablation line from coronary sinus into the vena cava to prevent atrial flutter.

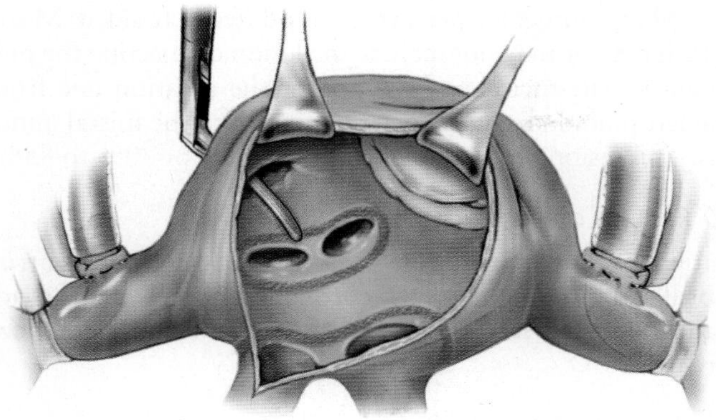

FIG. 13.6 After amputation of left atrial appendage, a lesion is created to the left pulmonary veins using the bipolar clamp.

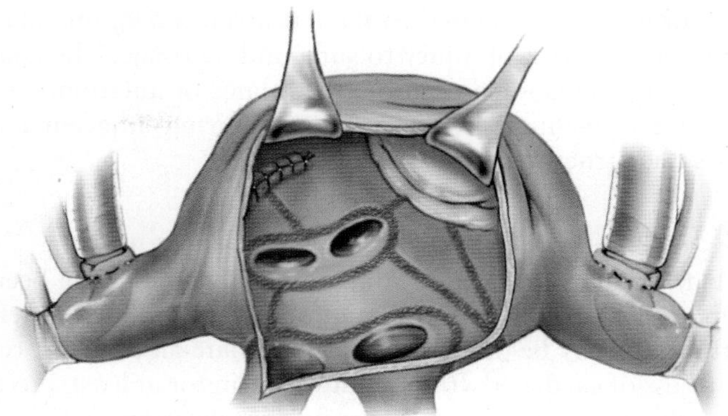

FIG. 13.8 Completed lesion set inside the left atrium.

fibrillation to prevent air embolism. The absence of a patent foramen ovale must be confirmed by transesophageal echocardiography in the operating room before instituting cardiopulmonary bypass. ⊘

⊘ Transmural Lesions

The bipolar radiofrequency clamp has the distinct advantage of increasing the likelihood of transmural lesions. The clamp needs to be applied a minimum of two times to increase the likelihood of transmurality. We apply cryoprobe for 2 to 3 minutes depending on the atrial tissue thickness. Discoloration of the endocardium should be apparent. ⊘

⊘ Bleeding from the Base of the Left Atrial Appendage

If the base of the appendage is ablated with the radiofrequency probe and then the appendage is amputated and oversewn, the ablated tissue may tear when the heart fills with blood and contracts. The appendage should be either surgically amputated or ablated with radiofrequency energy, not both, to avoid this complication. ⊘

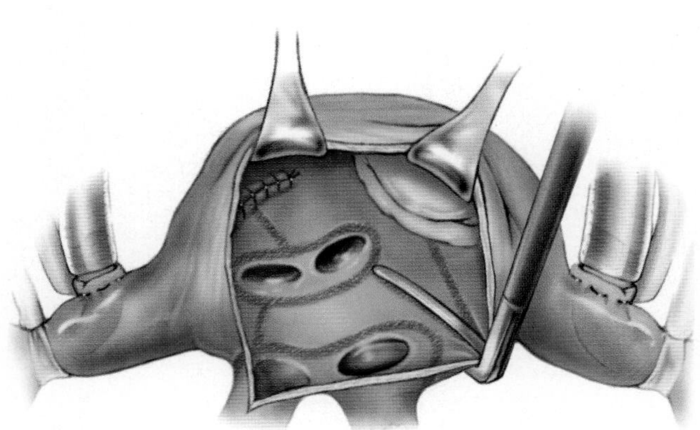

FIG. 13.7 Radiofrequency lesions within the left atrium (see text).

⊘ Thrombus in the Left Atrial Appendage

If thrombus is present in the left atrial appendage, it should be amputated. ⊘

⊘ Stenosis of the Pulmonary Vein Orifices

The healing process that takes place after radiofrequency ablation may lead to fibrosis and contraction of tissue. The lesions surrounding the orifices of the pulmonary veins should be well within the left atrium to avoid subsequent scarring and pulmonary vein stenosis. ⊘

⊘ Injury to the Valve Leaflet Tissue

The radiofrequency energy will damage the valve leaflet tissue. Therefore, care must be exercised when creating lesions extending onto the tricuspid and especially the mitral valve annulus. Because of this concern, some surgeons prefer to use a cryoprobe to make these lesions because cryoablation does not permanently damage leaflet tissue. It is also important to carry out these lesions before any valve repair or replacement procedure is performed. ⊘

⊘ Injury to the Circumflex Coronary Artery

In performing the ablation from the left pulmonary veins to the mitral annulus, care must be taken because the circumflex coronary artery underlies this area. Transmural lesions may injure this artery. For this reason, cryoablation may be preferable in this location. Alternatively, the risk of damaging the artery can be reduced by maintaining flow through the vessel during the ablation. This is accomplished by the administration of antegrade cardioplegic solution. ⊘

⊘ Injury to the Esophagus

Esophageal injury has been seen with dry radiofrequency ablation of the posterior left atrial wall. By lifting the cryoprobe when adhered to the left atrial tissue, one may minimize the risk of injury to surrounding tissue. The goal of any energy source used to create lines of ablation is to achieve transmural lesions without injuring adjacent tissues and structures. ⊘

⊘ Thrombogenic Foci

Ablation lines created by some energy sources have been reported to result in thrombus formation within the left atrium. It may be prudent to anticoagulate all patients, regardless of cardiac rhythm, with warfarin for at least 3 to 6 months to prevent this devastating complication. ⊘

The planned mitral valve procedure is now performed. Postoperative atrial arrhythmias are common and do not mean that the surgery has been unsuccessful. In general, these patients are maintained on amiodarone for 3 to 6 months postoperatively.

Freedom from atrial tachyarrythmia at 12 months is estimated around 80% to 90% in patients who undergo Cox-Maze IV procedure. Pulmonary vein isolation alone is the simplest ablation procedure with a success rate of 60% to 70%.

NB The bipolar radiofrequency clamps can be used to create the pulmonary vein encircling lesions on a beating heart. This procedure can be safely and quickly performed in patients with atrial fibrillation undergoing coronary bypass or aortic valve operations. NB

Many surgeons perform a modified left-sided Maze, which may or may not include the lesion connecting the pulmonary vein encircling lines and/or the ablation line from the left pulmonary vein encircling lesion to the mitral annulus. This lesion set has a higher success rate of 70% to 85%.

⊘ Failure of Procedure

Patients with enlarged left atria, longer duration of atrial fibrillation preoperatively, coronary disease, and/or advanced age are less likely to respond to a modified Maze procedure. ⊘

⊘ Postoperative Left Atrial Flutter

Because of concern regarding injury to the circumflex coronary artery, some surgeons omit the ablation line connecting the left pulmonary vein encircling lesion to the mitral annulus. This may allow left isthmus reentry to occur postoperatively, resulting in left atrial flutter, which can be difficult to control. ⊘

NB Left Atrial Appendage Excision

The left atrial appendage has several beneficial physiologic functions in patients who are in sinus rhythm. However, these are probably outweighed by the role that the appendage plays in thrombus formation in patients with atrial fibrillation. Excising the left atrial appendage during cardiac surgery in patients with atrial fibrillation removes the most important source of thromboembolism, and has been proposed as a stand-alone treatment for chronic atrial fibrillation. NB

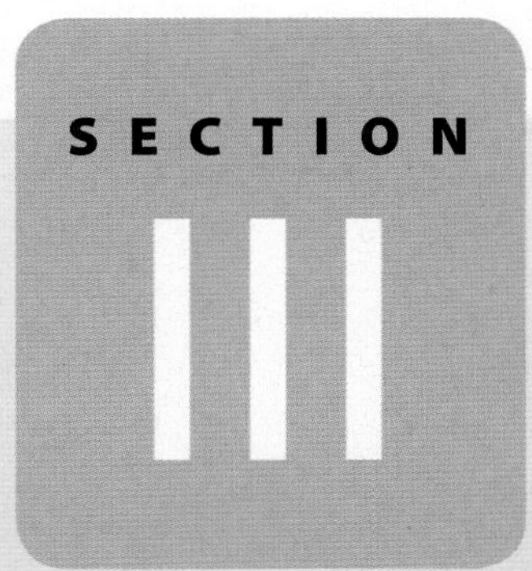

Surgery for Congenital Heart Defects

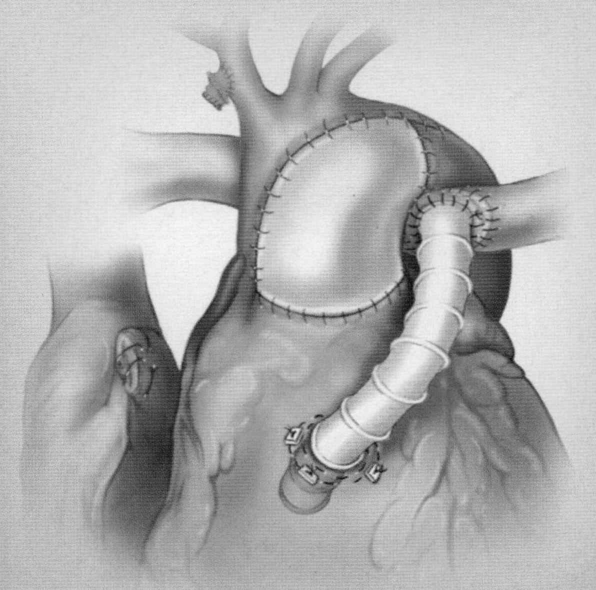

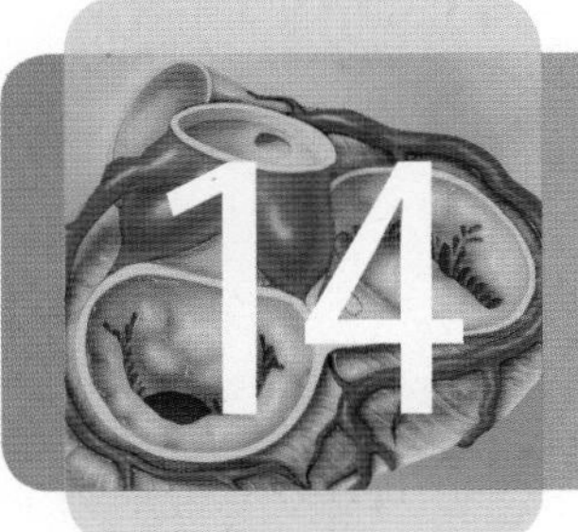

14 Patent Ductus Arteriosus

INCISION

The ductus arteriosus can be adequately exposed through a small left anterior thoracotomy. A limited left posterolateral thoracotomy through the third or fourth intercostal space partially dividing the latissimus dorsi muscle and preserving the serratus anterior muscle provides good exposure and is more commonly used. The skin incision can be quite short, especially in premature infants. If a right aortic arch and right ductus are present, a right thoracotomy approach must be used.

SURGICAL ANATOMY

The ductus arteriosus runs parallel to the aortic arch from the superior aspect of the origin of the left pulmonary artery and passes through the pericardium to join the medial margin of the aorta at an acute angle just opposite the origin of the left subclavian artery (Fig. 14.1). The left vagus trunk enters the thorax from the root of the neck in a groove between the left subclavian artery and the left common carotid artery, crosses the aortic arch and the ductus arteriosus, and continues downward. The recurrent laryngeal branch curves around the ductus arteriosus and extends back upward into the neck. The vagus nerve gives rise to many other small branches that are important tributaries to the pulmonary and cardiac plexuses. There are usually some lymph nodes buried in the hilum of the left lung that sometimes extend upward near the inferior margin of the ductus arteriosus. The left phrenic nerve enters the thorax medial to the vagus nerve and continues downward on the pericardium.

Technique for Exposing and Dissecting the Ductus Arteriosus

The left lung is retracted inferiorly and medially to expose the ductus arteriosus. The parietal pleura is divided longitudinally behind the vagus nerve if the intention is to retract the vagus nerve medially. Alternatively, a pleural incision may be made between the vagus and phrenic nerves when the vagus nerve is to be retracted laterally (Fig. 14.1). The incision of choice is extended superiorly along the left subclavian artery and inferiorly to the left hilum. The pleural edges are then suspended.

In an infant, the ductus is exposed by sharp dissection with scissors both from above and below. A blunt right-angled clamp or preferably a Waterson dissector/ Dennis–Browne is then carefully passed above and below the ductus to create a plane for its ligation or division. The ductus can most often be occluded by the application of a metal clip.

NB Recurrent Laryngeal Nerve Location with Medial Retraction

To facilitate dissection and exposure of the posterior aspect of the ductus arteriosus, many surgeons prefer that the vagus nerve and its recurrent laryngeal branch be reflected medially on the pleural flap (Fig. 14.2). The surgeon should be aware that traction of the nerve toward the pulmonary artery causes the recurrent nerve to lie along a diagonal course behind the ductus arteriosus. Therefore, care must be taken to ensure that the recurrent nerve is not injured during dissection. Alternatively, the vagus nerve and its branches can be isolated and retracted laterally to ensure their protection during the process of dissection of the posterior wall of the ductus. NB

⊘ Complete Exposure of the Ductus

Special care should be taken when dissecting near the angle between the pulmonary artery and the ductus arteriosus because the ductus is particularly susceptible to injury. A lappet of pericardium usually covers the ductus anteriorly. It should be dissected free to ensure complete exposure of the ductus (Fig. 14.3). Similarly, it is essential to separate the cranial aspect of the ductus from the transverse aortic arch—this maneuver more clearly demonstrates the angle that the clip will need to follow so as not to either impinge upon the arch or only partially occlude the ductus (Fig. 14.4). ⊘

Technique for Dividing and Ligating the Ductus Arteriosus

The vagus and recurrent laryngeal nerves are identified so that they are not divided inadvertently. Two heavy

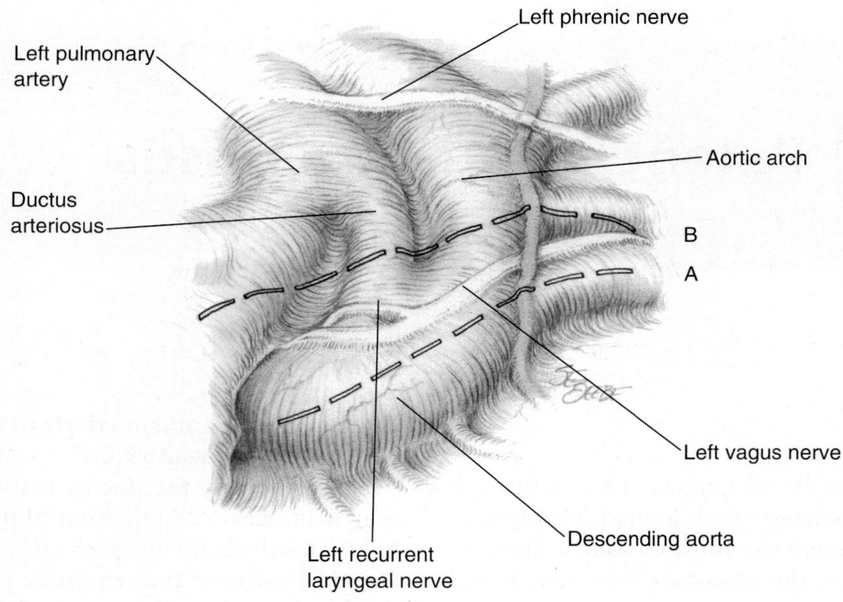

FIG. 14.1 Surgical anatomy of the ductus arteriosus. **A:** This incision line is used if the vagus nerve is to be retracted medially. **B:** This incision line is used if the vagus nerve is to be retracted laterally.

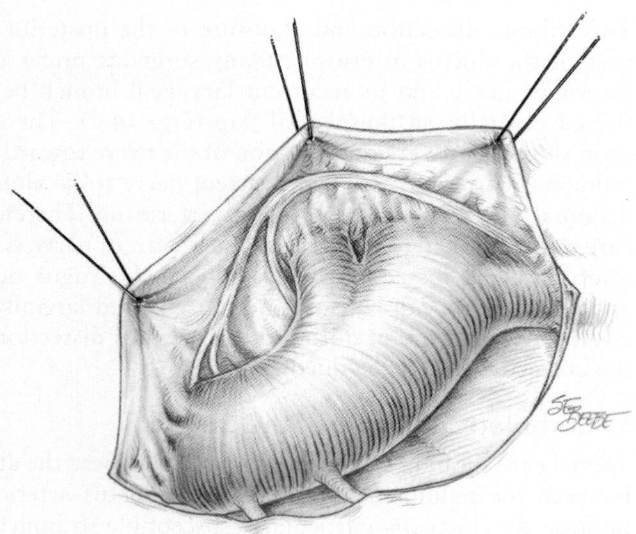

FIG. 14.2 Medial reflection of the vagus nerve on the pleural flap.

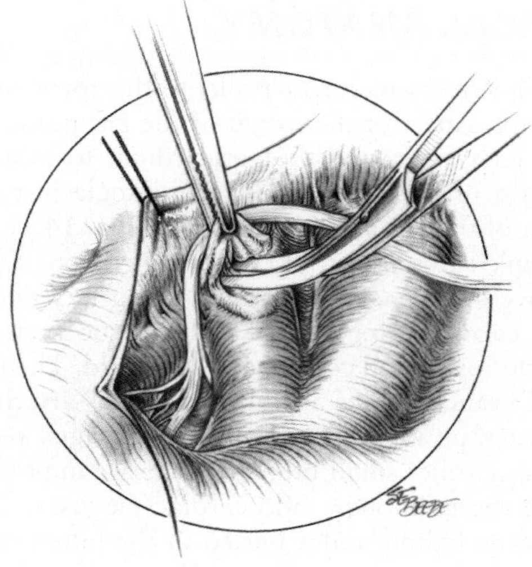

FIG. 14.3 Dissecting the lappet of pericardium to ensure complete exposure of the ductus.

Ethibond sutures are individually passed behind the ductus, which is then securely ligated (Fig. 14.5). Some favor using a 5-0 or 6-0 Prolene taking occasional adventitial bites circumferentially around the ductus to secure the tie. A purse-string suture of 4-0 Prolene may be placed between the ligatures to secure complete occlusion of the ductus (Fig. 14.5, inset).

Alternatively, the ductus is divided between clamps and oversewn with fine, nonabsorbable sutures (Fig. 14.6). This technique is particularly useful when the ductus is exceptionally short and large. Another option is to occlude the ductus with one or two metal clips. This latter technique is especially applicable to premature infants and is the most commonly practiced.

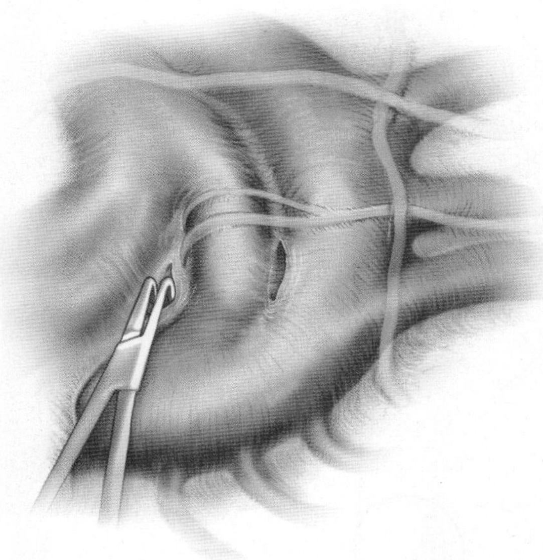

FIG. 14.4 Using a Waterston dissector to expose and separate the transverse arch from the cranial aspect of the ductus, and freeing the recurrent nerve from the inferior aspect.

⊘ Injury to the Recurrent Laryngeal Nerve during Ligation of the Ductus Arteriosus

The surgeon must always pay special attention to the recurrent laryngeal nerve. It can easily be divided during ductus mobilization. It can also be caught in the ligature, metal clip, or ductal clamp. ⊘

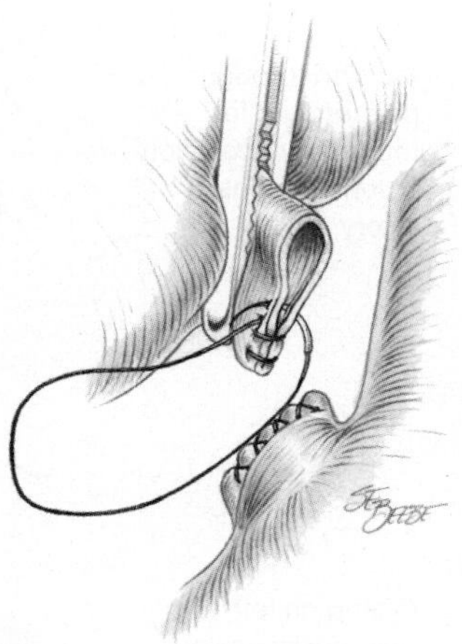

FIG. 14.6 Dividing the ductus arteriosus between clamps and oversewing it with fine, nonabsorbable sutures.

⊘ A Ductus Arteriosus Tear

The ductus arteriosus is liable to be injured and torn any time during dissection, ligation, or division, resulting in massive hemorrhage. Digital pressure over the ductus usually controls the bleeding and provides adequate exposure in a dry field. The aorta can then be temporarily clamped above and below the ductus while the torn ductus is oversewn with nonabsorbable sutures. The pulmonary artery end of the ductus can be similarly oversewn. Occasionally, this end of the ductus, if completely severed, may retract medially and its

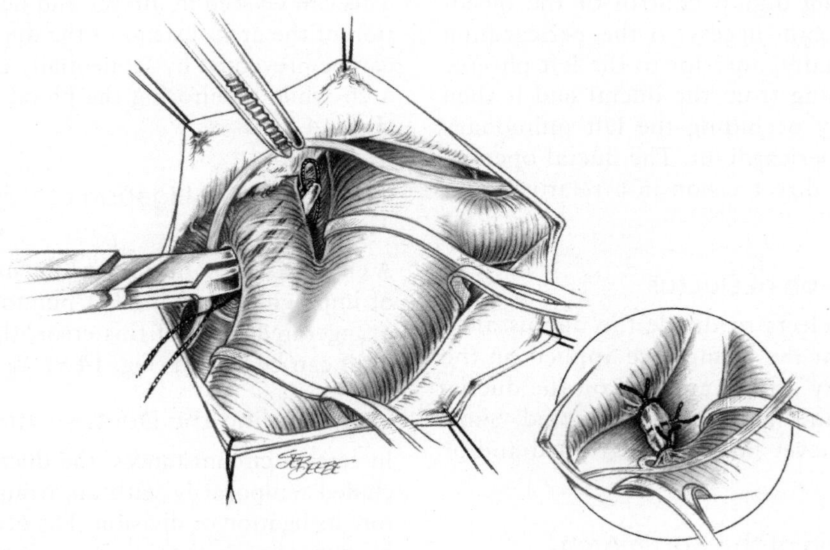

FIG 14.5 Ligation of the ductus. Inset: Securing the occlusion with purse-string sutures.

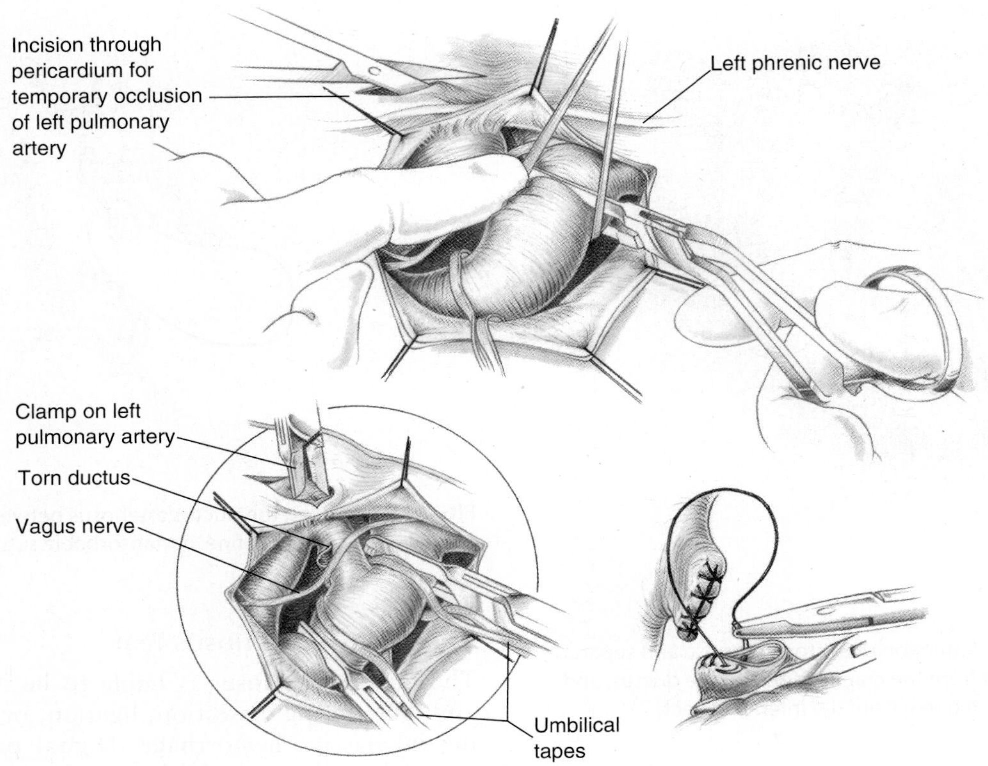

FIG. 14.7 Control of bleeding from and management of the torn ductus arteriosus.

exposure may become impossible. Under these circumstances, while continuing digital control of the bleeding, the surgeon must gain access to the pericardium by incising it longitudinally, anterior to the left phrenic nerve. Control of bleeding from the ductal end is then achieved by temporarily occluding the left pulmonary artery from within the pericardium. The ductal opening is then oversewn under direct vision in a relatively dry field (Fig. 14.7). ⊘

NB Clamping for Division of Ductus

Whenever the surgeon elects to divide the ductus arteriosus, it is essential that the clamps are applied on the aorta and the pulmonary artery, and not on the ductus itself, which is friable and liable to be disrupted. Similarly, the ductus must never be directly gripped and/or pulled. NB

⊘ Inadvertent Ligation of the Aortic Arch

The ductus arteriosus and aortic arch must both be identified. Occasionally, the ductus is very much larger than the arch, which may be underdeveloped and hypoplastic. This can be seen in infants and neonates. Inadvertent ligation of the arch instead of the ductus is a catastrophe that can be prevented by sequentially occluding the ductus and arch while monitoring the blood pressure in the left arm (Fig. 14.8). ⊘

⊘ Inadvertent Ligation of the Left Pulmonary Artery

A clip placed too far toward the mediastinum runs the risk of impinging upon the left pulmonary artery; in the most exaggerated form of this error, the left pulmonary artery itself can be ligated (Fig. 14.9). ⊘

⊘ Occluding the Ductus Arteriosus

In certain circumstances, the ductus arteriosus can be occluded temporarily with an atraumatic tissue forceps before its ligation or division. The occurrence of hypotension, bradycardia, or changes in oxygen saturation suggests that the patient has a ductal-dependent congenital anomaly and needs further diagnostic studies. ⊘

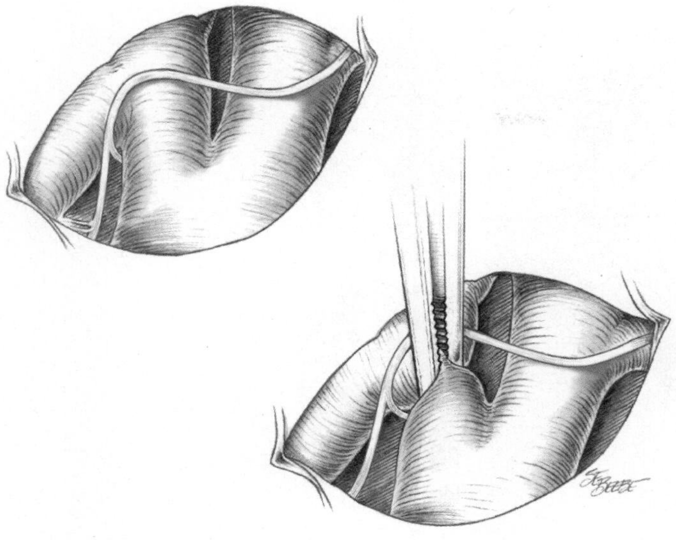

FIG. 14.8 Temporary occlusion of the ductus arteriosus to prevent the inadvertent ligation of the aortic arch.

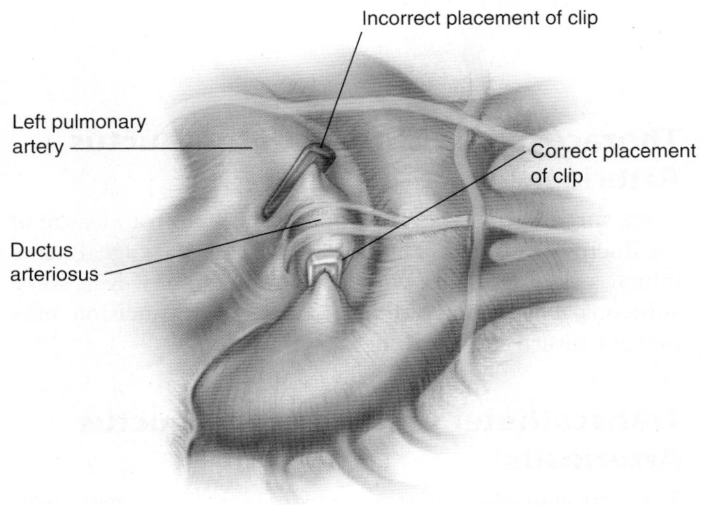

FIG. 14.9 Placement of a clip too proximal can cause narrowing (or complete occlusion) of the left pulmonary artery.

Closure of the Ductus Arteriosus in Premature Infants

The ductus arteriosus is visualized through a short, left lateral thoracotomy in the fourth intercostal interspace. The parietal pleura over the descending thoracic aorta is incised. Minimal dissection with scissors or a fine-tipped clamp is needed above and below the ductus. Occlusion of the ductus with a metal clip is the preferred method in premature infants. A medium or medium-large metal clip is selected depending on the size of the ductus. The clip applier is positioned over the ductus arteriosus, directing the tips of the clip slightly inferiorly and away from the wall of the descending aorta and orienting the clip parallel with the aorta (Fig. 14.10). The ductus is then occluded with the metal clip. There is no need to pass an instrument around the ductus.

⊘ Erosion or Cutting by the Clip

If the ends of the clip are adjacent to the descending aorta or distal aortic arch, the clip may cut into these structures, resulting in immediate or delayed bleeding. ⊘

⊘ Scissoring of Metal Clip

Some clip appliers may cause the two sides of the metal clip to miss each other and cut through the ductus rather than occlude it. The surgeon should test the clip applier with a clip away from the operative field to verify proper closure of the clip before using the applier on the ductus itself (Fig. 14.11). ⊘

⊘ Tearing of Ductus with Tip of Instrument

The scissors or clamp used to create an adequate opening above and below the ductus for clip placement should have a rounded, smooth tip. The surgeon must inspect the instrument to verify that there is not a burr at or near the tip that could tear the delicate ductal tissue. ⊘

Completing the Operation

Rib blocks have been most effective in reducing postoperative thoracotomy pain. A long-acting local anesthetic agent is injected near the neurovascular bundle at least two interspaces above and two below the level of the incision. The chest tube is brought through the skin and muscle opening and introduced through the fifth or sixth intercostal space. Heavy braided sutures are passed around the ribs above and below to reapproximate the opening. The muscle layers, subcutaneous tissues, and skin are closed around the chest tube, which is connected to an underwater seal suction system. When the skin closure reaches the chest tube, several vigorous sustained ventilations are administered by the anesthesiologist. The chest tube is then withdrawn with the lungs inflated. A chest x-ray obtained in the operating room confirms reexpansion of the left lung and absence of pneumothorax.

⊘ Bleeding Caused by Intercostal Injections

In patients with coagulopathies or who are anticoagulated, rib blocks should be avoided to prevent extrapleural hematomas or intrapleural bleeding. Many premature infants

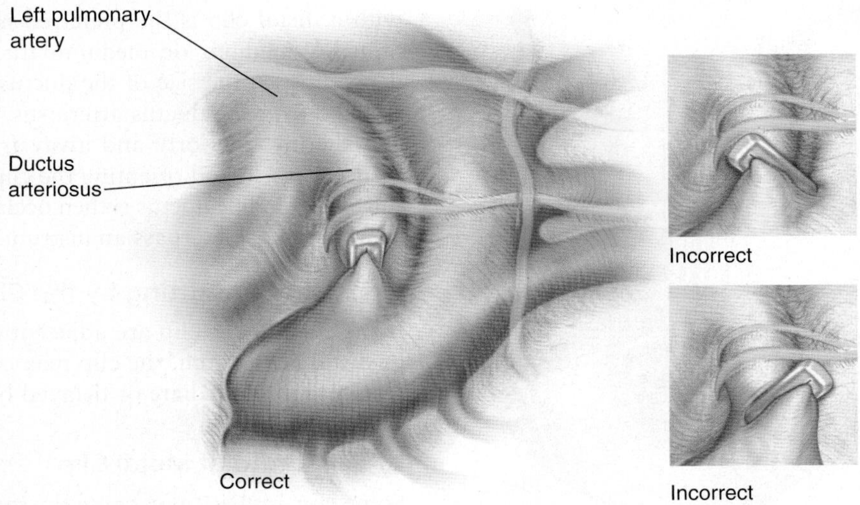

FIG. 14.10 It is important to place the clip completely across the ductus, parallel with the aorta, so as to not angle cranially (and the tips entrap the transverse aortic arch), or angle inferiorly or incompletely clip the ductus (as shown). The ideal placement of the clip allows distance from the recurrent nerve and also a "ductal bump" of tissue on the descending aorta (thus not causing a coarctation).

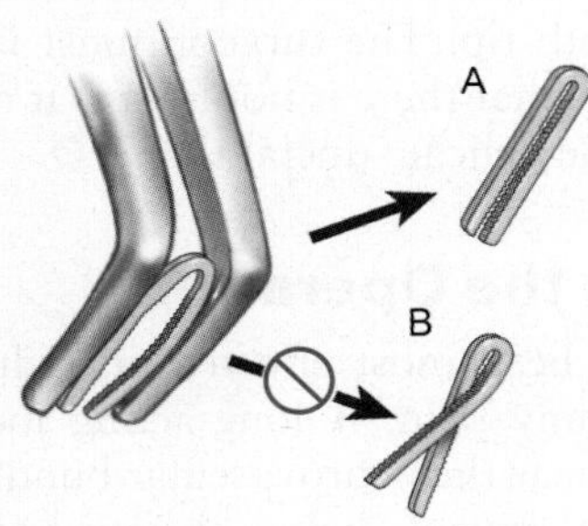

FIG. 14.11 Surgeon must test the clip applier to verify symmetric closure of the metal clip components **(A)**, to avoid using an applier that scissors the clip **(B)**.

have thrombocytopenia and should not receive intercostal injections. ⊘

⊘ Placement of Pericostal Sutures

The suture should hug the top of the rib to avoid injury to the intercostal artery or vein. ⊘

⊘ Injury to the Lung

If injury to the lung is noted, the chest tube should be left in place on suction for 12 to 24 hours. ⊘

Thoracoscopic Closure of the Ductus Arteriosus

Some surgeons use thoracoscopic techniques for closure of the ductus arteriosus. The risk of recurrent laryngeal nerve injury is slightly higher with this approach; however, some surgeons feel that avoiding a thoracotomy incision may prevent future chest wall deformities.

Transcatheter Closure of the Ductus Arteriosus

Transcatheter closure of a small patent ductus arteriosus with a coil or occluder device can be accomplished satisfactorily and avoids surgery in selected patients.

Calcification of the Ductus Arteriosus

The ductus may be calcified and/or aneurysmal, and simple ligation or division may not be feasible. Under these circumstances, it may be easier and safer to close the ductal opening through the left pulmonary artery under direct vision with the patient on cardiopulmonary bypass (see later).

⊘ Friable Tissues

If the tissues are friable, the patch can be sewn into place with interrupted pledgeted sutures. ⊘

ANTERIOR APPROACH TO CLOSURE OF THE PATENT DUCTUS ARTERIOSUS

A median sternotomy incision is used for infants and children with a patent ductus arteriosus undergoing repair of other congenital heart defects. This approach is also useful in adults with calcified and noncalcified as well as aneurysmal ducts.

Technique in Infants and Children

Before the initiation of cardiopulmonary bypass, the ascending aorta is retracted slightly to the right and the main pulmonary artery is retracted gently downward. The ductus is then dissected free of the left pulmonary artery and the aortic arch using scissors or a fine-tipped clamp. The ductus is encircled with a 2-0 braided suture and ligated or occluded with a metal clip at the onset of cardiopulmonary bypass (Fig. 14.12).

⊘ Flooding of the Pulmonary Circulation

With the initiation of cardiopulmonary bypass, flooding of the pulmonary circulation and low systemic blood pressure are likely to occur unless the ductus is occluded. All children undergoing cardiopulmonary bypass are evaluated for the presence of a patent ductus either by echocardiogram, direct inspection, or both. ⊘

⊘ Tearing of Ductal Tissue

The ductal tissue is friable, and care must be taken to prevent the suture or clip from cutting through the ductus. This results in bleeding that may be difficult to control, especially on the aortic side. ⊘

⊘ Stenosis of the Left Pulmonary Artery

The tie or clip should be placed far enough away from the origin of the left pulmonary artery to prevent narrowing of this vessel. This can result from external compression by the ligature or clip or from extrusion of ductal tissue into the lumen of the left pulmonary artery. ⊘

Technique in Adults

Closure of a patent ductus arteriosus in an adult can be safely accomplished through a median sternotomy on cardiopulmonary bypass. The patient is cooled systemically for 5 to 10 minutes to allow a brief period of very low perfusion. During low flow, the main pulmonary artery is opened longitudinally. The opening of the ductus is identified, and an appropriately sized Foley catheter is passed into the aorta (Fig. 14.13). After inflating the balloon

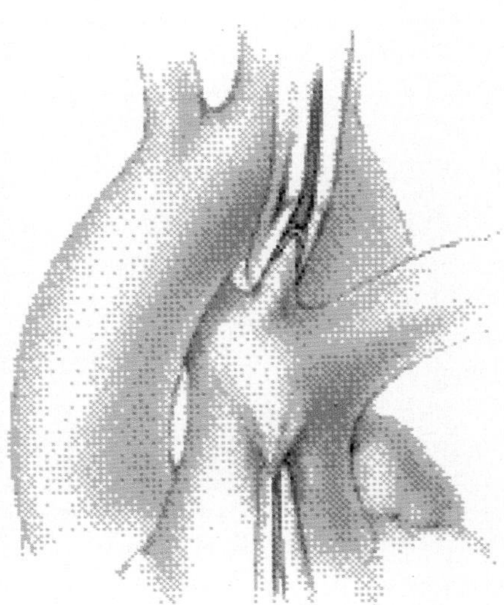

FIG. 14.12 Exposure and occlusion of the ductus arteriosus from the anterior approach.

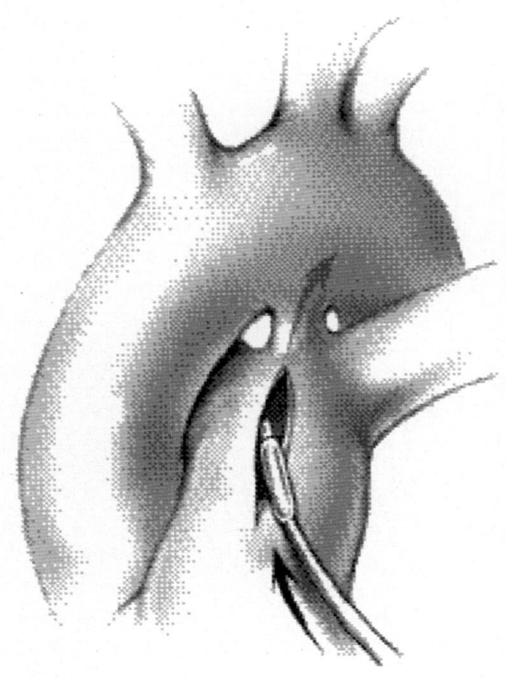

FIG. 14.13 Opening the main pulmonary artery and placing a Foley catheter in the ductus arteriosus.

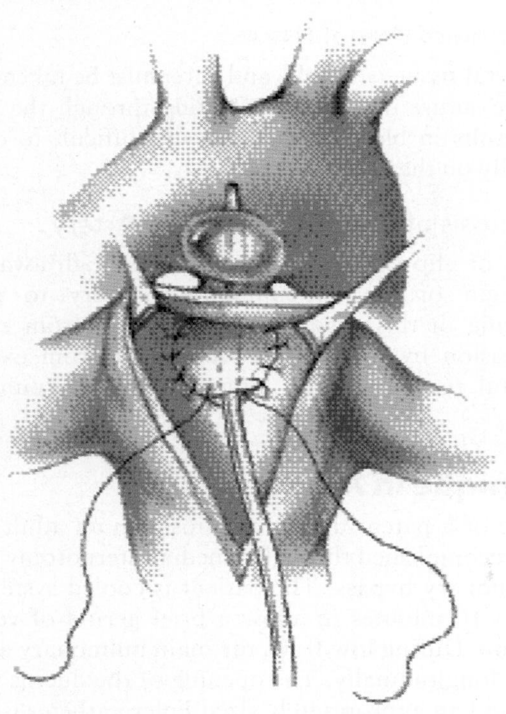

FIG. 14.14 Completing a patch closure of the pulmonary side of the ductus arteriosus with an inflated Foley balloon.

with saline, the flow through the ductus is controlled by placing traction on the Foley catheter (the connector end of the catheter must be occluded to prevent the backflow of blood). Cardiopulmonary bypass flow can be increased while a patch of autologous pericardium treated with glutaraldehyde, Gore-Tex or hemashield is sewn away from the edges of the ductal orifice using 5-0 monofilament suture (Fig. 14.14). Just before placing the last one or two stitches, the pump flow is turned very low while the Foley balloon is deflated, the catheter is removed, and the final stitches placed. Full flow is resumed, and the pulmonary arteriotomy is closed. The patient is weaned off cardiopulmonary bypass when systemic rewarming is completed.

⊘ Flooding of the Pulmonary Circulation

During cooling, the ductal flow must be occluded to prevent runoff of the aortic cannula flow into the pulmonary arterial bed. This is accomplished with forceful digital pressure on the distal main pulmonary artery. ⊘

⊘ Air Embolism through the Ductus Arteriosus

When the pulmonary artery is opened, some flow must be maintained through the aortic cannula to prevent air embolism. In addition, the patient may be placed in Trendelenburg position to prevent this complication. ⊘

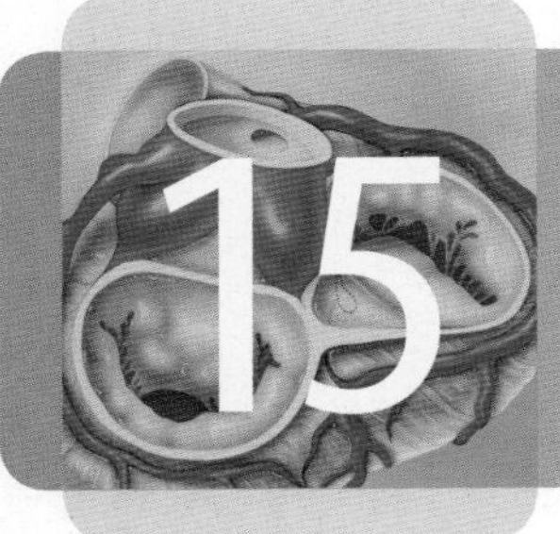

15 Coarctation of the Aorta

More than 50% of infants with a coarctation of the aorta become symptomatic during the first month of life. Associated cardiac anomalies accompany this lesion in more than 75% of patients. In neonates, infusion of prostaglandin E_1 prevents or reverses constriction of the ductal tissue. An open ductus improves lower body perfusion by allowing right-to-left shunting into the descending aorta. By relaxing the aortic end of the ductus, prostaglandin E_1 often results in a larger lumen at the coarctation site. Surgery can then be safely delayed until the left ventricular function, which is often poor, improves and any signs of low cardiac output syndrome, such as renal insufficiency, resolve. Older children may present with upper-body hypertension and/or signs and symptoms of decreased lower-extremity perfusion.

INCISION

In patients with an isolated aortic coarctation, the involved area can be adequately exposed through a fourth intercostal left posterolateral thoracotomy. For any patient undergoing coarctation repair through a thoracotomy, it is paramount in the morning of the operation to rule out fever and also to allow the patient to cool passively during the anesthetic preparation; mild hypothermia may mitigate the risk of spinal cord injury during the operation. Infants with associated lesions may be better served with a complete repair on cardiopulmonary bypass through a median sternotomy using a period of deep hypothermia to resect or augment the coarcted segment. Even in infants with no other cardiac anomalies, the aortic arch may be hypoplastic. These patients should undergo patch augmentation of the entire arch and proximal descending aorta under deep hypothermia (see Chapter 29).

SURGICAL ANATOMY

A coarctation of the aorta affects the junction of the aortic arch, descending aorta, and ductus arteriosus in more than 98% of patients. It can, however, occur anywhere along the course of the aorta.

The left vagus nerve enters the thoracic cavity from the root of the neck between the left subclavian and left common carotid arteries, crosses the aortic arch, and continues downward anteromedial to the descending aorta, traversing the ligamentum arteriosum. The recurrent laryngeal nerve has its origin in the vagus nerve, curves around the ligamentum arteriosum, and continues back upward into the neck (Fig. 15.1). There may be poststenotic dilation just distal to the coarctation. In older patients, the poststenotic dilation may be more pronounced and there may be extensive enlargement of collateral vessels about the shoulder and back muscles. This may include the intercostal arteries, whose walls may be paper thin and friable.

EXPOSURE OF THE COARCTATION

The left lung is retracted inferiorly and anteriorly, often with placement of a so-called "Kirklin tent" to help in exposure. The parietal pleura is divided longitudinally over the left subclavian artery and descending thoracic aorta across the coarctation segment. The pleural edges are then suspended (Fig. 15.1). The left subclavian artery, aortic arch distal to the left carotid artery, and the descending aorta are mobilized from the root of the neck to a distance well below the coarctation. Vessel loops may be passed around the aorta and the subclavian artery to facilitate exposure (Fig. 15.2).

⊘ Protection of the Vagus and Recurrent Laryngeal Nerves

The left vagus nerve and its recurrent laryngeal branch may be injured during mobilization. ⊘

⊘ Enlarged Intercostal Arteries

The intercostal arteries are usually enlarged. They have extremely thin walls and can cause troublesome bleeding if traumatized. ⊘

⊘ Bleeding from Aortic Branches

Bronchial arteries may occasionally arise from the posterior surface of the aorta and the left subclavian artery. They can be inadvertently torn during mobilization and dissection. ⊘

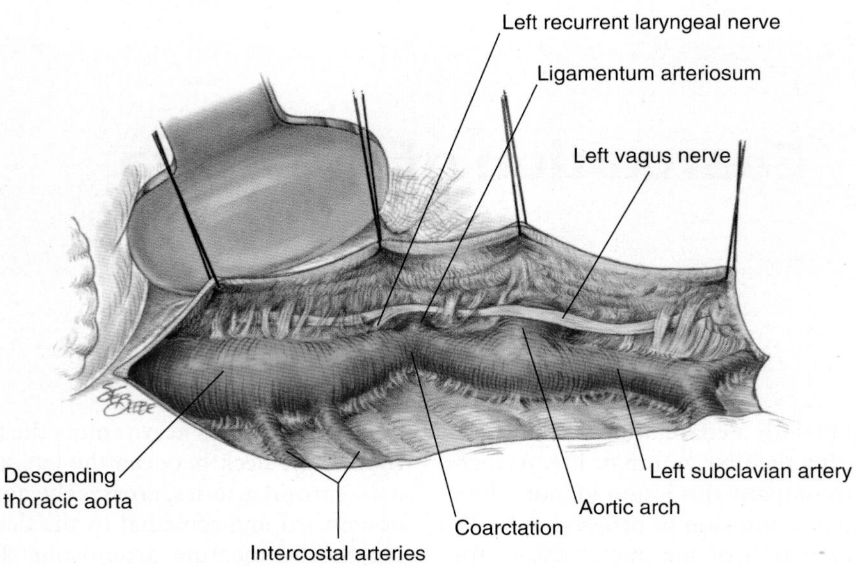

FIG. 15.1 Surgical anatomy of a coarctation of the aorta.

COARCTECTOMY

Whenever possible, a coarctectomy is the procedure of choice. It entails removal of stenosed or hypoplastic segments of the aorta and of abnormal ductal tissue in neonates. Appropriate clamps are selected, usually a straight vascular clamp for the descending aorta and a curved clamp to be placed across the left subclavian artery and distal arch. The descending aorta is clamped first and then the proximal clamp is applied. The ductus arteriosus or ligamentum arteriosum is ligated or clipped on the pulmonary artery side and divided to give the aorta additional mobility. The coarcted segment is excised, with attention paid toward making the proximal aortotomy on a bevel to increase the anastomotic surface, and the two clamps are now carefully maneuvered to bring the aortic ends together. The anastomosis is accomplished with a running Prolene suture (Fig. 15.3). The distal clamp and then the proximal clamp are removed, and the anastomosis is inspected for hemostasis as well as the absence of constriction or torsion.

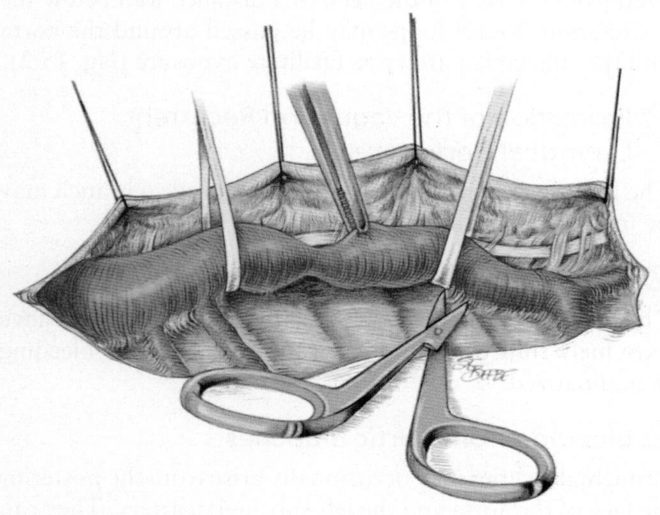

FIG. 15.2 Exposure of a coarctation.

NB Use of Approximator

A combination of straight and spoon-shaped atraumatic clamps with an approximator is useful. This allows the clamps to remain immobile while the aortic ends are being sutured together without tension. The operative field is not obscured by the assistant's hands, which is especially important in neonates. Alternatively, the assistant surgeon has the critical responsibility of holding the two ends of the aorta together so that a satisfactory anastomosis can be completed. NB

NB Placement of Clamps

The clamps should be positioned far enough away from the excision lines to provide adequate aortic cuffs for suturing. The aortic wall is elastic and will retract after each end is transected. At least 5 mm in neonates or 1 cm in older children is required to secure a satisfactory anastomosis. NB

⊘ Residual Coarctation

Inadequate resection of a coarctation may leave the patient with residual disease (Fig. 15.4). ⊘

⊘ Preserving the Maximal Diameter of the Lumen

The aortic anastomosis should incorporate the widest lumen of the aorta to prevent any local constriction. The

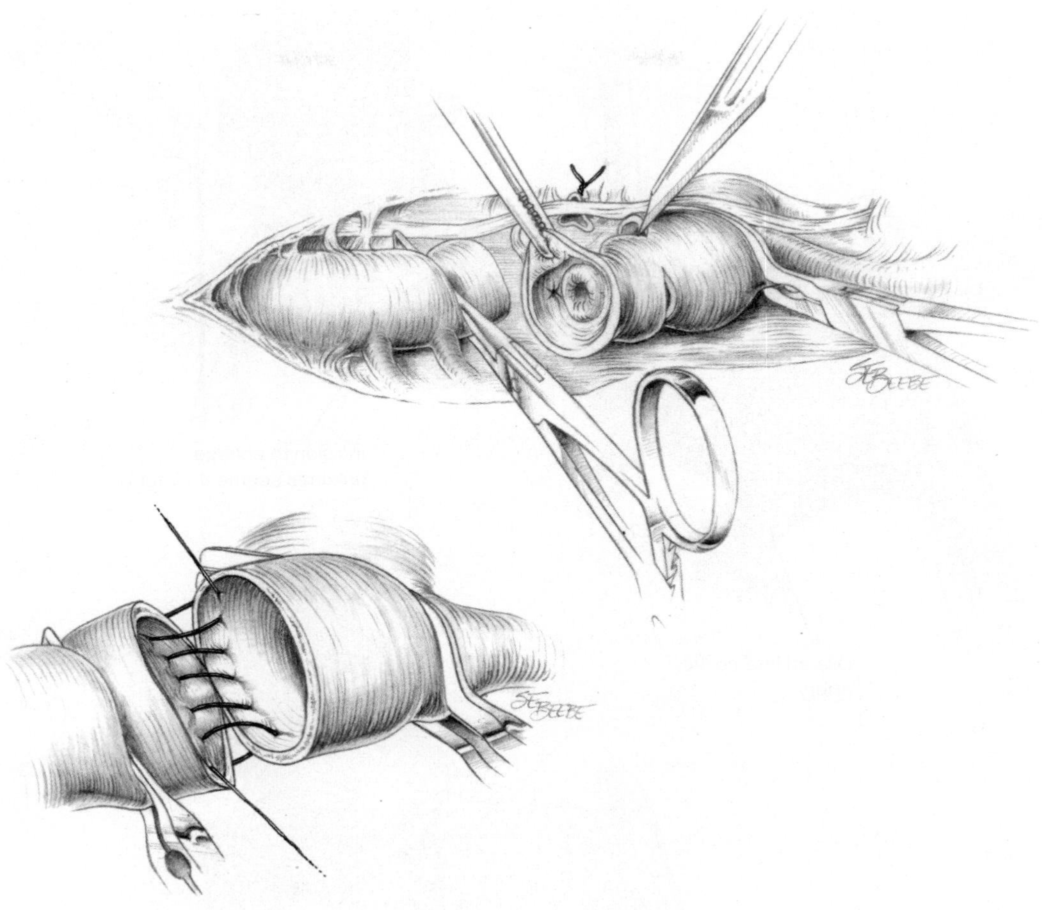

FIG. 15.3 Technique for a coarctectomy.

proximal opening can be enlarged, if necessary, to conform with the poststenotic dilation of the lower aortic segment (Fig. 15.5). ⊘

NB Intercostal Arteries

The first set of intercostal arteries is often located close to the distal extent of the coartation. They can usually be preserved and temporarily occluded with small bulldog clamps during the resection and anastomosis. The distal aortic clamp is placed below the first intercostal vessels (Fig. 15.5). However, if their division is required for full mobilization to perform and extended end-to-end anastomosis, this should be pursued. NB

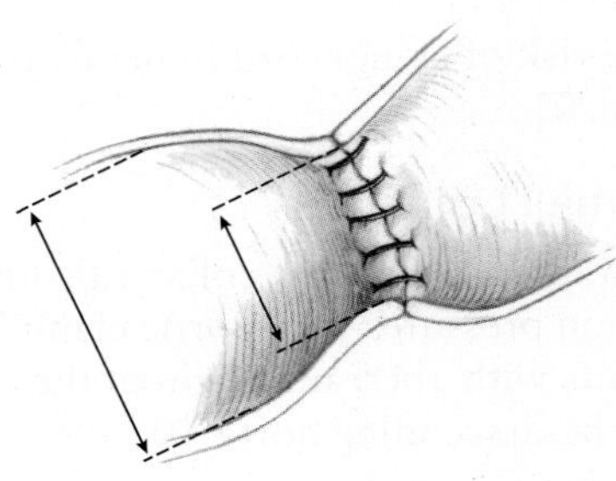

⊘ FIG. 15.4 Inadequate resection in a coarctectomy.

⊘ Interrupted Sutures in Neonates

Although continuous suturing provides better hemostasis and functions quite satisfactorily in most cases, interrupted suturing in the neonate is used by some surgeons to reduce the possibility of recurrent stenosis. Alternatively, the posterior layer is completed with a continuous technique, and the anterior layer is approximated with interrupted sutures. Some surgeons use absorbable suture, such as polydioxanone (PDS), which at least theoretically should ensure better growth at the site of the anastomosis. ⊘

⊘ Hemostasis

There may be bleeding along the suture line requiring additional sutures. Often, adventitial U-stitches are effective. It may be advisable to temporarily reapply the proximal clamp so that the sutures can be placed and tied without tension on the anastomosis. ⊘

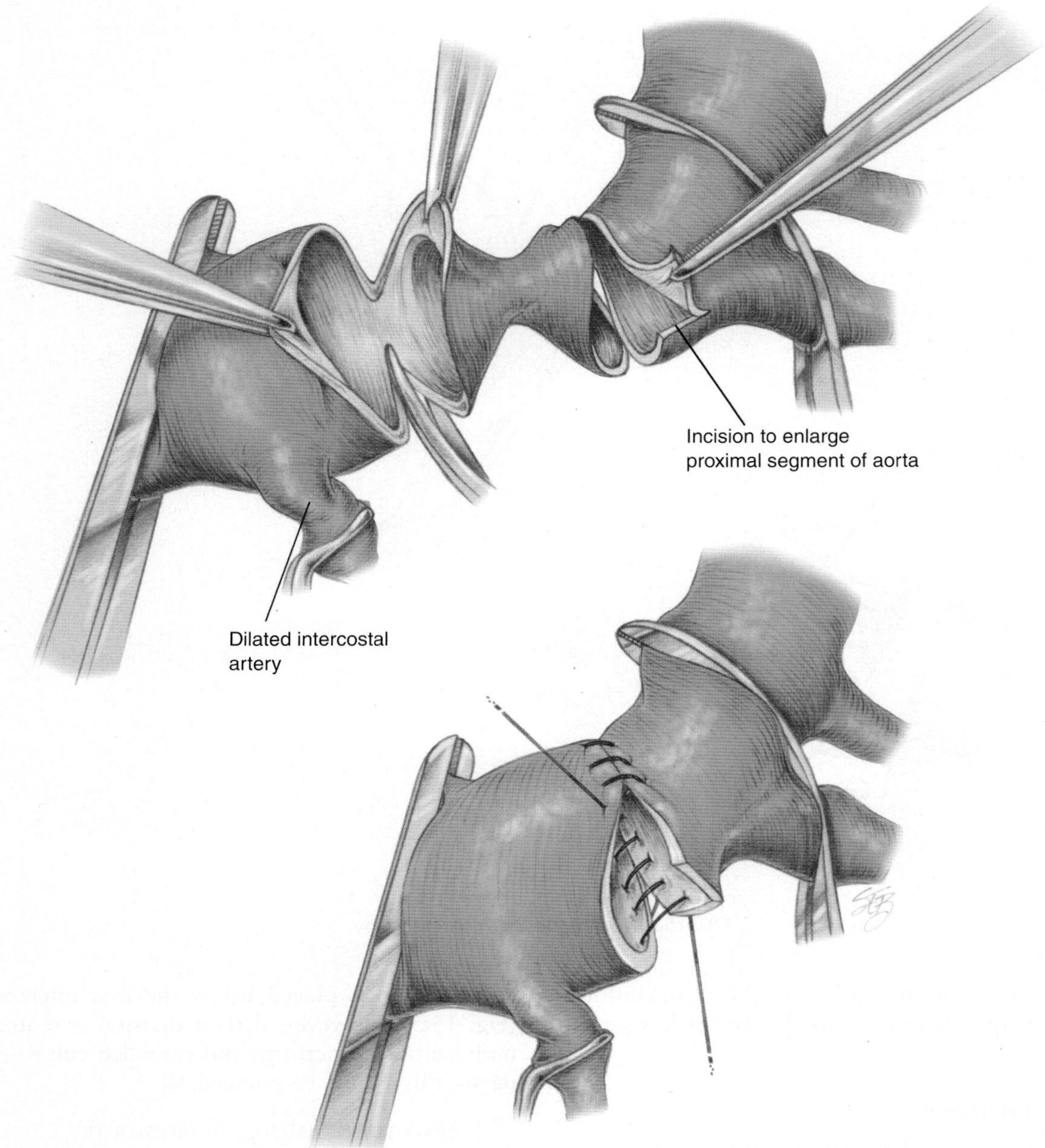

FIG. 15.5 Enlarging the proximal aortic segment to ensure the maximal lumen diameter.

⊘ Spinal Cord Ischemia

Paraplegia is a devastating complication of surgical repair of coarctation of the aorta. Factors associated with spinal cord injury are longer cross-clamp time, higher body temperature, and lower distal aortic pressure during the procedure. ⊘

NB Intraoperative Mild Hypothermia

The core body temperature should be maintained at or below 35°C by keeping the room cold, using a cooling blanket, and/or chest irrigation with cold saline solution to minimize the risk of spinal cord ischemia during the cross-clamp period. NB

NB No or Small Collaterals

Patients with underdeveloped collaterals tend to have low distal perfusion pressures with aortic clamping. This is also seen in patients with aberrant origin of the right subclavian artery from the descending aorta. NB

NB Distal Circulatory Support

To avoid spinal cord injury, distal circulatory support should be used if a cross-clamp time over 30 minutes is anticipated, or if test clamping of the aorta results in a distal pressure of less than 50 mm Hg. Partial cardiopulmonary bypass is the preferred technique.

Technique with Partial Bypass

These patients should be monitored with right radial and femoral arterial lines. After full heparinization, the descending aorta below the anticipated clamp site is cannulated with an aortic cannula through a purse-string suture. The lung is retracted posteriorly and a longitudinal incision is made on the pericardium anterior to the phrenic nerve. A purse-string suture is placed on the left atrial appendage and a venous cannula is introduced into the left atrium during a Valsalva maneuver. Ventilation is continued and the venous flow is controlled by the perfusionist to maintain a normal pressure in the right radial artery and to keep the femoral pressure above 45 mm Hg. Following repair of the coarctation, the patient is weaned from bypass and the venous cannula is removed from the left atrium during a Valsalva maneuver. The heparin is reversed with protamine and the descending aortic cannula is removed.

⊘ Air Embolism

To prevent entry of air into the left atrium during placement and removal of the venous cannula, the anesthesiologist must perform a sustained inflation of the lungs until the purse-string suture is secured. ⊘

SUBCLAVIAN FLAP ANGIOPLASTY

This procedure may be useful in a neonate with a long-segment coarctaion. The left subclavian artery is well mobilized up to the origin of its branches in the root of the neck; all the branches are ligated (Fig. 15.6). The proximal clamp is placed across the aortic arch just distal to the left carotid artery, and the descending aorta is clamped with a straight clamp (Fig. 15.7A). Alternatively, a single curved clamp can be used (Fig. 15.7C). The left subclavian artery is

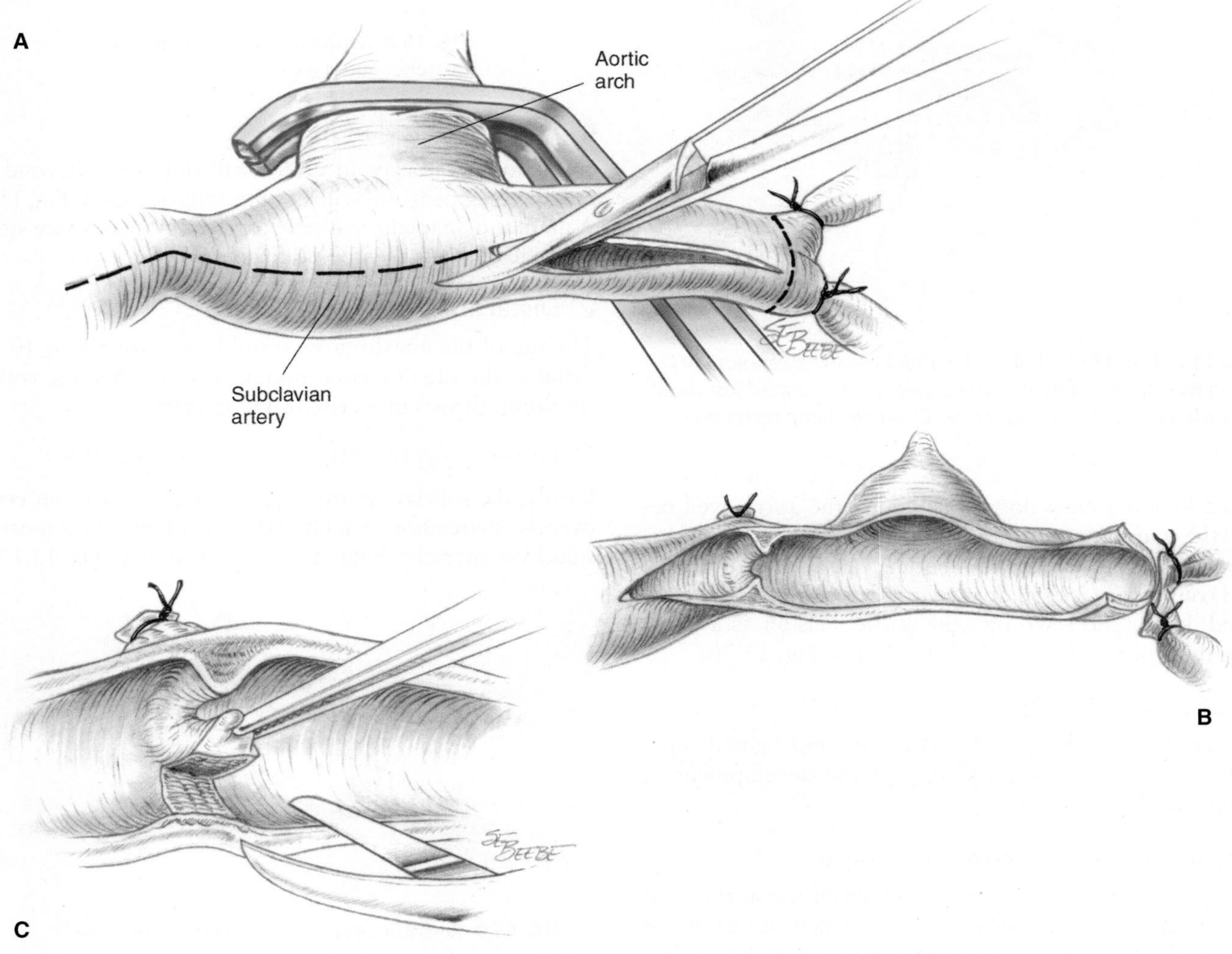

FIG. 15.6 A–C: Technique for a subclavian flap angioplasty: Preparing the subclavian flap.

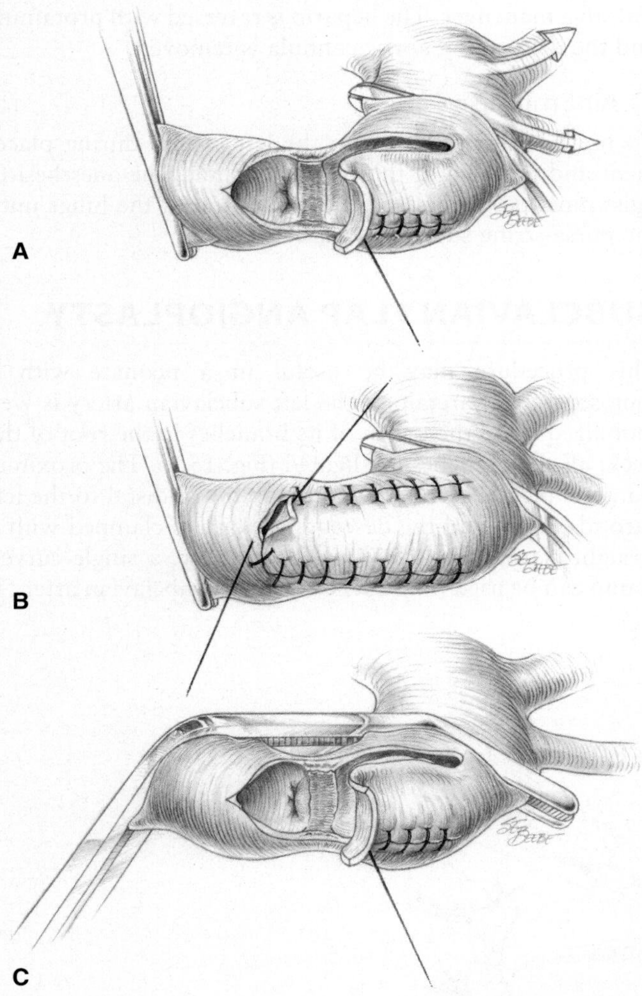

FIG. 15.7 **A and B:** Technique for a subclavian flap angioplasty using two clamps. Note that the upper clamp is placed just distal to the left common carotid artery. **C:** Single-clamp technique.

incised longitudinally downward along the aorta, well beyond the coarctation segment. Whenever a prominent coarctation ridge is present, it should be excised (Fig. 15.6C). The subclavian artery is then divided at the level of its branches, folded down, and sewn into the aortic incision as a patch using two continuous 7-0 Prolene sutures (Fig. 15.7B).

⊘ Subclavian Steal Syndrome

The vertebral artery must be identified and ligated separately to eliminate the possibility of the development of subclavian steal syndrome. ⊘

⊘ Resection of the Coarctation Ridge

The coarctation ridge within the lumen of the aorta must be excised, but not so deeply as to weaken the posterior aortic wall. Any perforation must be sutured with fine Prolene and tied on the outside (Fig. 15.8). ⊘

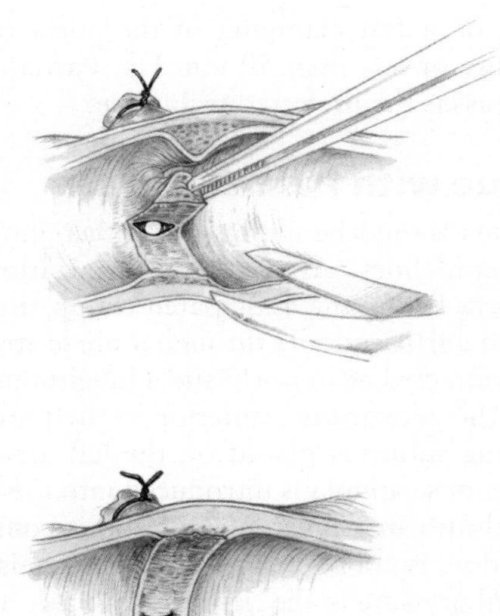

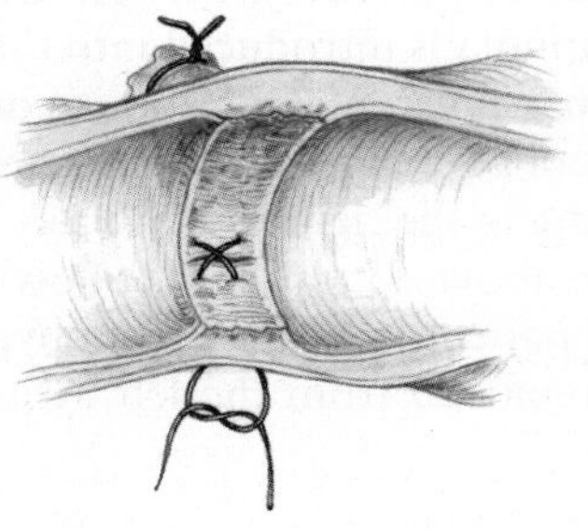

FIG. 15.8 Repairing a perforation in the posterior aortic wall.

⊘ Short Subclavian Artery

Too short a subclavian artery will not reach beyond the coarcted segment and will leave residual stenosis (Fig. 15.9). A diamond-shaped prosthetic patch angioplasty (see subsequent text) must then be performed. ⊘

⊘ Distal Stenosis

The toe of the anastomosis should be at least 8 to 10 mm distal to the site of coarctation. Otherwise, healing with its resulting fibrosis gives rise to recoarctation. ⊘

⊘ Positioning the Subclavian Artery Patch

Ideally, the subclavian artery patch must balloon out evenly over the coarctation. A kink at the heel of the anastomosis results from overstretching of the subclavian flap (Fig. 15.10). ⊘

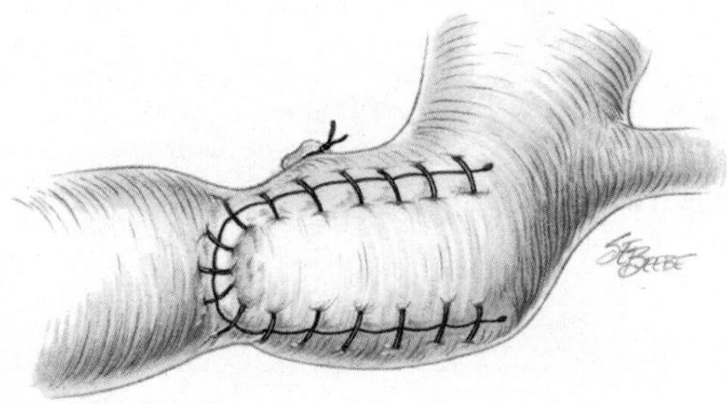

⊘ **FIG. 15.9** Persistence of residual stenosis when the subclavian artery is too short to reach beyond the coarcted segment.

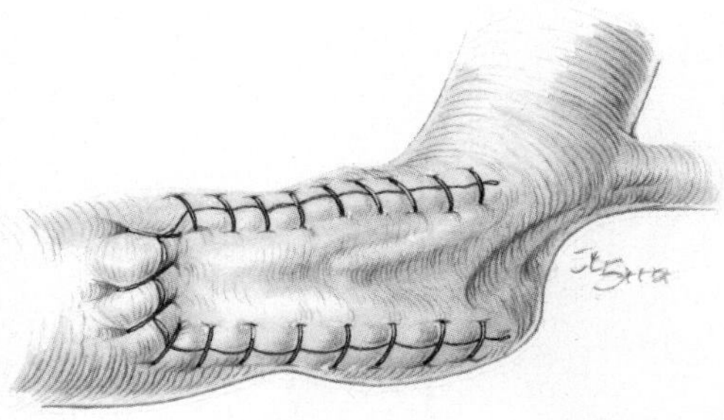

⊘ FIG. 15.10 A kink at the heel of the anastomosis resulting from overstretching of the subclavian flap.

⊘ Incision on the Subclavian Artery and the Aorta

The line of incision on the subclavian artery and the aorta should be straight along the lateral aspect of the both vessels. Any deviation interferes with a satisfactory anastomosis. ⊘

LONG-SEGMENT COARCTATION

If the coarctation segment is too long, a coarctectomy with an end-to-end anastomosis or subclavian flap angioplasty may not be feasible. One option in older children and adults is to resect the coarctation segment and replace this portion of the aorta with an adult-sized tube graft (Fig. 15.11, see Chapter 8).

An alternative to graft interposition is to roof the defect with a patch. This procedure is equally useful in cases of recoarctation of the aorta. The aorta is clamped above and below the coarctation segment as described previously. The aorta is then incised longitudinally across the lesion. The prominent coarctation ridge is excised, taking the usual precautions. A wide, diamond-shaped Gore-Tex, Hemashield, or pulmonary homograft patch is sewn to the aortic edges with a running 4-0 or 5-0 Prolene suture (Fig. 15.12).

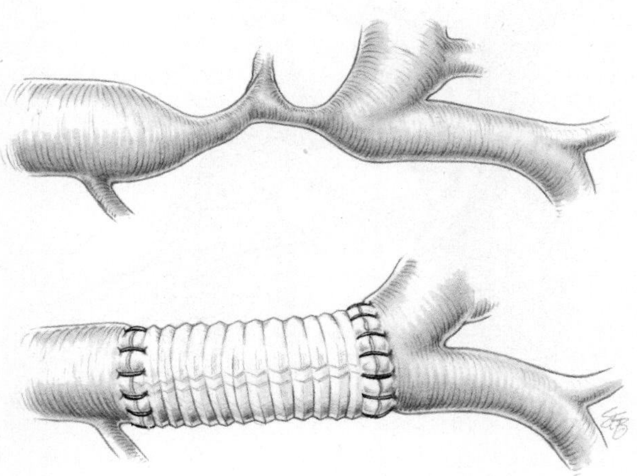

FIG. 15.11 Tube graft replacement for a long coarctation segment.

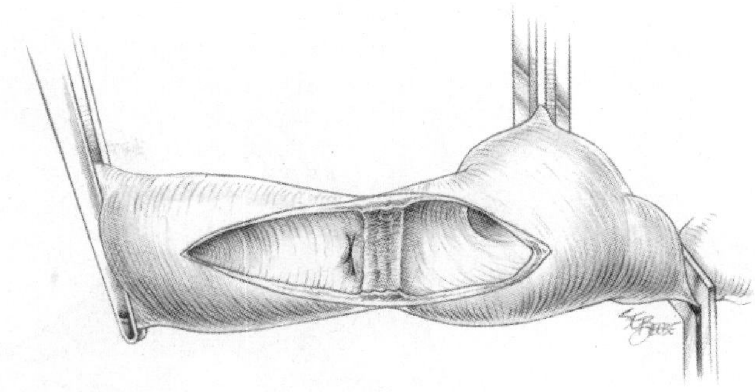

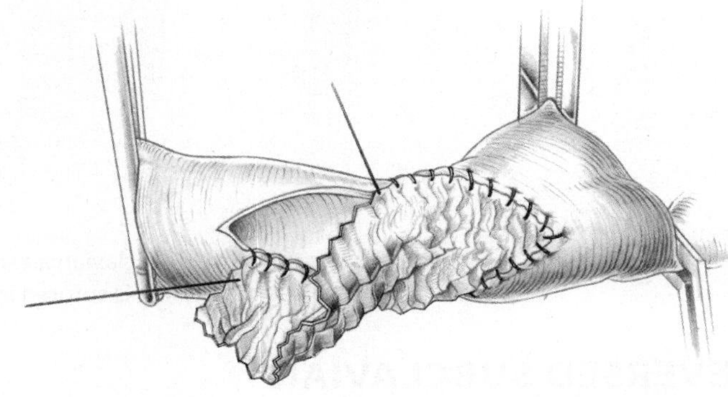

FIG. 15.12 Technique for a diamond-shaped patch angioplasty.

⊘ Recoarctation

Recoarctation can occur as the aorta grows. For this reason, the diamond-shaped patch must be very wide, resulting in a redundant, patulous bulge over the coarctation (Fig. 15.13). An aesthetically satisfactory patch often results in recoarctation. ⊘

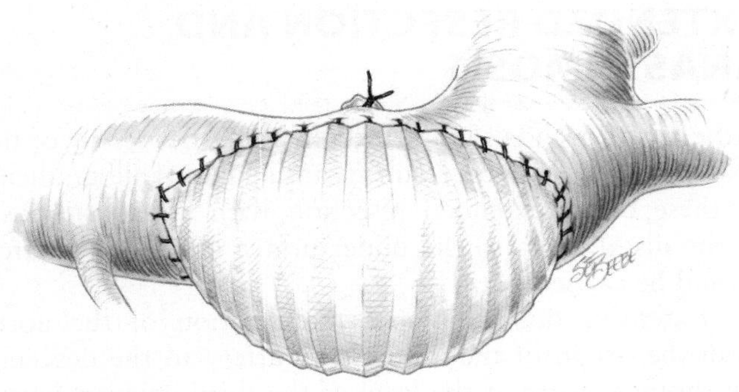

FIG. 15.13 Using an especially wide patch prevents recoarctation as the aorta grows.

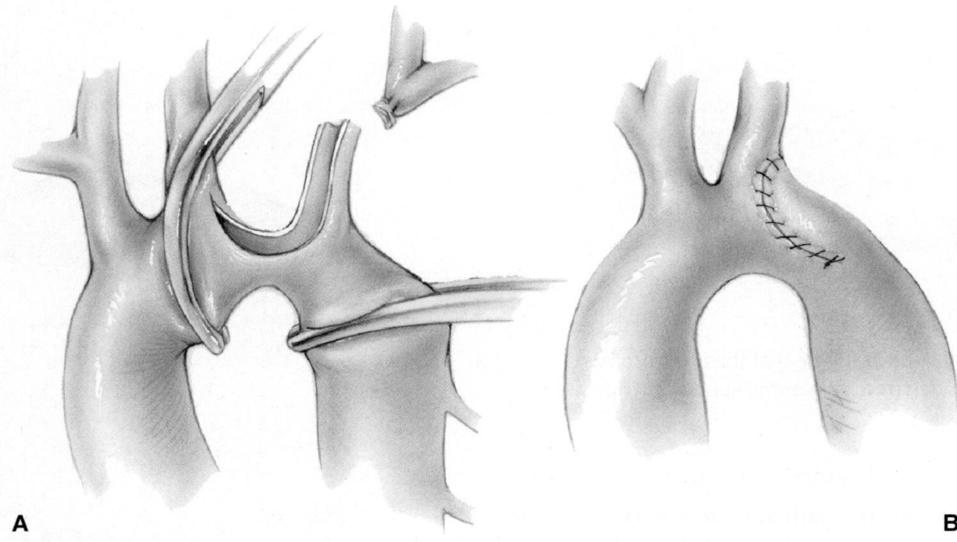

FIG. 15.14 A: The transected subclavian artery is opened medially across the roof of the aortic arch. **B:** The subclavian flap is sutured in place, augmenting the hypoplastic segment.

REVERSED SUBCLAVIAN ANGIOPLASTY

Hypoplasia of the aortic arch between the left carotid and left subclavian arteries can be treated by a reversed subclavian flap angioplasty. In patients with combined discrete coarctation and significant hypoplasia of the distal arch, this technique can be combined with a standard coarctectomy. The distal arch must be mobilized, as well as the origin of the left carotid artery and the portion of the arch just proximal to it. The left subclavian artery is ligated as in the standard subclavian flap angioplasty. One vascular clamp is placed across the left carotid artery and the aortic arch. The other clamp is placed on the descending aorta. The transected subclavian artery is opened medially onto the aortic arch, across the roof of the distal arch, and onto the base of the left carotid artery (Fig. 15.14A). The flap is then sutured in place with 6-0 or 7-0 Prolene sutures (Fig. 15.14B).

EXTENDED RESECTION AND ANASTOMOSIS

If the aortic arch is significantly hypoplastic, repair of the coarctation alone may result in an unacceptable gradient. In these cases, extended resection with an anastomosis of the distal aorta to the undersurface of the aortic arch should be carried out.

Extensive dissection and mobilization of the aorta from the origin of the innominate artery to the descending thoracic aorta at the level of the third or even fourth intercostal artery are carried out. Ligation and division of the ductus or ligamentum arteriosum facilitate the dissection. A curved vascular clamp is placed across the origin of the left subclavian and left carotid arteries as well as the proximal aortic arch just beyond the innominate artery. A straight clamp is placed across the descending aorta. The coarcted segment and ductal tissue are resected. An incision is now made inferiorly on the aortic arch while a second matching incision is made on the lateral aspect of the distal aorta (Fig. 15.15). The descending aorta is then anastomosed to the opening in the aortic arch with a running suture Prolene. Some centers advocate for the use of continuous near-infrared spectrometry (NIRS) cerebral monitoring throughout the case to confirm adequate cerebral bloodflow during the period of cross-clamping.

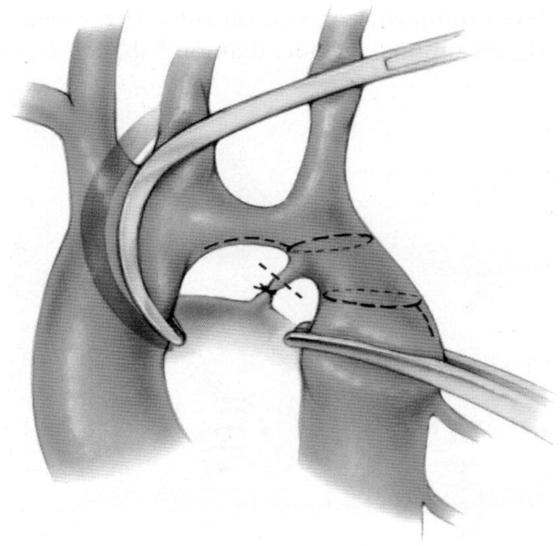

FIG. 15.15 Extended resection and anastomosis of the coarctation and hypoplastic arch. Note the improper placement of the clamp (shaded) (*shaded*) the innominate artery.

⊘ Occluding Innominate Artery

The arch clamp must not occlude or compromise flow to the innominate artery (Fig. 15.15). Monitoring the pressure in a right radial arterial line will allow this problem to be detected and quickly rectified. ⊘

⊘ Tension at the Anastomosis

Aggressive proximal and distal mobilization will avoid tension on the anastomosis; this will minimize the risk of suture line bleeding and the subsequent development of stenosis. ⊘

NB Division of Intercostal Vessels

It may be necessary to ligate and divide one set of intercostal arteries in order to adequately mobilize the descending aorta for a tension-free anastomosis. Sacrificing more intercostal vessels may increase the risk of spinal cord injury. NB

ALTERNATE TECHNIQUES

Most patients with recoarctation can be successfully treated with balloon angioplasty with or without stent placement. Balloon angioplasty is also an alternative to surgery for native coarctations in patients older than 3 months of age who have a discrete aortic narrowing.

Extraanatomic bypass grafts, such as those between the left subclavian and descending aorta or from the ascending to the descending aorta, are rarely used now. Even the most complex recoarctations can be dealt with directly using excision and an interposition graft or patching of the narrowed segment. If a left thoracotomy approach is deemed to be inadvisable, a median sternotomy with the use of cardiopulmonary bypass and deep hypothermia allows good exposure of the distal arch and proximal descending aorta (see Chapter 8).

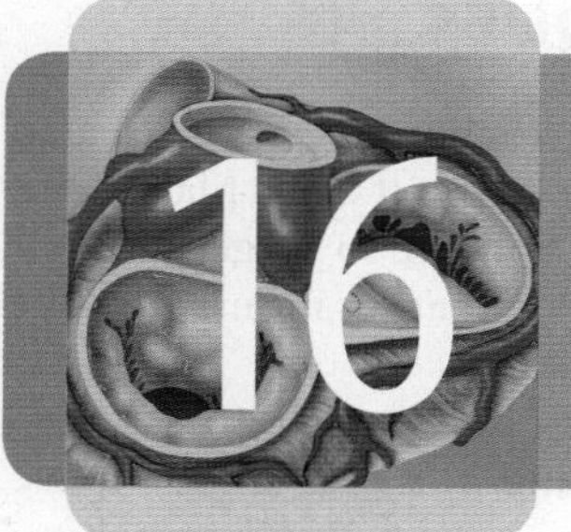

16 Pulmonary Artery Banding

Because most neonates undergo total correction for congenital heart defects, banding of the pulmonary artery is only indicated for specific subgroups of patients. These include patients with multiple muscular ventriculoseptal defects or ventriculoseptal defects complicated by other noncardiac congenital anomalies. Patients who present after 4 to 6 weeks of age with simple transposition of the great arteries may require preliminary pulmonary artery banding to prepare the left ventricle for an arterial switch procedure (see Chapter 25). Banding of the pulmonary artery is also performed in some patients with univentricular hearts and pulmonary overcirculation (see Chapter 30).

INCISION

Most surgeons use a median sternotomy because it allows the anatomy to be evaluated more accurately. A left thoracotomy incision is used in some patients, especially if the banding is performed in conjunction with the repair of a coarctation.

TECHNIQUE

Through a median sternotomy, the pericardium is opened longitudinally after resecting the thymus. (Removing the entire thymus in this surgery makes dissection at reoperation easier.) A patent ductus arteriosus, if present, is first ligated (see Chapter 14). The main pulmonary artery is dissected free from the aorta and the origin of the right pulmonary artery is identified. A band of Silastic 3- to 4-mm wide is placed around the proximal pulmonary artery and tightened until the pressure distal to the band is approximately one-third systemic with an arterial oxygen saturation no less than 75% on 50% inspired oxygen (Fig. 16.1). The constriction site on the band is made permanent with stainless steel clips or interrupted sutures. The band is then secured to the adventitia of the pulmonary artery at various intervals with interrupted 6-0 or 5-0 Prolene sutures (Fig. 16.1, inset).

Through a left thoracotomy, the pericardium is incised anterior and parallel to the phrenic nerve. The main pulmonary artery is isolated, and the Silastic band is passed around it and narrowed as described previously.

⊘ Damage from the Band

The pulmonary artery may be tense and its wall thin and friable. Regular suture material or a narrow band may cut through and produce hemorrhage that is difficult to control. ⊘

⊘ Difficulty Passing the Band around the Pulmonary Artery

It may be easier and safer to initially pass the tape around both the aorta and pulmonary artery through the transverse sinus and then between the aorta and pulmonary artery. ⊘

⊘ Troublesome Bleeding

Small adventitial vessels on the aorta and pulmonary artery may give rise to troublesome bleeding; they must be identified and cauterized. ⊘

⊘ Excessive Banding

The degree of banding must not be too constrictive because this will result in unacceptable cyanosis and possible hemodynamic collapse. ⊘

⊘ Inadequate Banding

Many times, the tightness of the band is limited by the hemodynamic response of the patient. Patients with subaortic narrowing may not tolerate adequate constriction of the band. To limit the pulmonary blood flow in these patients, ligation of the pulmonary artery or a Damus–Kaye–Stansel anastomosis and shunt procedure may be required (see Chapter 30). ⊘

NB Early Reoperation to Adjust Band

It is not uncommon to leave the operating room with a suitable band, only to have the patient develop signs that the band is too tight or too loose in the early postoperative period. In this case, reoperation may be required. If the band is too loose, the patient may grow into it. The surgeon must weigh the risk of reoperation with that

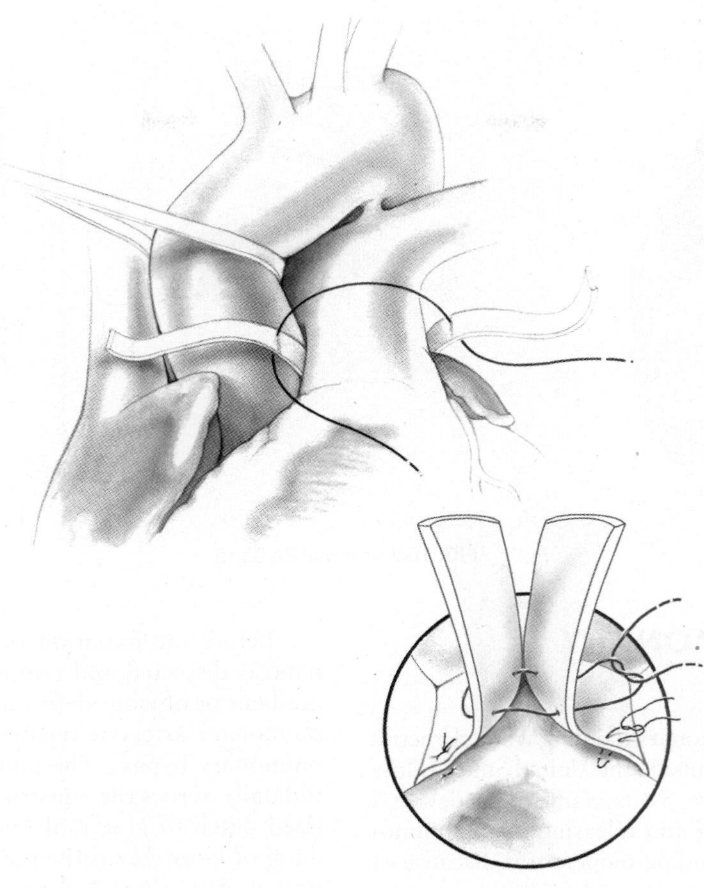

FIG. 16.1 Technique for placement of a pulmonary artery band. The band is tightened with interrupted sutures. Securing the band to the adventitia of the pulmonary artery **(Inset)**.

of continued pulmonary overcirculation, possible pulmonary vascular disease, and failure to thrive. NB

⊘ Placing the Band Too Proximally

If the band is placed too proximally, the sinotubular ridge of the pulmonic valve will be distorted. To adequately relieve the gradient during the debanding procedure, the sinus portion(s) of the pulmonary root often needs to be patched. This may result in an incompetent pulmonic valve. This is especially problematic when an arterial switch or Damus–Kaye–Stansel procedure is planned at the second stage. ⊘

⊘ Band Migration

The band should be sewn to the adventitia of the proximal aspect of the main pulmonary artery (Fig. 16.1, inset). This precaution prevents the band from migrating distally, narrowing the pulmonary artery at its bifurcation and obstructing the right, left, or both branches. ⊘

After the optimal band constriction has been achieved, it is secured and the pericardium is approximated with multiple interrupted sutures. The median sternotomy or thoracotomy is then closed in the usual manner.

If the procedure requires the use of concomitant cardiopulmonary bypass to repair other lesions (e.g., arch reconstruction), the use of an internal pulmonary artery band is recommended, owing to the difficulty of properly adjusting the band during the initial period immediately off bypass. In this procedure (Fig. 16.2), a small disc of thin-walled Gore-Tex is used, whose diameter is that of the main pulmonary artery. A punch is taken from the center of this disc, whose diameter is roughly the size of a shunt appropriate for the baby by weight. A transverse, partial pulmonary arteriotomy is made halfway between the pulmonary root and the bifurcation, and through this partial incision, the backwall of the Gore-Tex "washer" is sewn using a running Prolene. As this is continued anteriorly, the Gore-Tex is included in between the two edges of the cut pulmonary artery. This technique has the advantage of (1) a controlled source of pulmonary blood flow and (2) eliminating the possibility of either band migration or pulmonary valve damage.

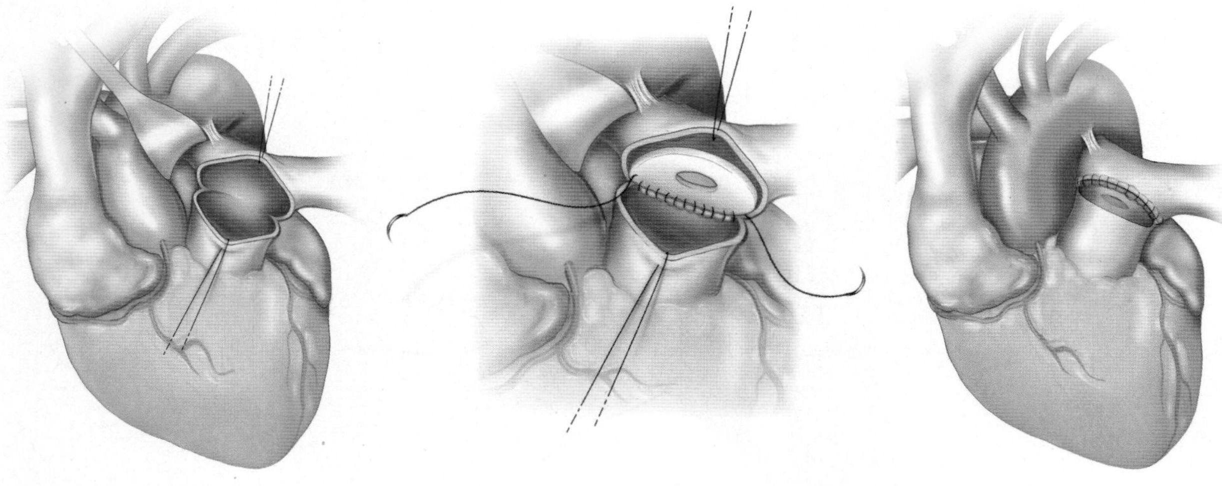

FIG. 16.2 Internal PA Band

ADJUSTABLE PULMONARY BAND DEVICE

An implantable device for pulmonary banding with telemetric control is currently available outside the United States (Flow Watch, EndoArt S.A., Lausanne, Switzerland). This device is capable of repeated narrowing and releasing of the pulmonary artery at the bedside, avoiding reoperation. Because of its elliptic shape, there usually is no need for reconstruction of the pulmonary artery when the device is removed.

PULMONARY ARTERY DEBANDING

When total correction of the cardiac anomaly is undertaken, the pulmonary artery band must be removed. It may be necessary to reconstruct the pulmonary artery to eliminate any gradient across the band site. When a Silastic band has been in place for a short time, simple removal of the band often results in no gradient.

Before the initiation of cardiopulmonary bypass, the band is dissected and removed (Fig. 16.3A). If a pressure gradient or obvious deformity is noted at the band site, the pulmonary artery is repaired with the patient on cardiopulmonary bypass. The pulmonary artery is incised longitudinally across the constricted segment. An appropriately sized patch of glutaraldehyde-treated autologous pericardium or Gore-Tex is then sewn onto the defect with a continuous 5-0 or 6-0 Prolene suture (Fig. 16.3B).

⊘ Persistence of the Gradient

Inadequate enlargement of the main pulmonary artery may be responsible for persistence of the gradient across the site of the band. ⊘

Alternatively, the portion of the main pulmonary artery involved in the banding can be resected and an end-to-end anastomosis performed between the proximal main pulmonary artery and the confluence of the right and left pulmonary arteries (Fig. 16.3C).

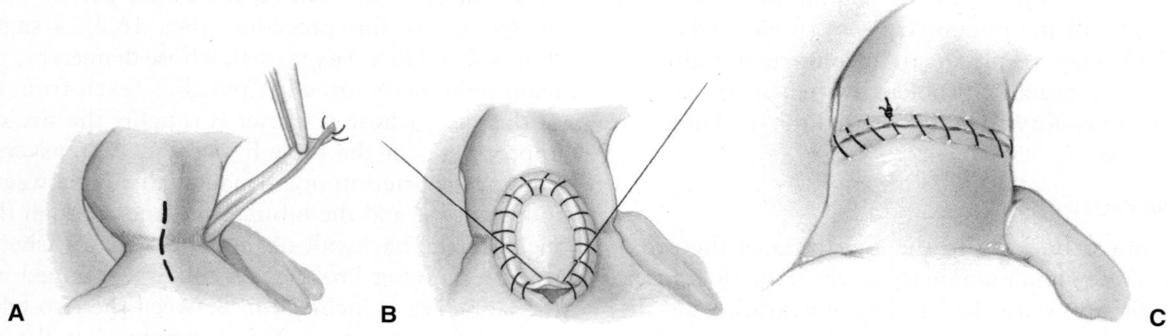

FIG. 16.3 Technique for pulmonary artery debanding. **A:** Removal of the band. **B:** Incision and patch enlargement of the pulmonary artery. **C:** Resection of the constricted segment and an end-to-end anastomosis of the pulmonary artery.

⊘ Constriction of Anastomosis

All fibrotic tissue must be excised to prevent stenosis at the anastomotic site. ⊘

⊘ Pulmonary Valve Insufficiency

When the band has caused distortion of the sinotubular ridge, patching anteriorly into one sinus only often causes valvular insufficiency. If the patient will not tolerate pulmonary valve incompetence, the pulmonary artery can be transected and all three sinuses patched as described for supravalvular aortic stenosis (see Chapter 24). ⊘

NB Incorporation of the Band into the Pulmonary Artery

With the passage of time, the band may burrow through the wall of the pulmonary artery to become subendothelial. The band can be divided anteriorly but left *in situ* and the pulmonary artery enlarged with a patch angioplasty. Resection with an end-to-end anastomosis may also be used when this situation is encountered. NB

Occasionally, the band may migrate distally to the pulmonary artery bifurcation and cause distortion of its branches. The incision on the pulmonary artery is then extended distally onto the left or both the left and right pulmonary artery branches as needed. The defect is closed with a pericardial patch (Fig. 16.4).

NB Sizing the Patch

The pericardial patch should be wide enough, particularly at its distal end, to prevent a residual gradient. NB

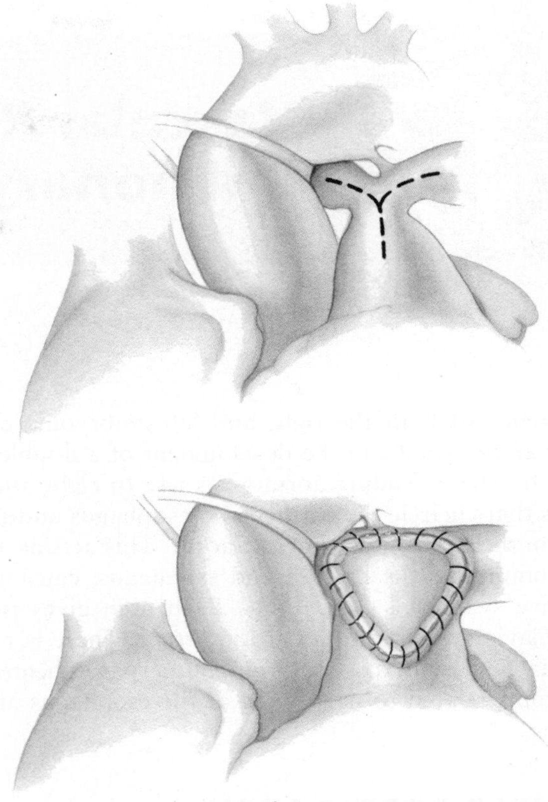

FIG. 16.4 Technique for patching pulmonary artery constriction at the bifurcation.

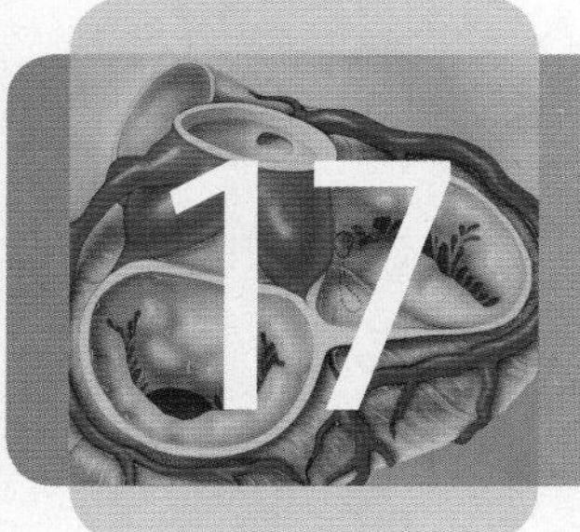

17 Vascular Ring and Pulmonary Artery Sling

Persistence of both the right and left embryonic dorsal aortic arches results in the development of a double aortic arch. The ascending aorta gives rise to right and left arches that encircle the trachea and esophagus and rejoin to form the descending thoracic aorta. This acts as a ring and compresses the trachea and esophagus, causing obstructive symptoms (Fig. 17.1). Each arch gives rise to a subclavian artery and a carotid artery. There is no innominate artery in this condition. Surgery is indicated for symptoms related to narrowing of the esophagus and/or trachea.

DOUBLE AORTIC ARCH

Incision

A left posterolateral thoracotomy in the fourth intercostal space is the approach most commonly preferred. A right thoracotomy can be used if the left aortic arch is dominant, which occurs rarely.

Technique

The left lung is retracted anteriorly and inferiorly toward the diaphragm to bring into view the area of the aortic arch and ductus arteriosus or ligamentum. The parietal pleura is incised longitudinally on the anterior surface of the descending aorta and left subclavian artery. The pleural flap containing the vagus nerve and its branches is retracted anteriorly; meticulous dissection is carried out to identify the local anatomy precisely. The surgeon should be aware that pulling the nerve toward the pulmonary artery causes the recurrent nerve to lie along a diagonal course behind the ductus or ligamentum, thereby increasing the risk of injury to the nerve.

The aorta and ductus or ligamentum are then mobilized by sharp dissection. The ductus or ligamentum is divided after ligating both ends.

The smaller (usually left anterior) aortic arch is dissected free and divided between clamps. The ends are then oversewn with 5-0 or 6-0 Prolene suture in two layers (Figs. 17.2 and 17.3).

NB Adhesions of the Esophagus and Trachea

Both the trachea and the esophagus must be dissected free of any adhesions and fibrous bands to ensure that narrowing of these structures is relieved. This entails freeing up the divided ends of the arch from the surrounding tissues. NB

⊘ Division of Ductus or Ligamentum

The ductus arteriosus or ligamentum must always be doubly ligated and divided. Otherwise, compression of the trachea and esophagus will persist because of the aortic arch

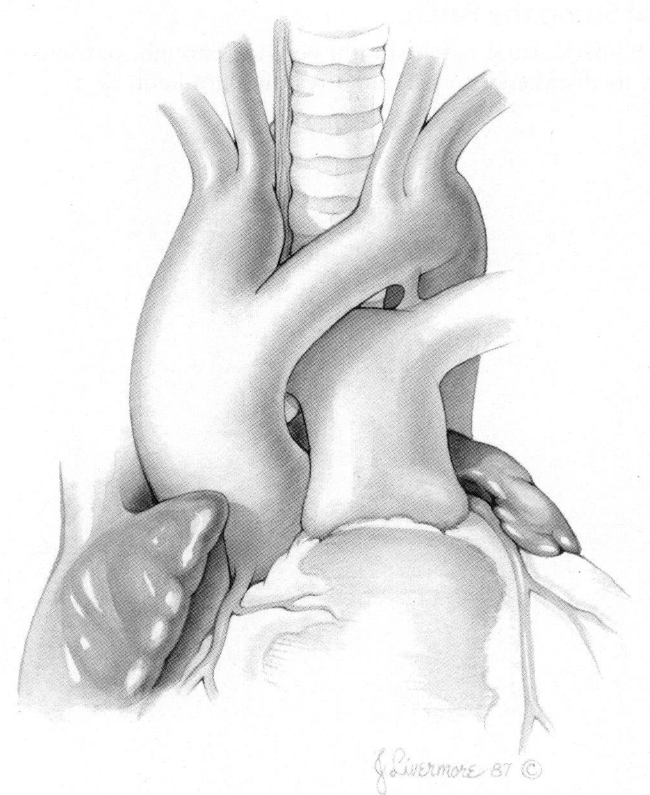

FIG. 17.1 Double aortic arch.

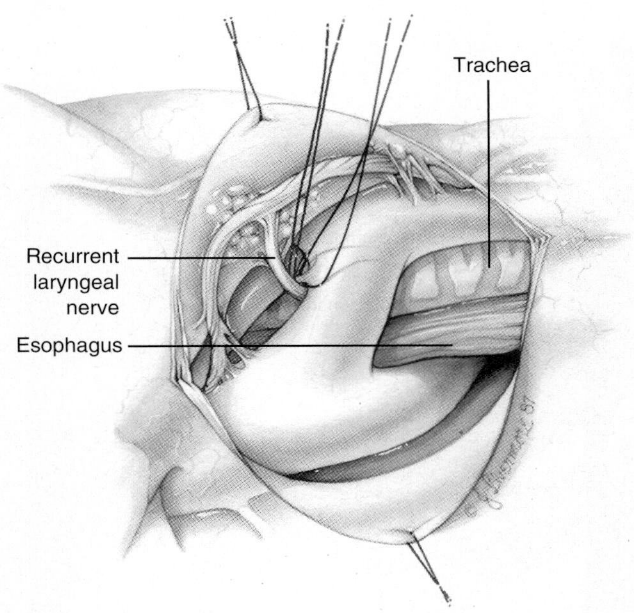

FIG. 17.2 Exposure of the left anterior arch. Note ties around ligamentum arteriosum.

being pulled downward toward the pulmonary artery. It is also important to resect any adjacent scar tissue that could contribute to postoperative tethering or scar. ⊘

⊘ Injury to the Recurrent Laryngeal Nerve

The vagus and recurrent laryngeal nerves are identified so that they are not inadvertently divided or traumatized. ⊘

⊘ Division of the Smaller Arch

The smaller of the two arches should be divided, otherwise a pseudocoarctation may develop. Therefore, both arches are dissected and the smaller one is identified. As a precaution, blood pressure cuffs should be placed on one leg and both arms and a trial occlusion of the smaller arch should be carried out to confirm the absence of a pressure gradient before dividing it. ⊘

⊘ Aortopexy

Some advocate tacking the suture line of the descending aorta toward the lateral chest wall fascia so as to open up the area of the ring "like a book" and thereby prevent postoperative impingement or scar. ⊘

PULMONARY ARTERY SLING

A pulmonary artery sling results when the left pulmonary artery arises from the right pulmonary artery and passes leftward between the trachea and esophagus to reach the hilum of the left lung. The ligamentum arteriosum extends from the superior aspect of the main pulmonary artery to the undersurface of the aortic arch. This creates a vascular ring that constricts the trachea but not the esophagus (Fig. 17.4). Hypoplasia of the distal trachea, with or without complete cartilaginous rings, is present in approximately 50% of these patients.

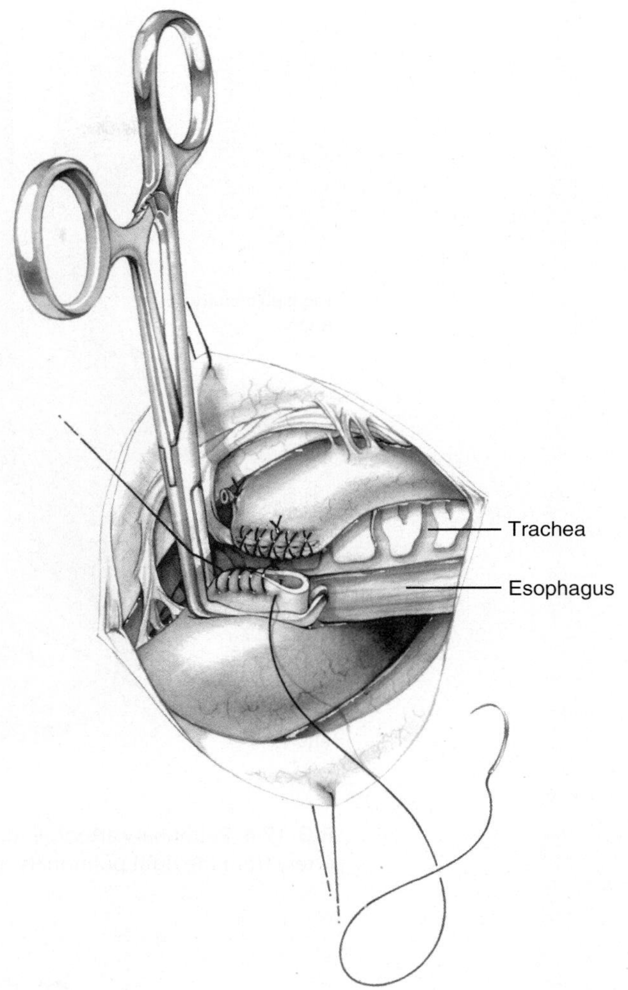

FIG. 17.3 Stepwise technique for division and oversewing ends of the left anterior arch.

Incision

Although this lesion can theoretically be approached through a left thoracotomy and repaired without the use of cardiopulmonary bypass, stenosis and occlusion of the left pulmonary artery have been seen with this technique. Most surgeons prefer a median sternotomy with cardiopulmonary bypass, especially if tracheal reconstruction is anticipated.

Median Sternotomy Technique

A standard median sternotomy incision is performed, and cardiopulmonary bypass is instituted with an ascending aortic cannula and single straight venous cannula in the

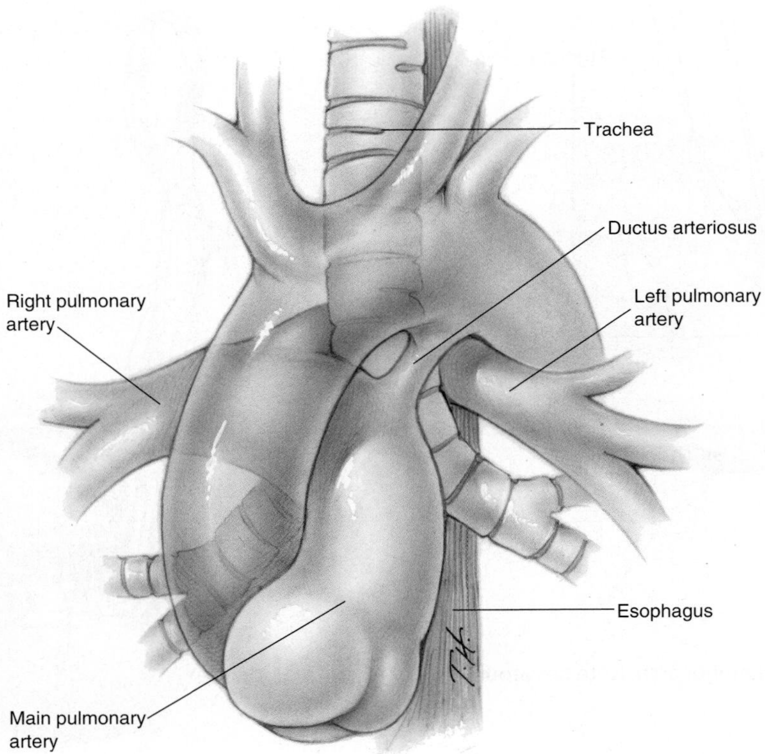

FIG. 17.4 Pulmonary artery sling. Note the origin of the left pulmonary artery from the right pulmonary artery and its course behind the trachea.

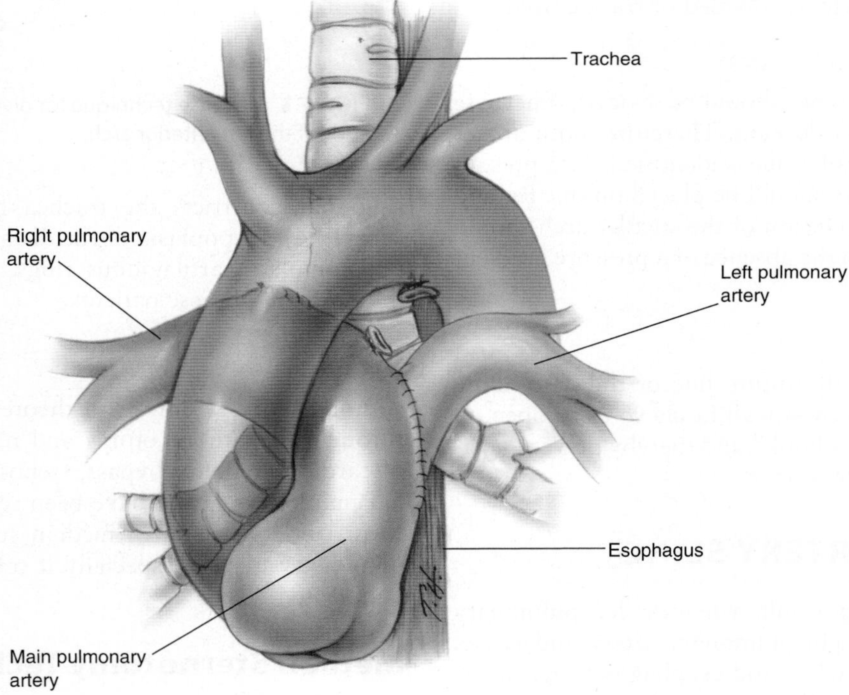

FIG. 17.5 Correction of a pulmonary artery sling. Note the division and reimplantation of the left pulmonary artery onto the main pulmonary artery in front of the trachea.

right atrium. The procedure is carried out with the heart beating.

The ductus or ligamentum arteriosum is doubly ligated and divided. The main, right, and left pulmonary arteries are extensively mobilized. With the aorta retracted leftward, the origin of the left pulmonary artery is identified and dissected free of the back of the trachea. The left pulmonary artery can now be detached from the main pulmonary artery and brought anterior to the trachea. The resultant opening in the distal main pulmonary artery is oversewn with a 6-0 Prolene running suture. The left pulmonary artery is reimplanted more proximally on the main pulmonary artery, using care to not twist or kink the left pulmonary artery. A generous arteriotomy is made at the appropriate site on the distal main pulmonary artery and the left pulmonary artery is trimmed obliquely to match this opening. The anastomosis is completed with a running 6-0 Prolene suture (Fig. 17.5). In certain circumstances, this may require an additional left pulmonary arterioplasty if the left pulmonary artery is hypoplastic.

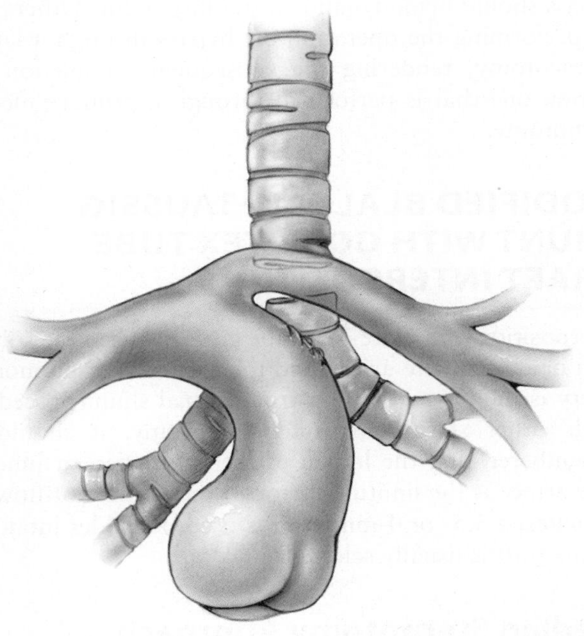

FIG. 17.6 Pulmonary artery sling with a stenotic distal trachea. The left pulmonary artery can be brought anteriorly between the divided ends of the trachea.

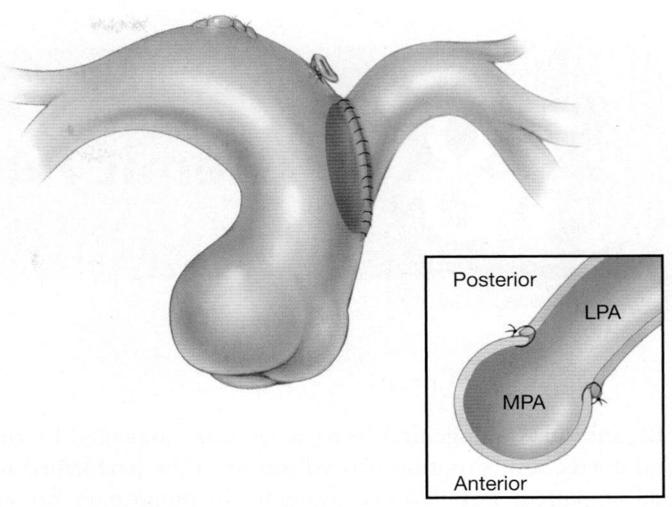

FIG. 17.7 Low/posterior insertion of the LPA.

NB If a stenotic segment of the trachea is present, the trachea may be transected, allowing the left pulmonary artery to be brought anterior to the trachea through the space between the two divided ends of the trachea (Fig. 17.6). Subsequently, the stenotic portion of the trachea is resected and the two ends are reanastomosed; occasionally, a full "slide" tracheoplasty is required for long-segment tracheal stenosis. The lie of the left pulmonary artery must be assessed, and if kinking or stretching is noted, the left pulmonary artery should be detached and reanastomosed more proximally on the main pulmonary artery. NB

NB When implanting the left pulmonary artery, it is important to place the anastomosis somewhat posteriorly and inferiorly along the main pulmonary artery; this reduces the chance of stenosis or issues of angulation at the anastomosis (Fig. 17.7). NB

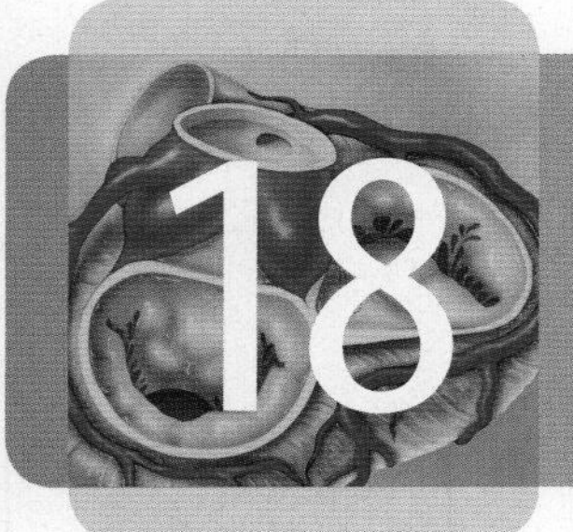

18 Systemic Pulmonary Shunting

Because most congenital heart defects are managed by total correction, shunting procedures are now performed in select patient populations. Systemic to pulmonary artery shunts offer excellent palliation in patients with anatomically complex cardiac anomalies, in whom definitive repair is best delayed. They are also indicated as a source of controlled pulmonary blood flow in the initial management of neonates with single-ventricle anatomy.

A common application of the systemic to pulmonary artery shunt is in the neonate with a ductal-dependent pulmonary circulation. The ability to keep the ductus arteriosus patent with an infusion of prostaglandin E_1 allows these patients to be stabilized and undergo surgery on a semiurgent basis in an unhurried manner.

TYPES OF SHUNTS

The Blalock–Taussig shunt was introduced in 1945. Classically, it consists of anastomosing the subclavian artery to the pulmonary artery on the side opposite the aortic arch. However, with some technical modifications, the subclavian artery can be anastomosed to the pulmonary artery on the same side as the aortic arch.

Other shunting procedures were subsequently introduced. They include the Potts shunt (descending aorta to the left pulmonary artery), Waterston shunt (ascending aorta to the right pulmonary artery), central shunt (interposing a graft between the ascending aorta and the main pulmonary artery), and the modified Blalock–Taussig shunt (interposing a Gore-Tex tube graft between the subclavian or innominate artery and the right or left pulmonary artery).

The Potts shunt was abandoned because it was cumbersome to perform, difficult to close, and could cause high flow and the early development of pulmonary vascular disease. The Waterston shunt lost favor because of the high incidence of injury to the pulmonary artery and the difficulty in controlling the amount of flow through the shunt. The classical Blalock–Taussig shunt is rarely used. Currently, some surgeons perform a central shunt or modified Blalock–Taussig shunt through a median sternotomy with the belief that the relative disadvantage of this approach requiring a redo sternotomy and dissection of adhesions for the next procedure is outweighed by the superior exposure and ability to place the patient on cardiopulmonary bypass should hemodynamic instability occur. Others prefer performing the operation off bypass through a lateral thoracotomy, rendering the subsequent completion operation one that is performed through a primary median sternotomy.

MODIFIED BLALOCK–TAUSSIG SHUNT WITH GORE-TEX TUBE GRAFT INTERPOSITION

Interposition of a Gore-Tex tube graft between the subclavian or innominate artery and the right or left pulmonary artery is the most commonly performed shunt procedure. With either sternotomy or thoracotomy, it should be remembered that the lumen of the subclavian or innominate artery is the limiting factor to the volume of flow. In neonates, a 3.5- or 4-mm graft is used; for older infants, a 5-mm graft is usually selected.

Median Sternotomy Approach

This approach has several advantages. The pulmonary end of the shunt can be placed more centrally, potentially allowing better and more uniform growth of both pulmonary arteries. The ductus arteriosus can be occluded at the conclusion of the procedure, preventing excessive pulmonary circulation in the early postoperative period. The ductus arteriosus can be ligated when a left thoracotomy approach is used but can rarely be accessed through a right thoracotomy. Finally, if the patient becomes unstable, cardiopulmonary bypass can be quickly initiated through a median sternotomy.

Incision

A standard median sternotomy with resection of the thymus is used.

Technique

After opening the pericardium, traction sutures are placed on the pericardial edges. The aorta and pulmonary arteries are dissected free using scissors or electrocautery on a low setting. Downward traction on the main pulmonary artery allows the ductus arteriosus to be identified and encircled with a tie or cleaned free of surrounding tissues in preparation for later metal clip closure. The innominate artery is dissected to allow application of a C-clamp. The right pulmonary artery is then dissected away from the posterior aspects of the ascending aorta and superior vena cava. It is mobilized circumferentially and the right upper lobe branch is identified.

NB Use of Heparin

If the shunt is being performed without cardiopulmonary bypass, light systemic heparinization (50 units/kg) is administered just before the clamp is applied to the innominate artery. NB

The Gore-Tex graft is trimmed obliquely. A fine vascular C-clamp is applied to the innominate artery so that the inferior aspect of the artery is centered in the excluded portion (Fig. 18.1). The handle of the clamp is then raised to position the inferior edge of the innominate artery anteriorly. A longitudinal incision is made in the artery, and a fine adventitial suture is placed on the superior edge of the

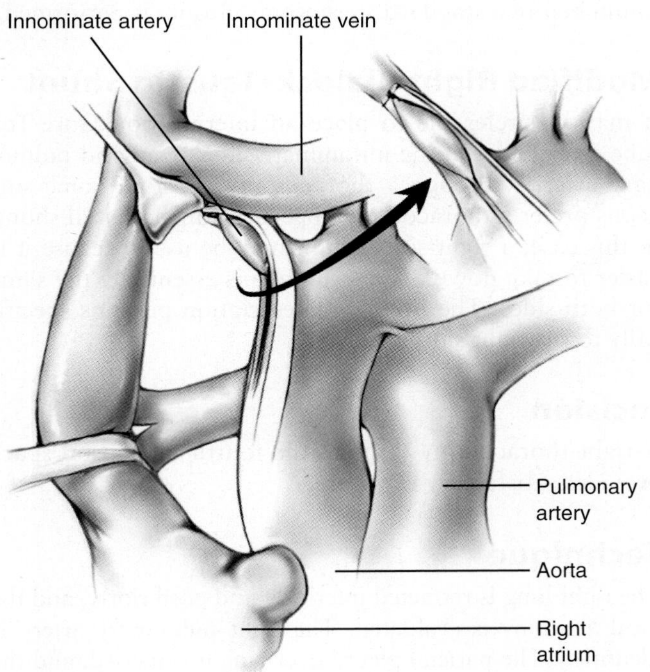

FIG. 18.1 Modified Blalock–Taussig shunt through a sternotomy: Placing a side-biting clamp on the innominate artery and rotating it to expose the inferior aspect of the artery. A vein retractor under the innominate vein improves exposure.

arteriotomy to keep the lumen open. The anastomosis is completed with Prolene suture (Fig 18.2).

With the other end of the graft occluded, the vascular clamp on the innominate artery is carefully removed and the anastomosis is checked for leaks. The length of the Gore-Tex graft is measured to just reach the superior aspect of the proximal right pulmonary artery. The graft is divided transversely at this site after placing a fine straight vascular clamp on the graft just below the innominate anastomosis. The right pulmonary artery is grasped with a fine C-clamp so that the cranial aspect is in the middle of the clamp. The clamp is then rotated so that a longitudinal incision can be made on the superior edge of the pulmonary artery. The arterial opening should be approximately two-third of the diameter of the graft lumen as the pulmonary artery stretches. The anastomosis is completed with a 7-0 Prolene (Fig. 18.3). The clamps are removed and hemostasis confirmed.

NB Centrally Located Shunt

The median sternotomy approach allows the pulmonary artery end of the shunt to be placed more centrally. The aorta must be mobilized and retracted leftward with a traction suture on the right side of the aorta, a vein retractor, or the back of the C-clamp itself (Fig. 18.3). NB

⊘ Coronary Ischemia

Care must be taken when applying traction to the aorta to prevent compression or kinking of the coronary arteries. If any electrocardiographic changes are noted or hemodynamic instability occurs, the traction suture, retractor, or clamp must be repositioned immediately. ⊘

⊘ Pulmonary Flooding

When the shunt is opened and flow through it confirmed, the ductus arteriosus, if present, should be occluded to prevent pulmonary overcirculation. Too much pulmonary blood flow may lead to systemic hypoperfusion and an inadequate diastolic blood pressure, resulting in coronary ischemia. ⊘

⊘ Hemodynamic Instability with Right Pulmonary Artery Clamping

Before incising the pulmonary artery, hemodynamic stability and systemic oxygenation with the C-clamp in place should be assessed. The clamp may interfere with ductal flow, and reapplying it more distally on the right pulmonary artery may rectify the problem. However, if desaturation or hemodynamic compromise persists after repositioning the clamp, the patient should be placed on cardiopulmonary bypass for support during this anastomosis. ⊘

⊘ Incorrect Length of the Tube Graft

Tension on the anastomosis owing to too short a tube graft may cause suture line bleeding and an upward pull on the

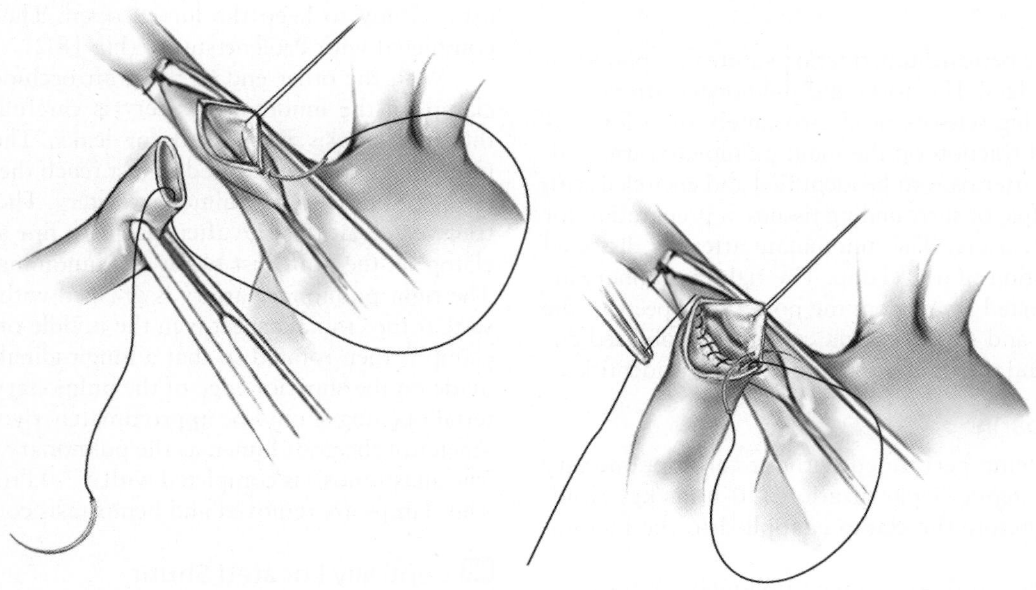

FIG. 18.2 Modified Blalock–Taussig shunt through a sternotomy: The end-to-side anastomosis of a Gore-Tex tube graft to the innominate artery. The inferior suture line is completed first.

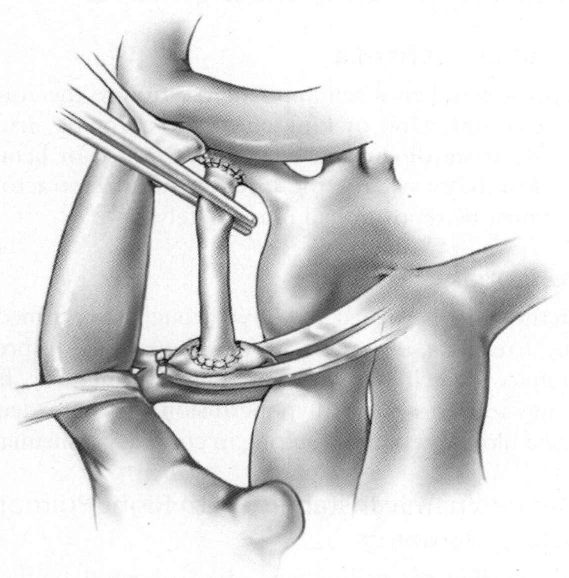

FIG. 18.3 Modified Blalock–Taussig shunt through a sternotomy: Completing the pulmonary artery anastomosis. The side-biting clamp has been placed so that the cranial edge of the right pulmonary artery is exposed.

pulmonary artery, which can lead to distortion or stenosis of the proximal right pulmonary artery. A graft that is too long may kink, thereby compromising flow through the graft. ⊘

If pericardial reapproximation is desired, a Gore-Tex pericardial membrane should be used in lieu of direct pericardial approximation since minor changes in mediastinal structures can cause compression and thrombosis of the shunt. A small chest tube is placed in the anterior mediastinum before a standard sternotomy closure is performed.

Modified Right Blalock–Taussig Shunt

It may be preferable to place an interposition Gore-Tex tube graft between the innominate/subclavian and pulmonary arteries through a thoracotomy incision. Some surgeons prefer a thoracotomy approach for the initial shunt. In this case, a right-sided shunt may be used because it is easier to take down. The technique is essentially the same for both sides. The following description pertains specifically to the right side.

Incision

A right thoracotomy through the fourth intercostal space provides satisfactory exposure.

Technique

The right lung is retracted inferiorly and posteriorly, and the local anatomy is evaluated. The right pulmonary artery is identified. The parietal pleura overlying it is incised, and the artery is mobilized medially toward the pericardium and distally to the hilum of the lung and proximally toward the mediastinum. Often the use of a blunt peanut dissector allows for mobilization without disruption of the pericardial edge. It is often helpful to ligate and divide the azygous vein, and also resect the lymphatic tissue that lies posterior and lateral to the superior vena cava, as this tissue will be in most direct path from the innominate artery to the right pulmonary artery.

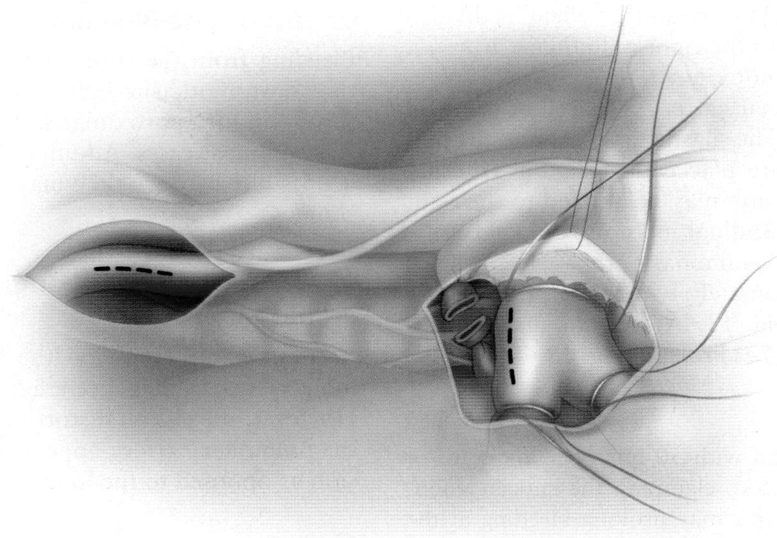

FIG. 18.4 Right-modified Blalock–Taussig shunt: Operative view of the hilum of the right lung and right subclavian artery with loose snares around the right pulmonary artery and its lobar branches.

NB Identification of the Right Pulmonary Artery

Sometimes the exact identity of the vessels within the hilum of the lung may not be clear. If there is any doubt as to the exact location of the pulmonary artery, it can be traced from within the pericardium through a short longitudinal incision on the pericardium, just anterior and parallel to the left phrenic nerve. NB

The right pulmonary artery, with its lobar branches having been clearly identified, is prepared for clamping or snaring with fine vascular elastic bands. The parietal pleura over the innominate or subclavian artery is incised, and the artery is mobilized and dissected free of its parietal sheath (Fig. 18.4).

A 3.5- or 4-mm Gore-Tex tube graft is used for neonates, and a 5-mm graft is rarely used for older patients. Because the size of the lumen of the innominate or subclavian artery is the limiting factor to the flow of blood, grafts larger than the subclavian artery do not necessarily increase the flow to the lungs and therefore are not responsible for pulmonary flooding, if it occurs.

The distal end of the graft is trimmed obliquely. An appropriate segment of the subclavian artery is excluded within a delicate vascular clamp. A longitudinal incision is then made in the artery. A fine adventitial traction suture on the anterior edge of the arteriotomy will keep the lumen of the artery open.

The anastomosis is started near the toe with a 7-0 Prolene suture and completed as a continuous anastomosis (Fig. 18.5).

With the other end of the graft temporarily occluded with fine, atraumatic forceps, the vascular clamp on the subclavian artery is loosened to detect a gross anastomotic leak that may require additional suture reinforcement. A cross-clamp is then reapplied to the graft. The length of the Gore-Tex tube graft is meticulously evaluated; it is divided

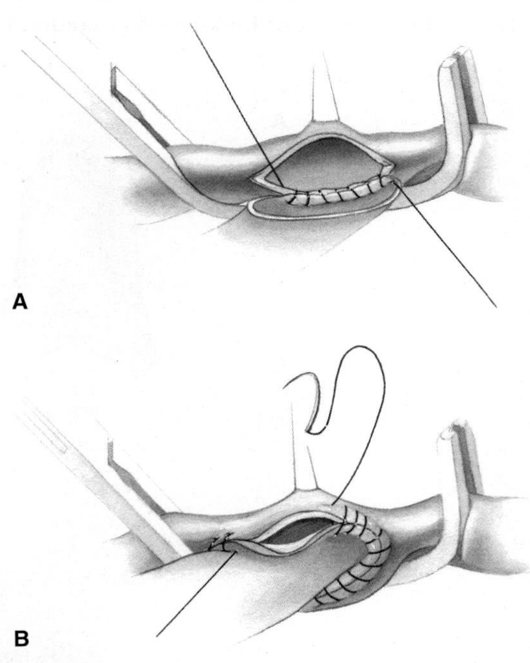

FIG. 18.5 **(A and B)** Left-modified Blalock–Taussig shunt: Stepwise technique for anastomosing a Gore-Tex tube graft to the left subclavian artery.

transversely at the appropriate site so that when its divided end is in close apposition to the right pulmonary artery, it is under no tension and is not kinked.

The main right pulmonary artery is snared or clamped as proximally as possible. The silastic tapes around the pulmonary artery branches are placed on traction. Alternatively, a fine vascular C-clamp may be applied to the right pulmonary artery. A longitudinal incision is made on the cranial aspect of the right pulmonary artery. The arterial opening should be approximately two-thirds of the diameter of the graft lumen (Fig. 18.6A) and the anastomosis completed with a running 7-0 Prolene (Fig. 18.6B).

NB Use of Heparin

Light systemic heparinization with 50 units per kilogram of body weight is initiated before clamping the subclavian/innominate artery. Although this may prolong bleeding at the anastomotic site, it lessens the risk of early graft thrombosis. NB

⊘ Too Short a Tube Graft

Tension on the anastomosis owing to too short a tube graft not only causes suture line bleeding but also pulls upward on the pulmonary artery, narrowing the lumen for distal flow and may result in early closure of the shunt. Too long a tube can lead to twisting or kinking due to redundancy. ⊘

⊘ Suture Line Bleeding

Bleeding from the suture line is not uncommon. Packing the anastomotic site lightly with Surgicel or Gelfoam and thrombin for approximately 5 minutes will achieve hemostasis in most cases. Additional sutures should be avoided, if possible, because they may jeopardize the lumen of the shunt. ⊘

⊘ Transverse versus Longitudinal Incision on the Pulmonary Artery

A transverse incision on the superior aspect of the pulmonary artery has been advocated by some surgeons. However, the risk of distortion and subsequent stenosis of the pulmonary artery appears to be greater with this incision as opposed to the longitudinal opening. ⊘

⊘ Right Aortic Arch

When a right arch is present, it can make the approach for a modified Blalock–Taussig shunt from a thoracotomy difficult. In such situations, consideration should be given to creating a central shunt (using a side-biting clamp on the greater curvature of the ascending aorta). More often, a central approach is used via median sternotomy. ⊘

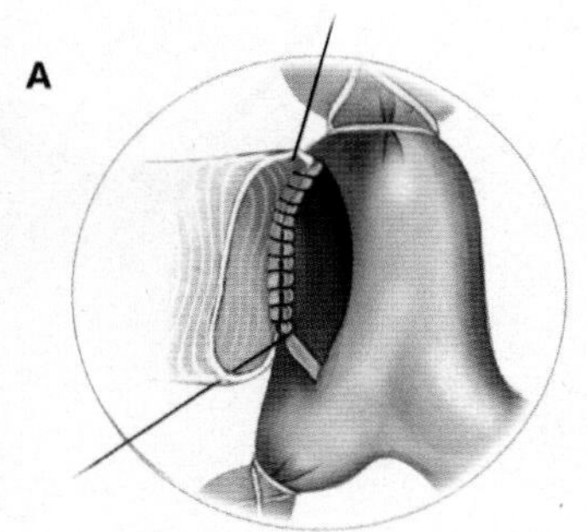

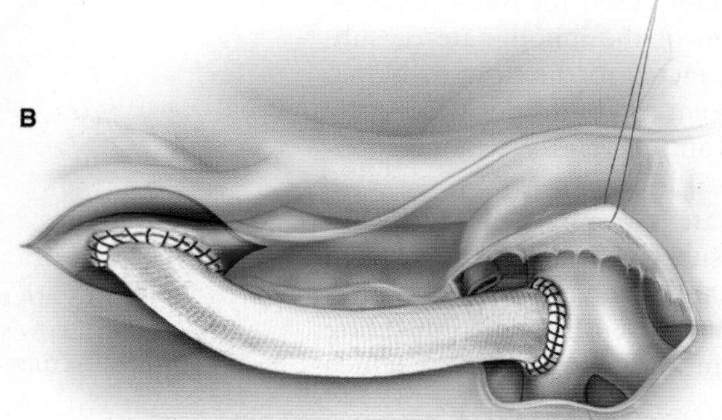

FIG. 18.6 Right-modified Blalock–Taussig shunt. **A:** Anastomosing the Gore-Tex tube graft to the right pulmonary artery. **B:** Graft interposition between the right subclavian and right pulmonary arteries.

⊘ Aberrant Right Subclavian Artery

An aberrant retroesophageal right subclavian artery is a relative contraindication toward performing the operation via right thoracotomy. If this approach is deemed necessary, the subclavian area of origin is more distally located than with a left aortic arch. ⊘

⊘ Right Recurrent Laryngeal Nerve

The right recurrent laryngeal nerve surrounds the right subclavian artery and can be quite close to the area chosen for the proximal shunt placement. Extreme care must be used not to damage the nerve with placement of the partial occluding clamp, given the space constraints of a small thoracotomy and the deep angulation of the clamp. ⊘

At the end of the procedure, a small chest tube is inserted and the thoracotomy is closed in the usual manner.

CENTRAL SHUNT

This procedure entails interposing a tube graft between the main pulmonary artery and ascending aorta. It provides an alternative technique when other shunts have failed or in cases where the branch pulmonary arteries are very small. The approach is through a median sternotomy.

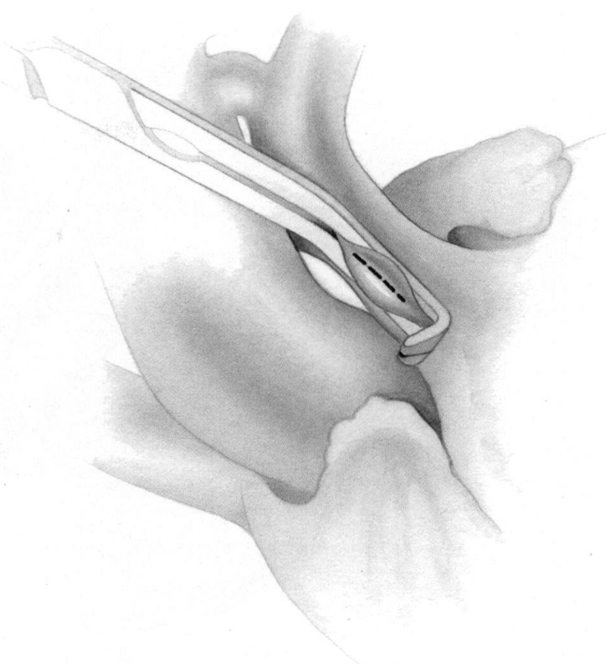

FIG. 18.7 Central shunt: Isolation and incision of the pulmonary artery.

Technique

The ascending aorta and main pulmonary artery are dissected free of each other. A small side-biting clamp is placed on the main pulmonary artery. A vertical pulmonary arteriotomy is made (Fig. 18.7). A 3.0, 3.5- or 4-mm Gore-Tex tube graft (with or without ringed reinforcement) is cut transversely and anastomosed to the pulmonary artery with continuous 7-0 Prolene suture. The Gore-Tex graft is now clamped with a fine straight vascular clamp close to the pulmonary anastomosis and the pulmonary artery clamp is removed. A side-biting clamp is now applied to the left lateral aspect of the ascending aorta and a small opening is made with a knife blade. This is enlarged to the appropriate size with an aortic punch. The other end of the Gore-Tex tube graft is cut obliquely and anastomosed to the aorta with 7-0 Prolene suture (Fig. 18.8). Air is removed by unclamping the tube graft before tying down the suture on the aortic side of the anastomosis. The aortic clamp is removed as the last step. A good thrill should be felt.

⊘ Kinking of the Graft

A Gore-Tex tube graft that is too long or angled inappropriately at its junction with the aorta is likely to kink and lead to early shunt failure. In some cases, it may be simpler to not trim the tube graft following the pulmonary artery anastomosis. The Gore-Tex tube graft is gently pulled against the side of the aorta, and both the aorta and tube are marked where they meet comfortably. A 3.5- to 4-mm hole is created at the marked site on the graft and, with a partial occlusion clamp on the ascending aorta, an aortic punch is used to create a matching opening. A side-to side anastomosis is performed with 7-0 Prolene suture. The distal end of the graft is then transected 4 to 5 mm distal to the aortic anastomosis, and the end is oversewn with a 7-0 Prolene suture (Fig. 18.9). Alternatively, a ringed reinforced graft can be used, and in addition some oblique angulation can be placed on the proximal (aortic) end of the graft to afford a more "vertical" lie. ⊘

PROSTHETIC ASCENDING AORTA–RIGHT PULMONARY ARTERY SHUNT

Occasionally, the aortic arch anatomy may make interposition from the innominate to the right pulmonary artery problematic. In these cases, a graft may be placed from the ascending aorta to the right pulmonary artery.

NB Limiting Factor to the Pulmonary Blood Flow

In modified Blalock–Taussig shunt interposition with a Gore-Tex tube graft, the size of the subclavian or innominate artery is the limiting factor to the flow of blood to the lungs. In an ascending aorta–right pulmonary shunt, however, the diameter and length of the Gore-Tex tube graft are important factors regulating the pulmonary blood flow. Therefore, except on very rare occasions, a 3.0-, or 3.5-tube graft should be used to prevent pulmonary overcirculation. NB

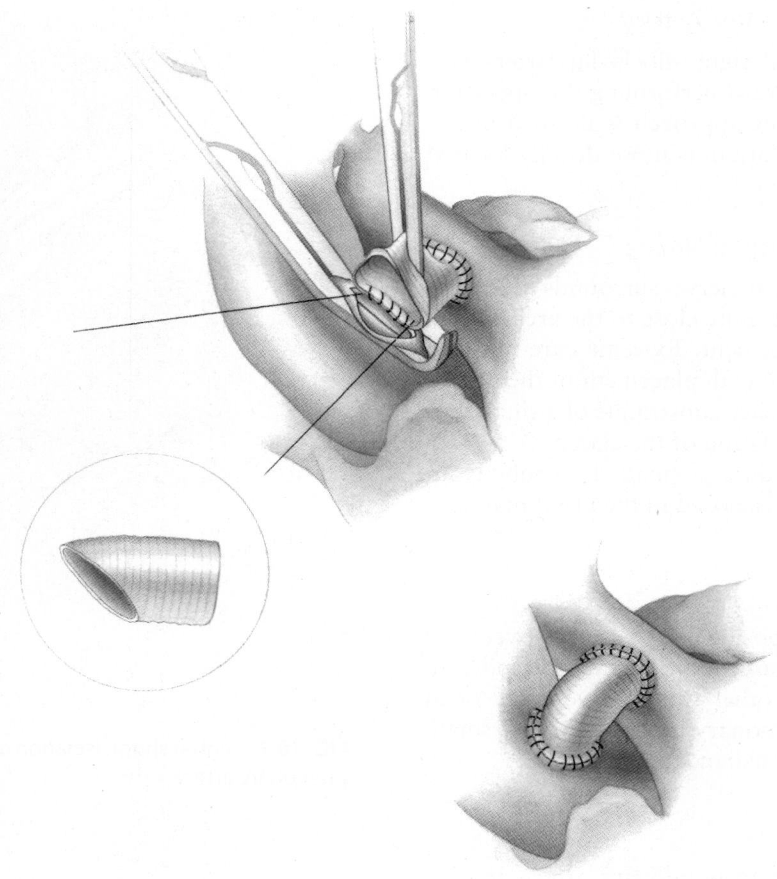

FIG. 18.8 Stepwise technique for creating a central shunt.

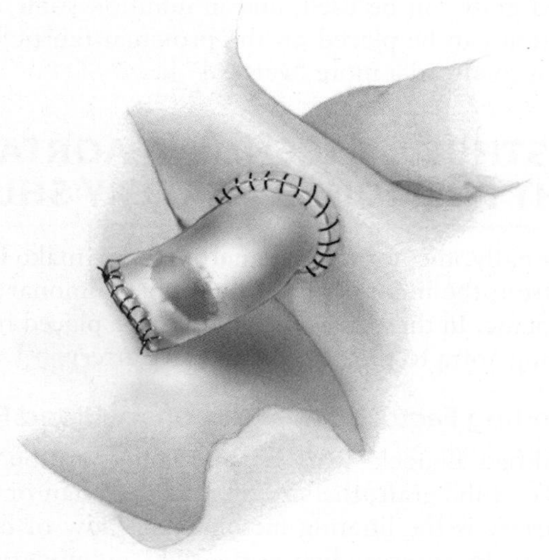

FIG. 18.9 Central shunt with a side-to-side aortic anastomosis and oversewing the end of the Gore-Tex tube graft.

Incision

A median sternotomy approach is used.

Technique

After removing the thymus, the pericardium is opened and traction sutures are placed. If the ductus arteriosus is patent, it is dissected free circumferentially for later closure after completion of the shunt. The right pulmonary artery is mobilized by gently retracting the aorta leftward and the superior vena cava rightward. The upper lobe branch of the right pulmonary artery is identified so that the shunt can be placed proximal to it. After systemic heparinization (50 units/kg), a C-clamp is placed on the proximal right pulmonary artery positioning the anterior portion of the artery in the center of the clamp. The appropriately sized Gore-Tex tube graft is cut transversely. A longitudinal arteriotomy is made in the pulmonary artery, approximately two-thirds of the diameter of the graft. A traction suture is placed on the inferior edge of the arteriotomy. A double-armed, 7-0 Prolene suture is used for a continuous running anastomosis. The graft is marked as is the ascending aorta. The graft may be cut obliquely to meet the opening on the ascending aorta without distortion. However, it is often advisable to create an opening on the aortic side of the graft matching the aortic opening and to perform a side-to-side anastomosis. This procedure is described as shown in Fig. 18.10.

After marking the graft, a fine vascular clamp is placed on the graft close to the pulmonary artery anastomosis. A small incision is made at the mark on the graft and enlarged to a size equal to the diameter of the graft with a 2.8-mm aortic punch. A side-biting clamp is now placed on the ascending aorta so that the marked area is centered in the clamp. A small incision is made and enlarged with the aortic punch. The end-to-side anastomosis is performed using a double-armed, 7-0 Prolene suture. If the ductus arteriosus is patent, it is now occluded with a heavy tie or metal clip. The pericardium is loosely approximated with a Gore-Tex pericardial membrane, a small chest tube is placed in the anterior mediastinum, and standard sternotomy closure is performed.

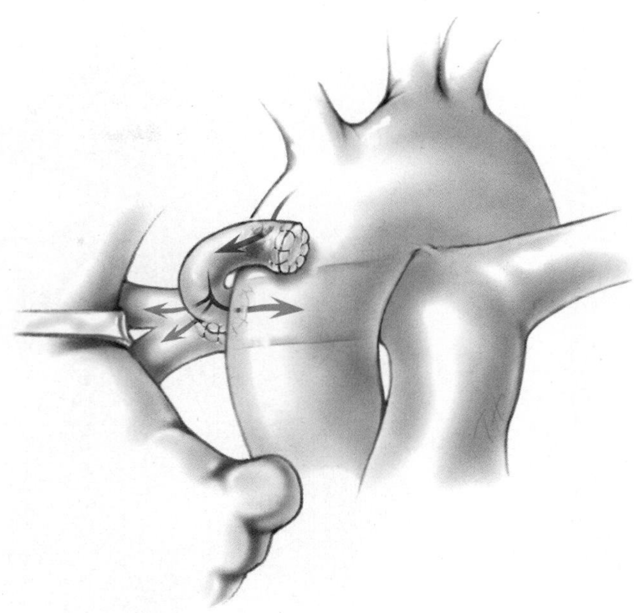

FIG. 18.10 Completed ascending aorta to the right pulmonary artery shunt: Note a circular patch closing the tube graft above the side-to-side aortic anastomosis.

⊘ Aortic Partial Occlusion

The side-biting clamp must be placed carefully on the ascending aorta, especially in neonates and infants with small aortas to avoid hypotension or myocardial ischemia secondary to compromised coronary flow. Before incising the aorta, the position of the clamp should be tested to ensure that no hemodynamic changes are going to occur. Multiple reapplications of the clamp from different angles may be required before a satisfactory placement is found. ⊘

⊘ Coronary Ischemia

It can be challenging to apply the partial occluding clamp while on cardiopulmonary bypass without causing coronary insufficiency. Should this occur, the procedure should be performed under cardioplegic arrest. Marking the future site of the central shunt on the ascending aorta is helpful so as to maintain orientation when the aorta is open and decompressed. ⊘

⊘ Thrombosis or Distortion of the Graft above the Aortic Anastomosis

The length of graft beyond the side-to-side anastomosis is crucial with this technique. If too much graft extends above the aortic anastomosis, there will be an area of relatively stagnant flow that may predispose to graft thrombosis. If too little graft remains, the suture line may distort or compromise flow into the graft from the aorta. If the graft has been cut too short, the end can be closed with a circular piece of Gore-Tex graft cut from extra graft material (Fig. 18.10). This prevents distortion and minimizes dead space. ⊘

⊘ Coronary Ischemia

It can be challenging to apply the partial occluding clamp while on cardiopulmonary bypass without causing coronary insufficiency. Should this occur, the procedure should be performed under cardioplegic arrest. Marking the future site of the central shunt on the ascending aorta is helpful so as to maintain orientation when the aorta is open and decompressed. ⊘

⊘ Melbourne Shunt

For patients with severe pulmonary atresia and confluent pulmonary arteries, it can be efficacious to transect the main (diminutive) pulmonary artery and anastomose this directly to the posterior aspect of the ascending aorta, thereby creating the equivalent of a central shunt without the use of prosthetic graft. Some suggest that this configuration maximizes pulmonary artery growth in part because of the growth potential (and lack of restriction) of the main pulmonary artery when compared with Gore-Tex (Fig 18.11). ⊘

CLOSURE OF SYSTEMIC PULMONARY SHUNTS

All these shunts should be dissected free and exposed for complete occlusion just after initiation of cardiopulmonary bypass, when contemplating complete correction of the anomaly or further palliative procedures.

Right-Sided Modified Blalock–Taussig Shunts

The aorta and superior vena cava are retracted away from each other, and the posterior pericardium is incised above the superior margin of the right pulmonary artery. The

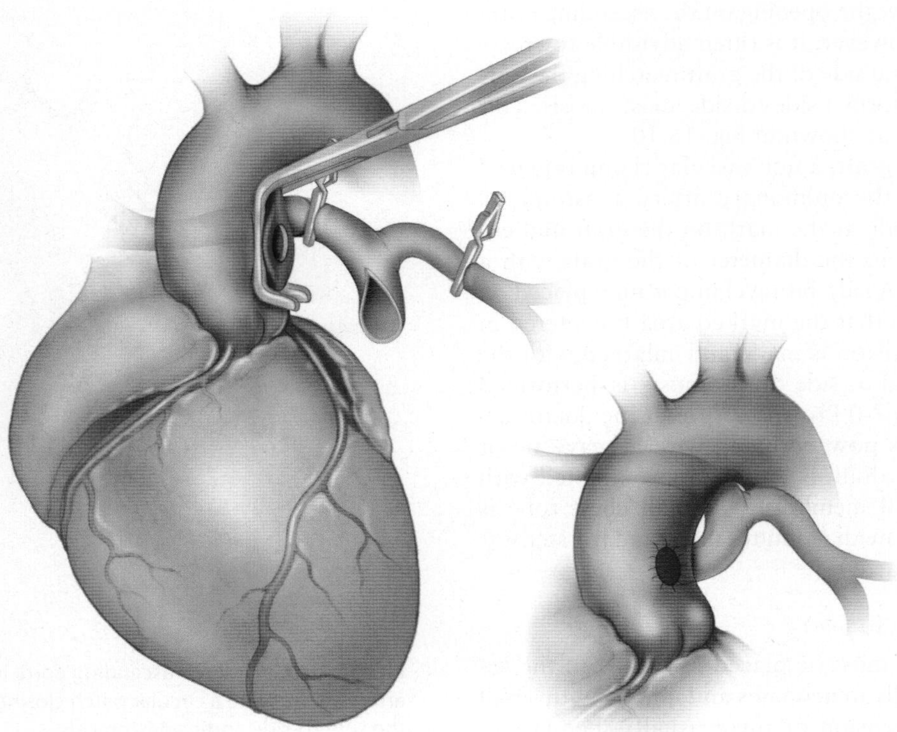

FIG 18.11 Melbourne shunt with anastomosis of the diminutive main pulmonary artery to the posterior aspect of the ascending aorta.

Gore-Tex tube graft is identified and occluded with one or two medium or medium-large metal clips just after the initiation of cardiopulmonary bypass (Fig. 18.12).

⊘ Dissection around the Right Pulmonary Artery

There are many adhesions and collateral vessels in this area. A minimal dissection to isolate the shunt should suffice. It is usually not necessary to pass a silk tie around the shunt. ⊘

⊘ Right Pulmonary Artery Stenosis

If significant stenosis is present at the insertion site of the shunt into the right pulmonary artery, the tube graft should be divided after the initiation of cardiopulmonary bypass. The transected end should be secured with at least two adequately sized metal clips or oversewn with a 6-0 or 5-0 Prolene suture. The residual Gore-Tex material should then be removed from the right pulmonary artery and this area is enlarged with an oval-shaped patch of autologous pericardium or pulmonary homograft. ⊘

⊘ Division of the Gore-Tex Shunt

Theoretically, as a child grows, an intact Gore-Tex tube graft may cause upward traction on the right pulmonary artery, which may lead to distortion and possible late development of pulmonary artery stenosis. If an adequate length of Gore-Tex tube graft can be dissected free without incurring excessive bleeding, the tube may be secured with two metal clips on each side and divided to prevent this potential late complication. ⊘

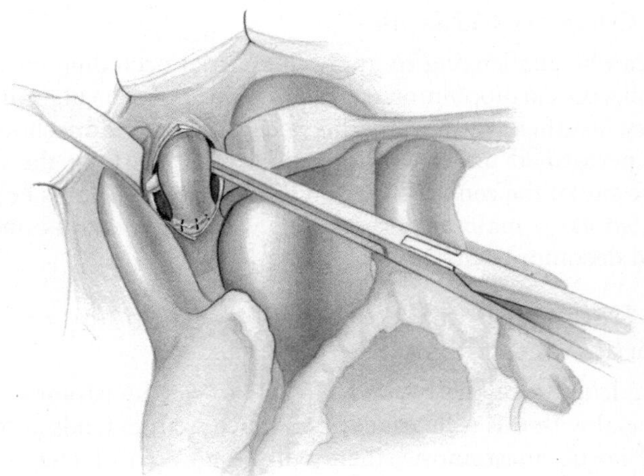

FIG. 18.12 Exposure of the right-modified Blalock–Taussig shunt.

⊘ Accessing the Gore-Tex Shunt

It is easiest to ligate the shunt if the surgeon can accurately develop a plane around the shunt. Using a scalpel and a sharp, fine dissector (e.g., Jacobson clamp), this plane is most easily found and developed so as to afford surrounding the shunt with a right-angled clamp without effort. ⊘

Left-Sided Modified Blalock–Taussig Shunts

Isolation of the left-sided shunt is somewhat more cumbersome and can be accomplished in many ways. Some surgeons prefer opening the left pleura. The Gore-Tex tube graft is then identified as it enters the left pulmonary artery (Fig. 18.13). It is minimally dissected free and doubly clipped, just before initiation of cardiopulmonary bypass. Alternatively, the left pulmonary artery is dissected free from within the pericardium, and the Gore-Tex tube graft is clipped just above its junction with the pulmonary artery.

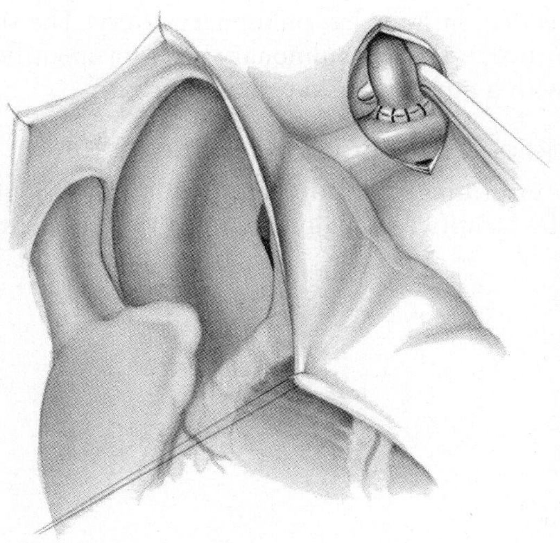

FIG. 18.13 Exposure of left-modified Blalock–Taussig shunt.

⊘ Clip Injury

Clips must be at least large enough to occlude the entire width of the graft. Smaller clips may pierce the graft and cause bleeding, in addition to closing the shunt incompletely. ⊘

Central Shunt

With the initiation of cardiopulmonary bypass, the Gore-Tex tube graft is occluded with a metal clip.

Prosthetic Ascending Aorta–Right Pulmonary Artery Shunt

The tube graft is carefully dissected free from the lateral aspect of the ascending aorta and occluded with a metal clip as cardiopulmonary bypass is commenced. Usually, the shunt tubing is divided while on bypass and the aortic and pulmonary ends are oversewn with a running 6-0 or 5-0 Prolene suture.

⊘ Aortic Injury

The Gore-Tex shunt is often very adherent to the side of the aorta. The correct plane for dissection must be identified, staying right on the Gore-Tex graft itself to avoid entry into the aorta. If the shunt cannot be safely dissected from the aorta, it should be occluded as much as possible with a vascular clamp or forceps when cardiopulmonary bypass is commenced and the dissection completed with the patient on bypass. ⊘

Waterston and Potts Shunts

Waterston and Potts shunts are no longer performed, but familiarity with the techniques of their closure is essential for the surgeon who operates on patients who have undergone these shunting procedures in the past.

Technique: Waterston Shunt

The easiest way to close a Waterston shunt is on cardiopulmonary bypass with the aorta cross-clamped. After administering cardioplegic solution, a small transverse aortotomy is made, and the shunt may be closed from within the aorta with a few interrupted sutures. The preferred method is to detach the right pulmonary artery from the aorta and oversew the defect in the ascending aorta with a running 5-0 Prolene suture. The defect in the pulmonary artery can be closed transversely by direct suture or preferably patched with a piece of autologous pericardium or pulmonary homograft.

⊘ Pulmonary Artery Distortion

If the shunt has created some stenosis or kinking of the right pulmonary artery, this should be reconstructed with an appropriate pericardial or homograft patch. ⊘

⊘ Flooding of the Pulmonary Circulation

The site of the shunt must be occluded with the initiation of cardiopulmonary bypass, or flooding of the lungs will occur. If this cannot be achieved with a vascular forceps or clamp, the right and left pulmonary arteries should be encircled before beginning cardiopulmonary bypass, and snared or clamped. ⊘

Technique: Potts Shunt

Closure of Potts shunt is performed on cardiopulmonary bypass with moderate hypothermia. The patient is placed in the Trendelenburg position, and with the heart decompressed, the perfusion pressure is temporarily reduced. A longitudinal incision is made on the main pulmonary artery and extended onto the left pulmonary artery. The site of a shunt orifice in the left pulmonary artery is identified and closed with a purse-string suture or patch.

⊘ Flooding of the Pulmonary Circulation

Before instituting cardiopulmonary bypass, the site should be identified by palpating for a thrill along the left pulmonary artery. The shunt flow can be interrupted or markedly reduced by digital pressure on this site. ⊘

⊘ Air Embolism through Aortic Opening

When the left pulmonary artery is opened, some flow must be maintained through the aortic cannula to prevent air embolism. ⊘

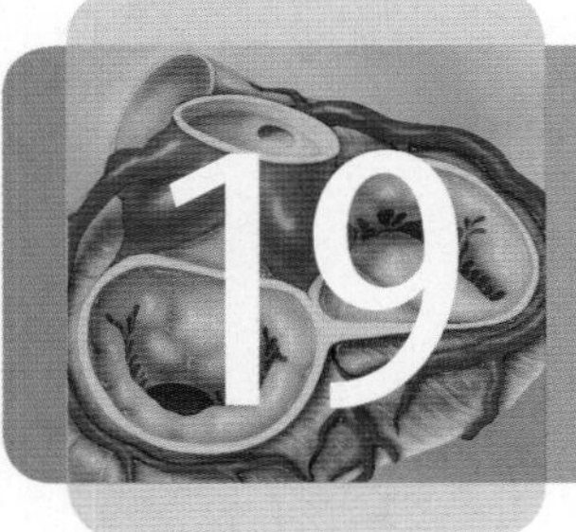

19 Atrial Septal Defect

Defects in the atrial septum are relatively common. They appear at various sites in the septum and can be associated with other congenital abnormalities. In addition, there is a real or potential slit-like opening, the foramen ovale, where the fossa ovalis flap disappears behind the superior septal limbus. Generally, the higher pressure in the left atrium keeps the fossa ovalis flap in apposition to the superior septal limbus, and therefore the opening remains closed. In 20% of the population, however, the foramen ovale is patent and has the potential to allow shunting under certain circumstances. When pressure in the right atrium increases, as in right-sided heart failure, the septum becomes stretched and allows the foramen ovale to enlarge with significant shunting at the atrial level.

The sinus venosus atrial septal defect occurs high in the atrial septum and extends into the orifice of the superior vena cava, which becomes malpositioned slightly toward the left. There is usually anomalous drainage from the right superior pulmonary vein associated with these defects (Fig. 19.1).

The fossa ovalis type, also known as the ostium secundum defect, is the most common variety. This defect occurs in the midseptum in the vicinity of the fossa ovalis and may be small or very large. Infrequently, the defect may occur low in the septum and extend into the orifice of the inferior vena cava, which also becomes malpositioned toward the left. This type of defect is sometimes referred to as a sinus venosus defect of the inferior vena caval type and may be associated with anomalous pulmonary venous drainage. Rarely, the whole septum may be absent, giving rise to a single common atrium.

A defect low in the interatrial septum that extends down to the level of the atrioventricular valve orifices is part of the atrioventricular septal defect complex (see Chapter 22).

SURGICAL ANATOMY OF THE RIGHT ATRIUM

Although the right atrium is morphologically molded into a single chamber, it is formed by two components: the sinus venarum and the right atrial appendage (sometimes referred to as the body of the atrium). Systemic venous return flows in from opposing directions through the superior and inferior venae cavae into the sinus venarum. This smooth-walled area is the most posterior portion of the right atrium and stretches between the orifices of the caval veins. From the viewpoint of the surgeon looking down into the right atrium, the sinus venarum is more or less horizontal with the superior vena cava entering from the left and the inferior vena cava (bounded by the eustachian valve) entering from the right (Fig. 19.2).

Just below and medial to the orifice of the superior vena cava arises a muscle bundle, the crista terminalis, which springs into prominence as it circles the orifice of the superior vena cava to the right lateral wall of the atrium and continues inferiorly toward the inferior vena cava, thereby forming the boundary between the sinus venarum and the atrial appendage. This muscle bundle is evidenced on the outside of the atrium by a groove, the sulcus terminalis. Lying subepicardially in the sulcus terminalis, just below the entrance of the superior vena cava, is the sinoatrial node, which may be vulnerable to injury from the various surgical incisions and cannulations commonly performed on the right atrium. The remainder of the right atrium is made up of atrial appendage, which begins at the crista terminalis and extends forward (upward from the surgeon's perspective) to surround the tricuspid valve and form an expanded chamber.

In contrast with the smooth-walled sinus venarum, the lateral wall of the atrial appendage is ridged with multiple narrow bands of muscle, the musculi pectinati. These bands arise from the crista terminalis and pass upward to the most anterior part of the atrium. Functionally, they supply the right atrium with enough pumping capacity to propel the venous inflow through the tricuspid valve into the right ventricle.

Just above the sinus venarum in the center of the medial wall is the fossa ovalis, a horseshoe- or elliptically shaped depression. The true interatrial septum consists of the fossa ovalis with variable contributions from the superior, anterior, and inferior limbic muscle bundles that surround it. The aortic root is hidden behind the anteromedial atrial wall between the fossa ovalis and the termination of the heavily trabeculated right atrial appendage. Segments of

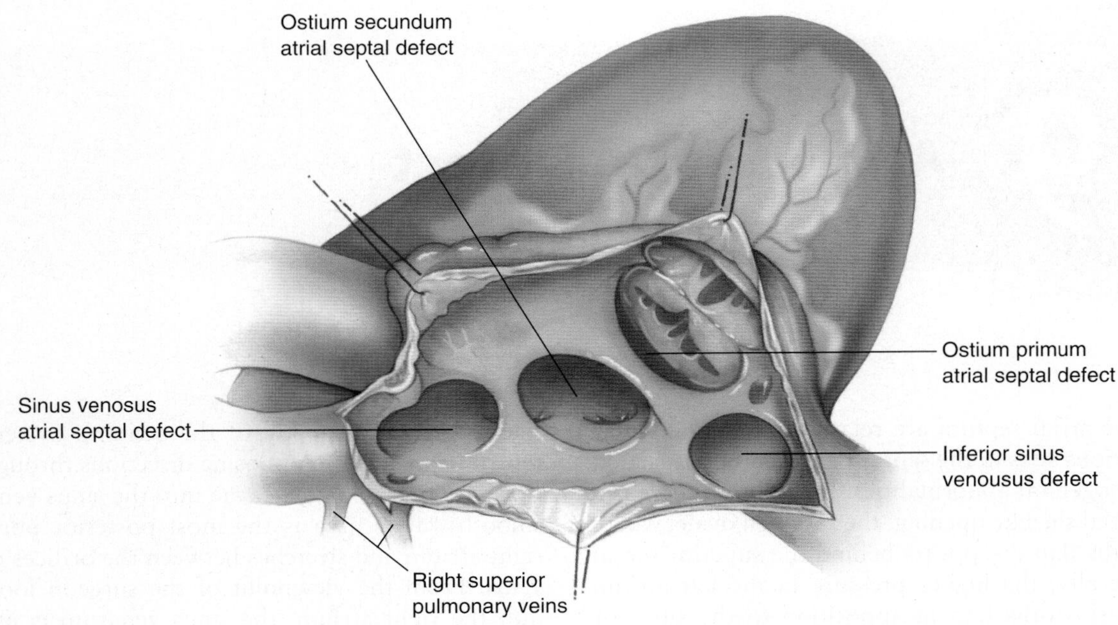

FIG. 19.1 Types of atrial septal defects.

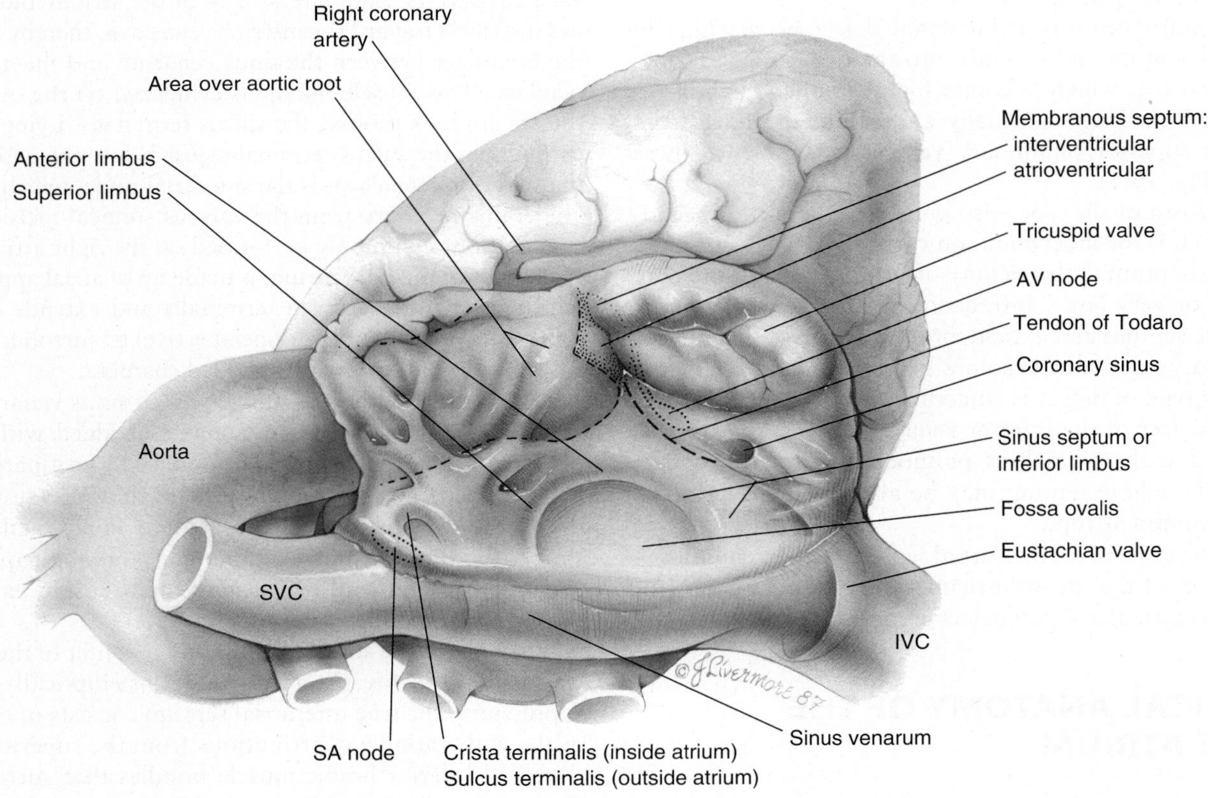

FIG. 19.2 Surgical anatomy of the right atrium. SVC, superior vena cava; SA, sinoatrial; IVC, inferior vena cava; AV, atrioventricular.

the noncoronary and right sinuses of Valsalva are in close apposition to the atrial wall in this area. Their location may be manifested by the aortic mound, which is a bulge above and slightly to the left of the fossa ovalis. The aortic valve here can be more clearly visualized if its continuity, through the central fibrous body, with the adjacent tricuspid valve annulus is taken into consideration.

Also, often invisible to the surgeon is the artery to the sinoatrial node, which can run through this same area. Although its origin and exact course are unpredictable, it takes a variable course toward the superior cavoatrial angle and the sinus node.

The tricuspid valve is located anteroinferiorly in the right atrium, where it opens widely into the right ventricle. The annulus of the tricuspid valve crosses over the membranous septum, dividing it into atrioventricular and interventricular segments. The membranous, or fibrous, septum is a continuation of the central fibrous body, through which the tricuspid, mitral, and aortic valves are connected. Immediately below the upper or atrioventricular section of the membranous septum lies the hidden atrioventricular node. It is situated at the apex of the triangle of Koch, the boundaries of which are the annulus of the septal leaflet of the tricuspid valve, the tendon of Todaro (running intramyocardially from the central fibrous body to the eustachian valve of the inferior vena cava), and its base, the coronary sinus. Anderson describes the tendon of Todaro as a fibrous extension of the commissure between the eustachian valve (of the inferior vena cava) and the thebesian valve (of the coronary sinus). Conduction tissue passes from the atrioventricular node as the bundle of His, below the membranous septum, and down into the muscular interventricular septum. The coronary sinus, draining the cardiac veins, is situated alongside the tendon of Todaro, between it and the tricuspid valve.

Incision

All forms of atrial septal defect can be approached through a median sternotomy. Many surgeons now use a lower ministernotomy approach or submammary right thoracotomy for simple secundum atrial septal defects. Others prefer the Brom modification of the median sternotomy incision to allow full exposure of the pericardial space with acceptable cosmetic results in female patients (see Chapter 1).

Cannulation

The ascending aorta is cannulated in the usual manner (see Chapter 2). The superior vena cava is usually cannulated directly, although it may be cannulated through the right atrial appendage. The inferior vena cava is cannulated through the atrial wall, just above the origin of the inferior vena cava. Tapes are then passed around both cavae. For those defects thought to be low in the atrial septum or for inferior sinus venosus defects, it is imperative to cannulate low on the inferior vena cava itself.

NB Aortic Cannulation with Minimally Invasive Approaches

The more distal ascending aorta is not easily accessible through a lower ministernotomy or submammary right thoracotomy. The aorta should be cannulated in its midportion where control of bleeding is relatively easy. Enough room should be left below the cannula to allow for deairing procedures. NB

NB Exposure of the Superior Vena Cava

A tie is placed on the right atrial appendage. Inferior traction on the appendage allows adequate visualization of the right superior vena cava for direct cannulation in most instances. If direct cannulation is not feasible, a straight venous cannula can be passed into the superior vena cava through a purse-string suture on the right atrial appendage. NB

⊘ Left Superior Vena Cava

The left superior vena cava cannot be cannulated through minimally invasive incisions. Preoperative echocardiography must determine the presence or absence of a left superior vena cava. ⊘

Myocardial Preservation

Cold cardioplegic arrest of the myocardium is achieved by infusion of cold-blood cardioplegia into the aortic root (see Chapter 3).

Alternatively, closure of a simple septum secundum–type defect can be accomplished safely without clamping the aorta by inducing ventricular fibrillation (see subsequent text). This approach is used with minimally invasive incisions because aortic cross-clamping in these cases may be difficult.

SINUS VENOSUS ATRIAL SEPTAL DEFECT

Sinus venosus atrial septal defects usually occur high on the septum close to the orifice of the superior vena cava and are associated with anomalous drainage of right upper lobe pulmonary veins into the superior vena cava and right atrium (Fig. 19.3). Approximately 10% of patients with this type of atrial septal defect also have a persistent left superior vena cava, which may be suspected from a large coronary sinus on the preoperative echocardiogram.

Technique

The superior vena cava is cannulated directly high above the entry site of the highest anomalous pulmonary vein or preferably at the innominate/caval junction.

The aorta is cross-clamped, and cardioplegic solution is administered into the aortic root (see Chapter 3). The vena caval snares are then snugged down. A longitudinal atriotomy is made starting at a point 0.5 to 1 cm posterior

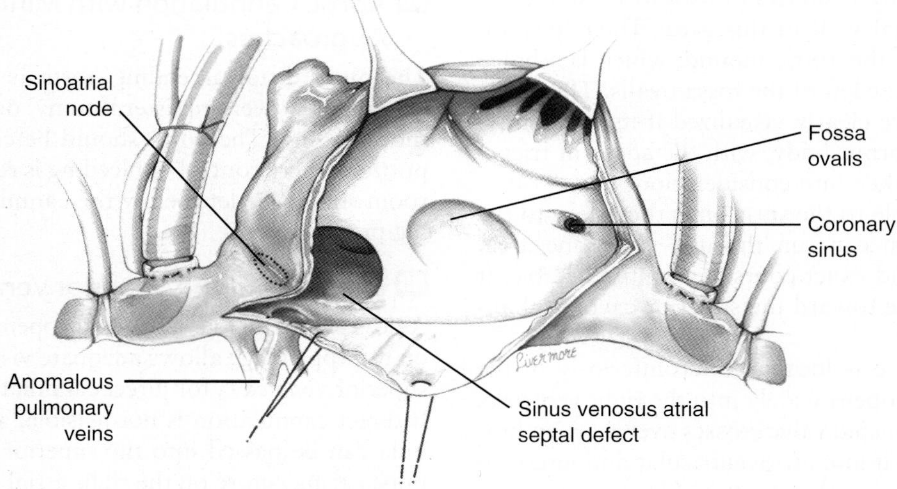

FIG. 19.3 Sinus venosus atrial septal defect and the superior extension of the atriotomy posterior to the sinoatrial node.

and parallel to the sulcus terminalis. The edges of the incision are then retracted to provide good exposure of the septal defect (Fig. 19.3). If additional exposure is required, the atriotomy is extended superiorly and posterolaterally across the superior vena caval–right atrial junction and onto the vena cava as far as necessary.

NB Drainage of Venous Return from a Left Superior Vena Cava

Although the venous return from a persistent left superior vena cava can be removed by pump suction, direct cannulation with a third venous cannula is the preferred approach. If an innominate vein is present and of adequate size, the left superior vena cava may be temporarily occluded with a snare. NB

⊘ Injury to the Sinoatrial Node

The superior extent of the atriotomy may have to be extended across the atriocaval junction onto the superior vena cava to provide adequate exposure. The sinoatrial node can be injured unless the atriotomy is extended well posterior to it. ⊘

⊘ Persistent Left-to-Right Shunt

It is important to ascertain that the tape around the superior vena cava is well above the level of the drainage of all the anomalous veins. Leaving a pulmonary vein draining into the superior vena cava results in a residual left-to-right shunt. ⊘

NB Difficult Exposure

The azygos vein, as it joins the superior vena cava, may at times obscure the surrounding structures. In this case, it may be ligated and divided to free up the superior vena cava and to provide better exposure of the anomalous pulmonary veins. NB

A patch of glutaraldehyde-treated autologous pericardium or Gore-Tex is cut to an appropriate size and shape after examining the extent of the defect. With a continuous suture of 5-0 or 6-0 Prolene, the patch is sewn around the orifices of the anomalous veins and across to the anteromedial margin of the atrial septal defect (Fig. 19.4).

⊘ Preventing Ostial Stenosis of Anomalous Veins

Sometimes it is necessary to place several sutures through the patch and the right atrial or superior vena caval wall around the openings of the anomalous veins before lowering the patch into position. Accurately placed sutures, well away from the anomalous vein orifices, will prevent subsequent stenosis. ⊘

⊘ Obstruction of the Pulmonary Venous Return

If the atrial septal defect is relatively small, it should be enlarged to prevent obstruction of the pulmonary venous return. In addition, the patch should be generous, creating a hood when the heart fills with blood and allowing unobstructed flow under the patch into the left atrium. ⊘

⊘ Injury to the Aortic Root/Valve

Care must be taken when enlarging the atrial septal opening, especially if the aortic root is enlarged or pressurized. The extension from the sinus venosus defect to the fossa ovalis should be kept posterior, and if possible a clamp should be placed through the sinus venosus defect or patent foramen ovale and used to lift the atrial septum away from the aortic root while incising the septum. Enlarging the atrial septal opening in this way also avoids injury to the sinus node artery. ⊘

The atriotomy is then closed. Occasionally, this can be done primarily with a continuous suture of 5-0 Prolene.

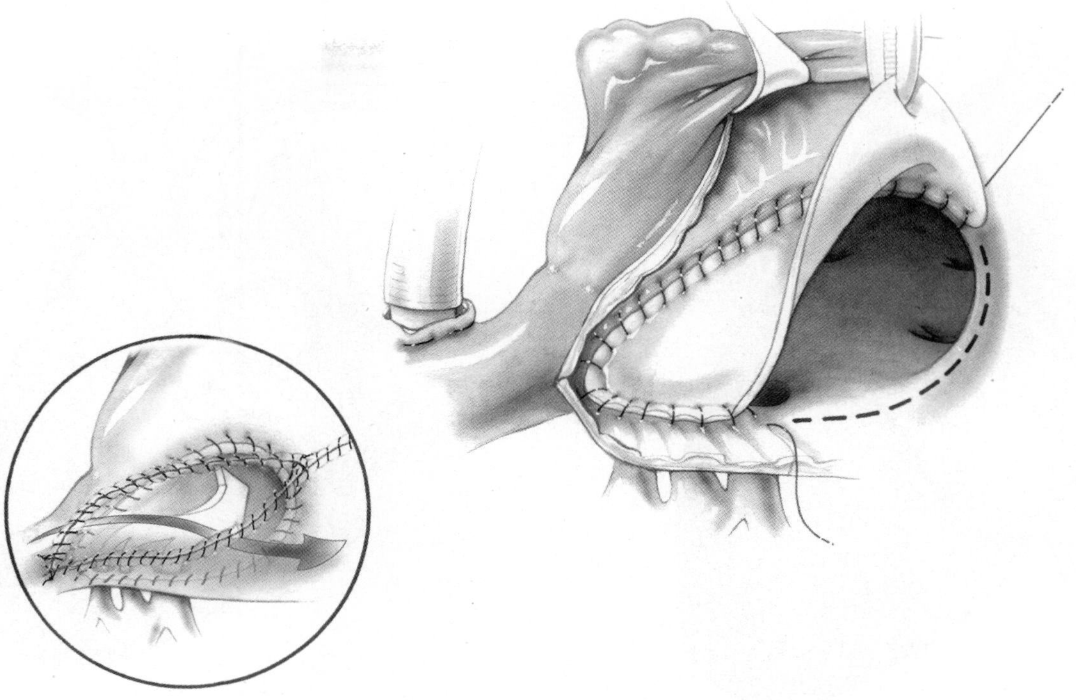

FIG. 19.4 First patch baffling anomalous pulmonary veins and closing the sinus venosus atrial septal defect. Inset: Second patch enlarging the superior vena caval–right atrial junction.

Most often, a second patch of pericardium is required to prevent narrowing of the superior vena caval–right atrial junction (Fig. 19.4, inset).

NB Air Removal

By having the anesthesiologist inflate the lungs before securing the septal patch, the left side of the heart is flooded with blood to displace any loculated air bubbles from within the pulmonary veins and left atrium. The patch is kept partially open with the tip of a forceps, while a sustained ventilation fills the left atrium with blood and the suture line is snugged down before the lungs are deflated. NB

⊘ Preventing Obstruction of the Superior Vena Cava

Often the atriotomy has been extended onto the superior vena cava for some distance for precise exposure of the anomalous pulmonary veins. Direct closure may cause narrowing of the superior vena cava and give rise to subsequent obstruction. Unless the superior vena cava is unusually large, it should be enlarged with a patch of pericardium (Fig. 19.4, inset). Alternatively, a V-Y atrioplasty can be performed if the right atrium is very large. ⊘

⊘ Sinoatrial Node Injury

As mentioned previously, the atrial and superior vena caval closure line is in close proximity to the sinoatrial node. The edges of the atriotomy should be handled with care to prevent conduction abnormalities from sinoatrial node injury. ⊘

The caval snares are removed following right atrial closure, the heart is filled, and the aortic clamp is removed. Standard deairing is performed, and the patient is weaned from cardiopulmonary bypass.

⊘ Cyanosis Following Cardiopulmonary Bypass

If decreased systemic oxygen saturations are noted after separation from cardiopulmonary bypass, consideration should be given to the existence of a right-to-left shunt. This may occur if a large azygos vein is included in the baffle of pulmonary veins to the sinus venosus atrial septal defect. Ligating the azygos vein will rectify this situation. ⊘

NB Caval Division Technique ("Warden")

Some surgeons use the technique of superior vena caval division and anastomosis of the proximal superior vena caval opening to the right atrial appendage for sinus venosus atrial septal defects; this technique is particularly effective if the entrance of several of the right pulmonary veins are high on the superior vena cava, making baffle placement without caval obstruction difficult. The superior vena cava is divided just above the highest anomalous pulmonary vein, and the distal opening of the superior vena cava is closed, taking care not to compromise the opening of the anomalous vein(s) (Fig. 19.5). The tip of the right atrial appendage is amputated, and it is additionally important that all of the pectinate muscles in the amputated right atrial appendage are excised (Fig. 19.5). Through a right atrial incision, a

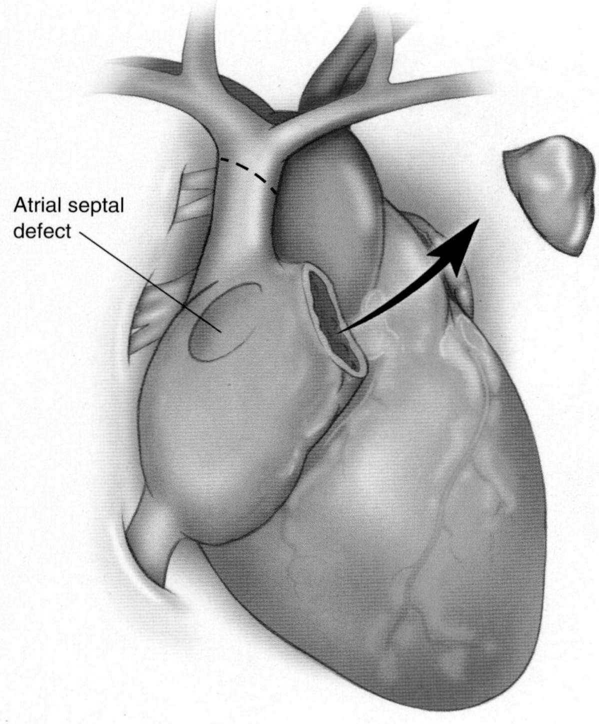

FIG. 19.5 The tip of the atrial appendage is amputated and the SVC is divided above the level of entry of the anomalous right pulmonary veins. It is important to resect all of the trabecular tissue within the atrial appendage so as to mitigate future systemic venous obstruction.

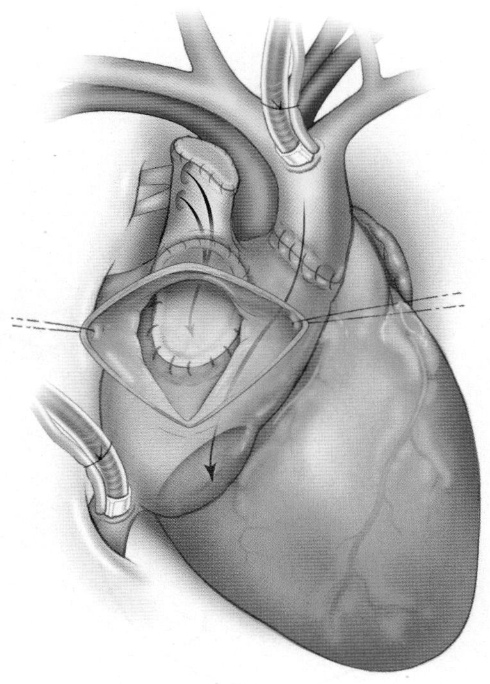

FIG. 19.6 Completed Warden procedure. Note the patch on the superior vena cava, which can be necessary at times so as not to have pulmonary venous obstruction that can occur with direct suture closure (if the entrance of the veins is close to the innominate–SVC junction). Arrows indicate the direction of flow of both the pulmonary and systemic venous return.

patch of pericardium or Gore-Tex is used to baffle the orifice of the superior vena cava to the sinus venosus defect (Fig. 19.6). This technique avoids a long incision and patch on the superior vena cava, especially when the anomalous veins enter high above the cavoatrial junction. The superior vena cava is then anastomosed to a mobilized portion of the right atrial appendage with care taken not to "purestring" the connection (Fig. 19.6). Often an additional patch augmentation of the caval-atrial anastomosis is required to reduce tension on the connection as well. NB

OSTIUM SECUNDUM ATRIAL SEPTAL DEFECT

Ostium secundum defects are the most common form of atrial septal defect. They are usually large and include the entire fossa ovalis (Fig. 19.7A).

Technique

The aorta is cross-clamped, and cardioplegic solution is administered into the aortic root (see Chapter 3). Alternatively, if a minimally invasive approach has been used, two pacing wires are secured on the anterior right ventricle and connected to a fibrillator to induce ventricular fibrillation. The vena caval snares are then snugged down. An oblique atriotomy is made and is extended toward the orifice of the inferior vena cava. The edges of the incision are retracted to provide good exposure of the septal defect.

Some smaller secundum defects can be closed directly. Sutures are placed at the superior and inferior ends of the defect and continued toward each other, incorporating the margins of the defect (Fig. 19.7B).

⊘ Depth of Sutures

The sutures must incorporate the thickened endocardium on both sides of the interatrial septum. The tissue of the fossa ovalis is usually too weak and friable to provide secure closure. Deep sutures should be avoided along the superior aspect of the defect because this area overlies the aortic root, as well as laterally to avoid narrowing the orifice of the right pulmonary veins (Fig. 19.2). ⊘

NB Using the Fossa Ovalis Flap to Close a Defect

Occasionally, the fossa ovalis flap is of sufficient size and quality to allow a tension-free primary suture closure,

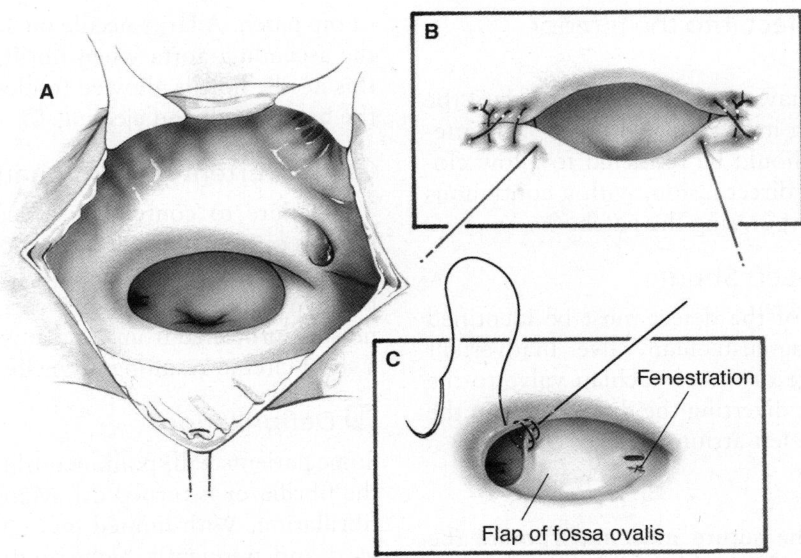

FIG. 19.7 **A:** Secundum atrial septal defect. **B:** Direct suture closure of a secundum atrial septal defect. **C:** Using the fossa ovalis flap to close the defect. Very small fenestrations of the flap can be primarily sutured.

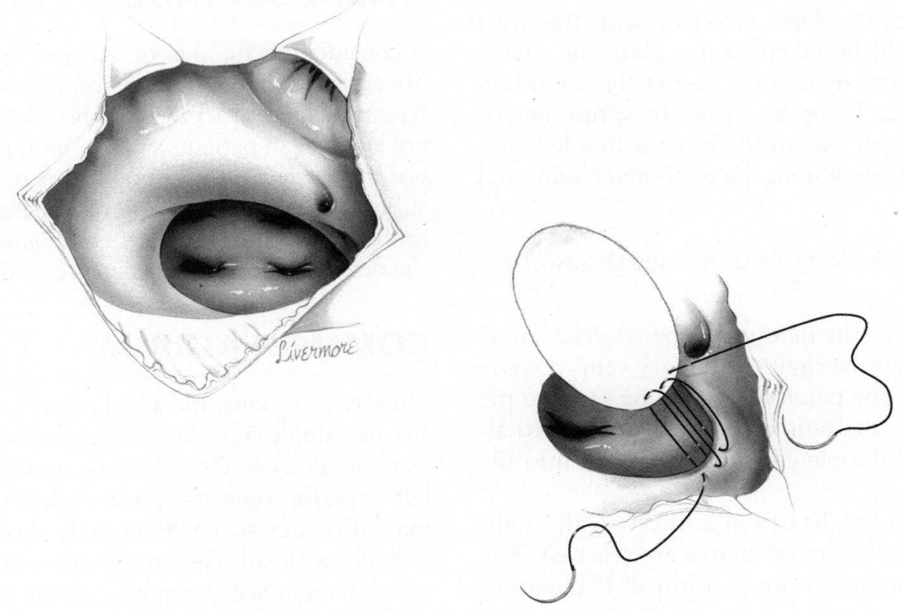

FIG. 19.8 Patch closure of a secundum atrial septal defect.

approximating the superior edge of the flap to the superior limbus (Fig. 19.7C). This is often the case in infants with a stretched patent foramen ovale. One must always check for fenestrations in the inferior aspect of the flap that could result in residual atrial septal defects. If fenestrations are present or the flap is thin and friable, patch closure should be undertaken. NB

Unless the size of the defect is small and the rim of the opening is quite strong, a patch of glutaraldehyde-treated autologous pericardium or Gore-Tex is used to close a secundum defect to eliminate any tension along suture lines. An appropriately sized patch is prepared and sewn into position with continuous sutures of 5-0 or 6-0 Prolene (Fig. 19.8).

⊘ Extension of the Defect into the Inferior Vena Cava

Occasionally, the defect may extend into the orifice of the inferior vena cava, making its exposure difficult. The inferior vena caval cannula should be retracted to allow closure of this margin under direct vision, with a continuous suture of 5-0 Prolene incorporating the patch. ⊘

⊘ Creating a Right-to-Left Shunt

The inferior free margin of the defect must be identified and distinguished from the eustachian valve. Inadvertent approximation of the edge of the eustachian valve to the patch will create a tunnel, diverting the drainage from the inferior vena cava into the left atrium. ⊘

⊘ Depth of Sutures

As with direct closure, the suture must incorporate the thickened endocardium on both sides of the septum and not the fossa ovalis tissue, which is often very thin and friable. ⊘

⊘ Air in Left Heart

The best way to prevent air embolism is to avoid introducing air into the left side of the heart. Whether the surgery is performed under cardioplegic arrest or with the heart fibrillating, care should be taken to not place the sucker through the atrial septal defect. By having the anesthesiologist inflate the lungs before securing the suture line or the patch closure, the left side of the heart is flooded with blood, displacing air from within the pulmonary veins and left atrium. ⊘

⊘ Right Pulmonary Vein Drainage into the Right Atrium

The posterior margin of the defect may be so deficient as to allow the drainage of the right pulmonary veins directly into the right atrium. The patch must then be sewn to the atrial wall, anterior to the pulmonary vein orifices, to allow diversion of their drainage behind the patch into the left atrium (Fig. 19.9). ⊘

After the septal defect has been addressed, the right atriotomy is closed and the caval snares are released. The heart is filled and ventilations are performed. If the aorta was clamped, the cross-clamp is removed, deairing accomplished, and cardiopulmonary bypass discontinued.

NB Minimally Invasive Approaches

When limited incisions are used, the aorta is generally not clamped. Two pacing wires are attached to the right ventricle and connected to a fibrillator after cardiopulmonary bypass is initiated. The caval tapes are tightened, and with the ventricle fibrillating, the right atrium is opened. A concerted effort is made not to place a sucker through the atrial septal defect, thereby preventing air from entering the left atrium. The lungs are inflated before tying the suture line of the patch. A large needle on a syringe is used to aspirate the ascending aorta when fibrillation is discontinued, and this needle hole is allowed to bleed for 1 or 2 minutes after the heart is full and ejecting. NB

⊘ Inadvertent Discontinuation of Fibrillation

The failure to continue ventricular fibrillation when the heart is open may result in ejection of air into the ascending aorta with disastrous consequences. The pacing wires must be sewn securely to the right ventricle. The cable connections must be protected from contact with metal, which can cause a short circuit, resulting in the loss of fibrillating current. ⊘

NB Defibrillation

Some patients will spontaneously regain sinus rhythm when the fibrillator is turned off. Many patients will require defibrillation. With limited incisions, small paddles must be used and frequently higher settings are required for successful defibrillation. Alternatively, external defibrillator patches secured on the patient's back and anterior chest wall before sterile draping may be used. NB

TRANSCATHETER CLOSURE OF ATRIAL SEPTAL DEFECTS

A considerable number of patients with atrial septal defects are currently undergoing placement of devices in the catheterization laboratory to close their defects. These procedures are effective in patients with secundum-type defects that are not too large and have good rims on all sides. Rarely, the surgeon may be called upon to operate for a complication in these procedures such as malposition or embolization of the device, or incomplete closure of the shunt.

COMMON ATRIUM

On rare occasions, the atrial septum may be absent, giving rise to a single common atrial chamber. Other lesions, such as anomalous systemic venous drainage with or without a left superior vena cava and endocardial cushion defects, may also coexist. Each anomaly should be managed individually with subsequent septation of the common atrium.

A patient with complete absence of the atrial septum, absence of the right superior vena cava, persistent left superior vena cava, and a cleft mitral valve (Fig. 19.10) underwent complete correction, taking into consideration the following guidelines.

Aortic cannulation is carried out in the usual manner. Tapes are passed around the left superior vena cava and inferior vena cava. Both inferior vena cava and left superior vena cava are cannulated directly. The aorta is cross-clamped, and cold-blood cardioplegia is administered into the aortic root. The snares around both vena cava are snugged down, and a traditional atriotomy (above and parallel to the sulcus terminalis) is then made.

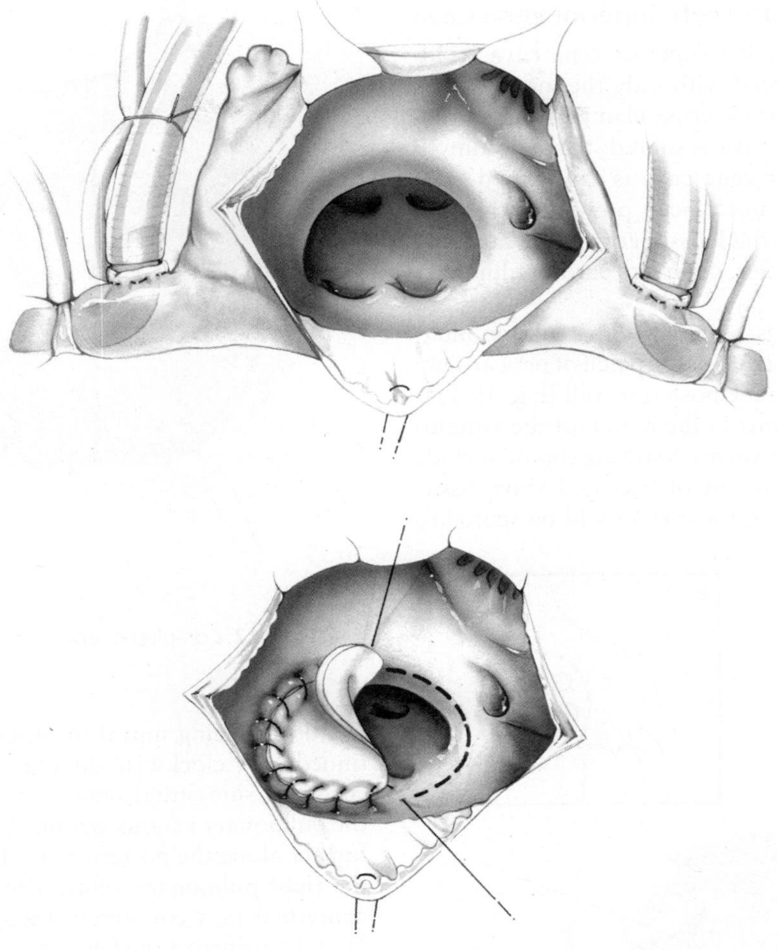

FIG. 19.9 Patch closure of an ostium secundum defect with malpositioned right pulmonary veins opening into the right atrium. The patch is sutured anterior to the orifices of the veins to reroute drainage into the left atrium.

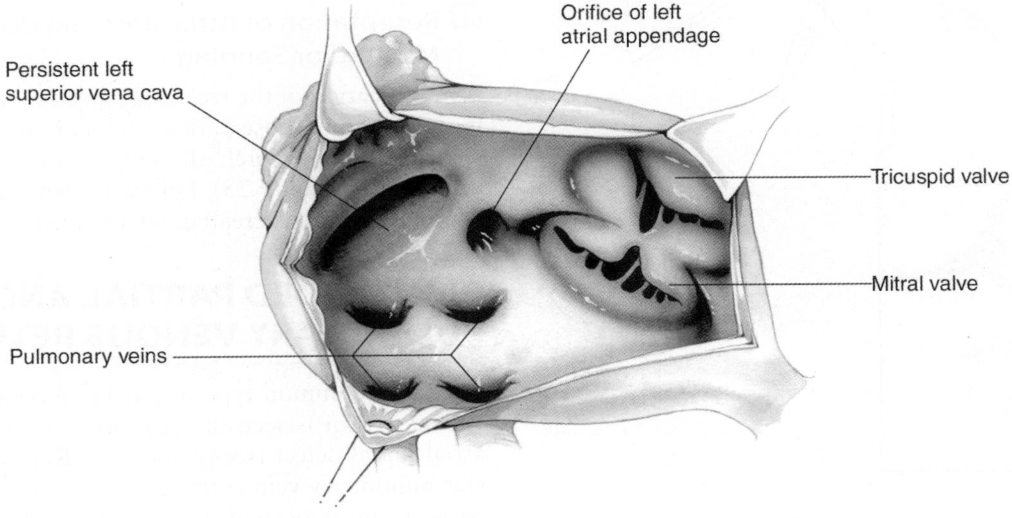

FIG. 19.10 Operative view of a single atrium with the absence of the right superior vena cava, persistent left superior vena cava, and cleft mitral valve.

NB Difficult Exposure of the Left Superior Vena Cava

If direct cannulation of the left superior vena cava is difficult, bypass may be initiated with only the inferior vena caval cannula. After the aorta is cross-clamped and cardioplegia is given, the inferior cava is snared, the atriotomy is made, and the left superior vena cava is cannulated from within the right atrium. If not placed previously, a snare can now be placed around the left superior vena cava and snugged down. In this manner, complete cardiopulmonary bypass is achieved. NB

The cleft mitral valve is repaired with multiple interrupted sutures (see Chapter 22). A large patch of pericardium or Gore-Tex is then sewn to the posterior wall (Fig. 19.11).

The septation should start in the region of the annulus between the atrioventricular valves. Suturing should include the annulus and a small amount of tricuspid valve tissue (Fig. 19.11C). The mitral valve leaflet should be spared to avoid producing mitral insufficiency. The suturing is continued in a clockwise direction around the orifice of the coronary sinus (that may be absent) so that it drains into the pulmonary venous atrium. The same suture is continued further along the posterior atrial wall around the orifices of the right pulmonary veins. The other end of the suture is continued in a counterclockwise direction below and behind the orifice of the left superior vena cava until the patch takes on the configuration of a septum (Fig. 19.12). The patch should be generous in size; if excess patch is present, it can be trimmed before suturing is completed. Otherwise, it may need to be augmented by sewing another patch to it.

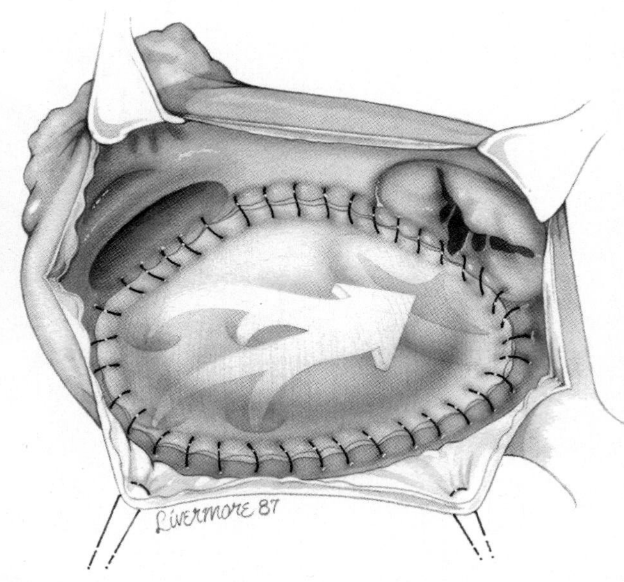

FIG. 19.12 Completed repair of the defect shown in Fig. 19.10.

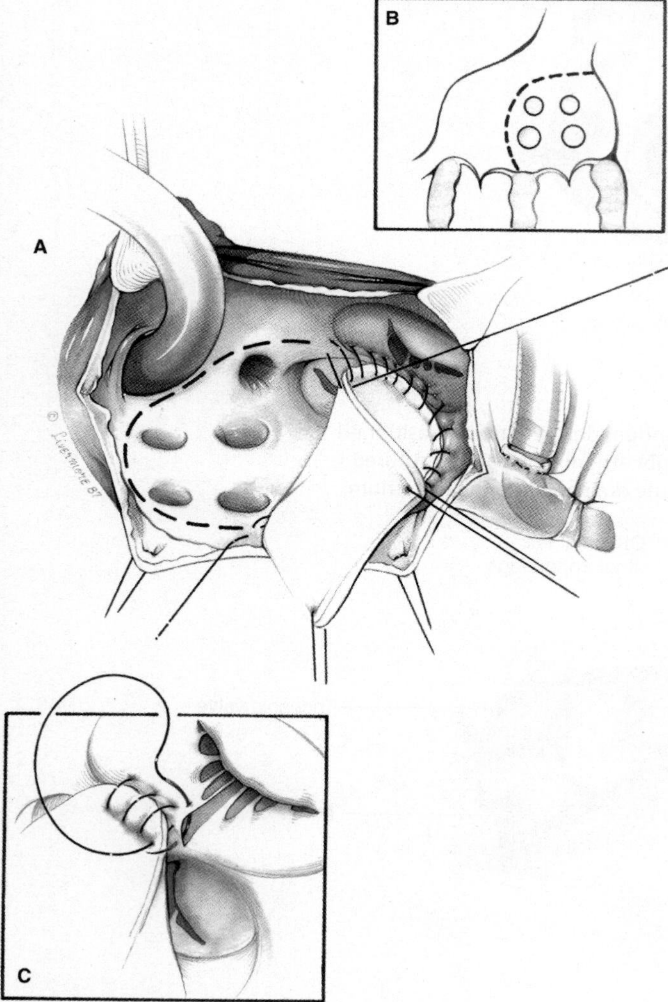

FIG. 19.11 A: Technique for repair of the defect shown in Fig. 19.8. B: Schematic illustration of repair. C: Suturing patch to tricuspid valve tissue.

NB Reseptation of Atria after Takedown of Mustard or Senning

A modification of the technique given in the preceding text may be used in those patients who are undergoing conversion from atrial switch anatomy to an arterial switch procedure (see Chapter 25). Following removal of the baffle, a common atrium is created, which must be septated. NB

RIGHT-SIDED PARTIAL ANOMALOUS PULMONARY VENOUS RETURN

The most common type of partial anomalous pulmonary venous return is seen in association with a sinus venosus atrial septal defect (see previously). Rarely, the right superior pulmonary vein enters the superior vena cava directly without an associated atrial septal defect. Repair of this anomaly requires creation of an adequately sized atrial septal defect and tunnel closure of the anomalous pulmonary vein to the left atrium (Fig. 19.4).

Scimitar syndrome consists of a large anomalous pulmonary vein draining the entire right lung or the right middle and lower lobes, passing inferiorly to enter the inferior vena cava just above or below the diaphragm. An intraatrial baffle technique can be used to tunnel the flow from the anomalous pulmonary vein orifice within the inferior vena cava up to an existing or surgically created atrial septal defect. Alternatively, the anomalous vein may be ligated at its entrance into the inferior vena cava, transected, and anastomosed directly to the left atrium.

NB Baffle obstruction

Intratrial baffle obstruction is not uncommon because of the acute angle that the pulmonary venous return must make within the inferior vena cava (Fig. 19.13). This obstruction can be mitigated in selected cases by performing a side-to-side type connection (Fig. 19.14). More recently, some have advocated repair via reimplantation through a right lateral thoracotomy off bypass NB.

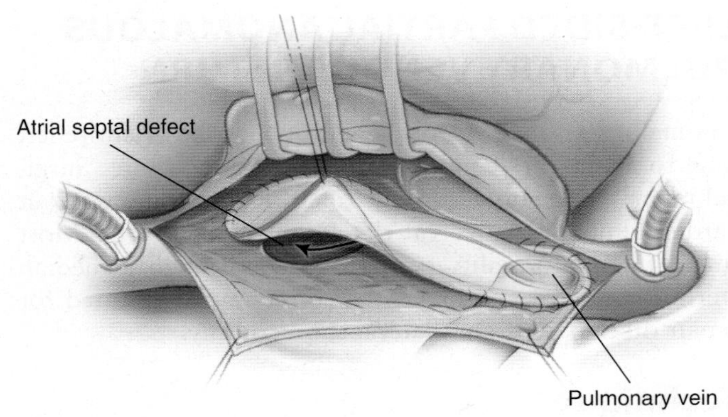

FIG. 19.13 Repair of Scimitar syndrome using a single patch. Note the acute angle that the pulmonary venous return must make as it enters near the IVC and is redirected through the more cranial atrial septal defect (which may require enlargement to afford unobstructed flow).

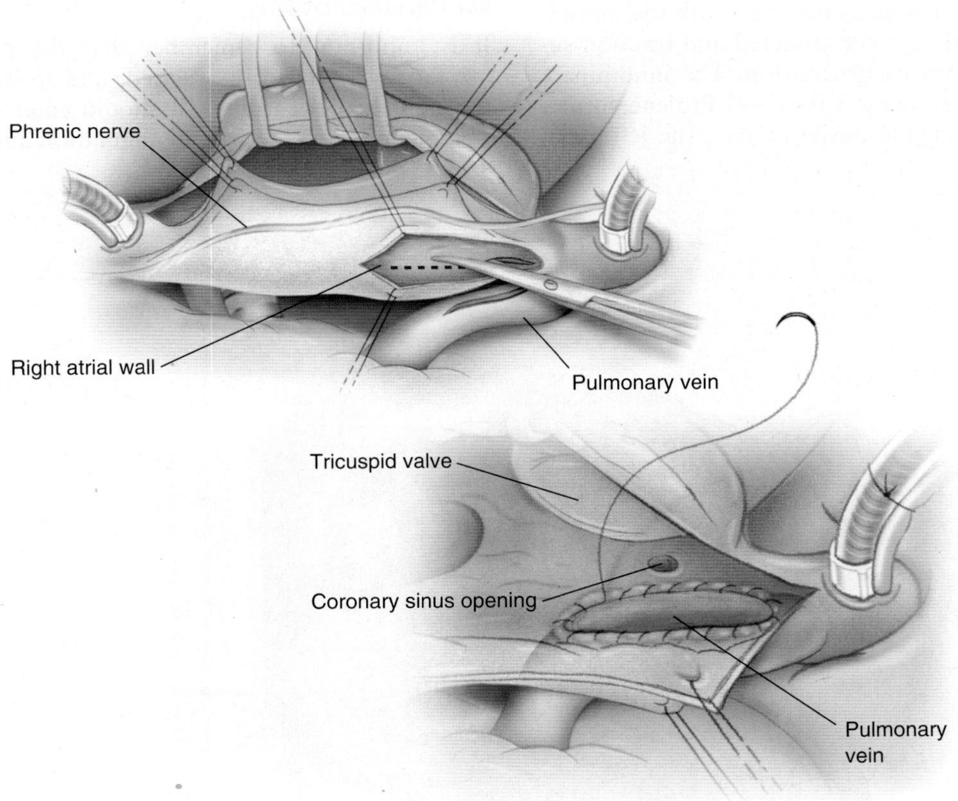

FIG. 19.14 Side-to-side repair of Scimitar syndrome. To reduce the acute angulation of pulmonary venous return with the single patch (Fig. 19.C), a side-to-side anastomosis along the posterior aspect of the right atrium makes for a larger connection, and one that is considerably closer to the atrial defect through which flow must be directed. Note the course of the phrenic nerve and how the anastomosis sits posterior. The patch connecting the new opening of the pulmonary venous drainage through the atrial septal defect is similar to that used in Fig. 19.C.

LEFT-SIDED PARTIAL ANOMALOUS PULMONARY VENOUS RETURN

Anomalous drainage from the left upper lobe or entire left lung to a vertical vein as an isolated lesion is rare. Surgical repair can be done through a left thoracotomy without cardiopulmonary bypass if the diagnosis is certain. Most often, this abnormality is approached through a median sternotomy. However, recently, some have advocated for repair off bypass via left lateral thoracotomy.

Technique

Standard aortic cannulation is used, and if there is no atrial septal defect, a single venous cannula can be placed in the right atrium. On cardiopulmonary bypass, the left vertical vein is exposed from the hilum to the innominate vein, and any systemic branches are ligated and divided. Opening the pericardium posterior to the phrenic nerve may facilitate exposure. The relationship of the left atrial appendage to the vertical vein is assessed before clamping the aorta and arresting the heart. A right-angle clamp is placed on the vertical vein at its junction with the innominate vein. The vertical vein is transected and traction sutures placed to maintain its orientation. The innominate end is oversewn with running 5-0 or 6-0 Prolene suture. A generous opening is made posteriorly on the left atrial appendage, and the vertical vein is now opened anteriorly. The vertical vein is anastomosed to the atrial appendage with running 6-0 or 7-0 Prolene, taking care to not twist or distort the vein (Fig. 19.15). Alternatively, the left atrial appendage can be amputated and the open end of the vertical vein anastomosed to the resultant opening. The heart is allowed to fill and the absence of kinking of the anastomosis ensured before standard deairing and cross-clamp removal.

NB Anastomotic Gradient

Intraoperative transesophageal echocardiography should confirm unobstructed flow from the left pulmonary veins into the left atrium. If a significant gradient is noted, anastomotic revision should be undertaken. NB

NB Maintaining Correct Orientation of Vertical Vein

Placing a bulldog-type clamp across the base of the vertical vein at the confluence of the pulmonary veins helps to prevent twisting of the vertical vein. NB

NB Pericardiotomy

It is important to remember that the pulmonary veins are largely posteriorly oriented, and in bringing the vein through the pericardium, it should enter posterior to the phrenic nerve so as to avoid angulation and kinking. NB

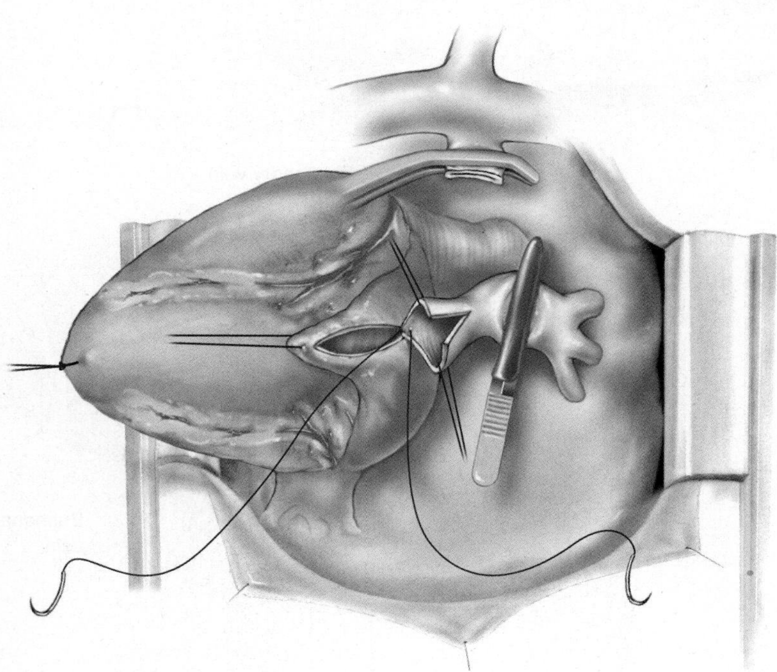

FIG. 19.15 Anastomosing vertical vein to left atrial appendage.

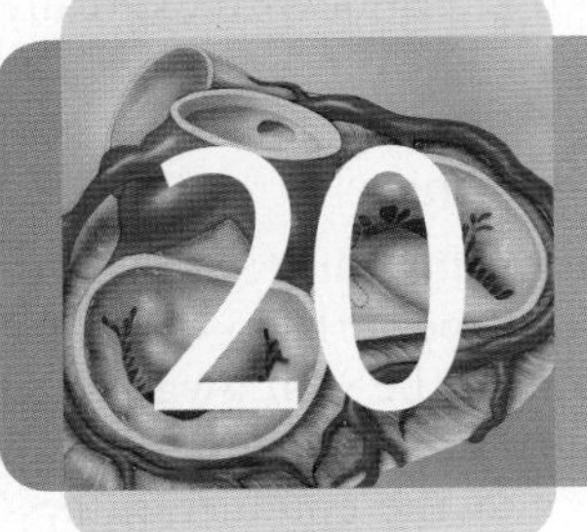

20 Total Anomalous Pulmonary Venous Connection

In a total anomalous pulmonary venous connection, there is no direct continuity between the pulmonary veins and left atrium. For the neonate to survive, there must be some mixing of circulation through a small atrial septal defect or a patent foramen ovale. The pulmonary veins converge to form a pulmonary venous confluence that in turn connects to the systemic venous system and right atrium. This confluence lies posterior to the pericardial sac behind the heart. The common pulmonary vein may rarely be atretic, a condition that results in death after a short time. Anomalous pulmonary venous connection may also be partial (see Chapter 19).

In approximately 25% of patients with total anomalous pulmonary venous connection, the drainage is directly into the right atrium or coronary sinus. The drainage in these cases is therefore exclusively intracardiac. In another 25% of patients, the drainage is through infracardiac connections, that is, the hepatic and portal veins. In 45% of patients, a common pulmonary venous channel drains into an anomalous vertical vein joining the innominate vein or superior vena cava, thereby reaching the right atrium in a supracardiac manner. In approximately 5% of cases, the drainage is mixed, occurring through all three or any combination of two of these connections. Very rarely, there is no connection to either atrium except through some collateral vessels, a condition referred to as common pulmonary vein atresia.

Two-dimensional echocardiography can usually delineate the anatomy and demonstrate any associated anomalies. Rarely is cardiac catheterization or magnetic resonance imaging necessary for patients who have not undergone previous cardiac surgery.

Some surgeons are now employing modifications of the sutureless technique in unoperated patients with pulmonary vein abnormalities or in patients who are at high risk for developing pulmonary vein stenosis. All of these techniques are based on the premise that anastomosing the left atrium to the pericardium surrounding the opening on the pulmonary veins and confluence, rather than to the edges of the veins themselves, will prevent the development of intimal hyperplasia and stenosis.

TECHNIQUE

Most patients are neonates with unstable cardiorespiratory status. Those who present with pulmonary venous obstruction are true surgical emergencies. In neonates, the procedure is usually carried out during a period of deep hypothermic circulatory arrest, although some have advocated performing the operation at mild to modest hypothermia. Continuous cardiopulmonary bypass using bicaval cannulation with aortic cross-clamping and moderate systemic hypothermia is used in older patients.

A median sternotomy is performed. The pericardium is opened, and the distal ascending aorta is cannulated. If hypothermic arrest is to be used, a single cannula is introduced into the right atrium through the right atrial appendage. Cardiopulmonary bypass is initiated, and the patient is cooled for 15 to 20 minutes. The aorta is cross-clamped, and cardioplegic solution is administered into the aortic root. Pump flow is discontinued, and after draining blood from the infant, the venous cannula is clamped and removed.

NB Ligation of the Ductus

The ductus must be dissected and occluded with a tie or metal clip before the initiation of cardiopulmonary bypass. **NB**

Intracardiac Type

A generous right atriotomy is made, somewhat below and parallel to the atrioventricular groove. The edges are retracted with fine sutures to provide maximal exposure. The inside of the right atrium is assessed carefully to delineate the precise anatomy. A patent foramen ovale or an atrial septal defect is always present. There may be a common pulmonary vein orifice opening into the right atrium, or the pulmonary veins may drain directly into the coronary sinus. In the latter case, the orifice of the coronary sinus is somewhat enlarged. The pulmonary venous return is rerouted into the left atrium by enlarging the atrial septal defect and using a pericardial patch to baffle the anomalous veins through the atrial septal defect.

⊘ Size of the Atrial Septal Defect

The defect in the septum must be large enough to allow an unobstructed flow of pulmonary venous return. Most commonly, it is enlarged by extending its inferior margin toward the inferior caval or common pulmonary vein orifice. ⊘

⊘ Cannulation

This type of repair may be performed a mild hypothermia, but it is important to cannulate the inferior vena cava low toward the diaphragm so as not to interfere with exposure of the coronary sinus. ⊘

NB Drainage into the Coronary Sinus

Whenever the common pulmonary vein returns to the coronary sinus, its orifice is extended superiorly to reach the atrial septal defect. This incision must be well away from the anterior margin of the coronary sinus to prevent damage to the atrioventricular node and the conduction system (Fig. 20.1). In addition, the incision in the roof of the

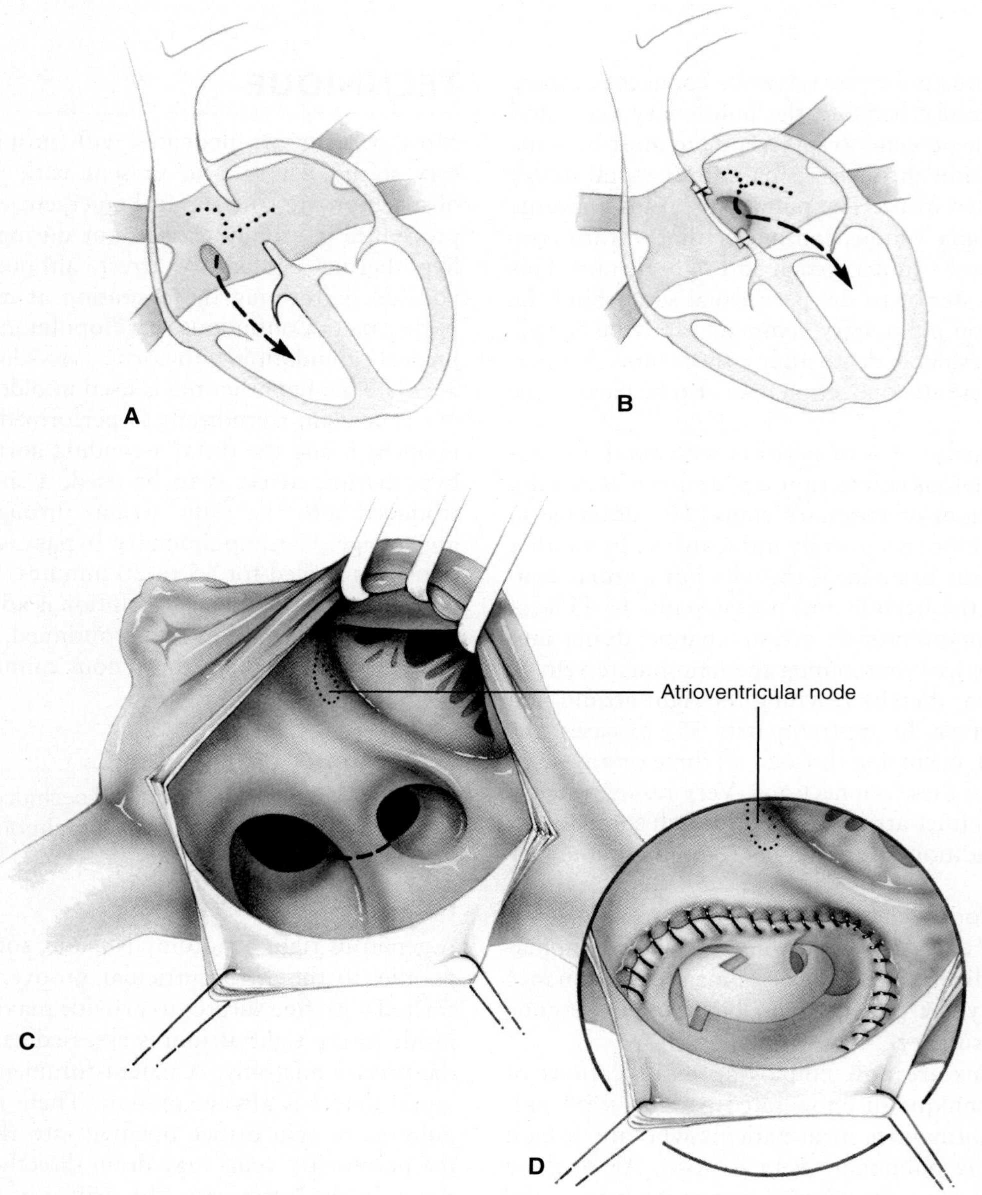

FIG. 20.1 Intracardiac type of total anomalous pulmonary venous drainage. A: Schematic illustration of the defect. B: Schematic illustration of the correction of the defect. C: Operative view of the extension of the atrial septal defect to incorporate the coronary sinus orifice. D: Correction of the anomaly by roofing the septal defect and rerouting the pulmonary venous drainage into the left atrium.

coronary sinus should be extended to the posterior wall of the heart, often, with further resection of the margins of the incision along the roof of the coronary sinus, thereby creating a V-shaped incision. The resulting defect in the atrial septum is closed with an autologous pericardial patch using 6-0 Prolene suture. NB

⊘ Suturing Inside the Coronary Sinus

The continuous suturing of the patch must incorporate the wall of the coronary sinus well below its anterior rim to avoid the conduction system. Alternatively, only very shallow bites of endocardium are taken along the anterior rim of the coronary sinus. ⊘

When the patch is satisfactorily sewn in place, the atriotomy is closed with a continuous 6-0 Prolene suture. The heart is filled with saline, the venous cannula is replaced, cardiopulmonary bypass is recommenced, and the patient is warmed. The aortic cross-clamp is removed, and the cardioplegic site is allowed to bleed freely.

Infracardiac Type

This type is usually associated with obstruction and represents a true surgical emergency. During the cooling phase of cardiopulmonary bypass, the heart is elevated upward and to the right to expose the anomalous descending vertical vein. A 5-0 Prolene suture is placed at the apex of the left ventricle to simplify retraction of the heart. The posterior pericardium is opened, and a vertical incision is made in the anomalous vein to decompress the pulmonary veins (Fig. 20.2). The heart is replaced in the pericardial well until complete cooling is achieved. A marking suture is placed on the tip of the left atrial appendage and reflected leftward to maintain its orientation. The aorta is cross-clamped, and cardioplegia is given. After emptying the circulating volume into the pump, the venous cannula is removed. The heart is again lifted out of the pericardial well, and the previous incision on the anomalous vertical vein is extended longitudinally along the length of the pulmonary confluence.

A matching incision is made on the posterior left atrial wall and is extended onto the left atrial appendage. The suture previously placed on the left atrial appendage helps to expose and position the left atrium for anastomosis. It is of paramount importance for the atriotomy to fall directly on the common pulmonary vein opening when the heart is allowed to resume its normal position.

The superior (rightward) aspect of the anastomosis is performed first with a continuous 7-0 Prolene suture. The inferior (leftward) aspect is similarly completed (Fig. 20.2C).

A small right atriotomy is now performed to close the atrial septal defect, usually a patent foramen ovale. If primary suture closure appears to compromise left atrial size, an autologous pericardial patch should be used (see Chapter 19). Cardiopulmonary bypass is started again, and the patient is warmed.

NB Enlargement of the Common Pulmonary Vein Opening

The vertical incision on the common pulmonary vein channel may be extended slightly onto the left upper pulmonary vein to allow for a larger anastomosis. However, some surgeons advocate a "no touch" technique, staying well away from individual pulmonary venous ostia to reduce the incidence of postoperative pulmonary vein stenosis. Therefore, it may be preferable to enlarge the anastomosis using the divided vertical vein (see subsequent text). NB

NB Vertical Vein Draining below Diaphragm

It is often useful to ligate and divide the vertical vein and use this tissue to create a wider anastomosis. After dividing the vertical vein at the diaphragm, it is opened longitudinally as described in the preceding text. This creates a hood-type opening of the pulmonary venous confluence, which is then anastomosed to a similar-sized opening on the posterior left atrium and left atrial appendage. NB

⊘ Anastomotic Leak

A secure, leakproof anastomosis must be ensured. Suture reinforcement in this area is most difficult and may disrupt or distort the anastomosis. ⊘

Supracardiac Type: Superior Approach

Another technique for dealing with the supracardiac type is the superior approach. The aorta is retracted leftward, and the dome of the left atrium is exposed. A marking suture is placed on the left atrial appendage and reflected leftward to maintain orientation. The posterior pericardium just superior to the dome of the left atrium is incised, and the pulmonary venous confluence is identified. A longitudinal incision is made along the entire length of the confluence and extended into a pulmonary vein orifice, if necessary, to create a patulous opening. A matching incision is made on the posterior aspect of the top of the left atrium, placing gentle traction leftward on the left atrial appendage (Fig. 20.3). The suture line is started at the leftward extent and carried along the superior edge of the atriotomy and the inferior edge of the venous confluence. It is completed by joining the two remaining edges.

NB Closure of the Atrial Septal Defect

A patent foramen ovale or a small atrial septal defect, which is invariably present, must be closed in the usual manner through a right atrial incision. NB

NB Ligation of the Ascending Vertical Vein

The ascending vertical vein is encircled with a heavy tie during cooling. After rewarming, this vein may be kept open as cardiopulmonary bypass is discontinued. This can serve as a pop-off if left atrial pressures are too high. After stable hemodynamics are achieved, the vein is ligated as far away from the venous confluence as possible. NB

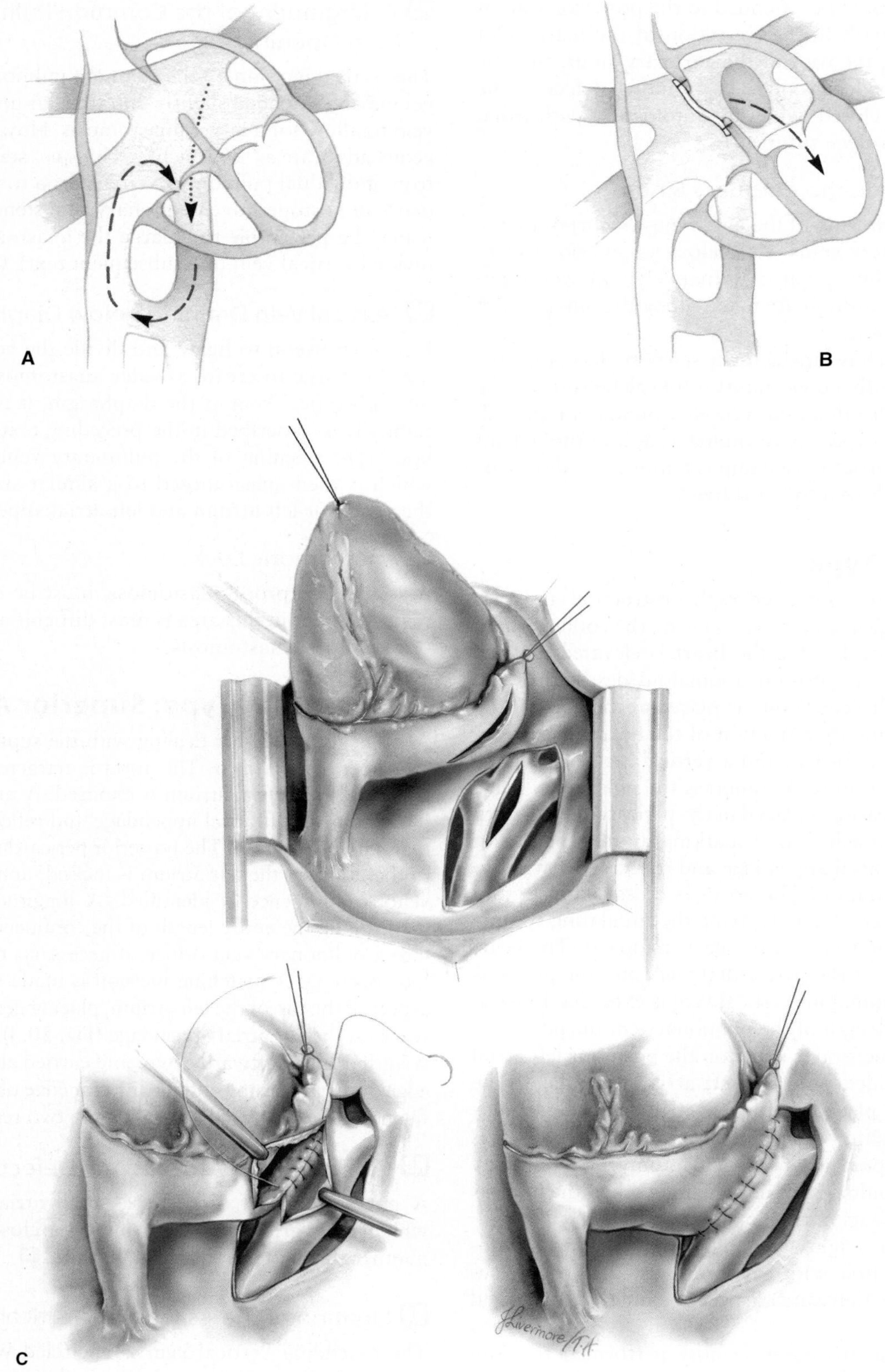

FIG. 20.2 Infracardiac type of total anomalous pulmonary venous drainage. **A:** Schematic illustration of the defect. **B:** Schematic illustration of the correction of the defect. **C:** Operative technique for the correction of the defect.

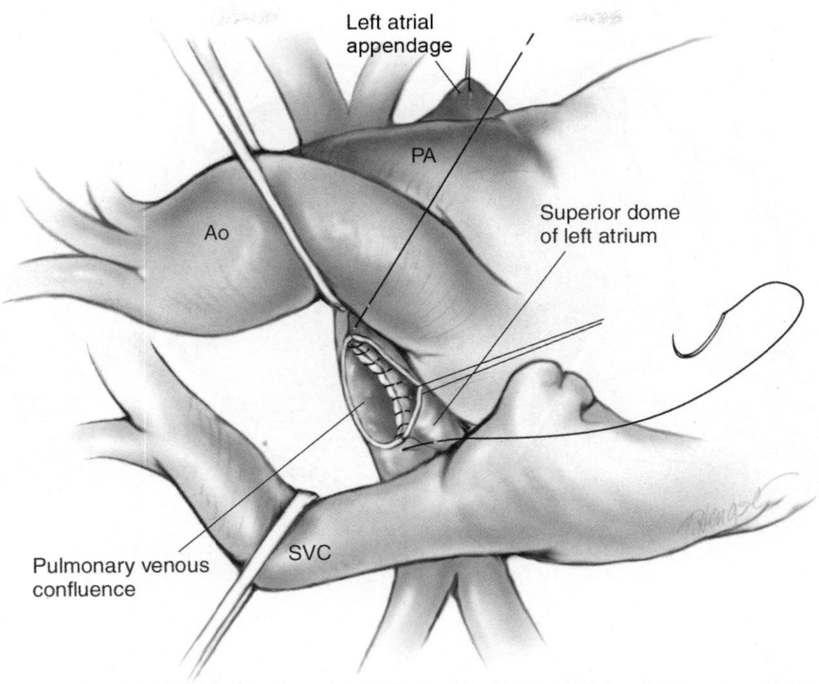

FIG. 20.3 Superior approach to the supracardiac type anastomosing the posterior aspect of the dome of the left atrium to the pulmonary venous confluence. Ao, aorta; PA, posterior aspect; SVC, superior vena cava.

PULMONARY VENOUS OBSTRUCTION

Pulmonary venous obstruction may occur as an isolated lesion, but most often is encountered following repair of total anomalous pulmonary venous connection. Occasionally, it is seen after other congenital heart procedures. The pathology involves a fibrous intimal hyperplasia with some medial hypertrophy. It may be limited to an anastomotic stenosis between the pulmonary venous confluence and the left atrium, or it may involve the ostia of one or more of the pulmonary veins themselves. The diagnosis is usually made with two-dimensional and Doppler echocardiography. Magnetic resonance imaging can be especially useful in visualizing patent pulmonary veins with atretic ostia.

Conventional Technique

An isolated anastomotic stenosis is approached through a right atriotomy and vertical incision on the atrial septum. The narrowed anastomosis is enlarged by removing as much of the tissue as possible between the posterior left atrium and the pulmonary veins (Fig. 20.4). If good adherence between these two structures is present, no suturing may be required. However, if there is any question about the integrity of the adhesions, the endocardium of the left atrial wall and pulmonary venous confluence should be reapproximated with a running 6-0 or 7-0 Prolene suture. If ostial stenosis of one or more pulmonary veins is present, it has been traditionally repaired by endarterectomy excision of the scar tissue or by incising and patching the pulmonary vein using pericardium, Gore-Tex, or atrial tissue. The results of these procedures have been disappointing with high rates of restenosis. More recently, a sutureless technique has been shown to have improved outcomes.

Sutureless Technique

The operation requires that the adhesions between the left atrium and pericardium be left intact. Circulatory arrest may be used, but some surgeons prefer bicaval cannulation. The superior vena cava is cannulated as high as possible and standard aortic and inferior vena caval cannulation is performed. Following aortic cross-clamping and cardioplegia delivery, a left atrial incision is made just posterior to the interatrial groove. The stenotic pulmonary venous ostia are identified. For right pulmonary venous involvement, as much scar tissue as possible is completely excised from the left atrium and by transecting the pulmonary veins beyond the narrowed area. Alternatively, incisions are made across the stenotic areas up to the pericardial reflection (Fig. 20.5A). A posteriorly based flap of pericardium is mobilized and sewn to itself and the

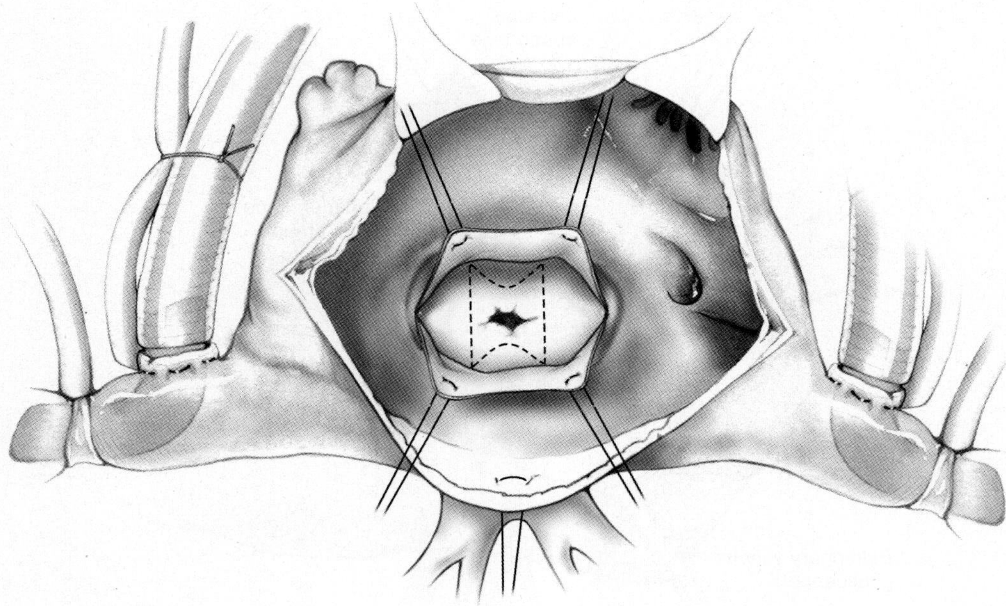

FIG. 20.4 Repair of anastomotic pulmonary vein stenosis through a right atriotomy and transseptal incision. Resection of scar tissue between the left atrium and pulmonary venous confluence results in an unobstructed communication.

right atrial wall above the left atrial opening, avoiding any sutures on the pulmonary venous tissue. This creates a neo-left atrial pouch, allowing unobstructed drainage of the open right pulmonary veins into the left atrium (Fig. 20.5B).

When left pulmonary veins are involved, the repair can be performed from within the left atrial cavity. A portion of left atrial wall is excised around the stenosed vein(s) (Fig. 20.5A). Through the resultant opening, the pulmonary vein(s) is dissected out to the left pericardium and divided beyond the stenosed segment (Fig. 20.6). If there are adequate pericardial adhesions, no suturing is required and the left pulmonary vein(s) drains into the left atrium through the closed posterior pericardial cavity. When pericardial adhesions are insufficient, the pericardium must be sutured to the left atrial wall away from the pulmonary venous ostium. This can be performed from inside the left atrium or from the outside by elevating the apex of the heart toward the right side. Alternatively, the left pulmonary veins can be dealt with from the outside by elevating the apex of the heart and opening the left atrium and stenotic pulmonary veins as described for right pulmonary vein stenosis. A pericardial flap is mobilized and sewn to itself and the left atrial wall as described in the preceding text.

NB Identifying Pulmonary Venous Ostia

The orifices of the stenotic pulmonary veins may be reduced to pinholes and can be difficult to identify. NB

⊘ Phrenic Nerve Injury

The suture lines for both the right-sided repair and the outside approach for left pulmonary vein repair come close to the phrenic nerves. Often in a reoperation, the course of the phrenic nerve cannot be appreciated from within the pericardial space. Therefore, it is best to open the pleural space(s) to check the location of the nerve before placing the sutures in the pericardium. Superficial bites over the nerve may be taken, or in some cases, the nerve with its pedicle can be mobilized away from the pericardium (Fig. 20.5B). ⊘

NB Sutureless Technique as Primary Procedure

Many have advocated for sutureless repair as a primary approach toward total anomalous pulmonary venous return, in particular for patients with heterotaxy syndrome, mixed total anomalous pulmonary venous return, and those with unusual orientation of the common confluence. Here, the development of a pericardial well around the confluence and veins affords an adjustment for orientation abnormalities. The plane between the pericardium and the pulmonary veins must be developed carefully, as this provides exposure to the veins as well as limits the borders ("well") of the "neo-atrium" (Fig. 20.7). NB

⊘ Bleeding

Suture line bleeding can be difficult to identify with the sutureless technique, in part because lifting the heart

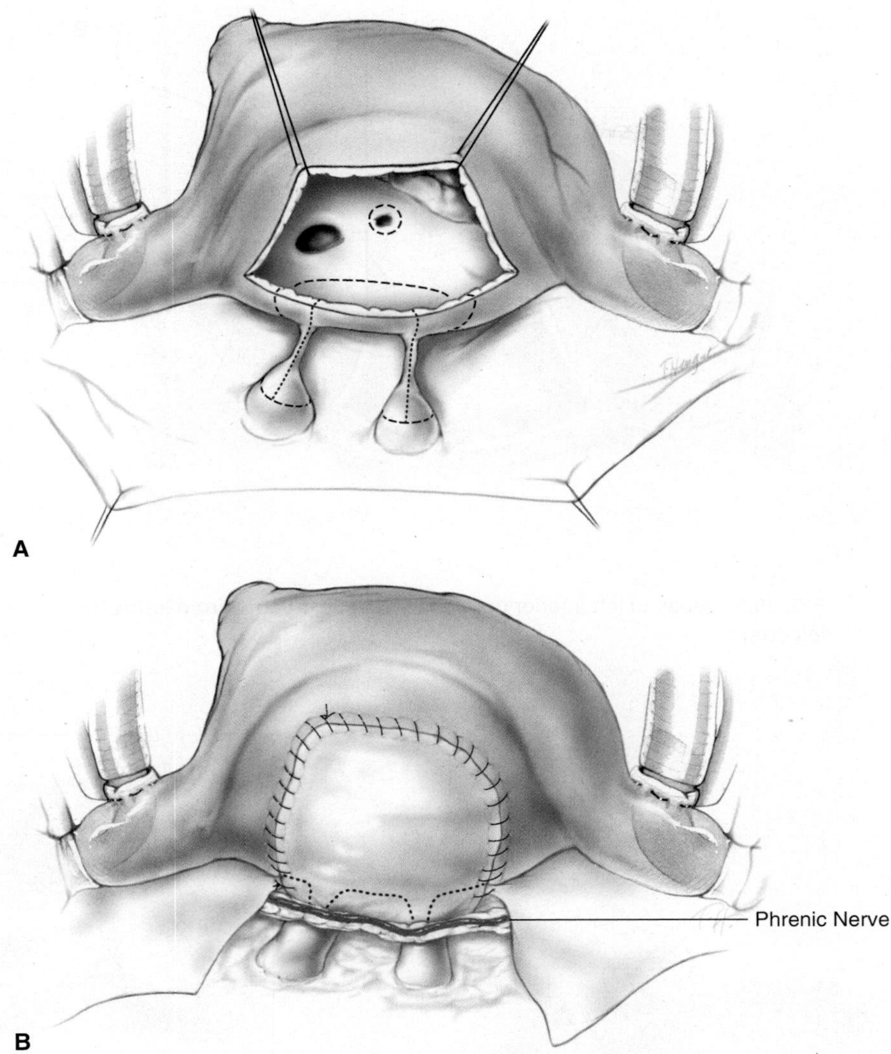

FIG. 20.5 Right-sided sutureless repair. **A:** Through a standard left atriotomy, the stenotic ostía are identified and the scar tissue either totally excised (*dashed lines*) or incisions made across the narrowed areas (*dotted lines*). **B:** Flap of pericardium sewn to itself and right atrial wall.

to inspect the suture line may tighten the anastomosis and mask the bleeding. In addition, inadvertent entry into the left pleural space, even if deemed trivial, can be the source of considerable hemorrhage and difficult to control. ⊘

COR TRIATRIATUM

Cor triatriatum is a rare defect in which the pulmonary veins drain into a common atrial chamber, usually located behind and above the true left atrium. This chamber is separated from the left atrium by a diaphragm. The upper chamber may or may not communicate with the right atrium through an atrial septal defect or foramen ovale.

Surgical Technique

Complete correction is usually performed on continuous cardiopulmonary bypass using bicaval cannulation. A transatrial or transseptal incision generally provides excellent exposure. The transatrial incision is extended across the right atrium and then across the atrial septum to the fossa ovalis (see Transatrial Oblique Approach section in Chapter 6). Retractors are placed beneath the edge of the atrial septum to inspect the left atrium. The entrance of

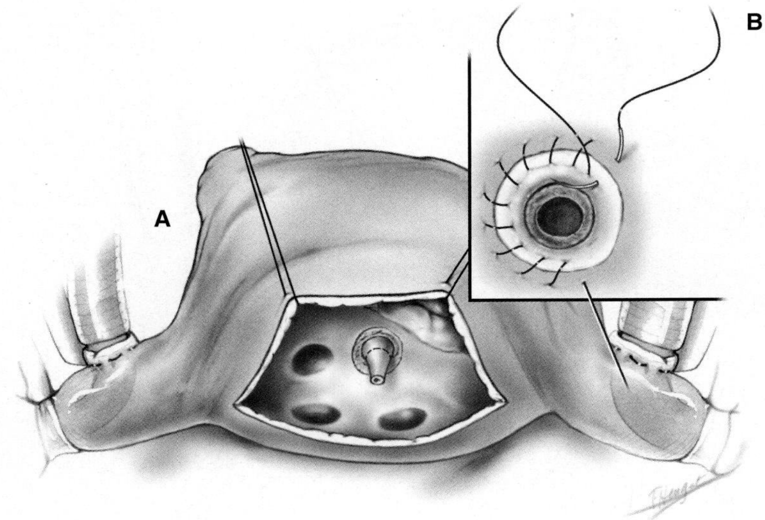

FIG. 20.6 Repair of left inferior pulmonary vein obstruction from inside the left atrium.

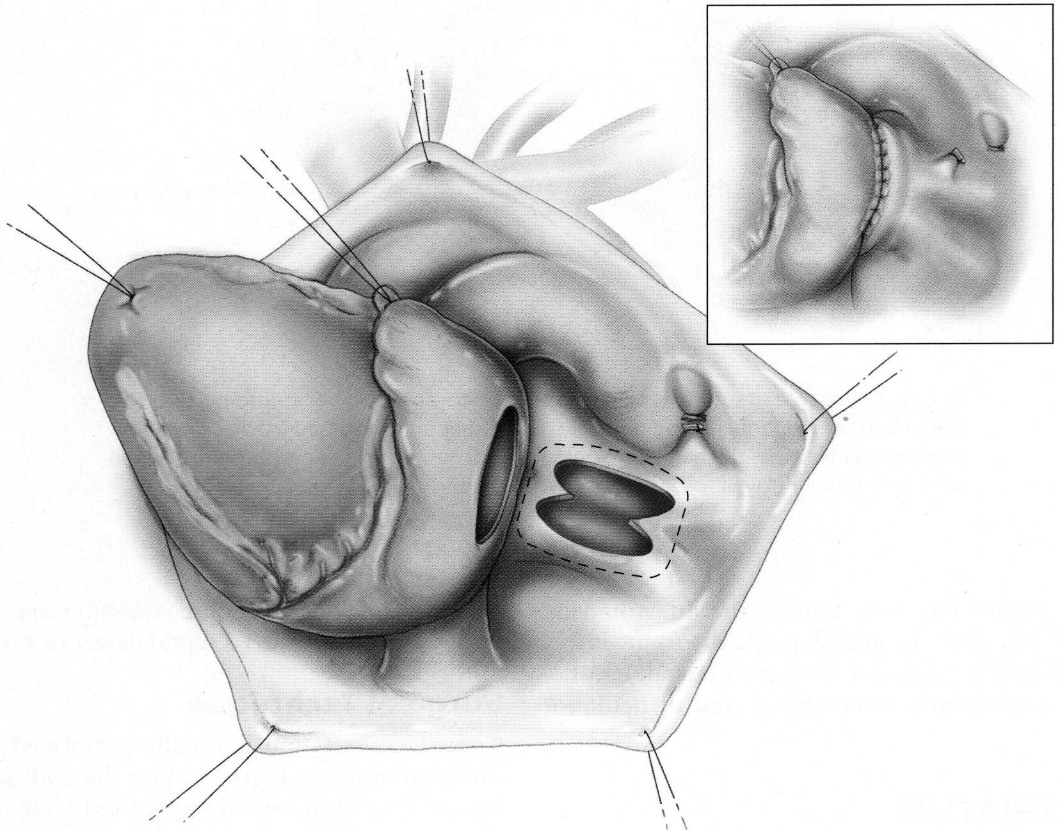

FIG. 20.7 The pulmonary vein confluence is opened into each of the vein orifices, but the "sutureless" connection is created between the left atrium and the area shown in the dotted line; this anastomosis is to the pericardium (not the underlying pulmonary vein tissue) that lies adjacent to the opening. Particular care must be made not to enter the left pleural space when opening the veins.

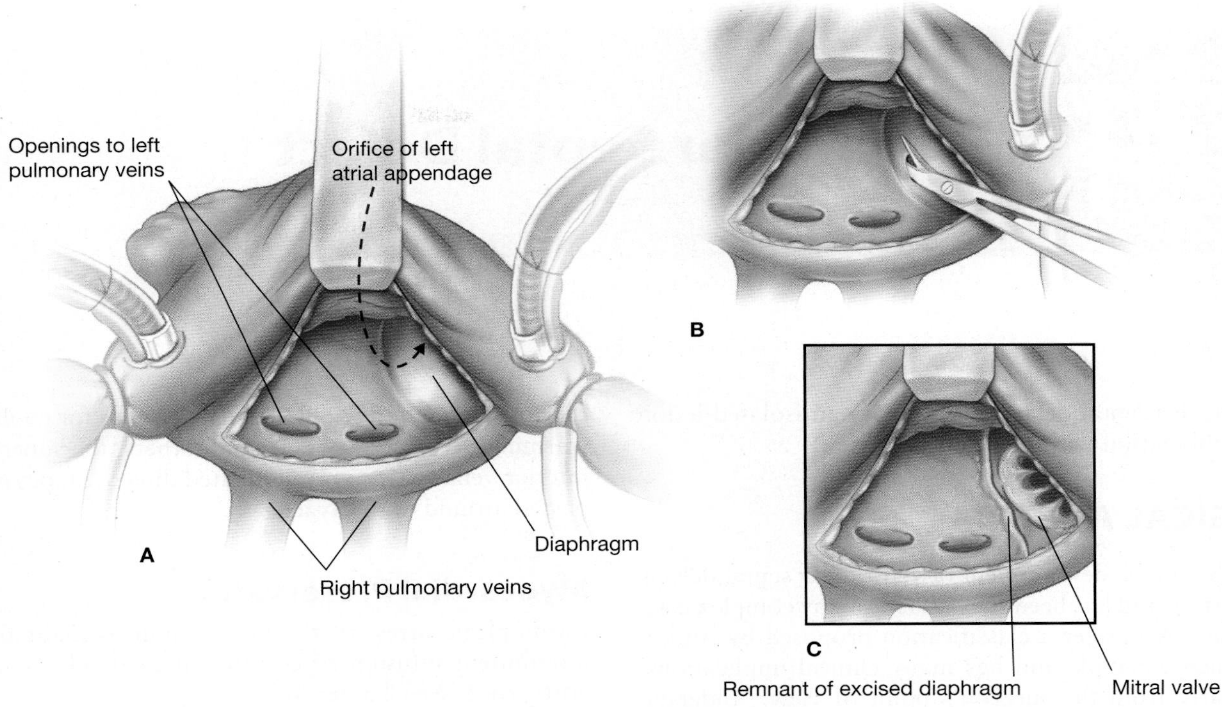

FIG. 20.8 With the first inspection of anatomy, it is important to delineate the location of the pulmonary vein orifices and the left atrial appendage. **A:** If the orifice of the appendage is easily visualized, the diaphragm may represent a supravalvar mitral ring. **B:** Removing the diaphragm to demonstrate the orifice of the appendage (the diaphragm separates the appendage from the veins) suggests this is cor triatriatum. **C:** Pulmonary veins, appendage, and mitral valve should all be visible at the end of the procedure.

all four pulmonary veins must be identified, as well as the left atrial appendage and mitral valve. The membrane is resected, taking care not to extend the incision outside the heart. This membrane can be densely adherent to the mitral valve apparatus (Fig. 20.8).

The incision on the atrial septum can then be closed primarily or more often with a patch of autologous pericardium prepared with glutaraldehyde using a running 5-0 or 6-0 Prolene suture. The incisions on the right superior pulmonary vein and right atrium are then closed with a running 5-0 or 6-0 Prolene suture. The patient is rewarmed, the aortic cross-clamp is removed, and deairing is carried out in the usual manner.

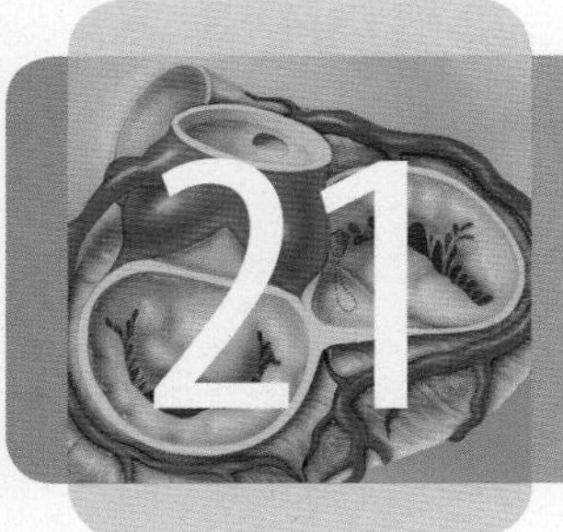

21 Ventricular Septal Defect

A ventricular septal defect can occur as an isolated lesion or in combination with other anomalies.

SURGICAL ANATOMY

The embryologic development of ventricular septal defects is interesting and has been the basis for many complex classifications. We prefer a classification proposed by Anderson, which is simple and has many clinical implications, particularly from the surgeon's point of view. Anderson divides ventricular septal defects into perimembranous, subarterial-infundibular, and muscular types.

The perimembranous variety of ventricular septal defects encompasses subgroups of defects that occur near the membranous segment of the interventricular septum and includes those septal defects commonly seen in tetralogy of Fallot and atrioventricular septal defects (Fig. 21.1). Because the path of the conduction tissue is intimately related to the inferior rim of these defects, an accurate knowledge of the surgical anatomy of this region is most helpful.

The atrioventricular node is situated in its usual position at the apex of the triangle of Koch, whose boundaries consist of the septal attachment of the tricuspid valve, tendon of Todaro, and the coronary sinus as its base (Fig. 21.2). The conduction tissue passes from the atrioventricular node as the bundle of His through the central fibrous body and the tricuspid annulus into the ventricular septum, following a course along the inferior rim of the defect toward the left ventricular side of the septum.

SURGICAL APPROACH

All forms of ventricular septal defects are approached through a median sternotomy although some have used right thoracotomy.

Cannulation

Cardiopulmonary bypass with moderate systemic hypothermia is used in most patients. In very small infants (<2 kg), deep hypothermic arrest using a single venous cannula through the right atrial appendage for cooling and warming may be preferred. In all others, the superior and inferior venae cavae are cannulated directly; tapes are then passed around both cavae.

Myocardial Preservation

Cardioplegic arrest of the myocardium is maintained by intermittent infusion of cold blood cardioplegia into the aortic root (see Chapter 3).

TRANSATRIAL APPROACH TO A VENTRICULAR SEPTAL DEFECT

Almost all the perimembranous and atrioventricular canal types of ventricular septal defects and many of the muscular variety can be exposed and closed through the right atrium. The subarterial-infundibular type is best approached through pulmonary arteriotomy.

The aorta is cross-clamped, and cardioplegic solution is administered into the aortic root. The venae caval snares are then snugged down. A longitudinal or oblique atriotomy is made, starting at a point 0.5 to 1 cm anterior and parallel to the sulcus terminalis, and is extended toward the orifice of the inferior vena cava. The edges of the incision are then retracted to provide a good exposure of the tricuspid valve and the triangle of Koch (Fig. 21.3).

⊘ Coexisting Patent Ductus Arteriosus

If a patent ductus arteriosus is present, it should be occluded before the initiation of cardiopulmonary bypass to prevent pulmonary overcirculation and suboptimal systemic perfusion (see Chapter 14). ⊘

⊘ Sinoatrial Node Injury

The sinoatrial node is vulnerable to injury from the snare around the superior vena cava. It can also be injured if the atriotomy is extended too far superiorly. ⊘

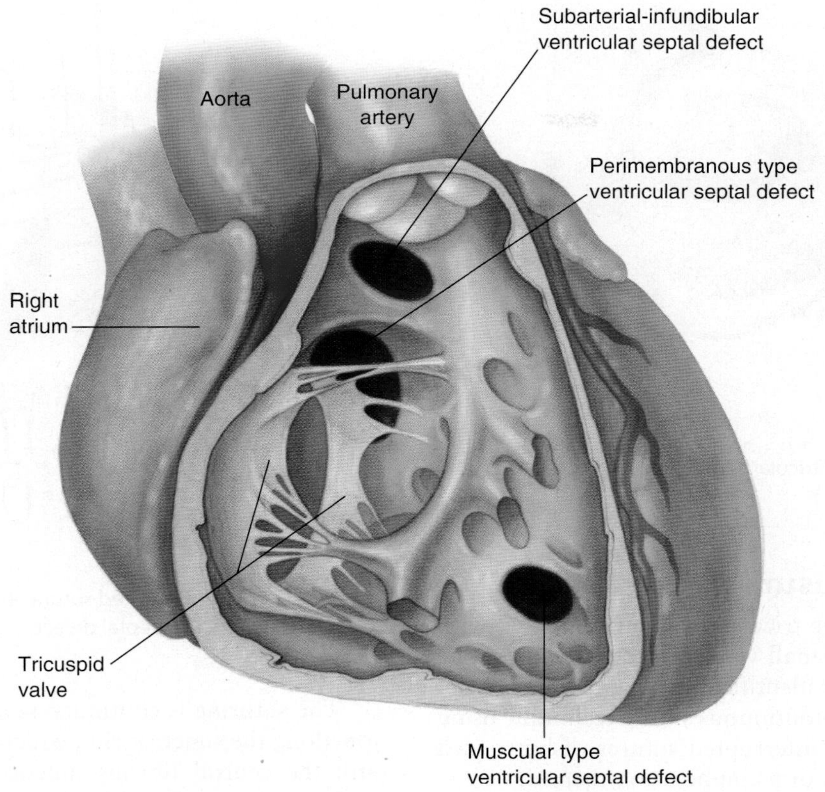

FIG. 21.1 Types of ventricular septal defects.

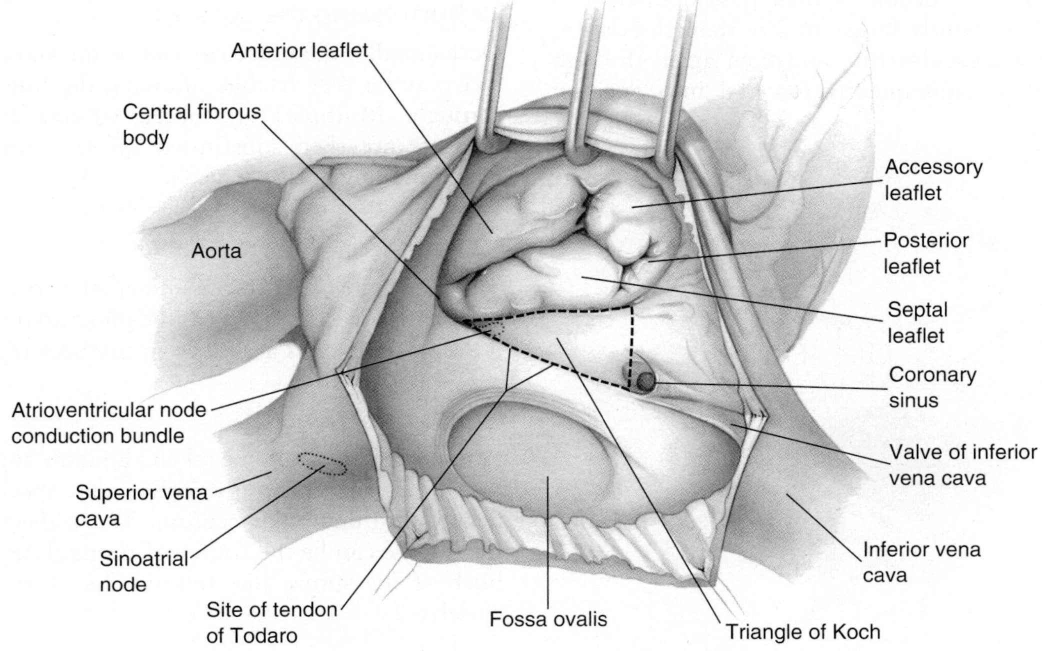

FIG. 21.2 Surgical anatomy of the right atrium.

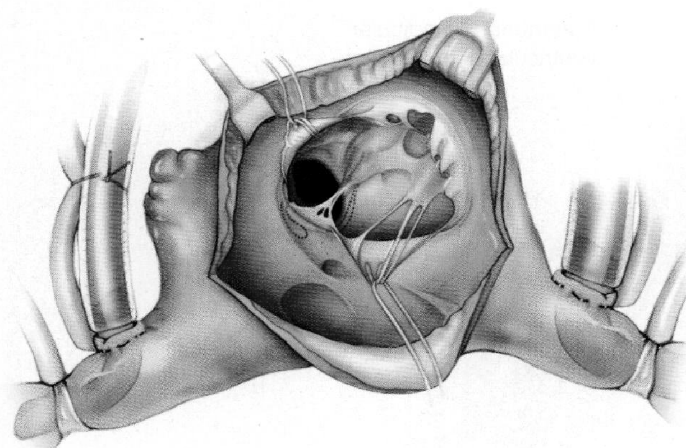

FIG. 21.3 Exposure of a ventricular septal defect by retracting the tricuspid valve leaflets.

Technique for Closure

The anterior leaflet of the tricuspid valve is retracted with a 6-0 Prolene suture or small vein retractor to expose the defect and its margins for identification (Fig. 21.3). The defect can be closed with a continuous suture technique using 5-0 Prolene, or multiple interrupted sutures of buttressed with Teflon felt pledgets, or a combination thereof.

Continuous Suture Technique

With a double-armed, half-circle needle of 5-0 Prolene, the suturing is started at the 12 o'clock position along the muscular rim. The needle is then passed through a patch of Gore-Tex slightly larger in size than the defect, again through the muscular rim, and then again through the patch, which is subsequently lowered into position (Fig. 21.4).

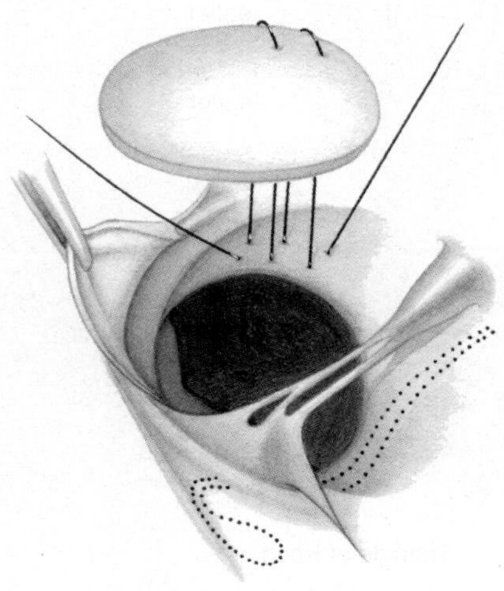

FIG. 21.4 Patch closure of a ventricular septal defect using a continuous suture technique.

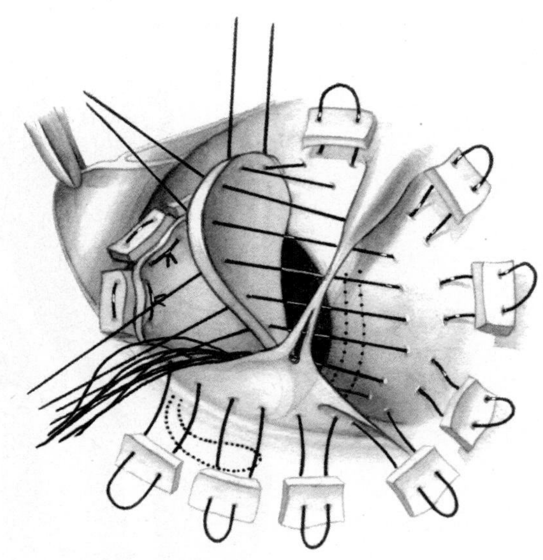

FIG. 21.5 Interrupted suture technique for closure of a ventricular septal defect.

The suturing is continued in a counterclockwise direction along the superior rim, which overlies the aortic valve, until the central fibrous junction of the septum, aortic root, and tricuspid annulus is reached. The needle is passed through the septal leaflet of the tricuspid valve. During the procedure, the placement of each stitch is facilitated by the assistant applying slight traction on the Prolene suture.

⊘ Buttressing the Sutures

Occasionally, the muscular rim of the ventriculoseptal defect may be very friable, allowing the fine Prolene to cut through. Multiple interrupted sutures buttressed with pledgets are then substituted for the continuous suture technique (Fig. 21.5). ⊘

⊘ Injury to the Aortic Valve

The aortic valve leaflets are immediately below the superior margin of the defect and can be punctured during suturing if deep needle bites are taken in this area (Fig. 21.6). ⊘

⊘ Residual defects

Particular care should be taken along the superior aspect of the defect adjacent to the aortic valve, specifically the area near the infundibular septum. The trabeculations within the muscle can be the source of residual defects; this is less likely if the suture line follows the aortic annulus quite closely. ⊘

NB Transitional Sutures

The junction of the tricuspid annulus, aortic root, and septum is a vulnerable area where a residual defect may occur.

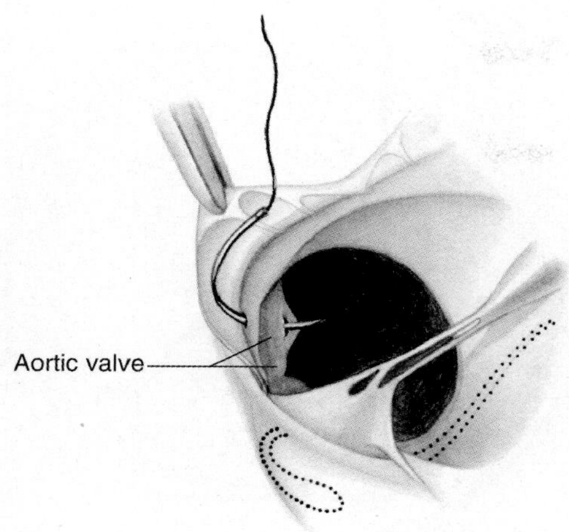

FIG. 21.6 Proximity of an aortic valve leaflet to the rim of the septal defect.

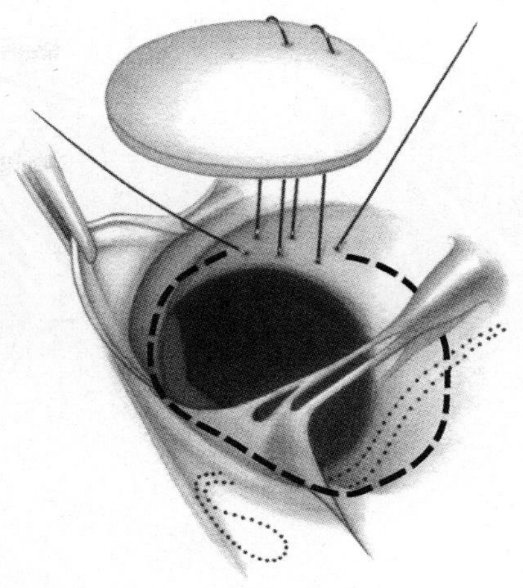

FIG. 21.8 Sutures are placed 3 to 5 mm from the rim of the defect inferiorly to avoid the conduction tract.

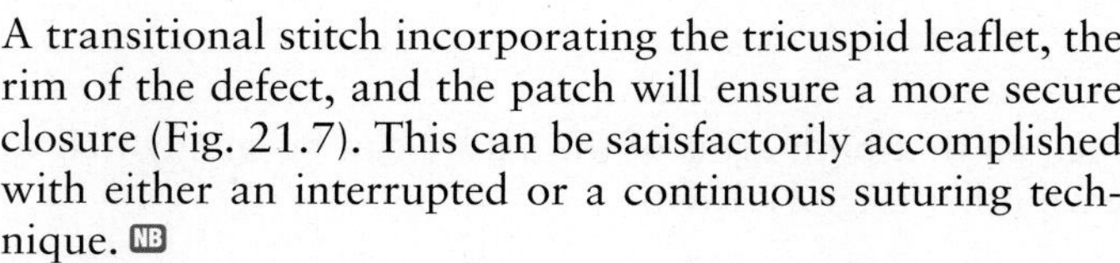

A transitional stitch incorporating the tricuspid leaflet, the rim of the defect, and the patch will ensure a more secure closure (Fig. 21.7). This can be satisfactorily accomplished with either an interrupted or a continuous suturing technique. NB

The other arm of the Prolene suture is then continued in a clockwise direction; superficial bites that include only endocardium are taken along the inferior rim of the defect, until the tricuspid leaflet is reached (Fig. 21.7). Alternatively, the other arm of the suture is continued, moving outward to a distance of 3 to 5 mm from the rim of the defect to avoid the underlying conduction tissue (Fig. 21.8).

⊘ Prevention of Heart Block

As already described, the bundle of His pierces the central fibrous body and the tricuspid annulus before penetrating the ventricular septum, where it follows a course along the inferior margin of the defect toward the left ventricular side of the septum. Because suturing along this course can be hazardous and culminate in heart block (Fig. 21.9A), shallow superficial bites are taken that include only the whitish endocardium close to the rim of the defect. In fact, the needle should be visible through the translucent endocardium (Fig. 21.9B). A more conservative and safer approach is to place sutures 3 to 5 mm from the inferior rim of the defect (Fig. 21.8). ⊘

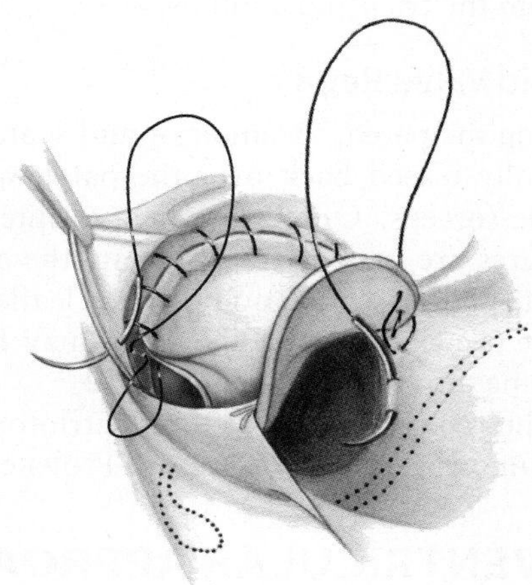

FIG. 21.7 Continuous suture technique for closure of a ventricular septal defect. Note upper needle passing through patch, muscular rim, and then tricuspid leaflet to complete transitional stitch.

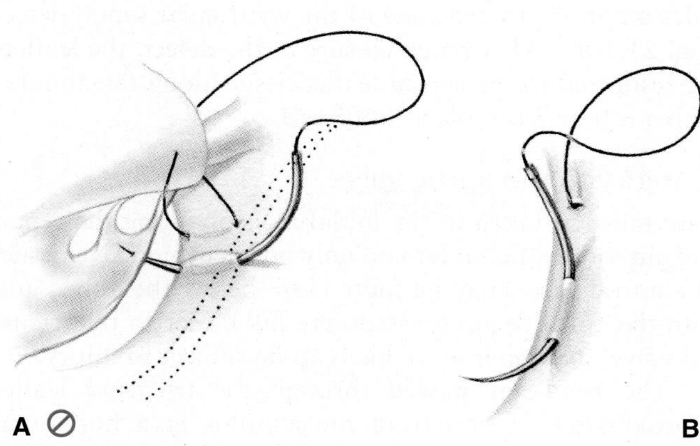

FIG. 21.9 **A and B:** Shallow bites of endocardium prevent the occurrence of heart block.

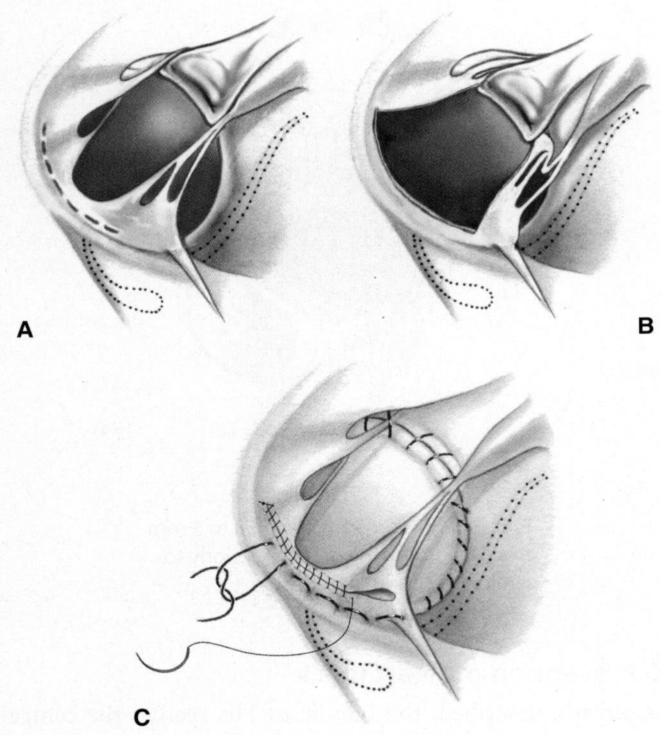

FIG. 21.10 **A:** Line of detachment of septal and anterior leaflet to provide improved exposure. **B:** Retraction of detached leaflets. **C:** Completing closure of ventricular septal defect and reattaching leaflets to annular rim.

NB Interference by Chordae Tendineae and Papillary Muscles

If the view of the ventricular septal defect is obscured by chordae tendineae or papillary muscles, the septal leaflet and a portion of the anterior leaflet of the tricuspid valve may be detached, leaving a 2- to 3-mm rim of tissue along the annulus (Fig. 21.10A). Retraction of these leaflets provides an unobstructed view of the ventricular septal defect (Fig. 21.10B). After patch closure of the defect, the leaflets are resutured to the rim of leaflet tissue along the annulus with a 6-0 or 7-0 Prolene suture. NB

⊘ Injury to the aortic valve

Care must be taken in the initial incision along the septal and anterior leaflet to remain only on tricuspid valve tissue. The aortic valve may lie quite close below the valve, and with the aorta decompressed may fall closer to the tricuspid valve, making it more likely to be subject to injury. ⊘

The needle is passed through the tricuspid leaflet approximately 2 mm from the annulus in a horizontal mattress fashion back into the right ventricle, taking a horizontal mattress bite of the patch before penetrating the leaflet once again. This maneuver is continued in a clockwise direction until the other arm of the Prolene suture is met, so that both arms of the suture can be snugly tied to each other (Fig. 21.10C).

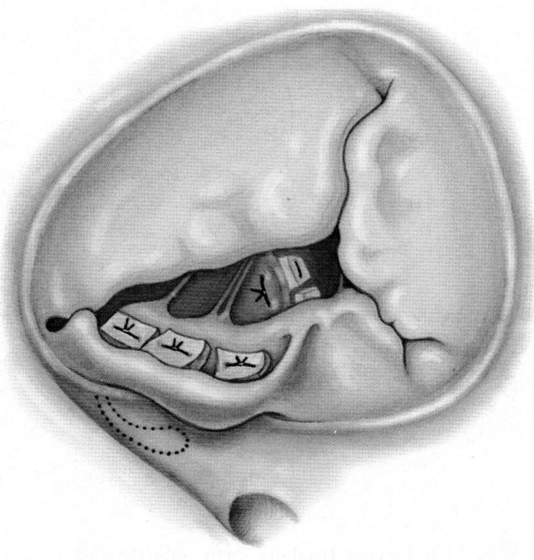

FIG. 21.11 Incorporation of excessive leaflet tissue in the suture line producing tricuspid valve insufficiency.

⊘ Buttressing the Sutures

The Prolene suture may cut through the thin, tricuspid leaflet tissue. The suture line can be buttressed with multiple pledgets or a strip of autologous pericardium. With the interrupted suture technique, pledgeted sutures are used. ⊘

⊘ Prevention of Tricuspid Insufficiency

Incorporation of excessive leaflet tissue in the suture line results in tricuspid insufficiency (Fig. 21.11). The suture line along the tricuspid leaflet should not exceed a distance of 2 mm from the tricuspid annulus. ⊘

NB Tricuspid Valve Repair

After securing the patch, the anterior and septal leaflet tissue is carefully teased back over the patch with a nerve hook or fine forceps. Often, one or two interrupted 6-0 Prolene sutures are used to approximate the anterior and septal leaflets and/or septal and posterior leaflets to ensure a competent tricuspid valve. The valve may be tested by injecting saline into the right ventricle. NB

When the repair is completed, the atriotomy is closed with a continuous suture of 5-0 or 6-0 Prolene.

TRANSVENTRICULAR APPROACH TO VENTRICULAR SEPTAL DEFECT

All septal defects, except those occurring near the left ventricular apex, can be closed through a right ventriculotomy. When there are associated lesions, such as infundibular

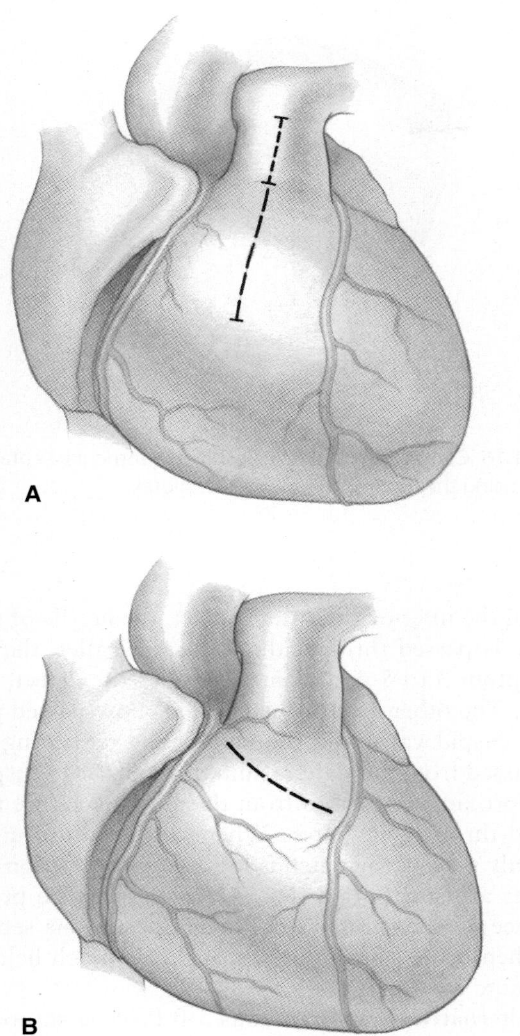

FIG. 21.12 **A:** Right ventriculotomy along entire length of infundibulum (*large dashed line*) and vertical pulmonary arteriotomy from annulus to confluence (*small dashed line*). **B:** Transverse right ventriculotomy.

stenosis (as in tetralogy of Fallot), a vertical ventriculotomy may be used. A transverse ventriculotomy has some theoretical advantages, especially when an aberrant coronary artery crosses the anterior wall of the right ventricle (Fig. 21.12).

⊘ Avoiding the Coronary Arteries

Every precaution should be taken to avoid dividing an aberrant coronary artery (Fig. 21.13). When the left anterior descending coronary artery originates from the right coronary artery, it courses across the anterior wall of the right ventricle. Its accidental division results in severe and often fatal myocardial dysfunction. If this unfortunate event occurs, the two severed ends of the vessel should be oversewn, and the left internal thoracic artery harvested

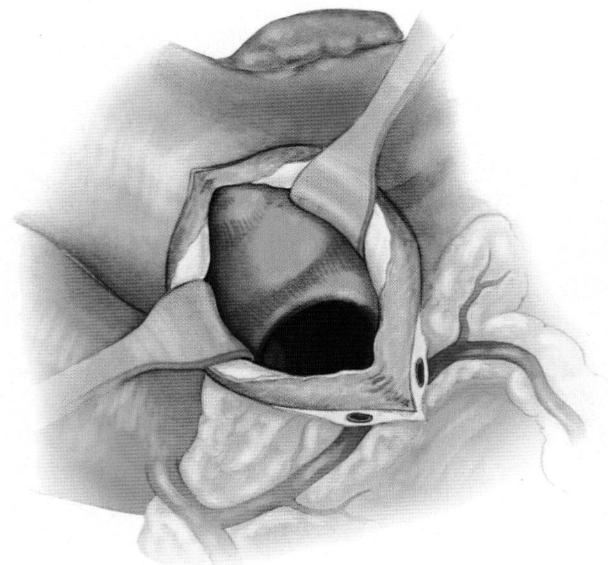

FIG. 21.13 Division of an aberrant coronary artery by a ventriculotomy.

and anastomosed to the more distal left anterior descending coronary artery (see Chapter 9). ⊘

NB Infundibular Hypertrophy Obscuring the Location of the Defect

Infundibular hypertrophy may obscure the location of the perimembranous type of defect. The hypertrophied muscle bands should be incised and/or excised to the extent needed to relieve the outflow tract obstruction. If visualization of the ventricular septal defect is still not adequate, the defect should be approached transatrially (see Chapter 23). NB

Interrupted Suture Technique

The technique for transventricular closure of the perimembranous ventricular septal defect is essentially the same as that described for the transatrial approach. The edges of the ventriculotomy incision are retracted with fine pledgeted sutures or vein retractors. The margins of the defect are inspected and interrupted fine pledgeted braided 4-0 or 5-0 double-armed sutures are started at the 12 o'clock position, along the muscular rim in an everting manner. Both needles are then passed through a patch of Gore-Tex slightly larger than the defect (Fig. 21.14). Slight traction on this stitch improves exposure and facilitates the placement of the next stitch (Fig. 21.15).

Suturing is continued in this manner in a counterclockwise direction along the superior rim (that overlies the aortic valve) until the central fibrous junction of the septum, aortic root, and tricuspid annulus is reached. The needle of the next stitch is passed through the tricuspid tissue close to the annulus, the muscular rim of the defect,

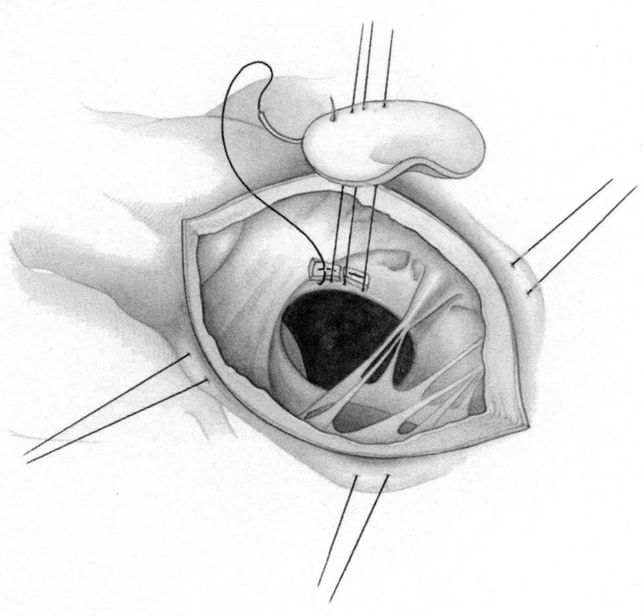

FIG. 21.14 Technique for closure of a ventricular septal defect by interrupted sutures.

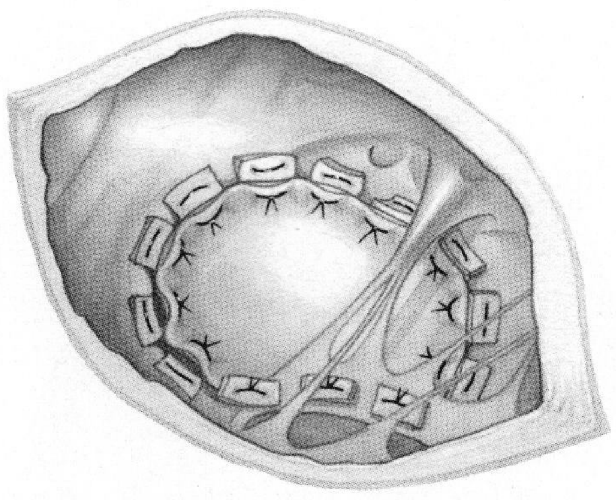

FIG. 21.16 Completion of patch closure of ventricular septal defect using the interrupted suture technique.

and the patch. The other arm of the needle is now passed through the tricuspid tissue and the patch. This is a true transitional stitch.

Suturing is then continued from the starting point in a clockwise direction, moving outward to a distance of 3 to 5 mm from the rim of the defect to avoid the underlying conduction tissue. Where the tricuspid annulus becomes part of the inferior rim of the defect, the needle of the next suture is passed through the tricuspid leaflet, the muscular septum 3 to 5 mm from the rim of the defect, and the patch. The other arm of the needle is now passed through the tricuspid valve and the patch. The remaining sutures are passed from the right atrium through the tricuspid leaflet approximately 2 mm from the annulus before they are passed through the patch. When all the sutures are satisfactorily placed, the patch is lowered into position and the sutures are snugly tied (Fig. 21.16). It may be preferable to place all the sutures first, tagging each one separately, and then bring each suture through the patch held by the assistant.

Alternatively, a continuous 5-0 Prolene suture can be used, sewing the patch to the ventricular side of the septal leaflet 1 to 2 mm from the annulus in the region of the tricuspid valve. When the septal defect has been satisfactorily repaired, the ventriculotomy is closed with two layers of continuous 5-0 Prolene suture (Fig. 21.17).

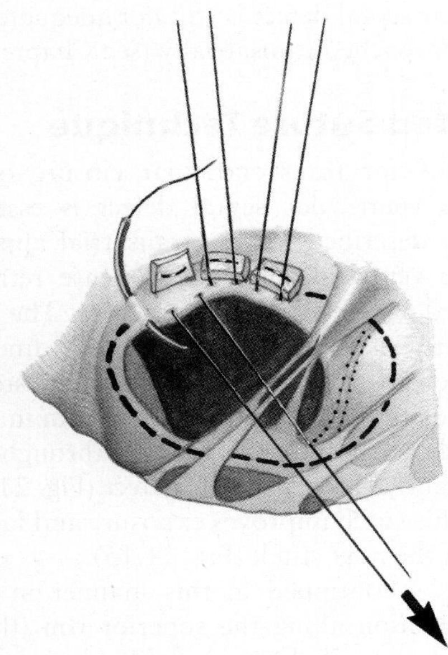

FIG. 21.15 Exposure is improved by gentle traction on the previously placed stitch.

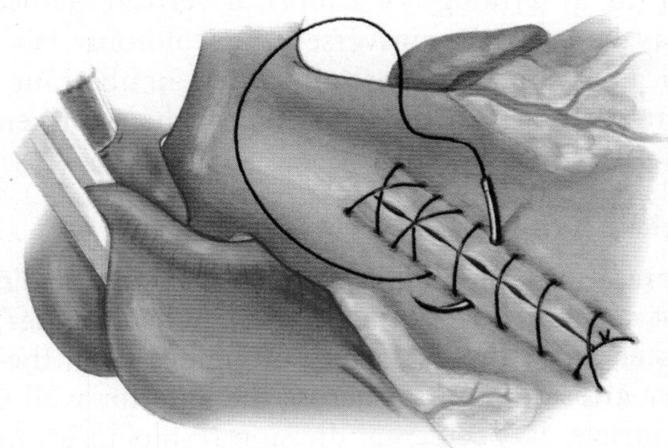

FIG. 21.17 Closure of ventriculotomy.

⊘ Injury to the Aortic Valve

The aortic valve leaflets are immediately below the superior margin of the defect and can be punctured during suturing if deep needle bites are taken in this area. Suturing in this area should therefore incorporate the crista marginalis, which holds sutures well. ⊘

⊘ Prevention of Heart Block

The bundle of His pierces the central fibrous body and the tricuspid annulus before crossing into the ventricular septum and following a course along the inferior margin of the defect toward the left ventricular side of the septum. Suturing along this course can be somewhat hazardous and may culminate in heart block. When using the interrupted suture technique, the safest approach is to place sutures 3 to 5 mm from the inferior rim of the defect. ⊘

⊘ Transitional Sutures

The junction where the tricuspid annulus forms the margin of the defect is also most vulnerable to a residual septal defect. Again, a transitional stitch incorporating the tricuspid leaflet, the muscular septum well away from the rim of the defect, and the patch (in that order) ensures a more secure closure. ⊘

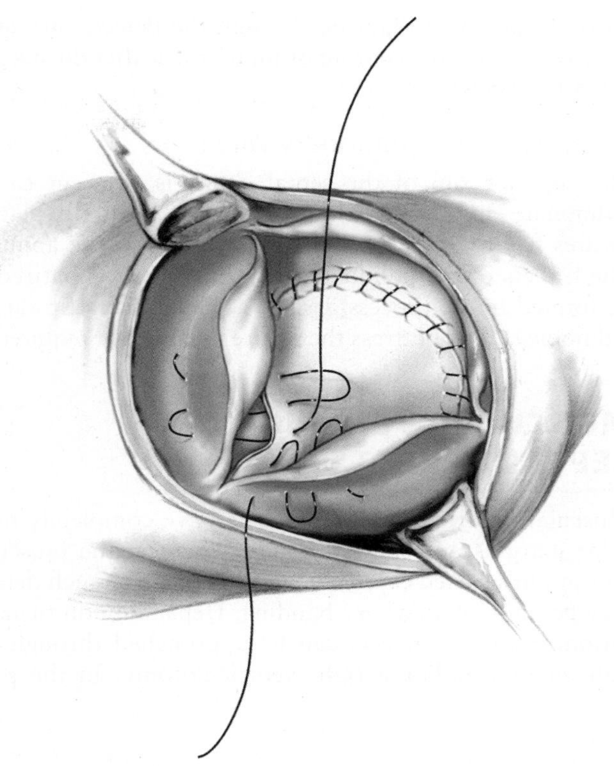

FIG. 21.18 Closure of a subarterial ventricular septal defect through the pulmonary artery.

SUBARTERIAL VENTRICULAR SEPTAL DEFECT

These defects may be associated with the development of aortic insufficiency. Even if small, these defects should probably be closed to prevent progression of aortic insufficiency and aortic valve leaflet damage.

Technique for Closure

A right ventriculotomy may be used; however, the transpulmonary approach is preferred. If there is significant aortic insufficiency, the aortic valve should be repaired before the ventricular septal defect is closed.

Standard cannulation is performed with a single venous cannula. Cardiopulmonary bypass is commenced, and moderate systemic cooling is begun. The aorta is cross-clamped, and cold blood potassium cardioplegic solution is infused directly into the aortic root.

The main pulmonary artery is opened transversely just above the commissures. A small vein retractor is then placed through the pulmonary valve to expose the ventricular septal defect. To further assess the degree of the aortic valve prolapse and insufficiency, blood cardioplegic solution is administered into the aortic root. All the aortic cusps may be visualized through the septal defect if it is at least moderate in size. In fact, one of the aortic valve leaflets may be prolapsing through and partially closing the defect. An autologous pericardial patch fixed with glutaraldehyde or patch of gortex is cut slightly larger than the defect and attached to the right ventricular aspect of the defect using 6-0 or 5-0 Prolene continuous suture. Superiorly, the patch must be secured to annulus of the pulmonic valve. In this area, the needle is brought through the patch and then passed through the base of the valve leaflet. The needle is then placed back through the leaflet and again through the patch. This weaving suture line is continued until the edge of the defect is seen apart from the pulmonary annulus. If the leaflet tissue is friable, the pulmonary artery side of the suture line can be reinforced with a thin strip of pericardium. When the suture line is completed, the sutures are tied snugly (Fig. 21.18).

The pulmonary arteriotomy is then closed with a running 5-0 or 6-0 Prolene suture. The aortic cross-clamp is removed after filling the heart, and deairing is carried out through the cardioplegic site. Transesophageal echo evaluation should confirm a competent aortic valve and complete closure of the ventricular septal defect.

⊘ Injury to the Aortic Valve

Because there is often a close association between the aortic and pulmonary valve annulus with this anomaly, care must be taken in placing the sutures along the superior aspect of the ventricular septal defect. A too deeply placed needle may incorporate the aortic leaflet tissue and result in significant aortic insufficiency. In addition, if one of the aortic leaflets is prolapsing through the defect, care must be taken to not incorporate or injure the leaflet during closure of the defect. ⊘

⊘ Injury to the Pulmonary Valve

The superior rim of the septal defect is adjacent to the pulmonary annulus. Closure of the defect entails placing sutures from within the pulmonary artery at the annulus. The leaflets of the pulmonary valve can be traumatized or perforated in the process. Use of a pericardial strip on the pulmonic side to buttress the suture line may be required. ⊘

MUSCULAR VENTRICULAR SEPTAL DEFECTS

Muscular ventricular septal defects have completely muscular margins and may occur anywhere in the muscular septum. In selected cases, the first approach to such defects may be pulmonary artery banding. Depending on their location, muscular defects can be approached through the right atrium and/or a right ventriculotomy. In the past, a limited left ventriculotomy near the apex was used to close muscular defects in the more distal portion of the septum. However, because of significant operative mortality and morbidity secondary to left ventricular dysfunction, this approach is rarely used. Many muscular ventricular septal defects can be located and closed through a right atriotomy using a small right-angled clamp or coronary artery probe passed through the foramen ovale into the left ventricle to demonstrate the defect, or by excluding the apex of the right ventricle in the region of the defect with a large patch. Apical muscular ventricular septal defects can be closed in the cardiac catheterization laboratory using transcatheter closure devices. Recently, intraoperative closure of muscular ventricular septal defects with a device (under echocardiographic guidance) has been found to be especially advantageous in patients too small to undergo transcatheter techniques who have defects difficult to approach through standard incisions. As newer devices become available, the management of patients with multiple muscular ventricular septal defects may evolve toward primary repair using hybrid surgical–catheter techniques and away from preliminary pulmonary artery banding.

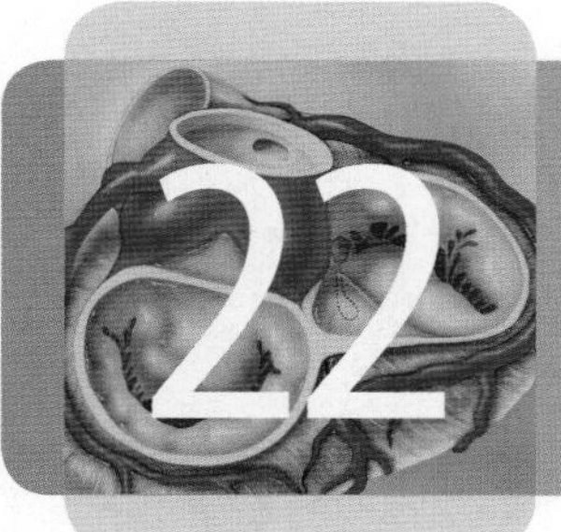

22 Atrioventricular Septal Defect

This anatomic complex has been referred to as an *atrioventricular canal*. The septal defect includes the inferior segment of the atrial septum and the superior segment or the inflow portion of the interventricular septum. The atrioventricular valves are developed in an abnormal, but varied manner.

In all but the mildest forms, there is a common atrioventricular valve, which is made up of six leaflets of variable size and shape attached to normally or abnormally located papillary muscles by chordae tendineae. This common atrioventricular valve can be subdivided into mitral and tricuspid components or segments, each with three leaflets. The leaflets constituting the tricuspid valve are designated right superior, right inferior, and right lateral, and those comprising the mitral valve are designated left superior, left inferior, and left lateral (Fig. 22.1).

It is of clinical and anatomic significance that in normal hearts, the anterior mitral leaflet contributes to one-third, and the posterior leaflet contributes to two-thirds of the annulus of the mitral valve. In an atrioventricular septal defect, this ratio is reversed; the posterior (left lateral) leaflet contributes to one-third and the bileaflet anterior cusp (the left superior and inferior leaflets together) contributes to two-thirds of the mitral valve annulus (Fig. 22.2).

From the clinical point of view, however, there are partial, intermediate, and complete forms of atrioventricular septal defects. In the partial form, there exists an ostium primum type of interatrial septal defect. Here the atrioventricular valves are attached to the crest of the interventricular septum, and there is usually no interventricular communication below the valves. The anterior leaflet of the mitral valve, which has a cleft of varying degree, is considered to form part of a trileaflet mitral valve (Fig. 22.1B). In most patients, the mitral valve is competent.

The intermediate form is similar to the partial form of atrioventricular septal defect. The main distinguishing feature is the incomplete attachment of the atrioventricular valves to the ventricular septum. This results in usually multiple small interventricular communications. Varying degrees of underdevelopment of the leaflet tissues may also be present.

The complete form of atrioventricular septal defect, as its name implies, is a defect in both the lower atrial and upper ventricular septum. The configuration and details of the attachment of the atrioventricular leaflets to the ventricular septum are quite variable.

Rastelli reviewed atrioventricular canal specimens obtained at autopsy at the Mayo Clinic and proposed a classification of atrioventricular septal defects that essentially focuses on the shape, size, location, and details of the attachments of the left superior leaflet. In type A, which is commonly seen, the left superior leaflet is over the left ventricle and its chordal attachment is to the crest of the ventricular septal defect (Fig. 22.3A).

In type B, which is rare, the chordal attachment of the left superior leaflet is to an abnormally located papillary muscle on the right ventricular aspect of the interventricular septum (Fig. 22.3B). In type C, which is seen quite often, the left superior leaflet is large and bridges the ventricular septal defect and right ventricle. Its chordal attachments are variable (Fig. 22.3C). It is a matter of the degree of overriding of the left superior leaflet on the ventricular septum that determines the type of defect.

NB Unbalanced Atrioventricular Septal Defect

Approximately 10% of patients have unbalanced atrioventricular septal defects. If the common atrioventricular valve is located more over the right ventricle, the left ventricle and other left-sided structures may be underdeveloped. When the common atrioventricular valve sits predominately over the left ventricle, a hypoplastic right ventricle with or without pulmonary outflow tract obstruction is usual. NB

OSTIUM PRIMUM ATRIAL SEPTAL DEFECT

The ostium primum type of atrial septal defect is part of the atrioventricular septal defect complex, sometimes referred to as a partial form of the atrioventricular canal. Clinically, a large ostium primum that is usually nonrestrictive is seen, but there is also always a cleft in the anterior leaflet of the mitral valve (Fig. 22.4). The mitral valve in these cases should be considered a trileaflet structure, and this should be kept in mind whenever a repair is attempted.

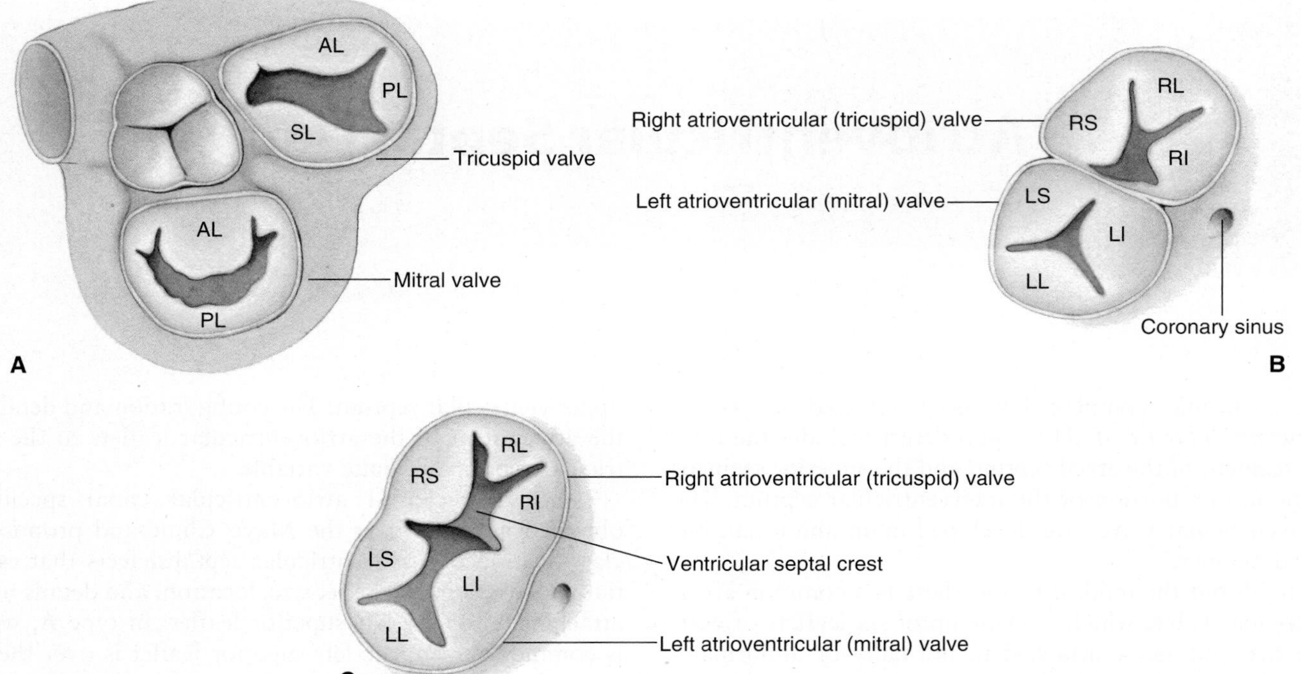

FIG. 22.1 Mitral–tricuspid valve relationship. **A:** In the normal heart, the mitral and tricuspid valve annuli are not in direct contact with each other. They are connected only by the fibrous skeleton of the heart as it encircles the aortic annulus. **B:** Partial atrioventricular septal defect (ostium primum atrial septal defect). The mitral and tricuspid valve annuli are fused, but there is no interventricular communication between the left and right sides of the heart. **C:** Complete atrioventricular septal defect. AL, anterior leaflet; PL, posterior leaflet; SL, septal leaflet; LS, left superior; RS, right superior; RL, right lateral; RI, right inferior; LI, left inferior; LL, left lateral.

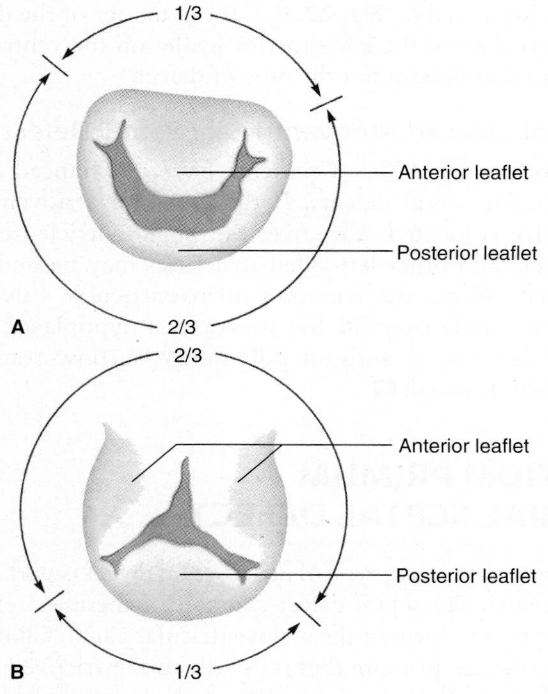

FIG. 22.2 **A:** Normal mitral valve annular configuration. **B:** Mitral valve annular configuration in an atrioventricular septal defect.

Incision

This form of atrial septal defect is usually approached through a median sternotomy. A right submammary thoracotomy incision can also be used (see Chapter 1).

Cannulation

The ascending aorta is cannulated in the usual manner (see Chapter 2). The superior and inferior vena cavae are cannulated directly; tapes are then passed around both cavae. A vent is placed through the right superior pulmonary vein and positioned in the left atrium proximal to the mitral valve. (The correct position can be obtained after the heart is opened.)

Myocardial Preservation

Cold cardioplegic arrest of the heart is achieved and maintained by intermittent infusion of cold blood cardioplegic solution into the aortic root (see Chapter 3).

Technique

A generous atriotomy is made from the base of the right atrial appendage to near the site of the inferior vena cava cannulation, parallel with the atrioventricular groove. The

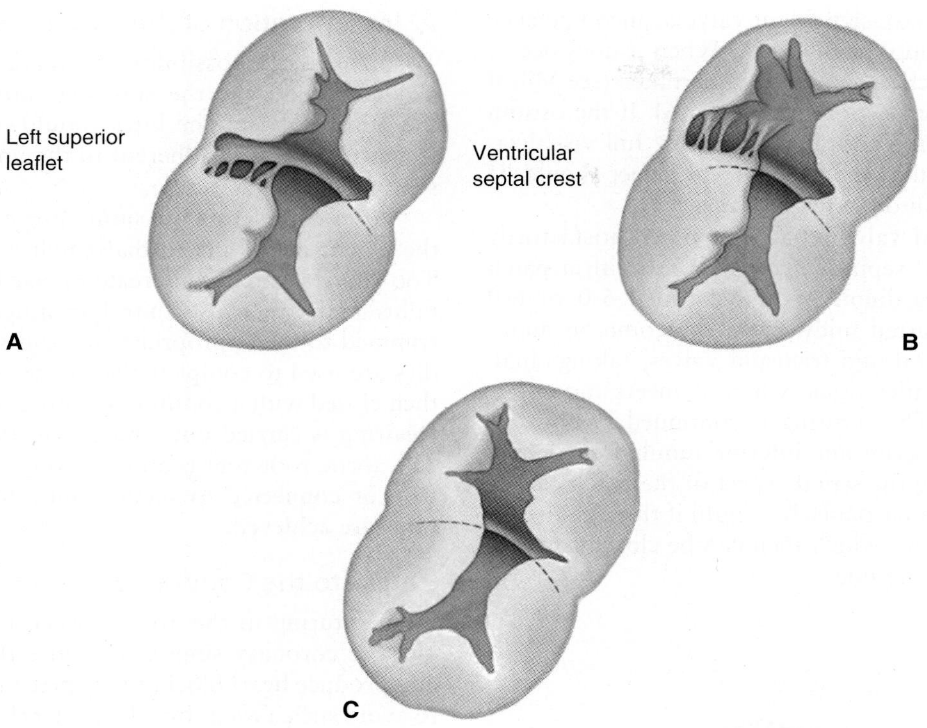

FIG. 22.3 Rastelli classification of atrioventricular septal defects. **A:** Type A. **B:** Type B. **C:** Type C.

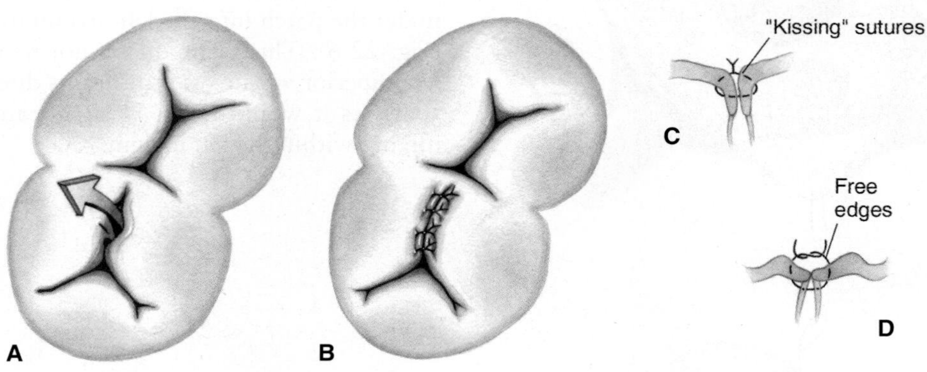

FIG. 22.4 **A:** Regurgitation through the cleft. **B:** Repair of the cleft. **C:** "Kissing" edges of the cleft. **D:** Free edges of the cleft.

atriotomy edges are retracted with fine sutures that are sometimes pledgeted. The presence and severity of mitral regurgitation must be carefully assessed. This may be carried out by simply injecting saline forcefully through the mitral valve. The cleft on the anterior leaflet of the mitral valve should be closed even if there is no valve incompetence at the time of surgery because these valves often become insufficient over time. This can be accomplished by approximating the "kissing" edges of the cleft starting at the annulus with three or four interrupted 6-0 Prolene sutures (Fig. 22.4).

⊘ Closure of the Cleft

Care must be taken to approximate only the kissing edges of the leaflet tissue, which are not the same as the free edges of the cleft (Fig. 22.4C, D). Incorporation of an additional extent of the leaflet to secure a better repair usually results in valvular insufficiency. The edges of the cleft are strong and quite fibrotic in older patients and consequently hold sutures well. In infants, the valve tissue may be somewhat friable. In these cases, horizontal mattress sutures reinforced with pericardial pledgets can be used to close the cleft. ⊘

It is unusual to have significant valvular incompetence in the ostium primum type of defect. When it does occur, aggressive reconstruction should be undertaken (see Mitral Valve Reconstruction section in Chapter 6). If the ostium primum defect is small and does not allow full visualization of the mitral valve, the atrial septal defect should be enlarged toward or into the fossa ovalis.

When the mitral valve repair has been satisfactorily completed, the atrial septal defect is closed with a patch of autologous pericardium. A double-armed 5-0 or 6-0 Prolene suture is started midway on the common annulus between the mitral and tricuspid valves, taking small bites of tricuspid leaflet tissue where it meets the mitral valve (Fig. 22.5B). The suturing is continued in both directions until the superior and inferior annuli are reached. The suture line along the septal aspect of the patch can be interrupted, which is particularly helpful if there is a small ventricular component, which then can be closed simultaneously with this suture line.

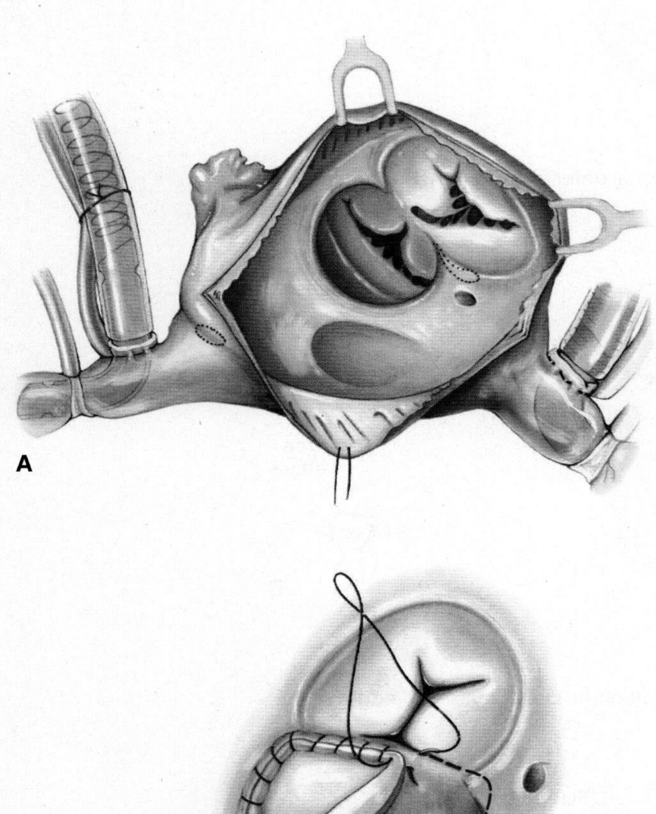

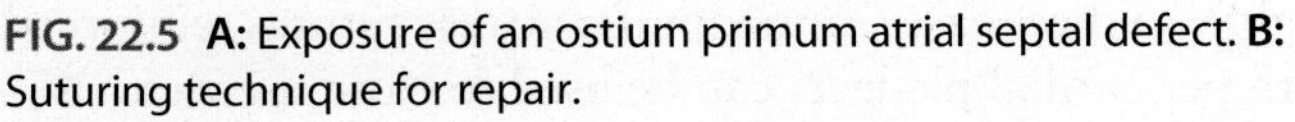

FIG. 22.5 **A:** Exposure of an ostium primum atrial septal defect. **B:** Suturing technique for repair.

⊘ Incorporation of the Mitral Leaflet

To prevent the possibility of creating or increasing mitral incompetence, the suturing should not incorporate the mitral leaflet. The bites should include tricuspid tissue just where it is adherent to the underlying ventricular septum. ⊘

After completing the suture line along the septal crest, the height of the pericardial patch is carefully measured. Too short a patch will create upward traction on the annulus and can cause mitral insufficiency. The patch is trimmed to the appropriate size and shape, and both needles are used to complete the suture line. The atriotomy is then closed with a continuous suture of 5-0 or 6-0 Prolene. Deairing is carried out, and the aortic clamp is removed. The aortic root vent is allowed to bleed into the operative field or connected to suction until good ventricular ejections are achieved.

⊘ Risk to the Conduction Tissue

Deep suturing in the area between the tricuspid annulus and the coronary sinus may injure the conduction tissue and produce heart block. Every precaution should be taken to avoid such a event by taking superficial bites of endocardium only (the needle should be visible through the tissue) in this region. The first several bites are near the mitral valve annulus (Fig. 22.5B). Alternatively, the right-hand side of the patch should be left a little longer and sutured around the orifice of the coronary sinus so that it drains under the patch into the left atrium to prevent heart block (Fig. 22.6). This technique is not to be used if there is a left superior vena cava that drains directly to the coronary sinus, as it would result in significant desaturation from mixing within the left atrium. ⊘

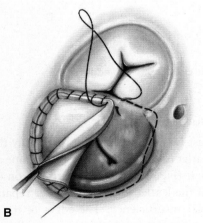

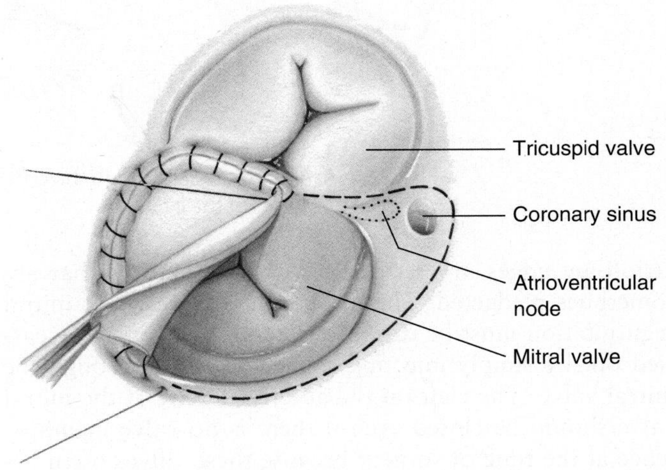

FIG. 22.6 Alternative suture technique for repair of an ostium primum atrial septal defect.

⊘ Preventing Hemolysis

A patch of autologous pericardium fixed in glutaraldehyde should be used. The use of Dacron or GORE-TEX may result in hemolysis if even a small mitral regurgitant jet hits the patch. ⊘

COMPLETE ATRIOVENTRICULAR SEPTAL DEFECT

The most crucial factor to consider when performing surgery for atrioventricular septal defect is competence of the mitral valve. A two-patch or single-patch technique can be used.

Cannulation

In small infants weighing less than 2 kg, hypothermic circulatory arrest allows optimal exposure. In most patients, however, direct cannulation of the superior vena cava and the inferior vena cava is carried out. Placement of the venous cannulas must not cause undue tension on the valvular apparatus. Aortic cannulation is performed as usual. When hypothermic arrest is used, a single venous cannula is placed through the right atrial appendage for cooling and rewarming and removed during the period of circulatory arrest. When continuous flow cardiopulmonary bypass is used, a vent is placed through the right superior pulmonary vein and positioned proximal to the mitral valve after the heart is opened.

Two-Patch Technique

A generous atriotomy is performed from just below the right atrial appendage down toward the inferior vena cava parallel with the atrioventricular groove. The edges of the atriotomy are retracted with fine sutures, sometimes buttressed with pledgets. Small leaflet retractors are used to provide additional exposure. The precise functional and pathologic anatomy is assessed. Saline is injected into the ventricles to assess the coaptation relationships between the inferior and superior leaflets. A 6-0 Prolene stay suture is used to approximate the left superior and left inferior leaflets at their coaptation point in the plane of the ventricular septum. This forms the landmark for the establishment of the future common annulus (Fig. 22.7). It is sometimes necessary to incise the left superior and/or left inferior leaflets up to the annulus for better exposure and a more secure closure of the ventricular septal defect. Any secondary chordal attachments to the ventricular septum that may interfere with closure of the defect are divided, although usually these attachments can be preserved and the patch secured on the right ventricular side of the crest below them. An appropriately sized, semicircular GORTEX patch is sutured with a double-armed 5-0 Prolene to the right ventricular aspect of the ventricular septum (usually starting in the middle). The first bite may be buttressed with a pledget (Fig. 22.7).

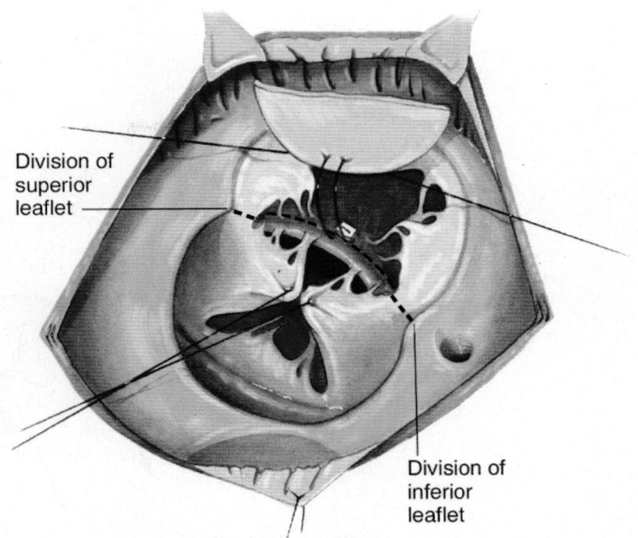

FIG. 22.7 Repair of a ventricular septal defect in a complete atrioventricular defect. Dotted line shows proposed division of the inferior and superior leaflets.

NB Division of Bridging Leaflets

When deciding where to incise the superior and inferior leaflets, the chordal attachments may help define the line of separation between left- and right-sided components. However, it is of paramount importance to have adequate left-sided leaflet tissue, so that often the leaflets are divided somewhat on the right ventricular side. NB

⊘ Prevention of Heart Block

The atrioventricular node lies in the atrial septum just anterior to the coronary sinus. The bundle of His extends from the atrioventricular node through the central fibrous body into the ventricles under the membranous part of the interventricular septum. Suturing of the patch to the ventricular septum should be well beyond the rim of the ventricular septal defect so as not to produce any conduction injury. ⊘

Gentle traction on the suture facilitates suturing in both directions until the superior and inferior annuli are reached. The needles are then brought out through the leaflets superiorly and inferiorly, and both ends of the suture tagged.

NB Height of the Interventricular Septal Patch

Resuspension of the valve leaflets at the appropriate level is important. Therefore, the height of the ventricular septal defect patch should correspond to the plane of the atrioventricular valve leaflets during the saline injection into the ventricles (Fig. 22.8). NB

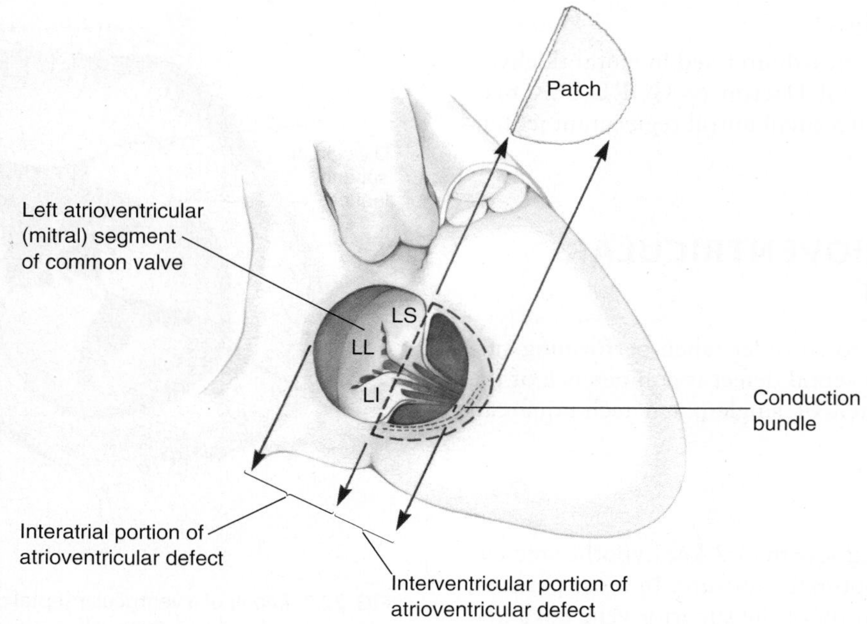

FIG. 22.8 Diagrammatic view of a complete atrioventricular septal defect from the right. The tricuspid or right half of the common valve and the remainder of the right side of the heart have been removed to show the dimensions for sizing the interventricular patch. The upper edge of the patch suspends the leaflets at the level of their annuli, and the lower edge extends below the muscular crest on the right side of the interventricular defect so that suturing will not injure the conducting bundle. LS, left superior; LL, left lateral; LI, left inferior.

A large patch of pericardium is then appropriately tailored to cover the atrial septal defect. The suture line that crosses the common atrioventricular valve incorporates leaflet tissue as well as the GORTEX patch used to close the ventricular septal defect. A continuous over-and-over suture is used if the leaflets have not been incised. If the leaflet tissue has been divided, particular care must be taken to incorporate both sides of the leaflet tissue, that is, left and right atrioventricular valve tissue, as well as the interventricular gortex patch and the interatrial pericardial patch. This is best accomplished with several horizontal mattress sutures of 6-0 Prolene passed first through the tricuspid leaflet component, then through the upper edge of the GORTEX patch, then through the mitral leaflet tissue, and finally through the inferior edge of the pericardial patch. All the sutures are placed and tagged separately, then the pericardial patch is lowered into place and the sutures tied.

⊘ Deformation of the Leaflet Anatomy

Overzealous incorporation of the atrioventricular leaflet tissue in suturing may shorten the height of the leaflet and produce valvular incompetence. ⊘

Once continuity of the ventricular and atrial patches has been established, the atrial patch is retracted into the right atrial cavity, and the cleft between the left superior and inferior leaflets is approximated with interrupted sutures bringing the kissing edges together. The left atrioventricular valve is tested for competence by injecting saline into the left ventricle (Fig. 22.9A). Regurgitant flow noted at the inferolateral and/or superolateral commissure may be controlled with pericardial pledgeted 5-0 or 6-0 Prolene horizontal mattress sutures placed at the corresponding commissure (Fig. 22.9B). Trivial central regurgitant flow can be accepted, but every effort should be made to achieve the most competent valve possible. Sometimes, a suture annuloplasty using a double-armed 5-0 Prolene suture along the mitral annulus from commissure to commissure achieves the best results. A pericardial pledget is placed at both ends of the double suture line, and the suture is tied over a Hegar dilator that corresponds to the Z-zero mitral diameter for the patient's size (Fig. 22.9C).

The correct height of the pericardial patch is then carefully gauged, and the patch is trimmed accordingly. The pericardial patch is sewn to the edges of the atrial septal defect, leaving the coronary sinus on either the left or right side, as described for repair of an ostium primum defect (Figs. 22.5B and 22.6). This is achieved by a continuous suture of 5-0 or 6-0 Prolene. Should the coronary sinus be left in the right atrium, care must be exercised to take superficial bites near the conduction tissue.

⊘ High Left Atrial Pressure

After separation from cardiopulmonary bypass, the left atrial pressure may be elevated secondary to mitral valve incompetence or left ventricular dysfunction. If the coronary sinus has been placed on the left atrial side of the patch, this will result in high coronary venous pressure, which may impair coronary arterial perfusion. ⊘

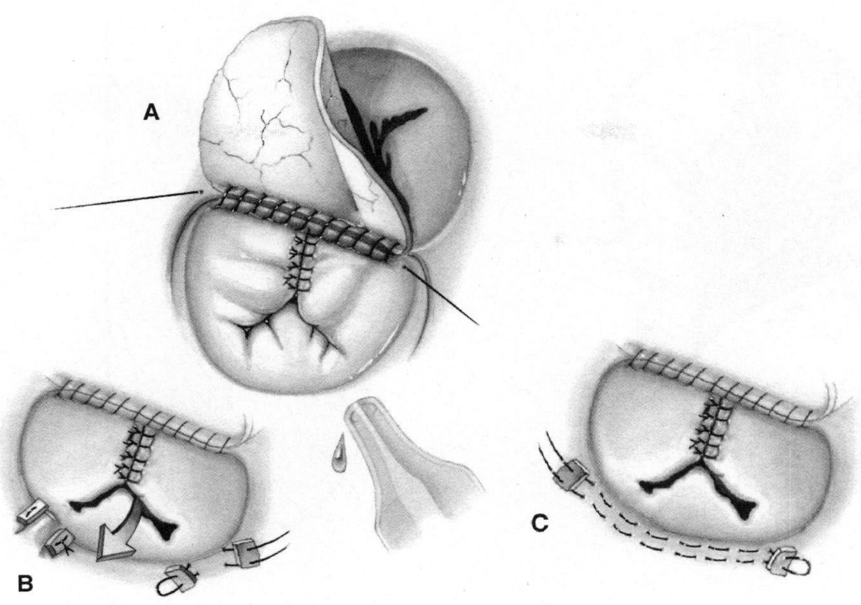

FIG. 22.9 **A:** Atrial patch with the completed suture line across the common atrioventricular valve. **B:** Mitral annuloplasty with pledgeted sutures at the commissures. **C:** Suture annuloplasty tied over appropriately sized Hegar dilator.

NB Valvular Competence

Residual moderate or severe valvular incompetence is not well tolerated. It is sometimes better to overcorrect and produce mild stenosis than to accept even mild mitral valve insufficiency. NB

⊘ Incorrect Height of Patches

A perfect valvular repair can be distorted, leading to mitral valve incompetence if either the ventricular or atrial septal patch is too tall or too short. ⊘

One-Patch Technique

Before cannulation, a large piece of pericardium is harvested, placed in glutaraldehyde, and rinsed in saline. After the right atrium is opened, the leaflets are assessed by filling the ventricles with saline. Coaptation of the superior and inferior leaflets overlying the ventricular septum is evaluated. A 6-0 Prolene suture is placed at the leading edges of the inferior and superior leaflets to determine the point of partition of the common atrioventricular valve into left- and right-sided valves.

The distance between the two points on opposite sides of the annulus where the ventricular septal crest meets the atrioventricular groove is measured. This determines the width of the patch at the annular level. If the patch is too wide, the left atrioventricular valve annulus will be increased, and this may lead to mitral regurgitation. If the left atrioventricular valve tissue is believed to be insufficient, then the width of the patch should be less than the measured distance between the two points on the annulus. This will reduce the size of the left atrioventricular valve annulus and help create a competent valve.

Leaflet incisions are nearly always required in the superior and inferior leaflets to allow placement of the pericardial patch. The leaflets should be incised in a line parallel with and overlying the ventricular septal crest, with the incision extending to the level of the annulus (Fig. 22.10).

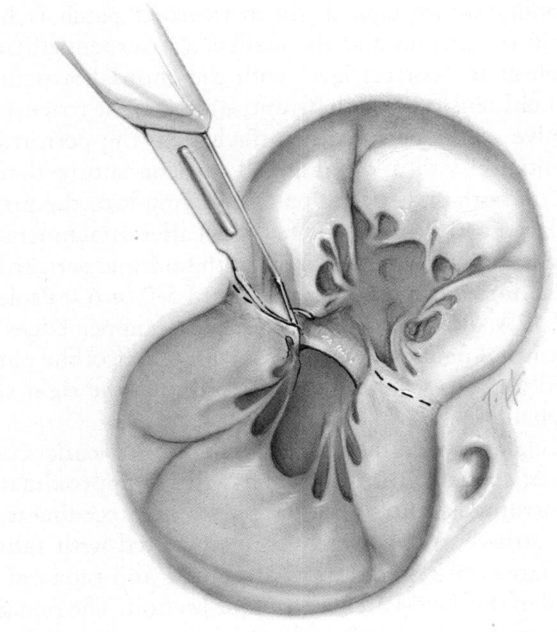

FIG. 22.10 Division of leaflets overlying the ventricular septal crest.

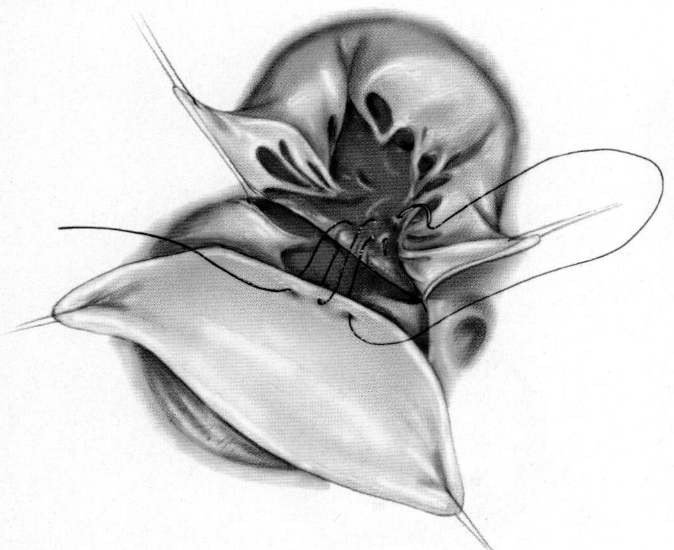

FIG. 22.11 Attaching a pericardial patch to the right ventricular aspect of the defect.

⊘ Inadequate Left-Sided Valve Tissue

The superior and inferior leaflets should be divided somewhat on the right ventricular side to ensure adequate left-sided leaflet tissue for a competent mitral valve. ⊘

The pericardial patch is attached to the right ventricular aspect of the defect beginning in the midportion with a running 5-0 Prolene suture. The suture line is continued, weaving in and out of the chordal attachments, until the annulus of the atrioventricular valve is reached both superiorly and inferiorly (Fig. 22.11). With the two ends of this running suture tagged, the pericardial patch is held up within the atrium and the leaflets are suspended from the patch at the correct level with the chordal structures under slight tension. The left-(mitral) and right-(tricuspid) sided valve components are reattached to the pericardial patch initially with a running 6-0 Prolene suture that is secured on both ends of the patch by tying it to the previously placed 5-0 Prolene stitch. The leaflet attachment to the pericardium is then reinforced with multiple pericardial pledgeted horizontal mattress sutures of 5-0 or 6-0 Prolene (Fig. 22.12A, B). Traction sutures on the upper edges of the pericardial patch allow the surgeon to deflect the patch back and forth to visualize the left and then the right side of the repair.

The cleft between the superior and inferior leaflet components of the left atrioventricular valve is approximated with interrupted sutures as described in the preceding text. The left atrioventricular valve is again tested with saline, and any areas of regurgitation are noted and repaired as discussed in the Two-Patch Technique section. The remainder of the pericardial patch is then secured to the atrial septal defect as described previously (Fig. 22.13).

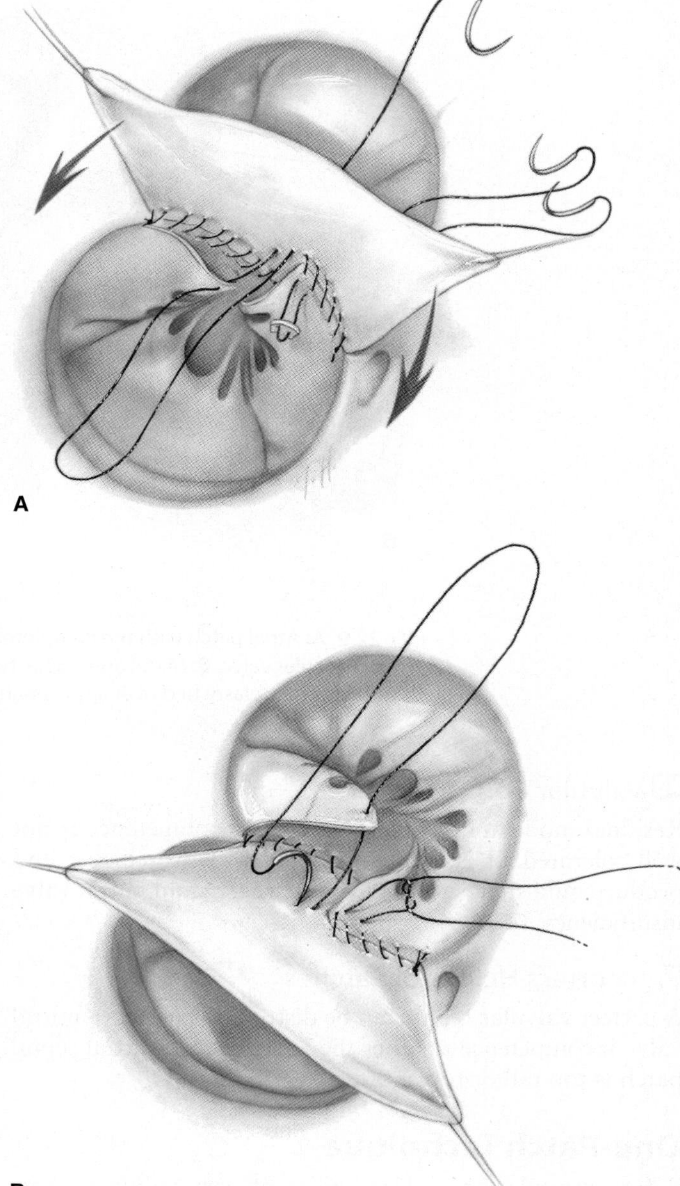

FIG. 22.12 Attaching mitral and tricuspid valve components to the pericardial patch. Running suture is completed inferiorly and interrupted reinforcing mattress sutures are placed from the left side through the mitral component, patch, and then tricuspid component and tied on the right side. **A:** Left-sided view. **B:** Right-sided view.

One-Patch Technique with Direct Ventricular Defect Closure

Recently, some surgeons have advocated direct suture closure of the ventricular septal defect in patients with complete atrioventricular septal defects. This technique involves the placement of interrupted pledgeted 5-0 polyester

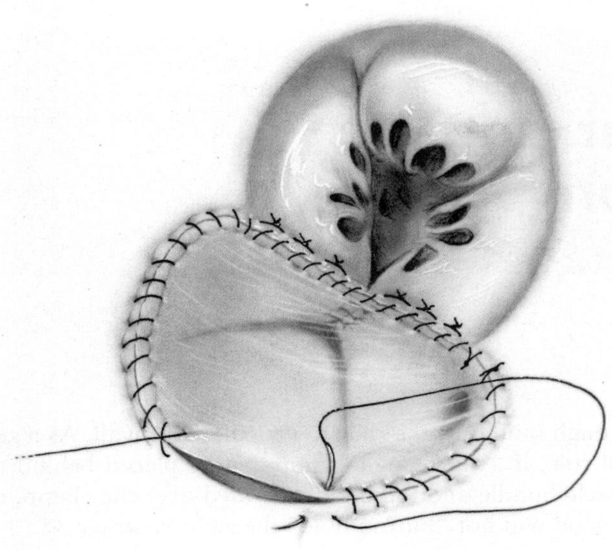

FIG. 22.13 The remainder of the pericardial patch is used to close the atrial septal defect.

sutures on the right ventricular aspect of the septal crest, avoiding the conduction tissue. These sutures are brought up through the superior and inferior bridging leaflets and then through the pericardial patch used to close the atrial defect. When deficient left-sided leaflet tissue is present, the sutures are placed more toward the right side to create a larger mitral valve. The cleft between the left superior and inferior leaflets is closed with interrupted 6-0 or 7-0 Prolene sutures. The septal sutures are tied securely, thereby closing the ventricular septal defect. The mitral valve is tested with saline, and if needed, annuloplasty sutures are placed as described in the preceding text. The pericardial patch is sewn into place with a continuous 6-0 Prolene suture, taking shallow bites between the annulus inferiorly and the coronary sinus to avoid the atrioventricular node.

NB Patient Indications

This simplified technique should be applied judiciously. If the ventricular septal defect is too deep, the tension required to pull the leaflets down to the septum may cause the sutures to pull through the muscle or may distort the valve and lead to unacceptable mitral insufficiency. At least theoretically, this direct closure of the ventriculoseptal defect could cause left ventricular outflow tract obstruction. A modification of this technique, closing the superior and/or inferior most extents of the ventricular septal defect directly and patching the other side or midportion of the defect may be useful. NB

Completion of the Operation

The right atriotomy is closed with a running 6-0 or 5-0 Prolene suture. If the operation has been performed on cardiopulmonary bypass, rewarming is begun during closure of the atrial septal defect component. After closing the right atrium, the heart is filled, the aortic cross-clamp is removed, and deairing procedures are performed. If the operation has been accomplished under circulatory arrest, the heart is filled with saline after closing the right atriotomy. Cardiopulmonary bypass is recommenced, the aortic cross-clamp is removed while deairing through the ascending aorta, and rewarming is carried out in the usual manner.

UNBALANCED ATRIOVENTRICULAR SEPTAL DEFECT

Patients with unbalanced atrioventricular septal defects to the right often have underdeveloped left-sided structures. Most of these patients are not candidates for biventricular repair and should undergo a Norwood-type initial procedure followed by staging to a completion Fontan operation (see Chapters 30 and 31). Patients with unbalanced atrioventricular septal defects to the left may tolerate a biventricular approach by leaving a restrictive atrial septal defect. Alternatively, they may be candidates for a one and one-half ventricle repair combining a septation procedure with a bidirectional cavopulmonary anastomosis (see Chapter 31).

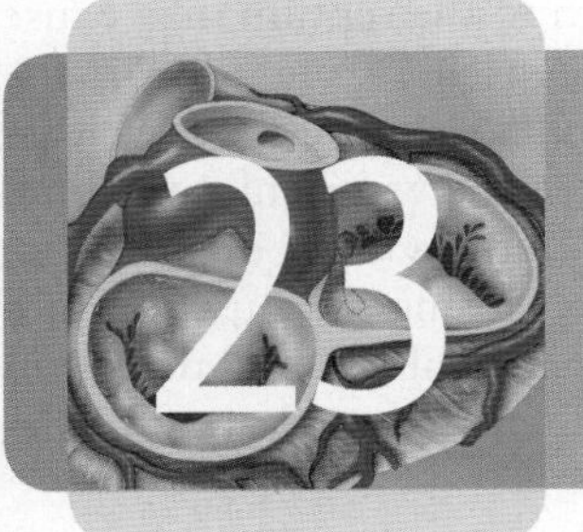

23 Right Ventricular Outflow Tract Obstruction

The right ventricular outflow tract includes the right ventricular outlet chamber (or the infundibulum); the pulmonary valve; the main, right, and left pulmonary arteries; and the peripheral pulmonary arterial branches. Obstruction can occur at a specific site or involve many segments of the right ventricular outflow tract. Obstruction of the right ventricular outflow tract is commonly associated with other cardiac anomalies.

DOUBLE-CHAMBERED RIGHT VENTRICLE

This consists of a hypertrophied muscle band creating obstruction between the inlet and infundibular portion of the right ventricle. An enlarged acute marginal branch of the right coronary artery often overlies the area of obstruction where an area of "dimpling" of the right ventricular free wall is also often present. Most often, a double-chambered right ventricle is associated with a perimembranous type of ventricular septal defect.

Technique for Repair

Cardiopulmonary bypass with bicaval cannulation is used. After aortic cross-clamping and cardioplegia delivery, a right atriotomy is performed. After identifying the papillary muscles of the tricuspid valve, the remainder of the obstructing muscle is resected until the fibrous "os infundibulum" is visible. Once this is resected, the pulmonary valve should be evident. The accompanying ventricular septal defect should now be apparent. This ventricular septal defect may be closed through the right atriotomy (see Chapter 21).

⊘ Misidentifying the Ventricular Septal Defect

The circular opening visualized if a right ventriculotomy approach is used may, on first examination, appear to be the ventricular septal defect. Care must be taken to identify the location of the tricuspid valve to avoid this mistake. ⊘

⊘ Creating a Right Ventriculotomy

In resecting the dense muscle bundles of double chamber right ventricle, it is important not to debride muscle through (and out) the right ventricular free wall. As a general rule, if a right angle clamp can be placed behind the muscle bundle and the bundle divided over the clamp, the surgeon will not "button hole" the right ventricle. ⊘

TETRALOGY OF FALLOT

An anatomic anomaly consisting of a ventricular septal defect, right ventricular outflow tract obstruction with resultant right ventricular hypertrophy, and dextroposition of the aorta was described by Fallot in 1888. These children usually present with mild to moderate cyanosis and may have intermittent hypoxic spells.

The anatomy must be accurately defined to plan the management of these patients. Echocardiography can demonstrate the presence of additional ventricular septal defects, can usually delineate the initial course of the right and left coronary arteries, and can size the main and proximal right and left pulmonary arteries. Cardiac catheterization is reserved for those patients in whom the echocardiographic diagnosis is incomplete, when aortopulmonary collateral vessels are suspected, or for patients with previous palliative procedures.

Staged Approach

Several centers have reported satisfactory results with complete repair of tetralogy of Fallot in neonates. However, as the long-term results of repair of tetralogy of Fallot become available, the significant problem of right ventricular failure and its causes are being elucidated. It is now believed that pulmonary regurgitation plays a major role in the development of right ventricular dysfunction. For this reason, some surgeons advocate a staged approach in patients who require surgery before 4 to 6 months of age. Patients who become symptomatic early in life or are ductal dependent tend to have small pulmonic valves and usually require a transannular patch. By performing an initial shunt procedure (see Chapter 18) and delaying definitive repair, the hope is that the native valve and/or annulus can be preserved.

In addition, 3% to 5% of patients with tetralogy of Fallot have an anomalous left anterior descending coronary artery arising from the right coronary artery. The course of the left anterior descending coronary artery across the right ventricular outflow tract may preclude an appropriate transannular incision. If these patients need surgery in the first few months of life, a shunt procedure is preferred. Some of these patients may be able to undergo a transatrial repair. However, many will require a right ventricular to pulmonary artery conduit as part of their repair, and this is best delayed as long as is possible and practical clinically.

Technique for Complete Repair

A median sternotomy provides excellent exposure. A generous patch of autologous pericardium is harvested, attached with metal clips to a piece of plastic, placed in 0.6% glutaraldehyde solution, and then rinsed in saline. Such treatment fixes the pericardium and thereby lessens the chances of aneurysmal dilation of the patch. If the patient has undergone a previous systemic to pulmonary shunt, it is dissected circumferentially to allow for closure with a metal clip at the initiation of cardiopulmonary bypass (see Chapter 18). In the absence of a shunt, minimal manipulation should be performed before cannulation to prevent hypoxic spells.

Besides confirming the anatomy with transesophageal echocardiography, an external examination of the heart is conducted. The surgeon looks for an anomalous coronary artery crossing the right ventricular outflow area, evaluates the size of the main and branch pulmonary arteries, and notes the distance between the aortic valve and the left anterior descending artery, which indicates the width of the right ventricular outflow tract. These observations help determine the surgical approach. A hypoplastic right ventricular outflow tract may favor the need for a right ventriculotomy or the probability of a transannular patch.

Standard bicaval and aortic cannulation is used to initiate cardiopulmonary bypass. A vent is placed through the right superior pulmonary vein into the left ventricle. Systemic cooling to 28°C to 34°C is achieved, the aorta is clamped, and cold blood cardioplegic solution is infused into the aortic root (see Chapter 3). In patients with discrete infundibular muscular obstruction and an adequate pulmonary annulus, the repair can be done through a transatrial approach.

Transatrial Technique

After achieving cardioplegic arrest, the tapes around the vena cavae are snugged down, and an oblique right atriotomy is made. The septal leaflet of the tricuspid valve is retracted to allow exposure of the ventricular septal defect and the right ventricular outflow tract. A right angle clamp is then used to identify hypertrophied muscle bands. With the clamp in place, each muscle band is divided with a no. 15 knife blade, cutting the band until the clamp is reached. The cut edge of the band can then be grasped with a forceps and resected with sharp scissors. When adequate resection of hypertrophied muscle has been completed, it should be possible to visualize the pulmonic valve (Fig. 23.1). A valvotomy can be performed by everting the leaflets and incising the commissures, if necessary. The annulus is sized with a Hegar dilator to ensure an adequate valve opening for the patient's size (see Appendix section).

⊘ Buttonholing of Anterior Right Ventricle

Care must be exercised when resecting muscle from the right ventricular outflow tract not to perforate the anterior wall. Checking outside the heart intermittently may be helpful. If a hole is created, it must be closed, usually with a pericardial patch (see subsequent text). ⊘

⊘ Resection near Ventricular Septal Defect

It is important to limit the resection of muscle along the anterior margin of the ventricular septal defect as this may compromise suturing of the patch to this edge. ⊘

The ventricular septal defect is closed with a patch of GORTEX cut slightly larger than the defect. This can be secured in place with a continuous suture or multiple interrupted horizontal mattress 5-0 braided sutures with felt pledgets (see Chapter 21).

Transventricular Technique

Some surgeons prefer a right ventriculotomy approach for patients with tetralogy of Fallot. The advantages include the ability to resect all obstructing muscle bundles under direct vision and to enlarge an underdeveloped infundibulum with a patch. The potential disadvantages include scarring of the right ventricle, which may give rise to ventricular dysfunction and dysrrhythmias. Even when a transventricular approach is used, every attempt is made to preserve the pulmonic valve leaflets and to avoid a transannular patch.

A vertical right ventriculotomy is made, and the edges are retracted with pledgeted sutures. The hypertrophied infundibular muscle bundles are incised and selectively excised as needed to open up the outflow tract (Fig. 23.2). The large malalignment type of ventricular septal defect can now be seen and is closed with a GORTEX patch using a continuous suture of 5-0 Prolene. With this technique, traction on the patch by the assistant facilitates placement of the next stitch. Suturing begins at the 1 o'clock position and continues clockwise around the tricuspid annulus, taking shallow bites of thickened endocardium up to the aortic annulus where the suture is tagged at the 8 o'clock position (Fig. 23.3).

NB Limiting Right Ventriculotomy

To better preserve long-term right ventricular function, the length of the ventriculotomy should be limited to that needed to open the hypoplastic portion of the infundibulum. NB

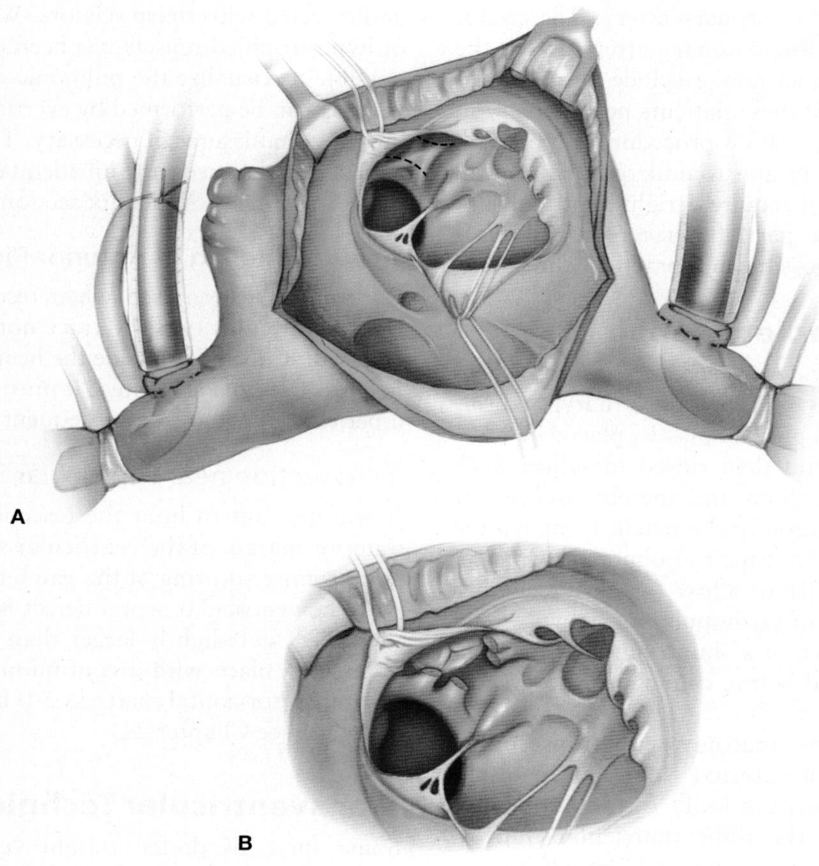

FIG. 23.1 **A:** Exposure of ventricular septal defect and right ventricular outflow tract through tricuspid valve. **B:** Infundibular resection is complete and pulmonic valve can be seen.

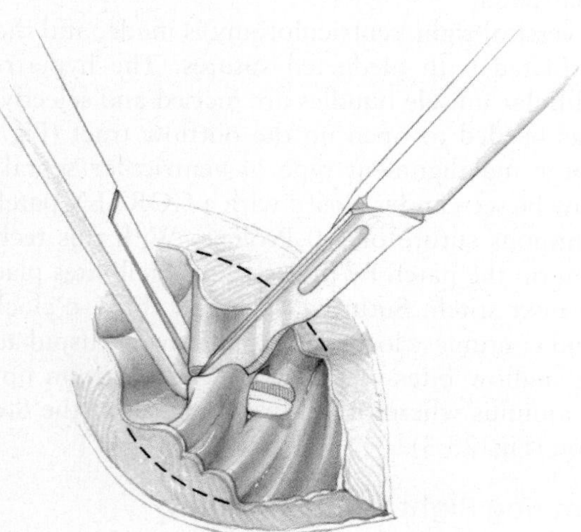

FIG. 23.2 Transection of muscle band. Dotted line shows resection lines to excise hypertrophied muscle.

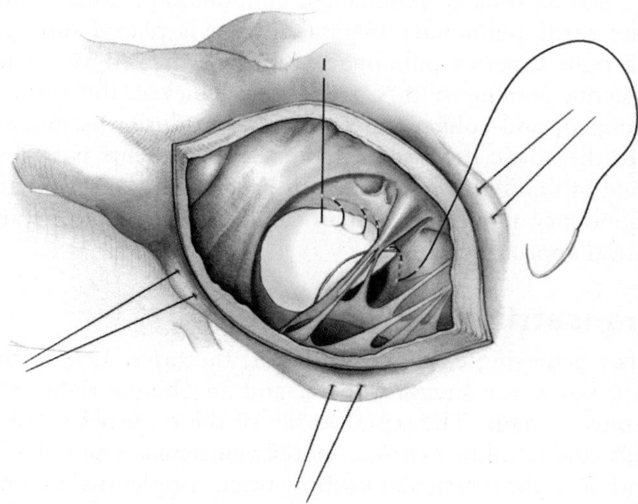

FIG. 23.3 Continuous suture technique for the closure of ventricular septal defect through right ventriculotomy.

⊘ Difficulty in Exposing Ventricular Septal Defect

If the right ventriculotomy must be extended to provide adequate exposure for closure of the ventricular septal defect, it is preferable to open the right atrium and close the ventricular septal defect through the tricuspid valve. Detachment of the anterior leaflet of the tricuspid valve may be useful to expose the outlet portion of the defect (see Chapter 21). ⊘

⊘ Extensive Resection of Muscle Bands

When a right ventriculotomy is performed, muscle resection can be more limited because the patch itself will open up the outflow tract. Aggressive muscle resection leads to more endocardial scarring that may contribute to right ventricular dysfunction. ⊘

⊘ Injury to the Aortic Valve

The aortic valve leaflets are immediately below the superior margin of the defect and can be punctured during suturing if deep needle bites are taken in this area (Fig. 23.4). Suturing in this area should therefore incorporate the crista marginalis, which holds sutures well. ⊘

The pulmonary valve and annulus are evaluated with Hegar dilators. Pulmonary valvotomy, if necessary, is carried out by bringing the pulmonary valve leaflets downward into the ventriculotomy.

Transpulmonary Approach to Pulmonic Valve and Annulus

Whether a transatrial or transventricular approach is used, evaluation of the pulmonic valve may be difficult working from below. In these cases, a separate vertical incision is made on the main pulmonary artery. Many surgeons prefer to use a transpulmonary approach to the pulmonic valve in all patients. After inspecting the valve and completing a valvotomy, if required, a Hegar dilator of the appropriate size is passed into the right ventricle (see Appendix section). If the annulus cannot be opened adequately with passage of sequentially larger dilators, the incision on the pulmonary artery is extended across the annulus only as far as necessary. This incision should be made through the anterior commissure of the pulmonic valve to reduce the amount of pulmonary insufficiency.

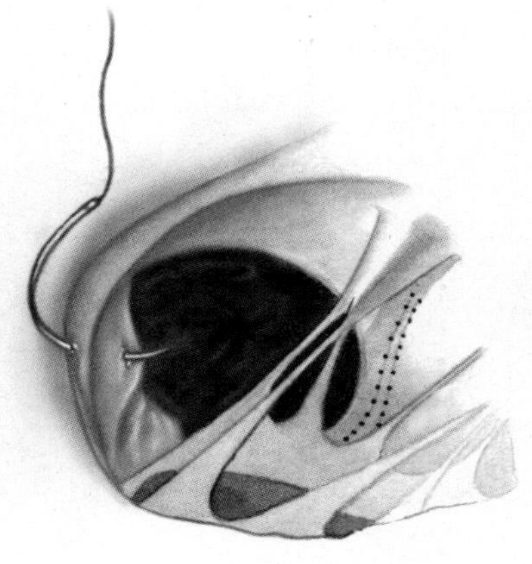

FIG. 23.4 Proximity of an aortic valve leaflet to the rim of septal defect.

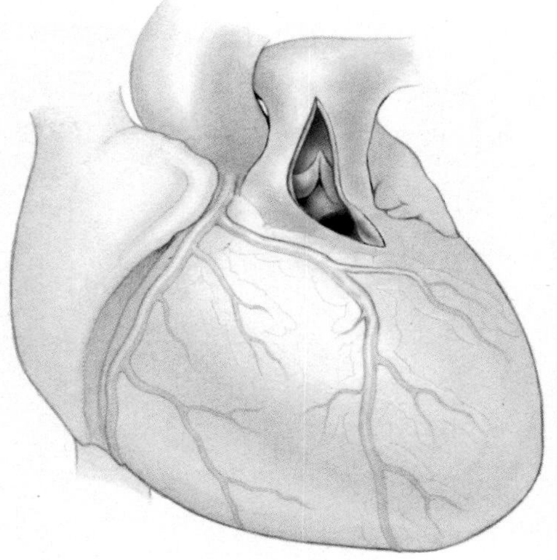

FIG. 23.5 Pulmonary arteriotomy extended across annulus onto infundibulum parallel to anomalous coronary artery.

NB Anomalous Coronary Artery

The transatrial-transpulmonary approach can be used in some patients with an anomalous coronary artery crossing the right ventricular outflow tract. In these cases, if transannular extension of the pulmonary arteriotomy is required, the incision must be made parallel to the anomalous vessel and an appropriately shaped patch used to maximize the opening of the right ventricular outflow tract (Fig. 23.5). NB

The orifices of the right and left pulmonary arteries are then evaluated. If stenosis of the takeoff of the left pulmonary artery is noted, the pulmonary arteriotomy can be carried out onto the left pulmonary artery as far as necessary to adequately relieve the stenosis. If narrowing of the right pulmonary artery is present, this may be best handled by extending the pulmonary arteriotomy onto the anterior surface of the right pulmonary artery behind the aorta. In this case, a separate rectangular patch is used to enlarge the opening of the right, or right and left pulmonary arteries (Fig. 23.6).

If the annulus is of adequate size, the pulmonary arteriotomy may be sutured primarily with a running 6-0 Prolene stitch, or closed with an appropriately sized patch of autologous pericardium to enlarge the main or left pulmonary arteries, as indicated. When used to enlarge the left pulmonary artery, the patch should be tailored with a squared-off end to provide optimal enlargement. The right ventriculotomy is then closed with an elongated oval patch

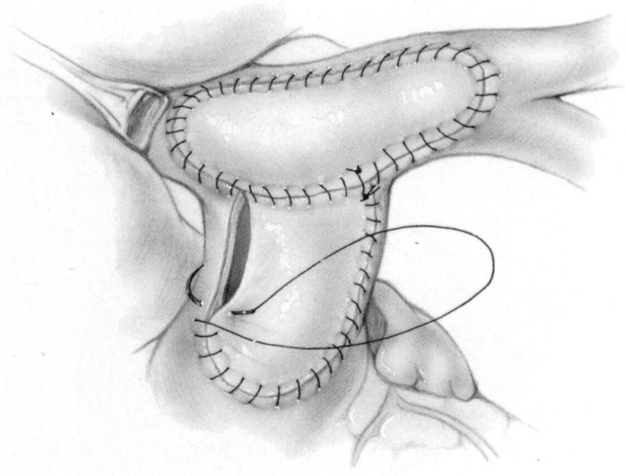

FIG. 23.6 Two-patch technique to enlarge the proximal right and left pulmonary arteries.

of autologous pericardium or Gore-Tex, using a running 5-0 Prolene suture.

If the infundibulum and annulus are hypoplastic, a transannular patch is required. Many surgeons use a patch with a monocusp valve made from pericardium, Gore-Tex, or excised from a large pulmonary homograft (Fig. 23.7A). The patch may extend only onto the proximal main pulmonary artery if the right and left pulmonary arteries are of adequate size (Fig. 23.7B). Often the distal main artery and the origin of the left pulmonary artery are small and the transannular incision is extended out onto the left pulmonary artery (Fig. 23.8A). The patch should be tailored in such a way that the new pulmonary artery dimension is equal to or slightly larger than the Z-zero value for the pulmonary valve based on the patient's body surface area (see Appendix section). When a monocusp is used, the patch is tailored so that the position of the valve leaflet is at the level of the patient's annulus (Fig. 23.7A and C). The patch is sewn into place starting at the distal pulmonary arterial opening, using running 6-0 or 5-0 Prolene suture. If a standard pericardial patch is used, it may be useful to place the correct size of a Hegar dilator into the new main pulmonary artery as the patch reaches the level of the pulmonary valve annulus. The patch can then be trimmed to fit snugly over the Hegar dilator at this level as it is being sewn into place (Fig. 23.8B).

As patching of the pulmonary artery and/or right ventricle is completed, systemic rewarming is begun. If an atrial septal defect or patent foramen ovale is present, it may be closed, and if the right atrium has been opened, may also be closed at the surgeon's discretion. Venting of the ascending aorta is carried out as the aortic cross-clamp is removed.

NB Surgery in Neonates

If complete repair of tetralogy of Fallot is performed on a neonate, the patent foramen ovale is generally left open. If pulmonary hypertension and/or right ventricular dysfunction occur in the postoperative period, right-to-left shunting at the atrial level can maintain left-sided filling pressures and adequate systemic cardiac output. The consequent desaturation is usually well tolerated. Because neonates may have little secondary right ventricular hypertrophy, only a limited resection of muscle from the right ventricular outflow tract is usually required. NB

At the end of cardiopulmonary bypass, pressures in the right ventricle, pulmonary artery, and left ventricle are measured directly or estimated by transesophageal echocardiography. The right ventricular pressure should be less

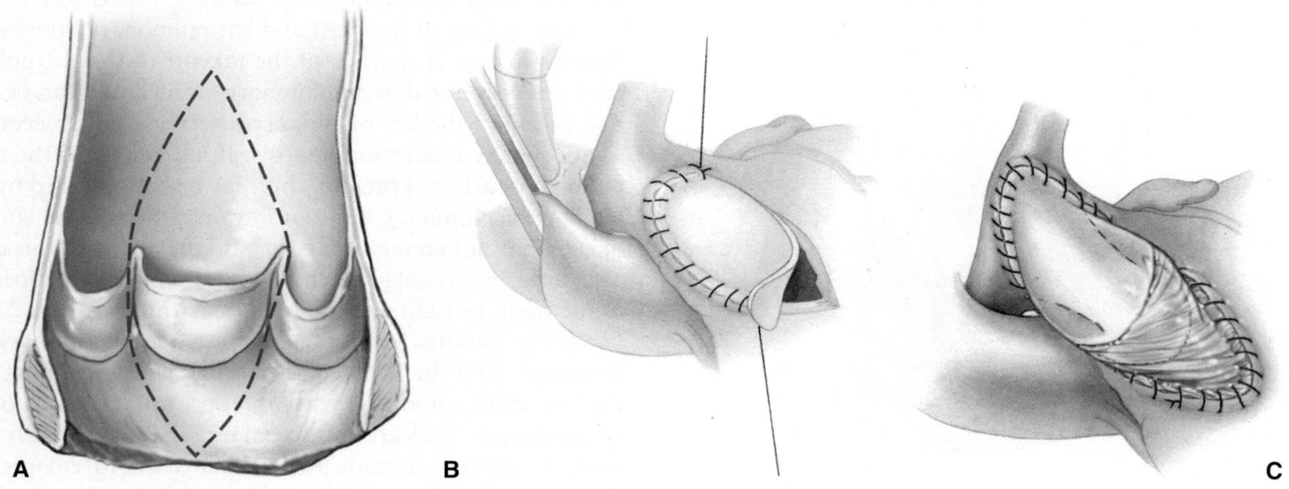

FIG. 23.7 Enlargement of pulmonary valve annulus. **A and C:** With a homograft monocusp patch. **B:** With a pericardial patch.

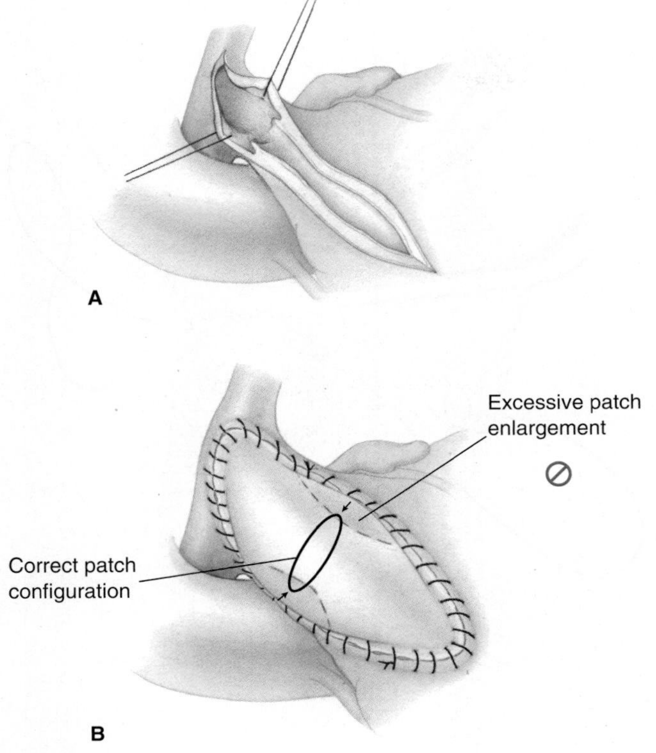

FIG. 23.8 Patch enlargement of the right ventricular outflow tract. **A:** Right ventriculotomy extended across annulus and onto left pulmonary artery. **B:** Correct patch configuration.

than 70% to 80% of left ventricular pressure. If the right ventricular pressure is greater than this and a transannular patch has not been placed, cardiopulmonary bypass should be recommenced and a transannular patch performed. If a transannular patch has been used, the site of obstruction should be localized by echocardiography or multiple pressure measurements proximal to, along the length of the patch, and distal to the right ventricular outflow tract patch. If a correctable obstruction is identified, cardiopulmonary bypass should be recommenced and the right ventricular outflow reconstruction should be revised. If the right ventricular pressure remains high despite these interventions and the patient is unstable, consideration should be given to creating a small atrial septal defect or a hole in the ventricular septal defect patch. This can be done on cardiopulmonary bypass during a brief period of aortic cross-clamping.

⊘ Poor Exposure of the Branch Pulmonary Arteries

Before placing the patient on cardiopulmonary bypass, the main and right pulmonary arteries must be dissected completely free from the aorta. This allows application of the aortic cross-clamp without limiting exposure or distorting the distal main pulmonary artery and origin of the right pulmonary artery. ⊘

⊘ Width of the Outflow Tract Patch

The width of the patch across the pulmonary annulus must be generous enough to eliminate most of the gradient between the right ventricle and pulmonary artery. It is better to accept a mild to moderate gradient than to create wide-open pulmonic insufficiency. The new annulus diameter should not be much greater than the Z-zero pulmonary annulus size for the patient (Fig. 23.8B). ⊘

⊘ Stenosis of the Distal Patch

The toe of the patch must be oval or square to minimize the risk of subsequent anastomotic stenosis. ⊘

PULMONARY ATRESIA AND VENTRICULA SEPTAL DEFECT

The intracardiac anatomy of pulmonary atresia and ventricular septal defect resembles that of tetralogy of Fallot, except that there is no connection between the right ventricular outflow tract and pulmonary artery. The anatomic subtypes range from those patients with well-developed pulmonary arteries connected to all bronchopulmonary segments, to those with hypoplastic pulmonary arteries in whom aortopulmonary collateral arteries are important sources of pulmonary blood flow, to the group of patients in whom no true mediastinal pulmonary arteries are present. In this last group of patients, all bronchopulmonary segments are supplied exclusively by aortopulmonary collateral arteries.

To plan the surgical approach in these patients, it is important to identify all aortopulmonary collateral arteries at the time of cardiac catheterization or computed tomography/magnetic resonance imaging. Smaller aortopulmonary collateral arteries may be embolized in the cardiac catheterization laboratory. Larger collateral vessels that supply a significant area of lung parenchyma must be detached from the aorta and anastomosed to a branch of the pulmonary artery, so-called unifocalization. Alternatively, unifocalization of collaterals to both lungs can be performed at one setting through a median sternotomy or clamshell incision with the option of connecting the unifocalized pulmonary arteries to the right ventricle with a homograft conduit with or without closure of the ventricular septal defect.

Patients with well-developed pulmonary arteries are usually dependent on a patent ductus arteriosus for adequate pulmonary blood flow. These infants require treatment with prostaglandin E_1 and a shunt procedure as a neonate (see Chapter 18). Complete repair can then be performed at 1 to 2 years of age.

Patients with hypoplastic, confluent pulmonary arteries may undergo an initial shunt procedure. However, better pulmonary artery growth may be achieved by early establishment of forward pulmonary blood flow from the right ventricle. This may be accomplished by performing a patch augmentation of the right ventricular outflow tract onto the main pulmonary artery across the atretic segment. Alternatively, a pulmonary artery homograft or GORTEX tube can be inserted between the right ventricle and pulmonary artery confluence using cardiopulmonary bypass, leaving the ventricular septal defect open.

⊘ Steal Phenomenon

If large aortopulmonary collateral arteries are not temporarily or permanently occluded before commencing cardiopulmonary bypass, a large amount of arterial blood return from the pump will run off through these vessels into the pulmonary arterial bed. This creates low perfusion pressure to vital organ systems including the brain and can lead to serious central nervous system deficits. ⊘

⊘ Ventricular Distention

If flow from the aortopulmonary collateral arteries cannot be completely controlled, the excessive blood return to the left ventricle causes left ventricular distention. Therefore, a vent placed through the right superior pulmonary vein into the left atrium and ventricle is usually required (see Chapter 4). ⊘

Complete repair in patients with absent true pulmonary arteries and large aortopulmonary collateral arteries can only be performed if adequate unifocalization of vessels supplying most of the bronchopulmonary segments has been achieved. The repair then consists of connecting the unifocalized segments, closing the ventricular septal defect, and placing a valved conduit from the right ventricle to this connection.

Technique for Complete Repair

Standard aortic and bicaval cannulation is performed. Before commencing cardiopulmonary bypass, any previously placed systemic to pulmonary artery shunts are dissected. As cardiopulmonary bypass is being initiated, the shunt is occluded, usually with one or two large metal clips. The intraventricular repair is carried out as for tetralogy of Fallot (see the preceding text). If the distance from the right ventricular outflow tract to the main pulmonary artery is less than 1.0 cm, the right ventriculotomy is extended across the atretic segment onto the main pulmonary artery (Fig. 23.8A). Any stenoses of the left and right pulmonary arteries are managed as described previously for tetralogy of Fallot. A rectangular graft of autologous pericardium or Gore-Tex or a monocusp patch is used to close the opening in the pulmonary artery and right ventricle, using running 5-0 or 6-0 Prolene suture and placing the stitches through the epicardial edges of the incised atretic connection between the right ventricle and pulmonary artery.

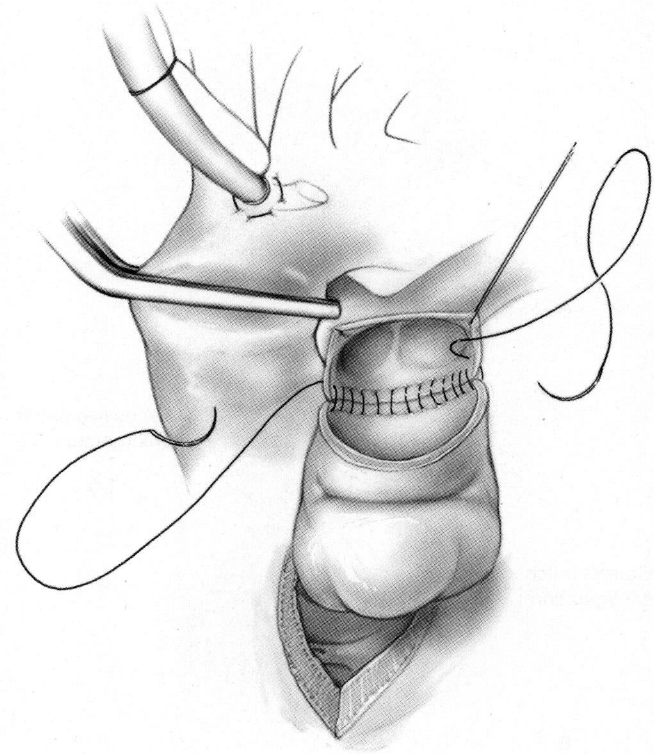

FIG. 23.9 Pulmonary homograft anastomosis to pulmonary artery.

⊘ Gradient across Transannular Patch

The patch must be sufficiently generous in the area of the atretic segment to ensure that an adequately sized Hegar dilator can pass through the completed pericardial tube graft that results from this anastomosis. ⊘

If the distance between the distal right ventricle and proximal pulmonary artery is too great, or if the pulmonary arteries are small, a homograft or bovine jugular valved conduit is used. In these cases, before aortic cross-clamping, the pulmonary artery confluence must be dissected free of the aorta. An appropriately sized aortic or pulmonary homograft is then prepared. The distal main pulmonary artery or pulmonary artery confluence is then opened, and the distal anastomosis performed in an end-to-end manner between the homograft and pulmonary artery, using a running 6-0 Prolene suture (Fig. 23.9). The proximal end of the homograft is then sewn directly to the upper margin of the right ventriculotomy incision. Suturing is begun at the heel of the anastomosis and continued on both sides of the homograft until one-third to one-half of the circumference of the homograft has been anastomosed to the right ventricular opening. A hood-shaped patch of autologous pericardium or Gore-Tex is then sewn to the anterior portion of the homograft circumference and to the remaining opening in the right ventricle, using running 5-0 or 6-0 Prolene suture. The remainder of the procedure is completed as for tetralogy of Fallot.

NB Hypoplastic Pulmonary Artery Confluence

Small confluent pulmonary arteries should be opened widely, extending the incision on the anterior surface of the left and right pulmonary arteries out to the hila of both lungs. A separate rectangular patch of autologous pericardium is then anastomosed to the edges of this opening, using running 6-0 or 5-0 Prolene suture. The distal end of the homograft is then anastomosed to an opening in the patch itself. Alternatively, a pulmonary artery homograft can be used, and the bifurcation portion of the homograft can be used to augment the hypoplastic pulmonary arterial confluence. NB

NB Tetralogy of Fallot with Anomalous Coronary Artery

Many patients with tetralogy of Fallot and an anomalous left anterior descending artery from the right coronary artery may require a valved conduit. The proximal graft is sutured to an opening in the right ventricle below the course of the anomalous vessel. Forward flow through the native pulmonary annulus may be preserved or eliminated. NB

⊘ Aneurysm of a Pulmonary Homograft

If distal pulmonary artery stenoses are present, the thin-walled pulmonary homograft or bovine jugular vein graft may dilate and even become aneurysmal. In patients with elevated pulmonary artery pressure, an aortic homograft may be more suitable. ⊘

NB Homograft Failure

Both aortic and pulmonary homografts may calcify and become stenotic. However, pulmonary homografts frequently remain unobstructed for a longer period of time. NB

NB Availability of Homograft Conduits

Many congenital heart defects require the use of a right ventricle-to-pulmonary artery conduit. Although homografts are generally preferred, their limited availability, especially in small sizes, is a significant problem. Several other types of valved conduits have been used, including composite bioprosthetic valved conduits, xenografts, autologous pericardial valved conduits, and bovine jugular vein conduits. The latter device has shown some promise, and is readily available in all sizes. When using a jugular valved conduit, care must be taken to not leave the conduit too long. These precautions, as well as careful rinsing before implantation, are necessary to prevent distal stenosis. In addition, some surgeons downsize larger homografts to create a two leaflet valved conduit approximately two-thirds the diameter of the original homograft. NB

ABSENT PULMONARY VALVE SYNDROME

Absent pulmonary valve syndrome occurs in approximately 3% of cases with tetralogy of Fallot (Fig. 23.10). Rarely, it can occur as an isolated lesion or in association with other cardiac anomalies. Characteristically, there is failure of development of the pulmonary valve leaflets. The pulmonary valve annulus is normal or somewhat small, but the central pulmonary arteries are massively dilated. Patients who present as neonates or infants have severe respiratory symptoms related to compression of the main stem bronchi by the aneurysmal central pulmonary arteries. These infants require urgent surgical attention. Older children may have few if any symptoms and can be operated on electively. Complete surgical correction consists of closure of the ventricular septal defect (if present), plication of the enlarged portions of the pulmonary artery, and placement of a homograft between the right ventricle and pulmonary artery.

Technique

A median sternotomy is performed, and most of the thymus gland is removed to aid in exposure of the central pulmonary arteries. A patch of pericardium is harvested and fixed with 0.6% glutaraldehyde solution. The aorta is then dissected free from the main and right pulmonary arteries,

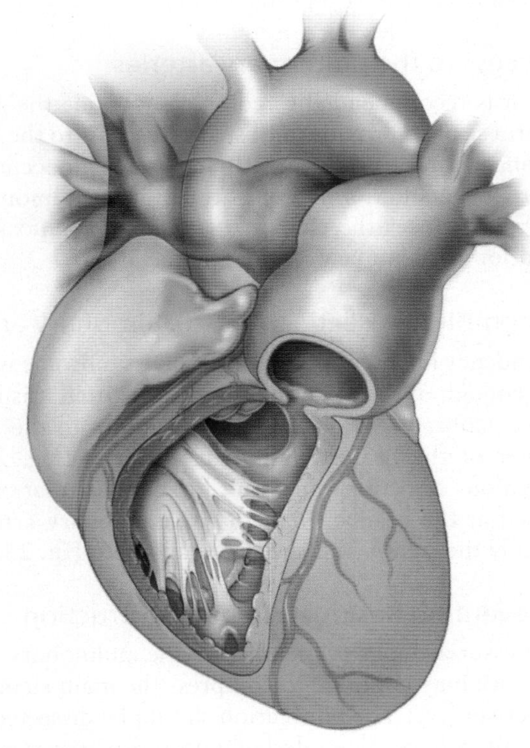

FIG. 23.10 TOF-APV heart.

and the pulmonary arteries are mobilized out to the hila of both lungs. Aortic cannulation is performed near the takeoff of the innominate artery on the right-hand side of the aorta to keep the cannula away from the operative site. Bicaval cannulation is performed, and cardiopulmonary bypass is established. Systemic cooling to 28°C–32°C is carried out. The aorta is cross-clamped, and cardioplegic arrest of the heart is achieved by infusion of cold blood cardioplegic solution into the aortic root. A high vertical right ventriculotomy is made that can be extended if the need arises. The hypertrophied infundibular muscles are divided and resected, although generally in absent pulmonary valve syndrome, little subpulmonary obstruction exists. This brings the ventricular septal defect into view and it is closed with a patch as described earlier. The abnormally enlarged main pulmonary artery is then dissected free posteriorly and incised just above the pulmonary valve annulus. This incision is brought through the main pulmonary artery.

The branch pulmonary arteries are reduced in caliber by removing a considerable portion of the anterior wall after full mobilization of the branches. Often there is early takeoff of the hilar branches and so the length of this resection can be limited. It is important to mobilize the remaining pulmonary artery tissue off of the underlying airway for the best result. When performing the reduction pulmonary arterioplasty, it is also important not to remove too much native tissue at the junction of the main pulmonary artery with the branches so as not to cause proximal obstruction from distortion (Fig. 23.11).

NB Access to the pulmonary arteries

Often it is recommended to completely divide the ascending aorta so as to provide unobstructed access to the branch pulmonary arteries. This greatly facilitates an accurate resection of the anterior aspect of the branch pulmonary arteries and reduces the chance of torsion or stenosis from angulation that can be obscured by the arch. NB

⊘ Incomplete resection of the pulmonary arteries

The tendency in absent pulmonary valve syndrome is not to resect enough of the pulmonary arteries. Often it is helpful to have calibrated Hegar dilators as guides to the proper diameter of the branch pulmonary arteries (Fig. 23.12). Overzealous resection can result in acute angulation (and stenosis) at the branch point of the pulmonary arteries—especially the right—and should be avoided (Fig. 23.11). ⊘

NB Preventing Residual Airway Obstruction

The pressurized posterior wall of the pulmonary artery confluence may continue to compress the main stem bronchi after surgery. The bifurcation should be dissected completely away from the underlying posterior structures, and any fibrous bands between the pulmonary artery and bronchi should be divided. NB

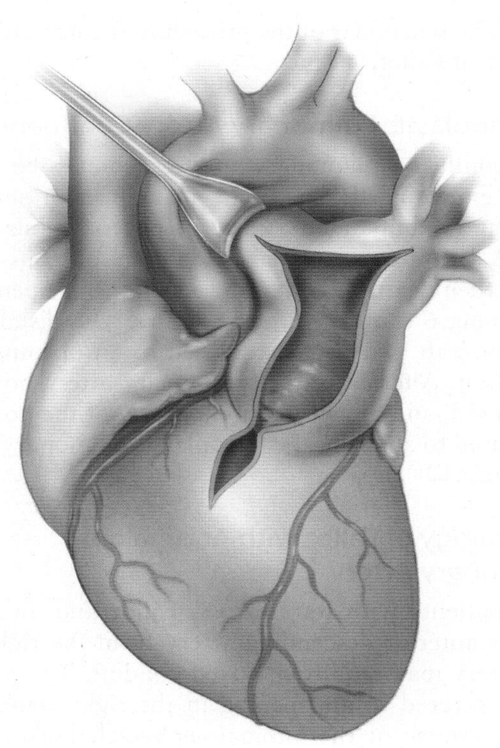

FIG. 23.11 Incisions for reduction pulmonary arterioplasty.

Alternatively, a Lecompte maneuver is performed transecting the ascending aorta and bringing the pulmonary confluence anterior to the aorta (see Chapter 25). Occasionally, a short segment of ascending aorta must be excised before the two ends are reapproximated. This technique requires extensive mobilization of the pulmonary arteries into the hila of both lungs and ligation and division of the ductus or ligamentum arteriosum. A reduction pulmonary arterioplasty is completed before placing the valved conduit from the right ventricle to the pulmonary artery confluence.

PULMONARY ATRESIA, INTACT VENTRICULAR SEPTUM

Patients usually present with cyanosis on the first day of life. Prostaglandin E_1 is begun to maintain patency of the ductus arteriosus. The diagnosis is made by echocardiography, which demonstrates the size of the right ventricular cavity, the size and competence of the tricuspid valve, the size of the pulmonary arteries, and the size of the interatrial communication. The size of the right ventricle in this anomaly ranges from diminutive to larger than normal. Ten percent of patients have major obstructions of one or more coronary arteries with fistulous communications from the right ventricular cavity to the distal coronary arteries. Cardiac

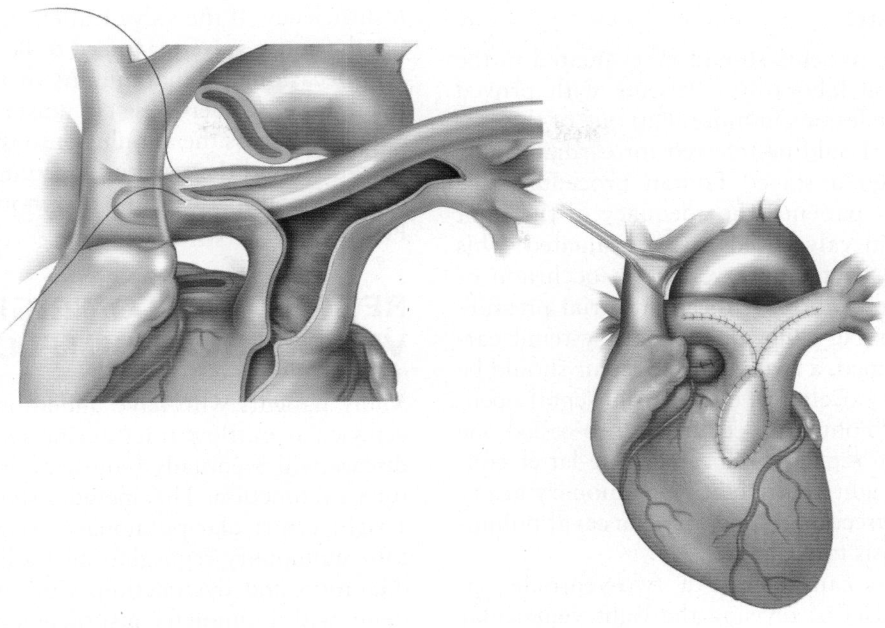

FIG. 23.12 Calibration and completion of reduction arterioplasty.

catheterization is required to identify these abnormalities of coronary circulation.

The initial management of these patients depends on the anatomy that is present. Patients with a small right ventricle whose tricuspid valve diameter is less than a z-score of –2.5 should undergo a modified Blalock–Taussig shunt. Similarly, patients with enlarged right ventricles and severe tricuspid regurgitation, and those with significant stenoses involving more than one of the three major epicardial coronary systems should also undergo a shunt procedure (see Chapter 18) with or without tricuspid valve exclusion (Starnes procedure).

Patients with larger right ventricles and competent tricuspid valves should undergo a procedure to open the right ventricular outflow tract. If the right ventricle is only mildly hypoplastic, a concomitant systemic to pulmonary artery shunt may not be required. However, most of these patients are best served by a combined outflow tract procedure and a modified Blalock-Taussig shunt.

Surgical Technique

A median sternotomy incision is used. A piece of pericardium is harvested and fixed with 0.6% glutaraldehyde. If use of a monocusp patch is planned, an appropriate pulmonary homograft piece is prepared. The aorta is cannulated, and a single straight or right-angled cannula is placed through the right atrial appendage for venous drainage. The ductus arteriosus is dissected and closed with a metal clip as cardiopulmonary bypass is commenced. Because a patent foramen ovale is always present, the aorta should be cross-clamped to prevent systemic air embolism, and cardioplegia used to protect the heart. Traction sutures are placed on the main pulmonary artery, and a vertical arteriotomy is performed. The pulmonary valve plate is visualized; if the infundibulum is patent and the annulus is of good size, a valvotomy or valvectomy may be performed. Otherwise, the incision is carried down across the atretic annulus and onto the right ventricle. The infundibular muscle should be resected toward a goal of providing a right ventricular "overhaul" and producing and unobstructed right ventricular outflow tract. The previously prepared patch of pericardium or monocusp patch is sewn into place, using a running 7-0 Prolene suture. The systemic to pulmonary artery shunt is constructed after removing the aortic cross-clamp (see Chapter 18). As the clamp is removed from the shunt, ventilation is begun, and cardiopulmonary bypass is discontinued. The patent foramen ovale is left open.

⊘ Postoperative Cyanosis

Right ventricular diastolic dysfunction increases right-to-left shunting at the atrial level across the patent foramen ovale. If transannular patching is performed without a shunt procedure, this may result in unacceptably low systemic oxygenation. If a shunt procedure is not performed, the ductus arteriosus can be left open and only temporarily occluded during cardiopulmonary bypass. Prostaglandin E_1 can be slowly withdrawn in the postoperative period and continued for as long as 3 to 4 weeks postoperatively, if required. If at the end of this period, inadequate oxygenation persists, the patient should be returned to the operating room for a systemic to pulmonary artery shunt. ⊘

Definitive Repair

By late infancy, these patients should be evaluated in the cardiac catheterization laboratory. Patients with proved significant obstructive lesions in more than one of the major coronary arteries should be referred for cardiac transplantation or undergo a staged Fontan procedure (see Chapter 31). In other patients, the adequacy of the right ventricle and tricuspid valve needs to be evaluated. This can be accomplished by temporary balloon occlusion of the interatrial communication. If the right atrial pressure remains below 20 mm Hg while an adequate systemic cardiac output is maintained, a two-ventricle repair should be tolerated. If temporary occlusion of the atrial septal opening is not tolerated, a Fontan procedure or a so-called one and one-half ventricle repair is indicated. The latter consists of combining a right ventricular to pulmonary artery connection with a bidirectional superior vena caval-pulmonary artery anastomosis (see Chapter 31).

For patients who can tolerate a two-ventricle approach, surgery consists of revising the right ventricular outflow patch if any residual obstruction is noted at the time of cardiac catheterization, and closing the interatrial communication and the systemic to pulmonary artery shunt. If the outflow patch is satisfactory, the atrial septal defect and shunt may be closed in the catheterization laboratory.

⊘ Tricuspid Regurgitation

If significant tricuspid regurgitation is present, a homograft valve should be placed in the right ventricular outflow tract and a tricuspid valve repair performed. ⊘

PULMONARY STENOSIS AND AN INTACT VENTRICULAR SEPTUM

Typically, the valve is dome-shaped with its three leaflets fused, leaving a tiny central opening. Occasionally, the leaflets are thickened and dysplastic and produce obstruction by their bulkiness. The pulmonary valve annulus may be hypoplastic; however, it often is of adequate size. Most of these patients can be managed in the cardiac catheterization laboratory by balloon valvuloplasty. However, occasionally, surgical intervention is required.

Technique for Repair

In neonates, pulmonary valvotomy may be carried out with or without cardiopulmonary bypass. Most often, it is preferable to perform a pulmonary valvotomy in all patients through a median sternotomy on cardiopulmonary bypass.

After initiation of cardiopulmonary bypass, a longitudinal incision is made on the anterior surface of the pulmonary artery. The commissures of the pulmonary valve are incised up to and including the annulus. The commissurotomy should be generous enough to produce some insufficiency. If the valve leaflets are thickened or dysplastic, the entire valve may need to be resected.

Occasionally, the annulus of the pulmonary valve is hypoplastic. Under these circumstances, the arteriotomy is extended across the annulus onto the right ventricular outflow tract and the resulting opening is closed with a patch of autologous pericardium or a monocusp, using 5-0 or 6-0 Prolene suture (Fig. 23.8).

REOPERATION ON RIGHT VENTRICULAR OUTFLOW TRACT

Many patients who have undergone surgery on the right ventricular outflow tract during repair of congenital heart disease will eventually require an intervention for outflow tract dysfunction. This includes stenosis of, or outgrowing a right ventricular-pulmonary artery conduit, and significant pulmonary regurgitation leading to right ventricular dilatation and dysfunction. Currently, asymptomatic patients with pulmonary insufficiency are being referred for treatment based on magnetic resonance image findings to prevent irreversible right ventricular dysfunction. The surgical management of these patients is centered on relief of any outflow obstruction and placement of a competent pulmonic valve.

Technique

Many patients have conduits or aneuysmal outflow patches, which may be positioned directly behind the sternum. A preoperative computed tomographic scan can define the anatomy and allow for institution of cardiopulmonary bypass through the femoral vessels before sternotomy in high-risk patients. Otherwise standard cannulation is performed. If no residual ventricular septal defect or atrial septal defect is present, the procedure is carried out on a warm, beating heart. Homografts or bovine jugular grafts are most often used to replace previous conduits, resecting all fibrotic and calcified tissue, and enlarging the right ventricular and/or pulmonary openings appropriately. Bovine pericardium or Gore-Tex is used to hood the proximal anastomosis. A bubble study should be performed to rule out intracardiac shunting if a beating heart approach is planned.

Patients with previous outflow tract patches often have thinning and scarring of the anterior surface of the right ventricle. These patients can undergo right ventricular remodeling by resecting or plicating the thinned out portion of the right ventricle as well as excising the previous patch that is often calcified. A double row of 4-0 Prolene sutures, reinforced with felt strips if needed, is used to reapproximate the anterior wall of the right ventricle (Fig. 23.13). In younger patients, a homograft valve in inserted (see preceding text). In older children and adults, a bioprosthesis is attached to the patient's annulus posteriorly with a running 4-0 Prolene suture. Anteriorly, a diamond-shaped

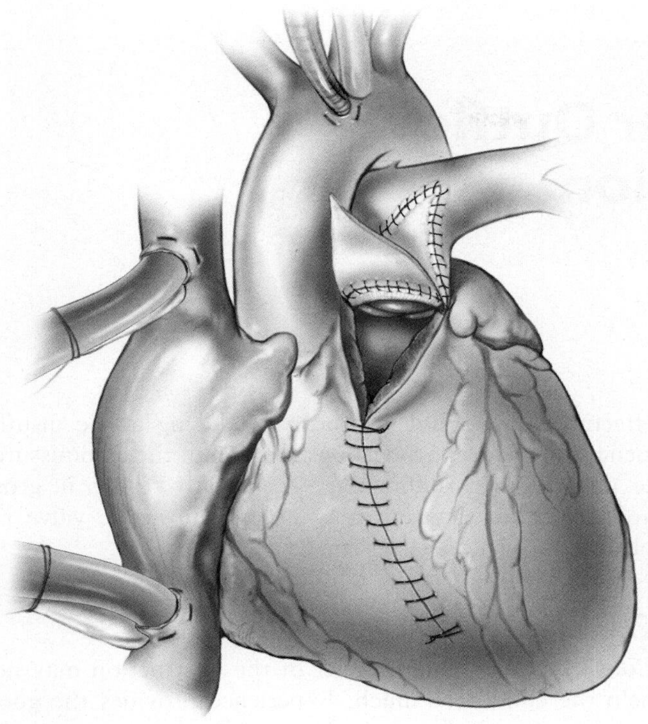

FIG. 23.13 Resection and reapproximation of anterior wall of the right ventricle, and placement of prosthetic valve in outflow tract.

patch of bovine pericardium or Gore-Tex is used to close the pulmonary artery opening with a running 5-0 Prolene suture. At the level of the valve, the patch is sewn to the prosthetic sewing ring by continuing the 4-0 Prolene valve suture, which is then secured (Fig. 23.13). The remaining portion of the patch is used to close the opening on the right ventricle, continuing the 5-0 Prolene stitch. The patient is now weaned from cardiopulmonary bypass and standard closure is completed.

NB Larger-Sized Prosthesis

Securing the prosthesis below the pulmonary annulus to the infundibular muscle posteriorly allows placement of a larger prosthesis. NB

NB Tricuspid Valve

Many patients with chronic pulmonary regurgitation and right ventricular dysfunction have at least moderate tricuspid insufficiency and should undergo a concomitant tricuspid annuloplasty (see Chapter 7). NB

NB Percutaneous Pulmonary Valve Implantation

Percutaneous implantation of pulmonary valves is an evolving field, and may allow some patients with right ventricular outflow tract dysfunction to avoid surgery. However, patients with large transannular patches are currently not candidates for this technology, and this approach does not allow for surgical right ventricular remodeling. NB

APPENDIX

Sizing the Pulmonary Outflow Tract

The internal diameter of the narrowest part of the pulmonary outflow tract is determined by passing calibrated Hegar dilators of increasing size through the pulmonary valve and into the pulmonary artery. Referring to the data from Rowlatt et al. (Rowlatt UF, Rimoldi HJA, Lev M. The quantitative anatomy of the normal child's heart. *Pediatr Clin North Am.* 1963;10:499–588.) allows the surgeon to determine if the annulus and/or right ventricular outflow tract is adequate for a given patient. With the diameters shown, only a 15% probability exists that the right ventricular-left ventricular pressure ratio will be more than 0.65.

Body Surface Area (m^2)	Diameter (mm)
0.15	5.9
0.20	7.3
0.25	8.4
0.30	9.3
0.35	10.1
0.40	10.7
0.45	11.3
0.50	11.9
0.55	12.3
0.60	12.8
0.65	13.2
0.70	13.5
0.75	13.9
0.80	14.2
0.90	14.8
1.0	15.3
1.2	16.2
1.4	17.0
1.6	17.6
1.8	18.2
2.0	18.7

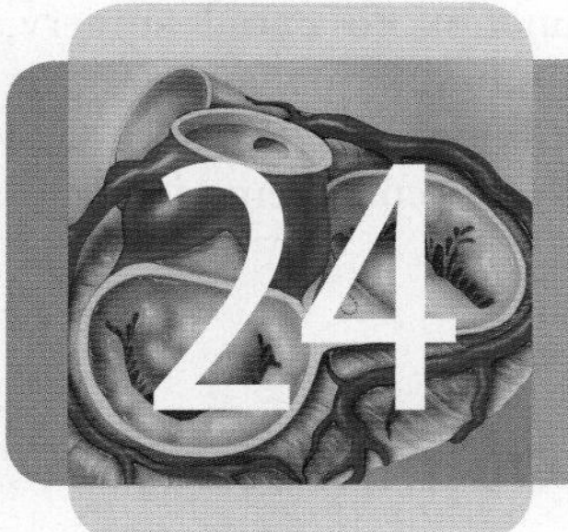

24 Left Ventricular Outflow Tract Obstruction

CONGENITAL AORTIC STENOSIS

Pathologic findings in congenital aortic stenosis can vary. The valve may be bicuspid, tricuspid, or unicuspid, and the commissures may be fused together in any combination. The functional orifice of the aortic valve, however, is usually between the left and noncoronary cusps, whereas the other cusp and commissures are fused and deformed to various degrees.

Infants or neonates with critical aortic stenosis may require urgent intervention. Neonates may present in extremis with marked metabolic acidosis. Infusion of prostaglandin E_1 may improve the circulation in these neonates by reopening the ductus arteriosus. It is critical in these cases to differentiate isolated, critical aortic stenosis from a form of hypoplastic left heart syndrome that requires a modified Norwood procedure (see Chapter 30). Although percutaneous balloon valvuloplasty for critical aortic stenosis in the neonate and infant is being performed with satisfactory results, surgery is still indicated for some patients.

Valvotomy Technique

A median sternotomy approach is used. Surgical valvotomy is performed on cardiopulmonary bypass. Cannulation is carried out with a standard aortic cannula and a single venous cannula in the right atrial appendage and a vent in the right superior pulmonary vein. Cardiopulmonary bypass is begun, and the ductus arteriosus is closed with a heavy tie or metal clip. The aorta is cross-clamped, and cardioplegic solution is administered (see Chapter 3). The aorta is incised transversely, the aortic valve is exposed, and its anatomy is studied closely. A no. 15 blade is used to incise the fused commissures to within 2 mm of the aortic annulus (Fig. 24.1).

⊘ Aortic Insufficiency

The purpose of the surgery is to relieve obstruction to the left ventricular outflow tract in these very sick infants as effectively as possible, without producing aortic insufficiency. Therefore, overzealous incision of the commissures or division of a rudimentary raphe only results in gross aortic insufficiency and may necessitate aortic valve replacement (Fig. 24.2). ⊘

⊘ Inadequate Relief of Obstruction

Conversely, inadequate relief of the obstruction may not help the child very much. Experience provides the good judgment required to incise to just the right extent at the precise area of a grossly deformed aortic valve. ⊘

NB Exposing the Aortic Valve

When the aorta is small, an oblique rather than transverse aortotomy provides better exposure of the aortic valve. NB

⊘ Awareness of Subvalvular Obstruction

It is of paramount importance to inspect the aortic subvalvular area and rule out the presence of a fibrous diaphragm or other forms of left ventricular outflow tract obstruction. A Hegar dilator of appropriate size can be used for precise evaluation of the valvular orifice and the left ventricular outflow tract. ⊘

⊘ Severely Deformed or Maldeveloped Aortic Leaflets

A satisfactory commissurotomy with long-lasting good results depends on how well the valve was formed initially. When there is severe deformity and maldevelopment of the aortic valve, surgical relief of left ventricular outflow tract obstruction is only temporary and palliative. These subgroups of patients should be followed closely so that a more definitive form of treatment can be performed before permanent left ventricular dysfunction ensues. ⊘

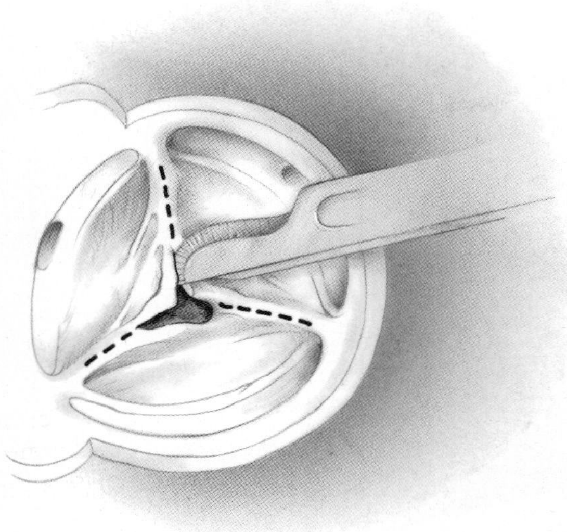

FIG. 24.1 Technique for aortic commissurotomy.

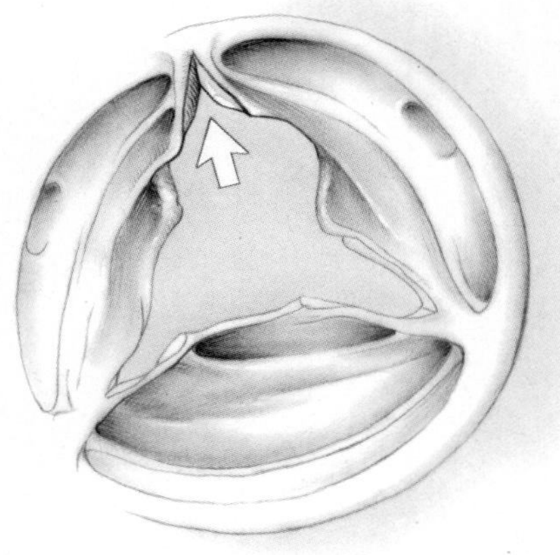

FIG. 24.2 Overzealous incision of the commissures, causing aortic insufficiency.

RESECTION OF THE SUBVALVULAR DIAPHRAGM

A fibrous, muscular, or membranous rim of tissue arising from the anterior two-thirds of the left ventricular outflow tract may be present within 1 cm below the aortic annulus. The aortic valve leaflets are retracted gently with narrow ribbon retractors. Often, exposure is greatly aided by placing three suspension sutures at each of the commissures, and three additional fine prolene sutures just below the nadir of each cusp on the left ventricular side, thereby producing a hexagonal opening that is unobstructed and requires no additional retraction from the surgical assistant (Fig. 24.3). The fibromuscular diaphragm is then excised with a no. 15 blade (Fig. 24.4A, B). This shelf of abnormal tissue can also be mobilized and enucleated in its whole circumference with an endarterectomy spatula.

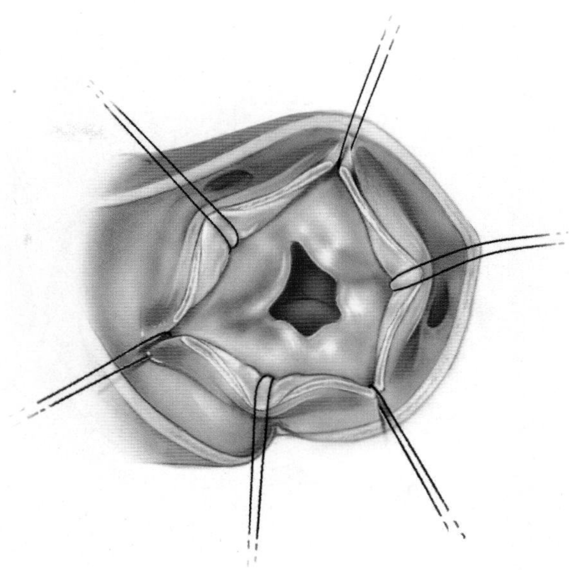

FIG. 24.3 Technique for exposure of the subaortic obstruction. Stay sutures are placed at the top of each commissure, as well as at the nadir of each aortic cusp. When retracted radially, these provide a view of the subaortic region, often obviating the need for additional retraction from an assistant.

NB Myotomy or Myectomy

A myotomy or a limited myectomy involving the bulging septum is recommended to prevent the possible persistence of a significant residual obstruction (Fig. 24.4C). This may also help to prevent recurrence of the membrane, the incidence of which is higher the younger the patient is when the initial surgery is performed. NB

⊘ Ventricular Septal Defect

A substantial segment of the abnormal fibromuscular tissue can be excised and removed from the septal area without producing a defect in the interventricular septum. If such a complication does occur, the defect must be identified and closed. Pledgeted sutures are essential to protect the friable muscular tissue. ⊘

⊘ Injury to Conduction Tissue

Only the white fibrous tissue should be mobilized and removed from the area immediately below the rightward half of the right cusp and the commissure between the right and noncoronary cusps. Otherwise, the conduction tissue may be injured resulting in heart block (Fig. 24.4B). ⊘

⊘ Valvular Insufficiency

Occasionally, the membranous tissue is adherent to the underside of the right coronary leaflet of the aortic valve. It must then be meticulously dissected free without damaging the aortic valve to avoid producing valvular insufficiency. ⊘

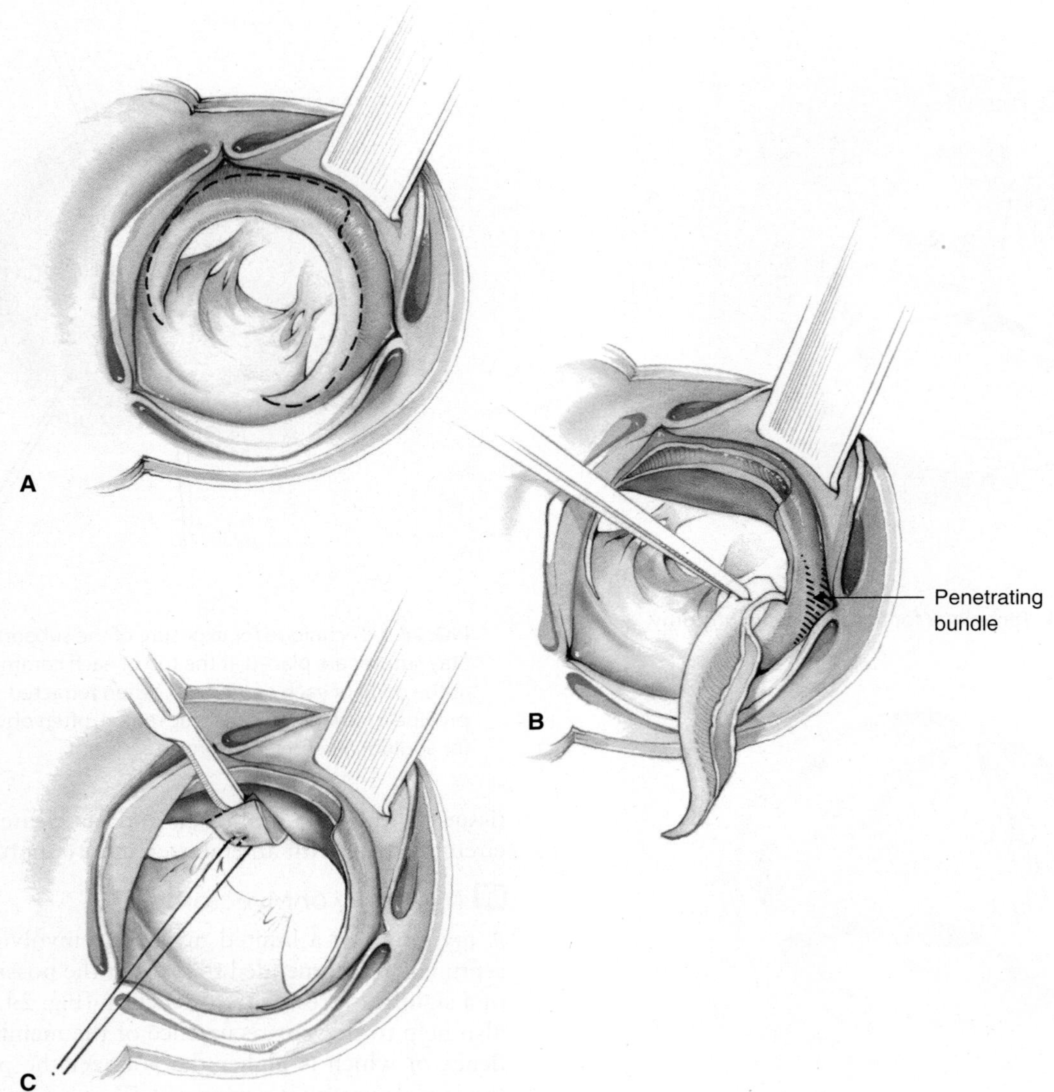

FIG. 24.4 Resection of a subvalvular diaphragm. **A:** Dashed line depicts the extent of resection. **B:** Only the white fibrous tissue is resected near the penetrating bundle. **C:** As an extra precaution against inadequate relief of an obstruction, a limited myectomy is also carried out.

⊘ Injury to the Mitral Valve

Occasionally, the lesion may extend and become adherent to the anterior leaflet of the mitral valve; in this case, it should be dissected free with the utmost care. Injury to the mitral valve near its annulus may result in an opening into the left atrium. ⊘

HYPERTROPHIC OBSTRUCTIVE CARDIOMYOPATHY

Hypertrophic obstructive cardiomyopathy is usually not a surgical lesion. Many patients respond to β-blockers or calcium channel blockers. Dual-chamber cardiac pacemakers may be useful in some patients. For severely symptomatic patients, ventricular septal myectomy is an established treatment. A relatively thick segment (1-cm deep by 1.5-cm wide) of septal wall extending downward to the base of the papillary muscles is excised and removed (Fig. 24.5).

NB Exposure of Hypertrophied Septum

Most surgeons use a transaortic approach. Exposure is facilitated by extending the aortotomy obliquely down to the noncoronary annulus and placing plegeted sutures just above the valve commissures. By placing traction on these sutures, the hypertrophied septum can be visualized. After the initial wedge resection, a small rake retractor can be placed into the septum and pulled upward toward the aortic annulus to allow visualization and resection of the apical portion of the septum. NB

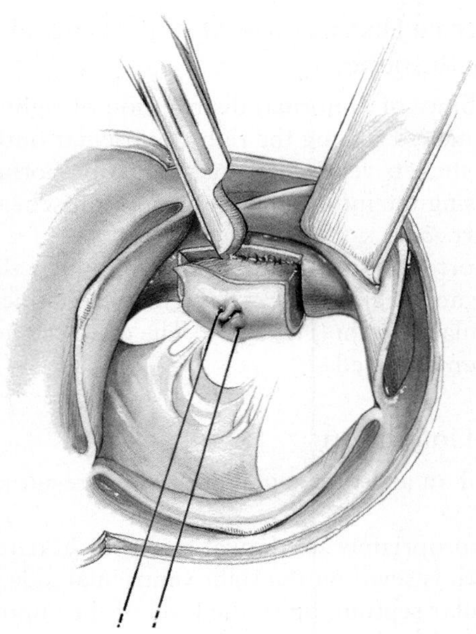

FIG. 24.5 Myectomy for idiopathic hypertrophic subaortic stenosis. Two longitudinal incisions, one below the commissure between the left and right leaflets and the other below the nadir of the right cusp are made. These are connected with an incision 1 cm below the valve, and a wedge of septal muscle is excised.

NB Surgery on the Mitral Valve

When systolic anterior motion of the anterior leaflet of the mitral valve is a significant component of the left ventricular outflow tract obstruction, an adequate septal myectomy usually resolves the abnormal motion of the anterior leaflet and any mitral regurgitation. However, some patients have associated abnormalities of the mitral subvalvular apparatus, which must be recognized and treated at the time of surgery. These include anomalous papillary muscle insertion directly into the anterior leaflet of the mitral valve and abnormal chordae tendineae attaching to the ventricular septum. If present, the abnormal chords are resected, and any areas of fusion of the papillary muscle(s) to the septum or free wall are divided. Occasionally, a valvuloplasty procedure to shift the coaptation level of the valve posteriorly may be required. This may involve anterior and/or posterior leaflet plication usually combined with an annuloplasty. A simple technique that may be effective is an Alfieri stitch placed 1 cm away from the free edges connecting the central portion of the anterior and posterior leaflets (see Chapter 6). Rarely, the mitral valve must be replaced with a low-profile prosthesis, resecting the entire anterior subvalvular apparatus. When combined with a myectomy, these techniques result in relief of the obstruction. NB

⊘ Flail Leaflet

All anomalous chords attached to the free edge of the anterior leaflet must be preserved to prevent a flail leaflet. ⊘

⊘ Embolism from Muscle Fragments Falling into the Ventricular Cavity

During the process of excising the hypertrophied muscle, fragments may fall into the left ventricular cavity, resulting in a subsequent embolism. This can be prevented to some degree by pulling on the desired segment to be excised with a 4-0 or 5-0 Prolene stitch (Fig. 24.5). A biopsy forceps may be used to resect muscle from the more apical portions of the septum. Care should be taken to remove all debris from within the left ventricular cavity. ⊘

NB Inadequate Exposure

Exposure may be inadequate through the retracted aortic leaflets. The obstructing muscle may then be removed through a left atriotomy working through the mitral valve. NB

NB Extent of resection

The myectomy can be considered complete when the mitral chordae and papillary support apparatus is clearly visualized through the left ventricular outflow tract. NB

LEFT VENTRICULAR TUNNEL OBSTRUCTION

When the left ventricular outflow tract is diffusely obstructed by a congenitally narrow tunnel, none of the aforementioned techniques are helpful to any significant degree. A left ventricular apical conduit to the ascending or descending aorta is an alternative, but not a favored one. The Rastan-Konno aortoventricular septoplasty, although a somewhat radical procedure, provides satisfactory results. In infants and children, a Ross-Konno procedure (replacing the aortic root with the pulmonary autograft, completing the ventriculoseptoplasty, and reconstructing the right ventricular outflow tract with a pulmonary homograft) is the operation of choice for this diagnosis.

Rastan-Konno Aortoventricular Septoplasty

Bicaval and aortic cannulations are made in the usual manner. On cardiopulmonary bypass with moderate cooling, the aorta is cross-clamped and cardioplegic arrest of the heart is achieved by the usual techniques (see Chapter 3). The aorta is incised anteriorly in a longitudinal direction. The incision is then extended downward under direct vision into the root of the aorta.

⊘ Direction of the Aortotomy

The direction of the aortotomy should be as far as possible to the left of the right coronary artery ostium, but not reaching the commissure between the right and left sinuses. This prevents injury to the ostium of the right coronary artery. ⊘

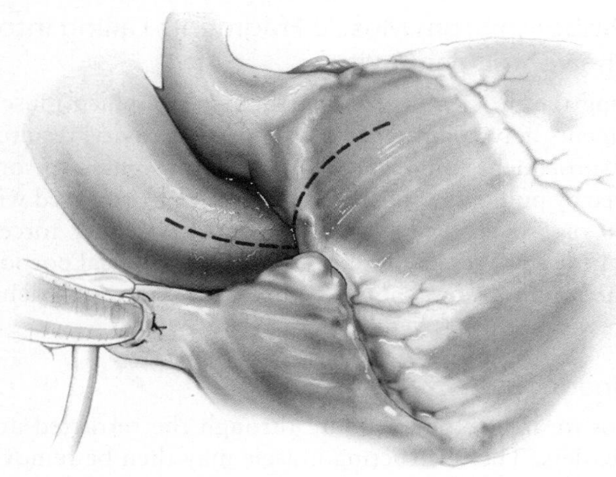

FIG. 24.6 Oblique incision on the aortic root and incision on right ventricle to expose the interventricular septum in the Rastan-Konno aortoventricular septoplasty.

The anterior surface of the right ventricular outflow tract is then incised obliquely downward from the aortic root for a distance sufficient to provide good exposure of the interventricular septum (Fig. 24.6). Alternatively, the right ventriculotomy is made first and then extended upward into the aortic root.

⊘ Injury to the Pulmonic Valve

The right ventricular outflow tract should be opened before cutting across the aortic annulus to ensure that the native pulmonic valve is not injured. Late pulmonary insufficiency is seen not infrequently following this procedure. ⊘

⊘ Abnormal Distribution of Right Coronary Artery Branches

The possibility of abnormal distribution of right coronary artery branches crossing the right ventricular outflow tract to supply the left ventricular mass must be borne in mind when incising the infundibulum to prevent ischemic injury to the heart. ⊘

The aortotomy is then continued obliquely downward across the aortic annulus onto the massively thickened interventricular septum (Fig. 24.7). The distorted aortic leaflets are then removed.

⊘ Septal Infarction

Division of an aberrant septal artery may result in a septal infarction. ⊘

An appropriately sized, oval Hemashield patch of generous width is sewn on the right ventricular side of the interventricular septum, up to the level of the annulus of the resected aortic valve (Fig. 24.8).

⊘ Reinforcing the Sutures on the Interventricular Septum

The interventricular septum is thick and friable; a continuous Prolene suture may tear through it, causing suture leaks and a resulting shunt across the septum. The suture line can be reinforced by buttressing the sutures over a strip of Teflon felt or pledgets on the left or right ventricular side (or both) of the septum (Fig. 24.8). Using interrupted sutures buttressed with pledgets results in surface-to-surface coaptation of the patch to the septum, thereby reducing the possibility of leaks (Fig. 24.8B). ⊘

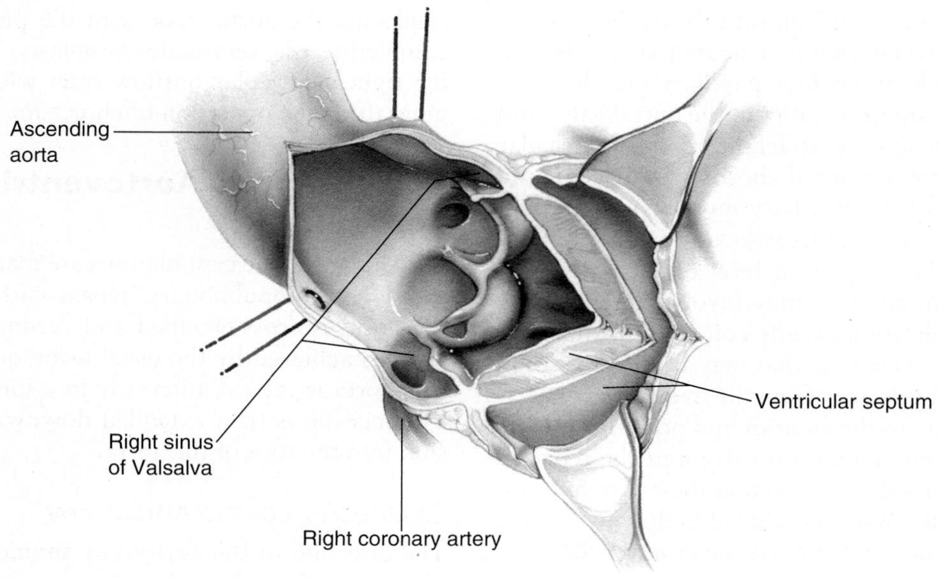

FIG. 24.7 Continuation of the oblique aortotomy on the interventricular septum.

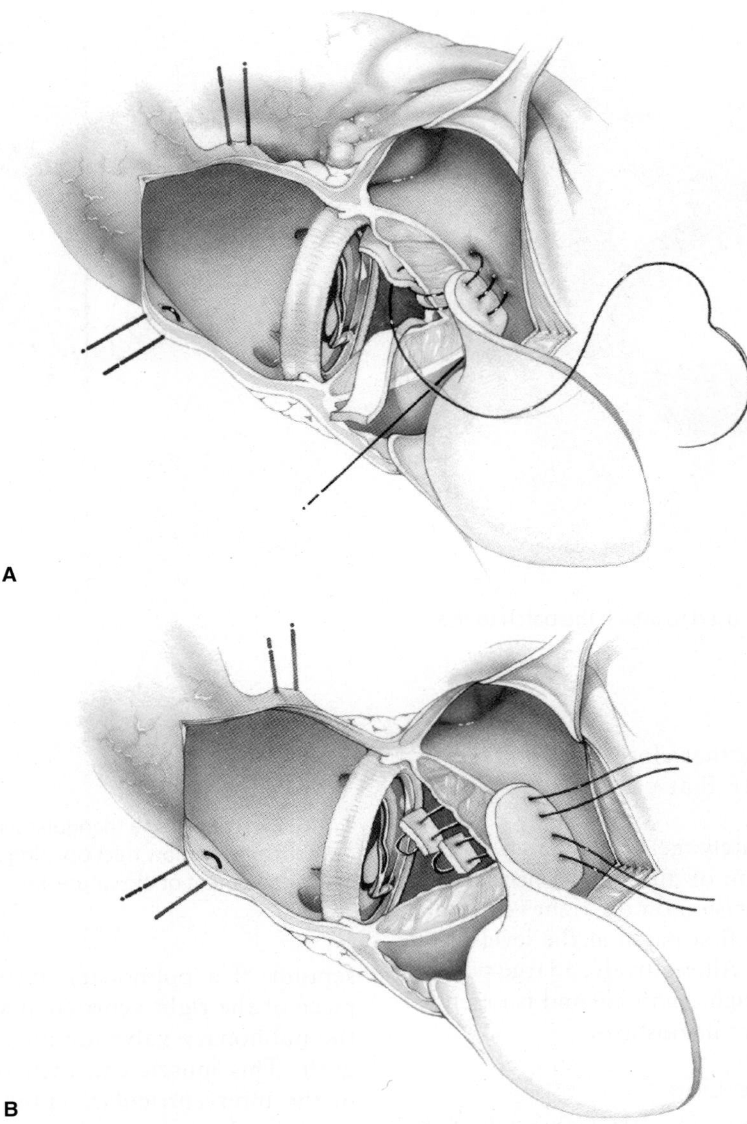

FIG. 24.8 Oval patch sewn on the right ventricular side of the interventricular septum, across the prosthetic ring and upward along the aortotomy.
A: A continuous suture line is reinforced with a strip of Teflon felt.
B: An alternate technique uses interrupted sutures buttressed with pledgets.

NB Maximizing the Enlargement

To maximize the left ventricular outflow tract enlargement, the Hemashield patch graft is sewn onto the right ventricular side of the septum. NB

Interrupted valve sutures are inserted into the aortic annulus and through the patch at the level of the annulus (see Chapter 5). After the sutures are inserted through the prosthetic sewing ring, the prosthesis is seated satisfactorily into position (Fig. 24.8). The prosthesis can be sewn to the Hemashield with either continuous or interrupted sutures.

NB Choice of Prosthesis

Because of their early calcification in children, stented tissue valves are not used. Low-profile disc or bileaflet mechanical valves are the preferred prostheses if a pulmonary autograft is not available or contraindicated. NB

NB Suture Line

A new continuous suture should be started at the valve sewing ring and should proceed so that the patch is laid onto the aortotomy incision. Therefore, the septal suture line is tied snugly at the level of the prosthesis. This

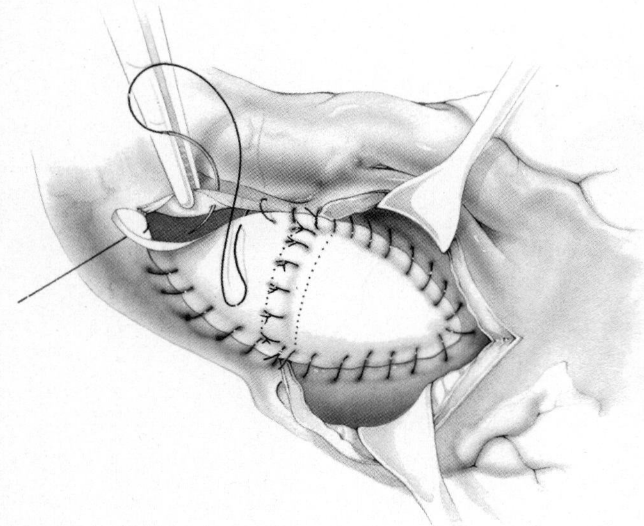

FIG. 24.9 A continuous suture is used to attach the patch to the aortotomy opening.

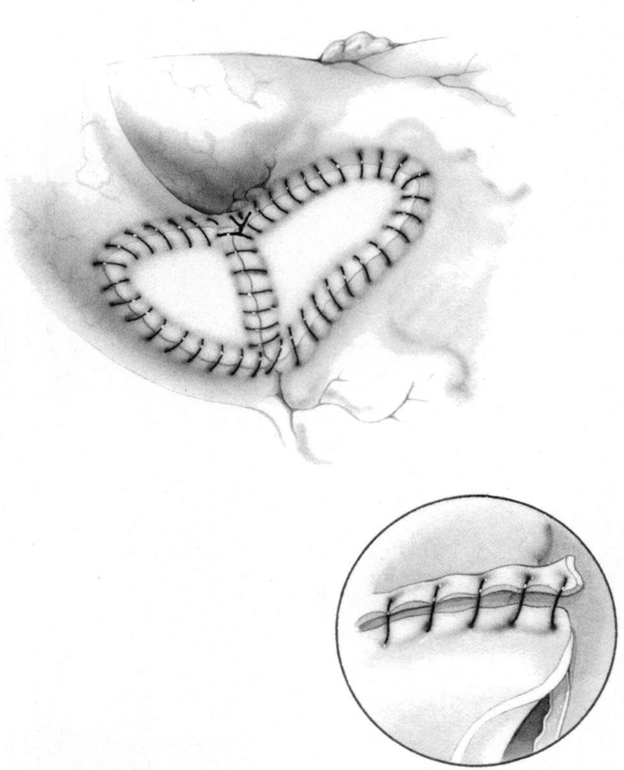

FIG. 24.10 Sewing a triangular patch to the edges of the right ventricular outflow tract opening and the aortic root. Inset: Reinforcement of the suture line with Teflon felt.

entails separating the suture that closes the interventricular septum from the suture that closes the aortotomy (Fig. 24.9). NB

A triangular, appropriately generous patch of Hemashield, bovine pericardium, or autologous pericardium is sewn to the edges of the incision on the right ventricular outflow tract and across the first patch at the level of the prosthetic valve (Fig. 24.10). Alternatively, a large pericardial patch is sewn onto the right ventricle and is extended over the aortic patch to secure hemostasis.

NB Reinforcing the Suture Line

The suture line can be reinforced with Teflon felt if the right ventricular wall appears to be thin and friable. NB

Once the aortotomy closure is completed, the heart is filled and standard deairing maneuvers are carried out (see Chapter 4).

NB Extended Aortic Root Replacement with an Aortic Homograft or Pulmonary Autograft

There are many problems associated with mechanical valves in infants and children. An alternative technique is to combine the concept of aortic root replacement with reimplantation of the coronary arteries and the concept of aortoventricular septoplasty. The aortic, right ventricular, and septal incisions are similar to those described earlier for the Rastan-Konno procedure. The coronary arteries are excised with a generous cuff of aortic wall and mobilized. The aortic valve and proximal ascending aorta are excised. If an aortic homograft is used, it is oriented so that the attached anterior leaflet of the mitral valve can be used to patch the incision on the ventricular septum. If a pulmonary autograft is used, a triangular piece of the right ventricular wall can be left attached to the pulmonary valve annulus when harvesting the autograft. This muscle can then be used to patch the defect in the interventricular septum. Aortic root replacement and reimplantation of the coronary ostia are completed as described in Chapter 5. The defect in the right ventricle is then closed with a piece of autologous or bovine pericardium. The patch is sutured to the edges of the right ventriculotomy incision and along the annulus of the valve of the homograft or autograft. NB

NB Orientation of the Aortic Homograft

When the anterior mitral leaflet is left attached to the aortic homograft and used to patch the ventricular septal defect, the homograft must be oriented in only one way. This may create complications for the reimplantation of the coronary ostia. Alternatively, the mitral leaflet can be excised and the ventricular septum enlarged with a triangular patch of Hemashield, which is then sewn to the annulus of the aortic homograft. If the anterior leaflet is used to close the ventricular septal defect, sometimes the arc of the aortic homograft is 180 degrees from the natural arc of the ascending aorta. In this situation, it is often helpful to divide the aortic homograft at the mid-ascending aorta and

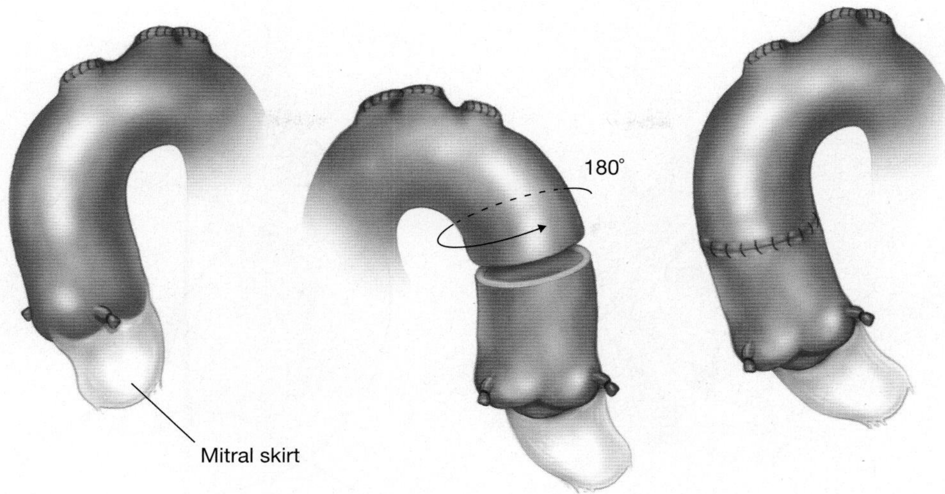

FIG. 24.11 If the mitral skirt of a homograft is used to extend the hood of an aortic homograft in the pulmonary outflow tract, it can sometimes make the graft angulated in the wrong direction for right ventricle to pulmonary artery continuity. In this case, it can be helpful to turn the distal homograft 180 degrees.

reverse the arc and reconnect with and end-to-end anastomosis (Fig. 24.11) NB

Modified Rastan-Konno Procedure

When there is diffuse long-segment tunnel stenosis with a competent aortic valve and adequately sized aortic annulus, a modified Rastan-Konno procedure is indicated.

Cardiopulmonary bypass with bicaval cannulation and aortic cross-clamping is used. An oblique incision is made in the infundibulum of the right ventricle below the pulmonic valve (Fig. 24.6). This is extended to the level of the aortic annulus just to the left of the right coronary ostium. A longitudinal incision is made in the ventricular septum extending from just below the aortic annulus at the commissure between the left and right coronary sinuses proximally on the septum past the area of obstruction. The thickened septal muscle is resected from the left ventricular outflow tract. An oval patch of Hemashield is then used to close the defect, placing horizontal, pledgeted, interrupted mattress sutures from the left ventricle through the septum and then the patch on the right ventricular side (Fig. 24.12). The opening on the right ventricle is then closed with a pericardial patch.

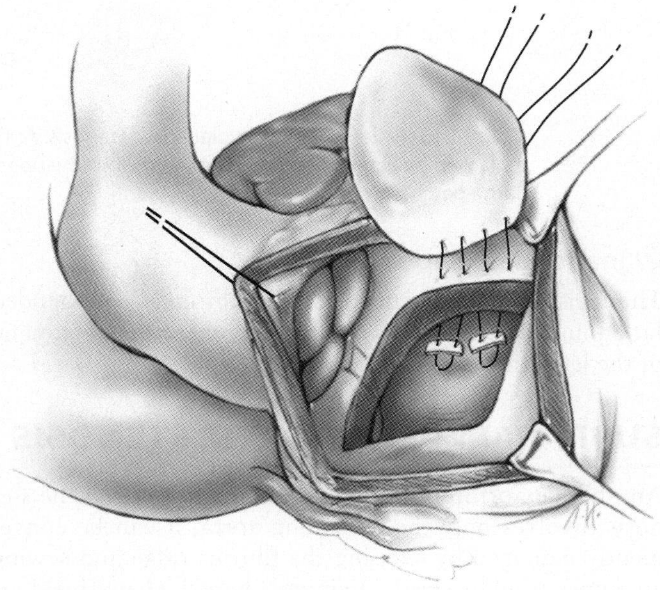

FIG. 24.12 Modified Rastan-Konno procedure: septal incision and placement of horizontal mattress sutures from the left ventricle to the right ventricle.

⊘ Aortic Valve Injury

Before making the septal incision, a small aortotomy to allow visualization of the aortic valve and annulus may be useful. A right-angled clamp passed through the aortic valve can identify the appropriate location for the septal incision. Alternatively, sometimes it is helpful to place a large needle from the left ventricular side across the septum to the right ventricular side at the base of the aortic valve, which then marks the superior-most extent of the Konno incision. ⊘

⊘ Injury to the Conduction System

The incision on the septum should be well to the left of the right coronary ostium to avoid the conduction system. ⊘

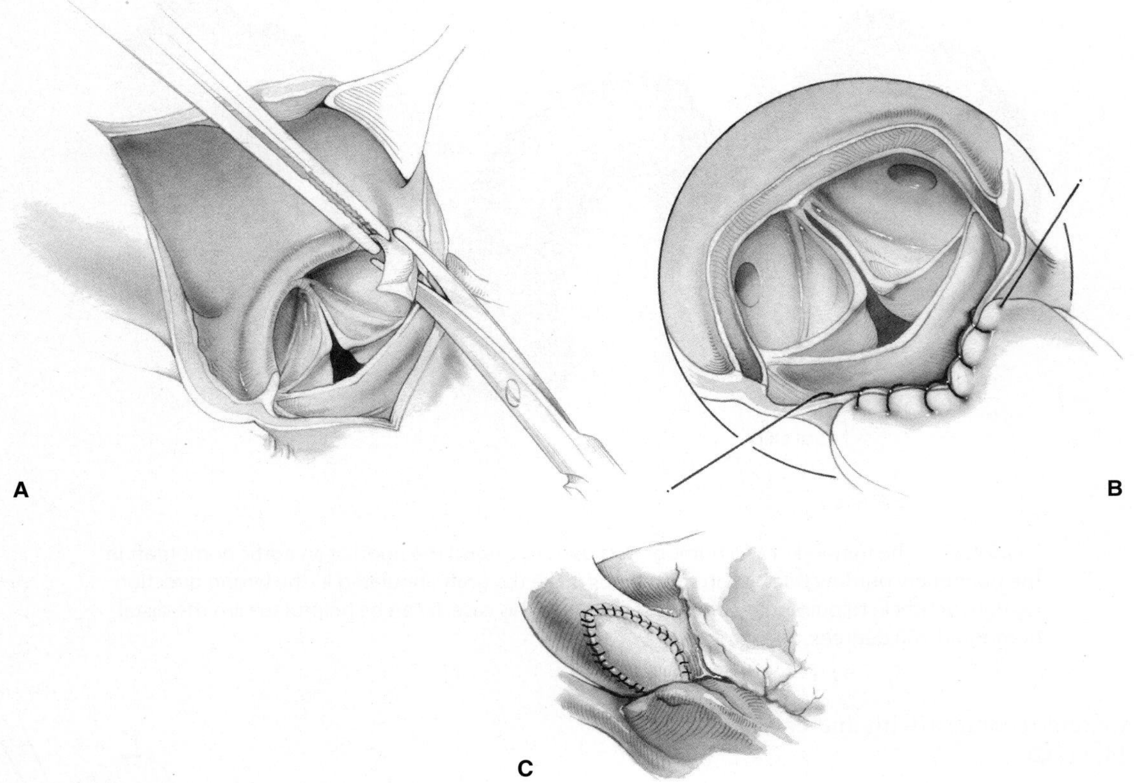

FIG. 24.13 Relief of supravalvular aortic stenosis. **A:** The shelf of fibrous tissue is excised. **B:** The aortic root is enlarged by extension of the aortotomy into the noncoronary sinus of Valsalva. **C:** The defect is covered with a large patch.

⊘ Inadequate Septal Opening

The incision on the ventricular septum must be extended far enough proximally to completely relieve the narrowing of the left ventricular outflow tract. ⊘

SUPRAVALVULAR AORTIC STENOSIS

An oblique aortotomy provides good exposure. If the stenosis involves only the ascending aorta, it can be conveniently managed by excising the fibrous ridge and sewing an appropriately sized, diamond-shaped Hemashield or Gore-Tex patch across the stricture to relieve the stenosis (Fig. 24.13). The type of supravalvular narrowing that is caused by a fibrous ridge usually extends onto the annulus and the commissures, however. This fibrous ridge must be meticulously excised to free the aortic leaflets.

⊘ Patch Enlargement of the Ascending Aorta

The supravalvular lesion may be extensive and affect major parts of the ascending aorta. This lesion may require extensive patch enlargement from the noncoronary sinus to the innominate artery. The width of the patch must be oversized, with allowance made for somatic growth, to prevent the late recurrence of stenosis (Fig. 24.14). Patients with William's syndrome may have long-segment narrowing of the entire ascending aorta, necessitating at times the replacement of the ascending aorta up to the innominate artery and possibly the aortic root as well. ⊘

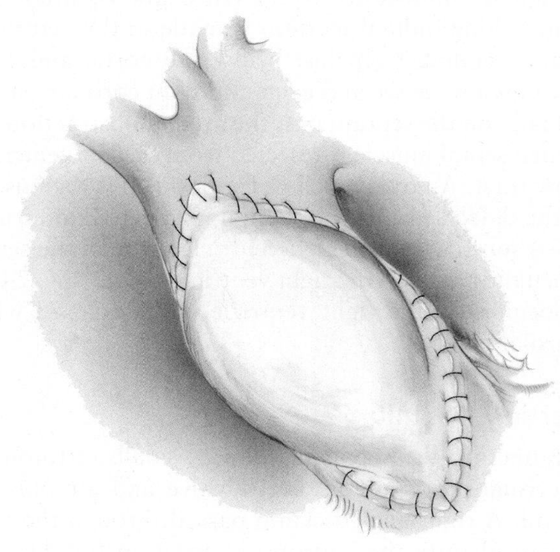

FIG. 24.14 Patch enlargement of the ascending aorta.

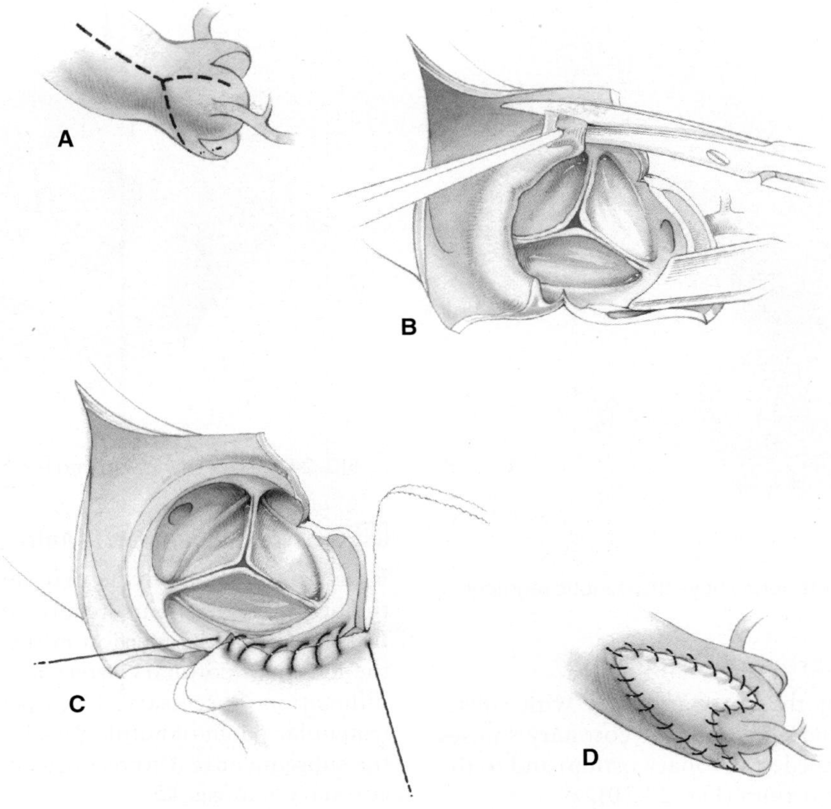

FIG. 24.15 Relief of an obstruction to the aortic sinuses. **A:** The aortotomy is extended down into the noncoronary and right sinus of Valsalva. **B:** The fibrous shelf is removed. **C and D:** Pericardium is incorporated as a patch to enlarge both aortic sinuses and the ascending aorta.

⊘ Injury to the Aortic Leaflets

While the fibrous ridge is being excised, the aortic valve leaflets must be protected. Injury to the aortic leaflets can produce aortic insufficiency. ⊘

⊘ Obstruction Extending into the Aortic Sinuses

At times, the fibrous ridge continues into, narrows, and distorts one or more of the aortic sinuses. After removing the ridge, the involved sinuses of Valsalva may need to be enlarged with a patch of glutaraldehyde-treated autologous pericardium or Hemashield to relieve the obstruction (Fig. 24.15). ⊘

⊘ Injury to the Left Coronary Artery Ostium

Removal of a fibrous ridge from the left coronary sinus region must be carried out carefully, always bearing in mind the possibility of injuring the left coronary ostium. ⊘

The degree of supravalvular obstruction may be so severe that a more extensive form of therapy is indicated. An effective procedure was devised by Brom with excellent results. In this technique, the aorta is completely transected just above the stenotic segment (Fig. 24.16). The lumen of the stenosic area is rarely larger than 6 to 8 mm in diameter, as measured with a Hegar dilator; by a simple calculation, the circumference of the stenosis is therefore approximately 18 mm, and the width of each segment between the commissures is 6 to 8 mm.

The aortic root, sinuses of Valsalva, and the coronary artery ostia are often dilated. A short, vertical incision is made down into the noncoronary sinus to the level of maximal width of the proximal aorta (Fig. 24.17). This improves exposure and allows close inspection of the lesion (Fig. 24.18). Similar incisions are made into the other two coronary sinuses; the stenotic lumen is now fully opened (Fig. 24.19).

⊘ Incisions into the Coronary Sinuses

Incisions into the coronary sinuses should never extend beyond the point of maximal width of the proximal aortic segment (Fig. 24.17). If these incisions are made deeper than this level, the patches will distort the base of the valve and give rise to aortic incompetence. ⊘

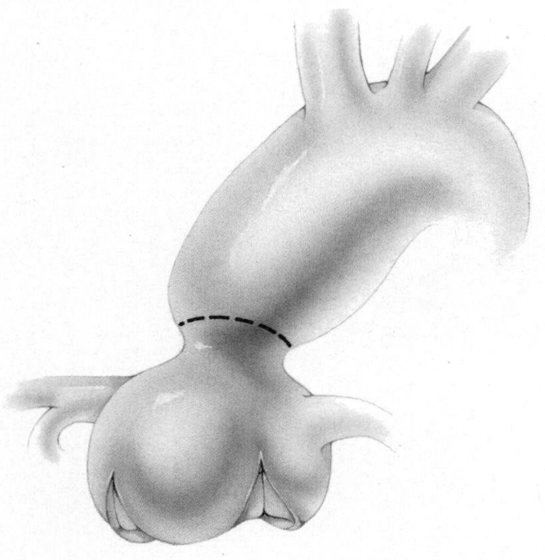

FIG. 24.16 Transection of the aorta above the stenotic segment.

⊘ Distortion of the Coronary Ostia

To prevent distortion of the coronary ostia with subsequent patch plasty, the incisions into the coronary sinuses should be to the right of the left coronary ostium and to the left of the right coronary ostium (Fig. 24.20). ⊘

NB Blood pressure control

Often patients with severe supravalvar aortic stenosis are "used" to much higher perfusion pressures of their coronary arteries, given that these have been under substantial afterload. This is important to keep in mind when weaning from cardiopulmonary bypass, so that the coronary arteries are not subject to relative hypotension (and ischemia). NB

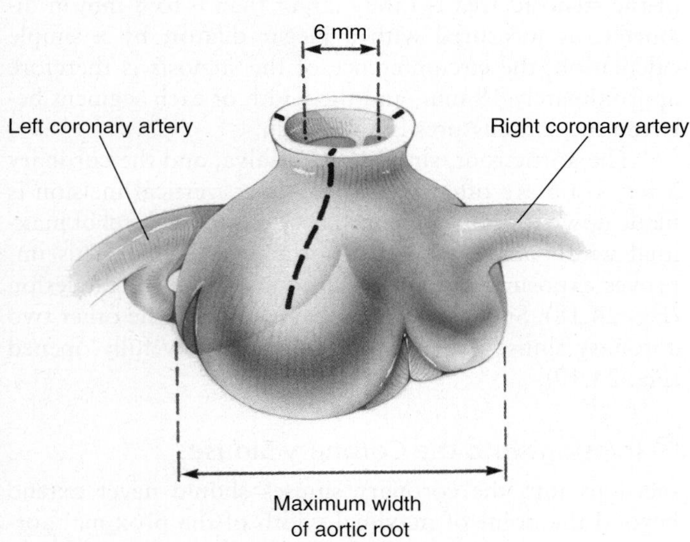

FIG. 24.17 Line of incision into the noncoronary sinus.

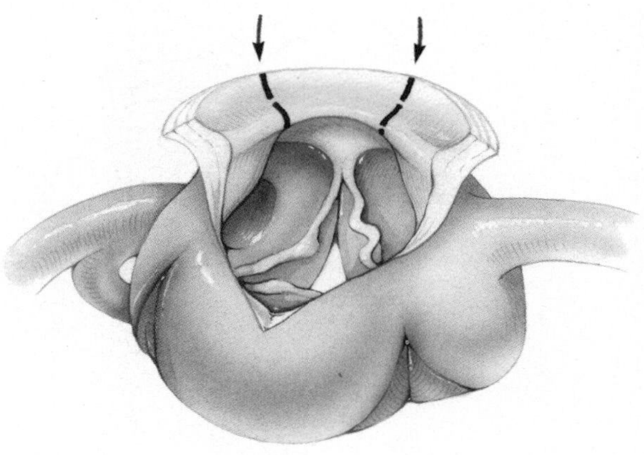

FIG. 24.18 Line of incision into the other two coronary sinuses.

NB Obstruction of Left Main Coronary Ostium

Rarely, the fibrous tissue may involve the left ostium and the orifice may remain stenotic after excision of the ridge. In these cases, the incision in the left sinus is carried onto the left main coronary artery and may be continued to its bifurcation if necessary. This opening is then closed with a triangular patch of autologous pericardium as described in the subsequent text to reconstruct the sinus and relieve the coronary stenosis. NB

The normal aortic valve annulus is measured with a Hegar dilator of appropriate size. The circumference of the annulus is approximately three times its diameter or Hegar size. For example, if the aortic annular diameter (Hegar size) is 24 mm, its circumference will be 24 mm × 3 or 72 mm. If the lumen of the stenotic segment is 6 mm (Hegar size), its circumference is 6 mm × 3 or 18 mm.

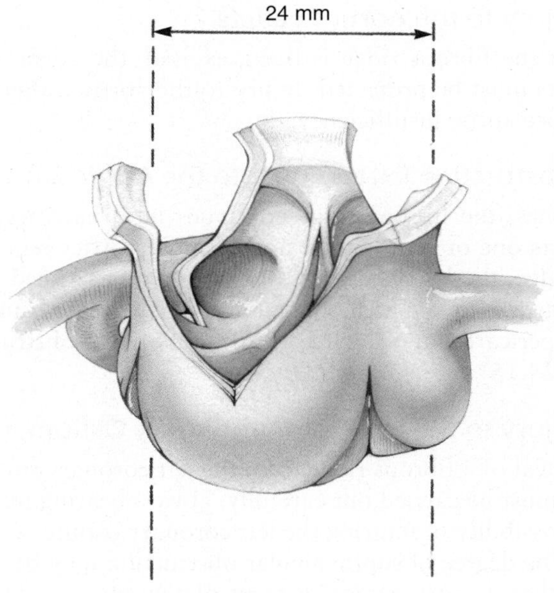

FIG. 24.19 Fully opened stenosis.

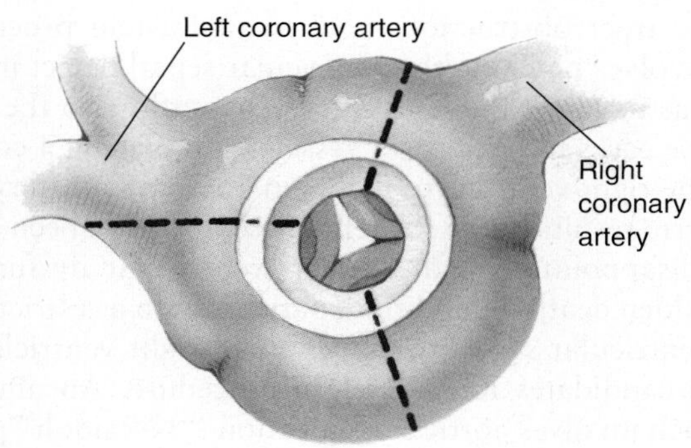

FIG. 24.20 Placement of incisions to prevent distortion of the ostia of the coronary arteries.

It is clear from these observations and calculations that the stenotic aortic segment must be enlarged by 54 mm (72 to 18 mm) for it to match the size of the aortic valve annulus. Because this enlargement must be made among the three commissures, each pericardial patch must be 54 mm/3, or 18-mm wide along its superior rim (Fig. 24.21).

Autologous, glutaraldehyde-treated pericardium is used to prepare triangular patches with specific measurements; in this example, an isosceles triangle with a base of 18 mm and a height commensurate with the distance between the stenotic segment and the maximal width of the proximal aorta (Fig. 24.21) is the necessary size. The pericardial patches are then sewn in place with Prolene sutures (Fig. 24.21).

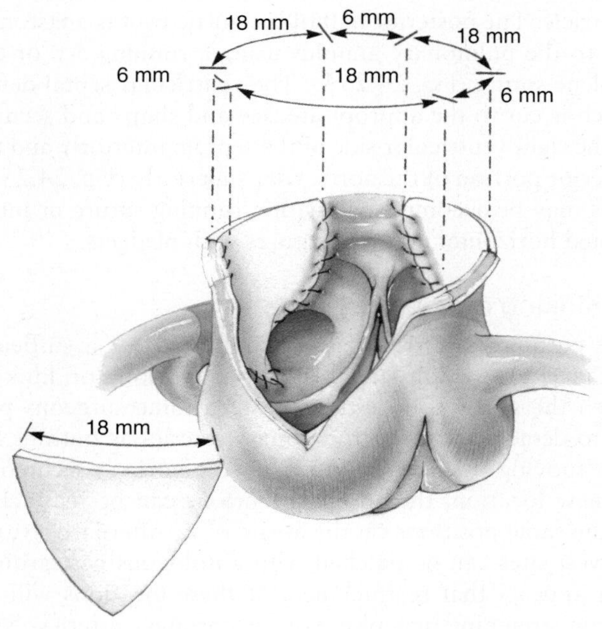

FIG. 24.21 An example of measurements needed for an accurate stenotic enlargement.

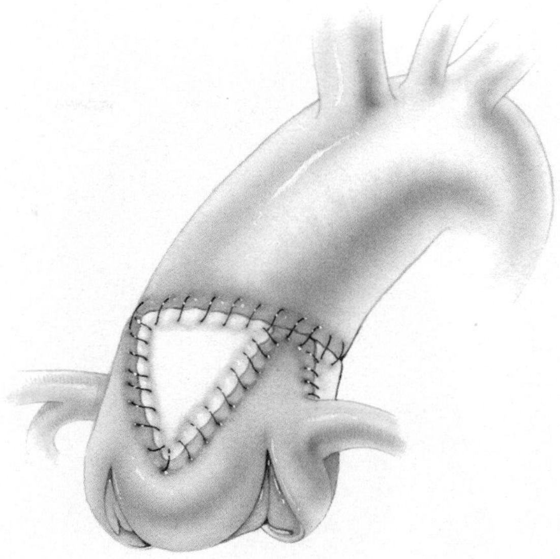

FIG. 24.22 Completed repair of the stenosis.

The two aortic ends are now anastomosed in an end-to-end manner with a continuous Prolene suture in a continuous suturing technique (Fig. 24.22).

NB Narrow Distal Aortic Segment

Occasionally, the lumen of the distal ascending aorta, just above the stenotic segment, may be small compared with the newly constructed proximal aorta. This discrepancy can be rectified by further resection of the distal aorta or a vertical incision into its lumen. NB

In select group of patients, it may be possible to perform end-to-end reconstruction of the aorta without the use of pericardial patches. The distal aorta is anastomosed to the aortic root by making appropriate counterincisions to provide three tongues of aortic tissue (Fig. 24.23).

NB Tension on the Anastomosis

The aorta must be well mobilized to provide adequate length, thereby minimizing any tension on the anastomosis. NB

MANAGEMENT OF LEFT VENTRICULAR OUTFLOW TRACT OBSTRUCTION ASSOCIATED WITH OTHER CARDIAC ANOMALIES

Interrupted Aortic Arch with Ventricular Septal Defect

Patients with interrupted aortic arch and ventricular septal defects often present with some form of left ventricular outflow tract obstruction. This may be at the valvar level

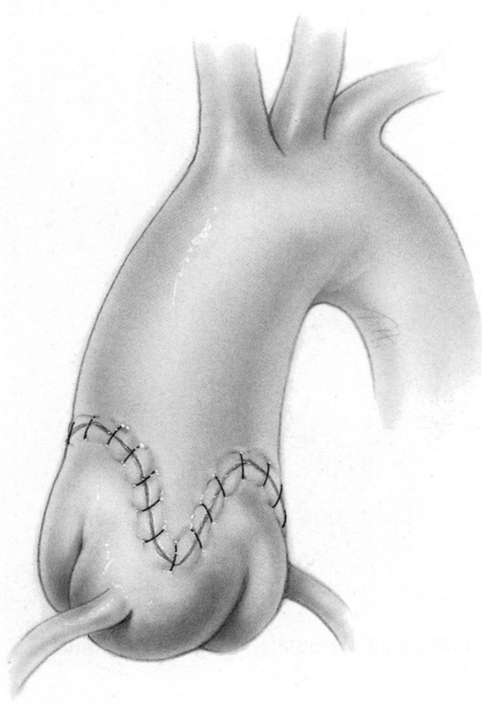

FIG. 24.23 Completed repair of the end-to-end reconstruction of the aorta.

with a bicuspid valve or small aortic annulus. The most common cause is posterior deviation of the conal septum.

Patients with adequate annulus size, but with subaortic diameters less than 4 mm are candidates for incision or resection of conal septal muscle before closure of the ventricular septal defect. Most frequently, this is accomplished through a right atriotomy approach, performing a myotomy or myectomy of the conal septum before securing the ventricular septal defect patch in place (see Chapter 21). A patch cut slightly smaller than the defect is attached to the left side of the conal septum, thereby pulling the septum anteriorly and opening the subaortic area.

NB Recurrent Obstruction

A significant number of patients undergoing surgery for this lesion require reoperation for left ventricular outflow tract obstruction. This may be secondary to valvar issues, or the development of a subaortic membrane or muscular narrowing. Therefore, these patients require close follow-up. NB

TRANSPOSITION OF THE GREAT ARTERIES WITH VENTRICULAR SEPTAL DEFECT AND LEFT VENTRICULAR OUTFLOW TRACT OBSTRUCTION

The traditional surgical repair for transposition of the great arteries with ventricular septal defect and left ventricular outflow tract obstruction has been a Rastelli procedure. This involves patching the ventricular septal defect in such a way as to direct the left ventricular outflow to the aorta (in these cases to both great vessels) and placing a conduit from the right ventricle to the main pulmonary artery. The long-term results of the Rastelli procedure have been somewhat disappointing with late left ventricular dysfunction and sudden death. In addition, patients with a restrictive or inlet ventricular septal defect or small right ventricle may not be candidates for a Rastelli procedure. An alternate approach involves aortic translocation ("Nikaidoh" procedure), which directly places the aorta over the left ventricle, eliminating the need for a large intracardiac prosthetic baffle.

Technique

Through a median sternotomy incision, cardiopulmonary bypass is achieved with distal aortic and bicaval cannulation. The ductus arteriosus or ligamentum is doubly ligated and divided. After cooling to 28°C, the aorta is cross-clamped and cardioplegia is administered into the aortic root. The aortic root is excised from the right ventricular outflow tract, leaving a 5-mm rim of attached muscle below the annulus (Fig. 24.24A). This maneuver is similar to the technique used to excise a pulmonary autograft (see Chapter 5). The pulmonary artery is transected just above the valve and the pulmonic valve leaflets are excised. The pulmonary valve annulus and conal septum are incised, carrying the incision into the ventricular septal defect (Fig. 24.24B). The continuity between the pulmonic and mitral annuli is now apparent. The aortic root is slid posteriorly, without rotation, into position over the left ventricle. The posterior half of the aortic root is anastomosed to the pulmonary annulus using a running 5-0 or 6-0 Prolene suture (Fig. 24.25A). The ventricular septal defect patch is cut to the appropriate size and shape and secured to the right ventricular side of the septum inferiorly and the anterior portion of the aortic root superiorly (Fig. 24.25B). This may be accomplished with a running suture or interrupted horizontal mattress sutures with pledgets.

⊘ Kinking of Coronary Arteries

The coronary arteries must be mobilized for a sufficient distance to prevent any distortion, tension, or kinking when the aortic root is translocated. Some surgeons prefer to detach one or both coronary arteries as buttons before moving the aortic root. After the aorta is secured in its new location, the coronary buttons can be reattached to the same positions on the aortic root. Alternatively, the harvest sites can be patched with autologous pericardium if it appears that reattachment at these locations will result in stretching or kinking of the coronary arteries. New implantation sites on the aortic root are then identified, and openings, using care to not injure the aortic valve leaflets. The anastomosis of the coronary button to the aorta

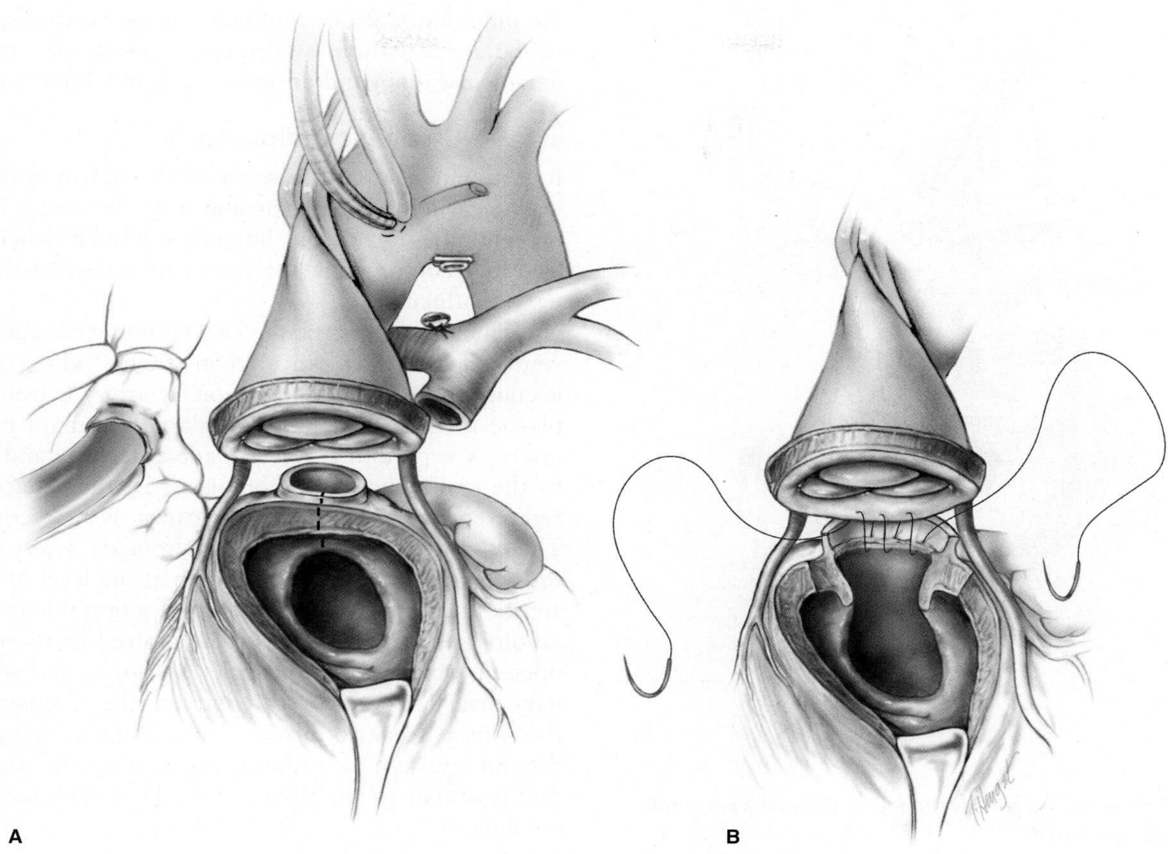

FIG. 24.24 **A:** The aortic root has been excised from the right ventricle and the proximal pulmonary artery divided. The dotted line shows location of conal septal incision. **B:** The pulmonary annulus is incised carrying the incision through the conal septum into the ventricular septal defect.

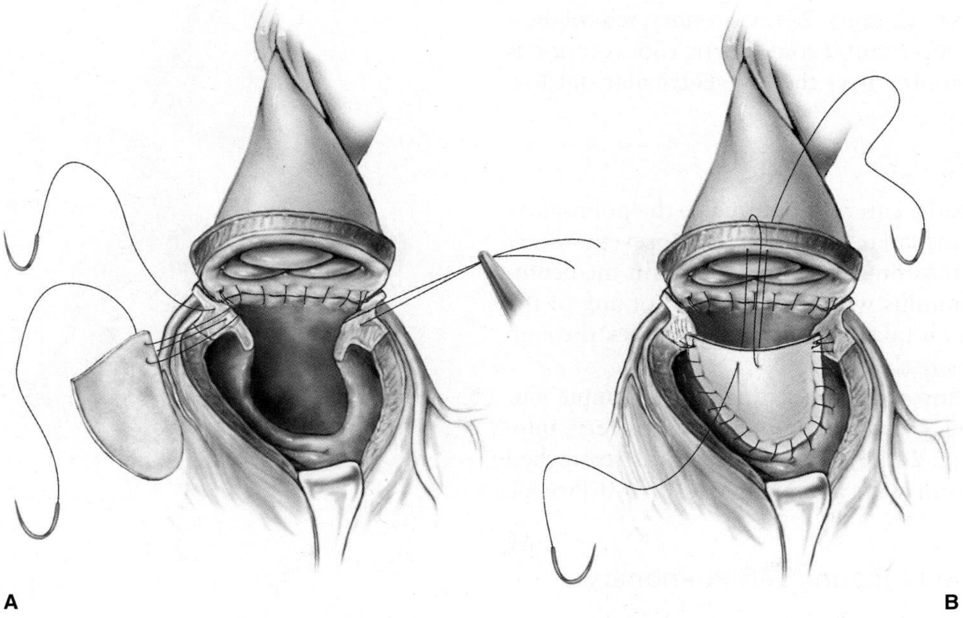

FIG. 24.25 **A:** Attaching posterior half of aortic root to pulmonary annulus. **B:** Securing patch to ventricular septal defect and anterior half of aortic root.

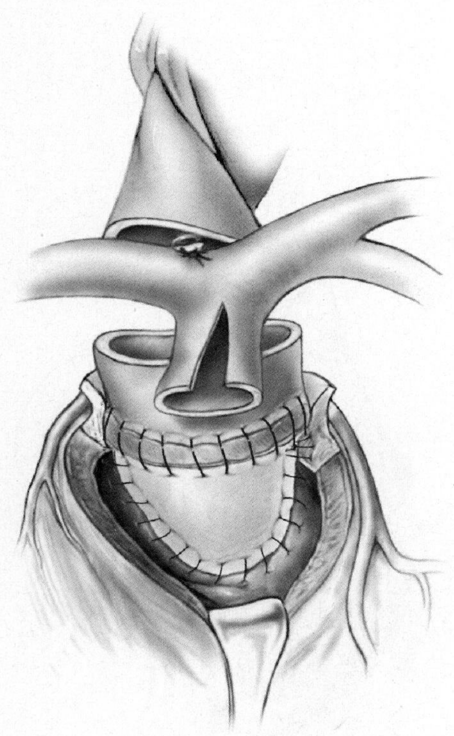

FIG. 24.26 The ascending aorta is divided to allow for a Lecompte maneuver to be performed.

is accomplished with a running Prolene suture. The techniques involved in mobilizing and reanastomosing the coronary arteries are similar to those used during the arterial switch procedure (see Chapter 25). Coronary reimplantation is particularly important if some aortic root rotation is required with positioning over the left ventricular outflow tract. ⊘

⊘ Aortic Insufficiency

The aortic root must be carefully sutured to the pulmonary annulus and the ventricular septal patch to prevent valvar insufficiency. The anastomosis should maintain the geometry of the aortic annulus without distortion of any of the leaflets. Care must be taken to not place sutures through the valve leaflets themselves. ⊘

The ascending aorta is transected, and a Lecompte maneuver is performed, bringing the pulmonary artery anterior to the aorta (Fig. 24.26). The aortic root is reattached to the ascending aorta with a running 5-0 or 6-0 Prolene suture.

NB Mobilization of Right and Left Pulmonary Arteries

The right and left pulmonary arteries should be completely mobilized out to the pericardial reflection. The ductus arteriosus or ligamentum also must be divided. This allows the pulmonary artery confluence to be positioned anterior to the aorta without any traction, which may stretch and narrow the main and/or one or both pulmonary arteries. NB

NB Length of Ascending Aorta

It is often necessary to resect a short segment of the ascending aorta before anastomosing it to the aortic root. This prevents the aorta from bulging anteriorly when pressurized and compressing the posterior aspect of the pulmonary confluence. NB

The aortic cross-clamp can be removed, and the right ventricular outflow tract reconstructed while rewarming is completed. The main pulmonary artery is usually hypoplastic in these patients. To enlarge the main pulmonary artery, a vertical incision is made anteriorly and extended to the confluence. If a homograft is not being used, the right ventricular outflow tract can now be reconstructed. The posterior half of the main pulmonary artery is sewn to the ventricular septal defect patch at the level of the aortic suture line (Fig. 24.27). A patch of glutaraldehyde-treated autologous pericardium is then sutured to the remaining opening on the right ventricle inferiorly, and the pulmonary artery superiorly, to complete the reconstruction. If the clinical scenario dictates (e.g., distance, angulation, or physiology), use of a homograft or a bovine jugular conduit is similar to any right ventricular to pulmonary artery conduit.

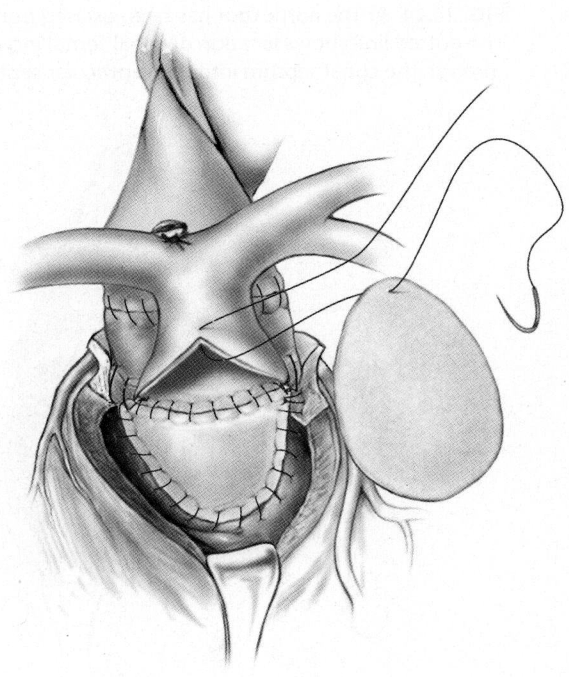

FIG. 24.27 Posterior half of enlarged main pulmonary artery is sewn to the septal patch at the level of the aortic suture line.

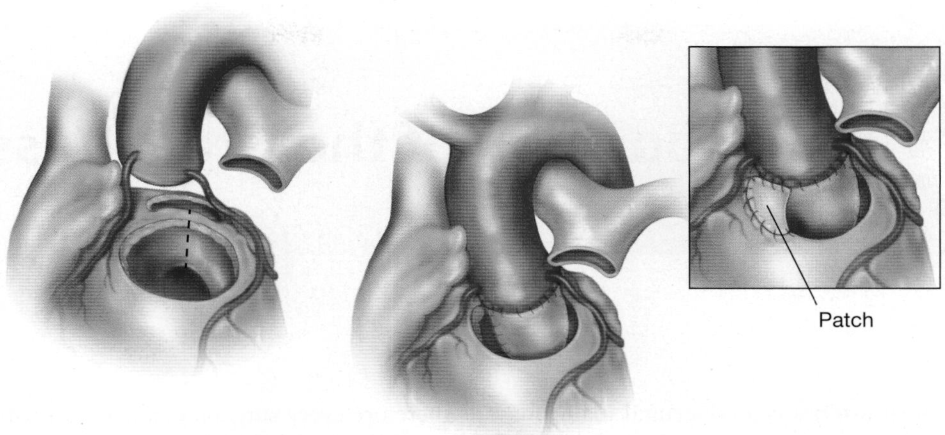

FIG. 24.28 In the Nikaidoh procedure, because the aortic root may be translocated inferiorly (with or without a VSD patch), it can create an awkward "triangle" deficiency along the rightward most aspect of the right ventriculotomy. To mitigate distortion of the proximal RV-PA conduit, it can be helpful to "close down" this area with a prosthetic triangular-shaped patch (shown as small, but may be quite considerable in size).

NB Conduit from Right Ventricle to Pulmonary Artery

Alternatively, a pulmonary homograft may be interposed between the right ventricular opening and the enlarged main pulmonary artery (see Chapter 27). Again, the posterior aspect of the homograft must be carefully sewn to the ventricular septal patch just at the aortic suture line to avoid injury to the aortic valve. NB

⊘ Injury to the Aortic Valve

When performing the posterior suture line connecting the main pulmonary artery to the right ventricular outflow tract, care must be taken to not injure the aortic valve. By suturing on the septal patch material itself, just below the aortic suture line, this complication should be avoided. ⊘

NB If using a conduit, sometimes the rightward aspect of the right ventriculotomy bordered by the translocated root can be closed with a triangle-shaped prosthetic patch so as to facilitate the proximal right ventricular to pulmonary artery conduit suture line (Fig. 24.28). NB

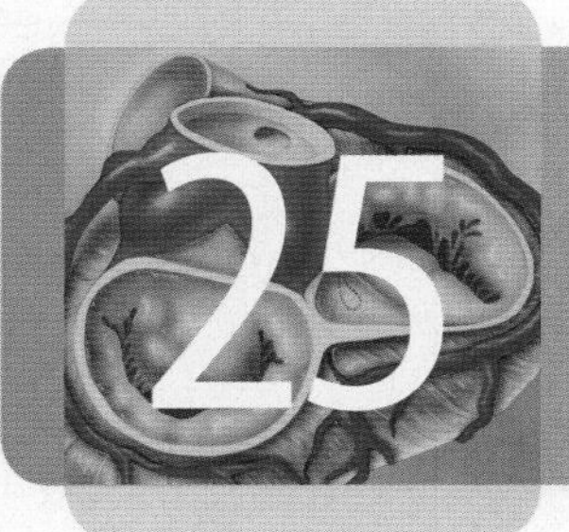

25 Transposition of the Great Vessels

Transposition of the great arteries is a congenital malformation in which the heart has atrioventricular concordance and ventriculoarterial discordance. Therefore, the clinical findings are an anterior aorta that originates from the morphologic right ventricle and a pulmonary artery that originates from the morphologic left ventricle. Other congenital defects can also be associated with transposition of the great arteries.

Today, anatomic correction of transposition of the great arteries with or without ventricular septal defect is the procedure of choice. When the interventricular septum is intact, the arterial switch operation must be performed while the left ventricle is still prepared to handle systemic pressures. After 2 to 3 weeks of age, changes in the left ventricular wall thickness and geometry may preclude a successful arterial switch procedure. If the left ventricular pressure is less than 60% systemic, a two-staged approach involving initial pulmonary artery banding with or without a systemic to pulmonary artery shunt followed by an arterial switch procedure when the left ventricle becomes prepared is required. Alternatively, a so-called atrial switch procedure (Senning or Mustard operation) may be undertaken.

The Senning and Mustard procedures were designed to achieve a rerouting of the venous returns in the two atria; this entails channeling the systemic venous return from the caval veins into the left atrium, across the mitral valve into the left ventricle, and through the pulmonary artery to the lungs. Similarly, pulmonary venous return from the pulmonary veins is directed into the right atrium across the tricuspid valve into the right ventricle, which functions as the systemic ventricle, pumping blood into the aorta. Except for the torn fossa ovalis, which is found if a palliative balloon septostomy has been performed, the surgical anatomy of both the right and left atria is essentially normal. The long-term follow-up of patients who have undergone a Senning and Mustard procedure has shown a high incidence of atrial arrhythmias and a significant rate of late right ventricular dysfunction. However, physiologic repair with one of these two procedures may be indicated in patients with transposition of the great vessels and associated pulmonary valve stenosis, nonresectable left ventricular outflow tract obstruction, or some abnormalities of the coronary arteries that may prohibitively increase the risk of anatomic repair. An atrial switch procedure may be part of the surgical approach in patients with some complex congenital heart lesions, and therefore every surgeon dealing with patients with congenital heart disease should have the Senning and Mustard procedures as part of his or her surgical armamentarium.

SURGICAL ANATOMY

In hearts with transposition of the great arteries, the right ventricular wall thickness is greater than normal at birth and increases progressively thereafter. If the ventricular septum is intact and no pulmonary stenosis exists, the left ventricular wall thickness does not increase after birth, and within 2 to 3 months, the left ventricle is relatively thin walled.

The aorta is most commonly directly anterior to the pulmonary artery, although occasionally, the great vessels are side by side with the aorta to the right. The coronary arteries usually arise from the aortic sinuses facing the pulmonary artery. Therefore, the nonfacing sinus is most often anterior. According to the Leiden convention, sinus 1 is on the right-hand side and sinus 2 is the next sinus counterclockwise to sinus 1, as viewed from the nonfacing, noncoronary sinus. Approximately 70% of patients have the left anterior descending and circumflex coronary arteries arising as a single trunk from sinus 1 and a right coronary artery from sinus 2 (Fig. 25.1A). The left anterior descending arises from sinus 1, and the right coronary artery and circumflex originate together from sinus 2 in approximately 15% of cases (Fig. 25.1B). Rarely, all three main coronary arteries arise from a single sinus, most commonly sinus 2. In some of these cases, the left anterior descending or left main coronary artery may be intramural.

Surgical Anatomy of the Right Atrium

Although the right atrium is morphologically molded into a single chamber, it is formed by two components: the sinus venarum and the right atrial appendage (sometimes referred to as the body of the atrium). Systemic venous return flows in from opposite directions through the superior and inferior venae cavae into the sinus venarum. This smooth-walled area is the most posterior portion of the right atrium and stretches between the orifices of the caval veins. From the viewpoint of the surgeon looking down into the right atrium, the sinus venarum is more or less horizontal, with the superior vena

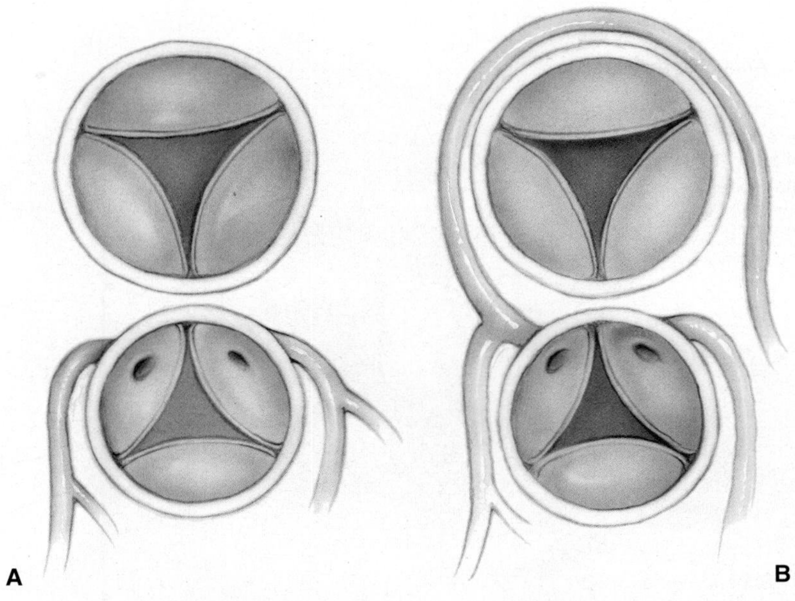

FIG. 25.1 **A–B:** Coronary artery configuration (see text).

cava entering from the left and the inferior vena cava entering (bounded by the Eustachian valve) from the right (Fig. 25.2).

Just below and medial to the orifice of the superior vena cava arises the crista terminalis, a muscle bundle that springs into prominence as it circles the orifice of the superior vena cava to the right lateral wall of the atrium and continues inferiorly toward the inferior vena cava, thereby forming the boundary between the sinus venarum and the atrial appendage. This muscle bundle is evidenced on the outside of the atrium by a groove, the sulcus terminalis. Lying subepicardially in the sulcus terminalis, just below the entrance of the superior vena cava, is the sinoatrial node, which may be vulnerable to injury from the various surgical incisions and cannulations that are commonly performed on the right atrium. The remainder of the right atrium is made up of atrial appendage, which begins at the crista terminalis and extends anteriorly (upward from the surgeon's perspective) to surround the tricuspid valve and form an expanded chamber.

In contrast to the smooth-walled sinus venarum, the lateral wall of the atrial appendage is ridged by multiple narrow bands of muscle, the musculi pectinati. These bands arise from the crista terminalis and pass upward to the most anterior part of the atrium. Functionally, they supply the right atrium with enough pumping capacity to propel the venous inflow through the tricuspid valve into the right ventricle.

Just above the sinus venarum in the center of the medial wall is the fossa ovalis, an elliptic or horseshoe-shaped depression. The true interatrial septum consists of the fossa ovalis with variable contributions from the superior, anterior, and inferior limbic muscle bundles that surround it. The aortic root is hidden behind the anteromedial atrial wall between the fossa ovalis and the termination of the heavily trabeculated right atrial appendage. Segments of the noncoronary and right sinus of Valsalva are in close apposition to the atrial wall in this area. Their locations may be manifested by the aortic mound, a bulge above and slightly to the left of the fossa ovalis. The presence of the aortic valve here can be more clearly visualized if one takes into consideration its continuity, through the central fibrous body, with the adjacent tricuspid valve annulus.

Also invisible to the surgeon is the artery to the sinoatrial node, which runs through this same area. Although its origin and exact location are unpredictable, the artery to the sinoatrial node takes a variable course toward the superior cavoatrial angle and the sinus node.

The tricuspid valve is located anteroinferiorly in the right atrium, where it opens widely into the right ventricle. The annulus of the tricuspid valve crosses over the membranous septum, dividing it into atrioventricular and interventricular segments. The membranous, or fibrous, septum is a continuation of the central fibrous body, through which the tricuspid, mitral, and aortic valves are connected.

Immediately below the upper or atrioventricular section of the membranous septum lies the hidden atrioventricular node. It is situated at the apex of the triangle of Koch, the boundaries of which are the annulus of the septal leaflet of the tricuspid valve, the tendon of Todaro (running intramyocardially from the central fibrous body to the Eustachian valve of the inferior vena cava), and its base, the coronary sinus. Anderson describes the tendon of Todaro as a fibrous extension of the commissure between the Eustachian valve (of the inferior vena cava) and the thebesian valve (of the coronary sinus). Conduction tissue passes from the atrioventricular node as the bundle of His below the membranous septum and

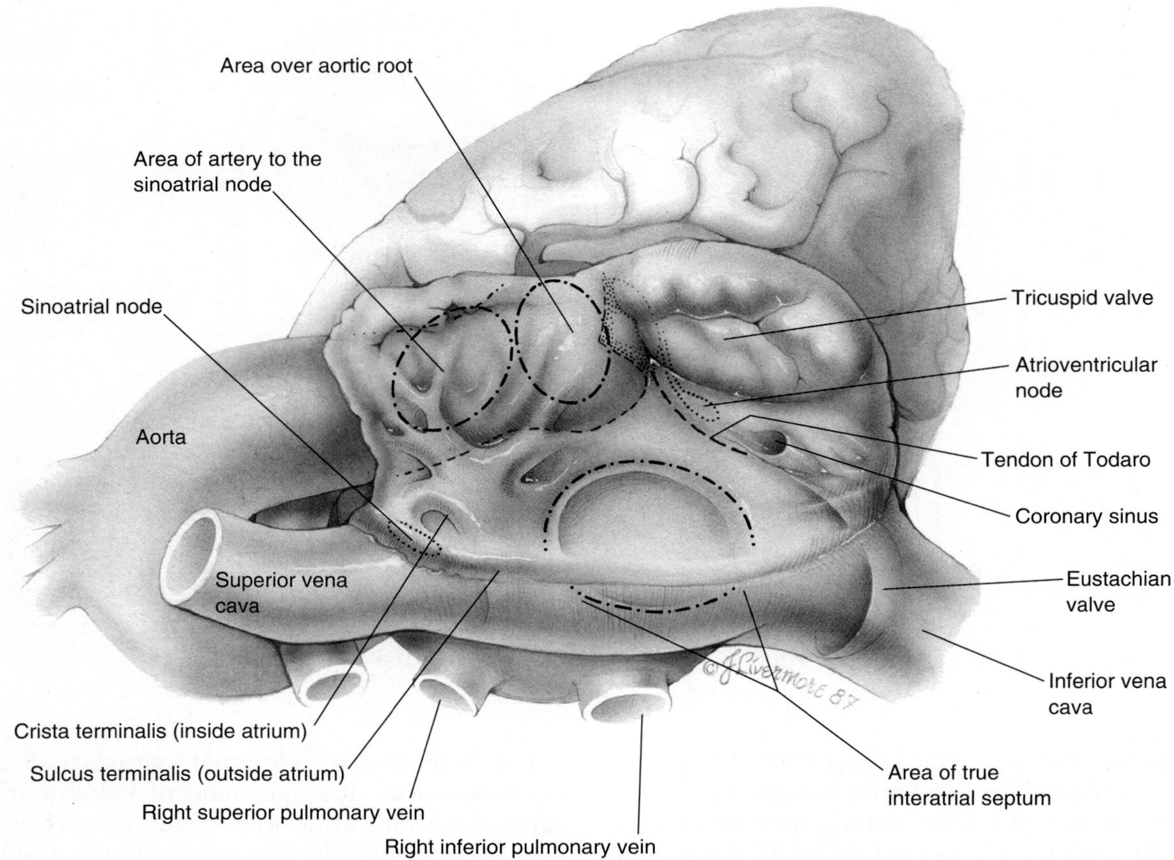

FIG. 25.2 Surgical anatomy of the right atrium.

down into the muscular interventricular septum. The coronary sinus, draining the cardiac veins, is situated alongside the tendon of Todaro, between it and the tricuspid valve.

THE ARTERIAL SWITCH OPERATION

Incision

A median sternotomy is performed, and the thymus is removed.

Preparation

A rectangular piece of pericardium is harvested and treated with glutaraldehyde. The relationship of the great vessels and coronary anatomy can be confirmed at this point.

Cannulation

The ascending aorta is cannulated as far distally as possible. Direct bicaval cannulation is carried out where possible, or single atrial cannulation for small weight babies. With initiation of cardiopulmonary bypass, the ductus arterious is occluded at its aortic end with a heavy tie or metal clip. The ductus arteriosus is later divided, oversewing the pulmonary artery side with 6-0 or 7-0 Prolene suture. A vent can be placed through the right superior pulmonary vein if necessary. During cooling, the ascending aorta is dissected free from the main pulmonary artery, and the right and left pulmonary arteries are extensively mobilized out to the first branches in the hilum of each lung. Most or all of the dissection is accomplished with an electrocautery on low current.

⊘ Flooding of the Pulmonary Bed

As soon as cardiopulmonary bypass is instituted, the ductus arterious must be occluded to prevent runoff of aortic cannula flow into the lungs. ⊘

NB Mobilization of the Pulmonary Arteries

It is essential to fully mobilize the branch pulmonary arteries beyond their hilar bifurcation so as to reduce tension on the Lecompte. NB

Transection of the Great Arteries

The aortic cross-clamp is applied just proximal to the aortic cannula. A dose of cold blood cardioplegic solution is

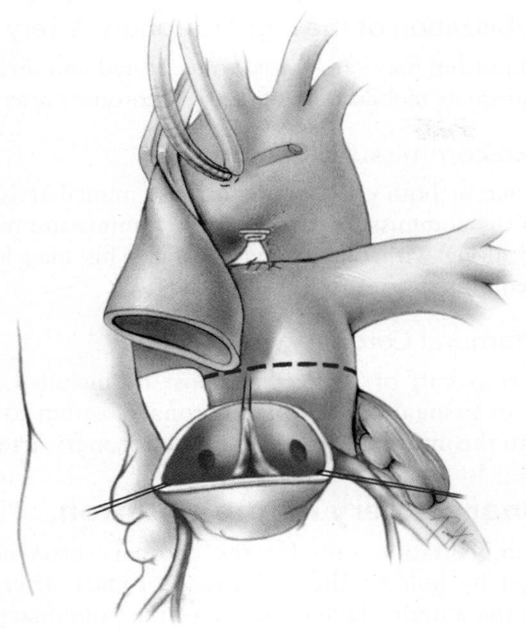

FIG. 25.3 The ascending aorta has been transected. Note the divided ductus arteriosus and line of transection on the main pulmonary artery.

administered through a needle into the ascending aorta at the mid ascending aorta. The aorta is then transected at this level, and traction sutures are placed just above the three commissures of the aortic valve and tagged (Fig. 25.3). The pulmonary artery is transected at the level of the takeoff of the right pulmonary artery, and traction sutures are placed at the commissures and tagged. The pulmonary valve is inspected to rule out significant abnormalities because this will be the new aortic valve.

NB Pulmonary Valve Abnormalities

The status of the pulmonary valve is usually defined by the preoperative transthoracic echocardiogram and intraoperative transesophageal echocardiogram. A sufficiently competent and nonstenotic valve must be confirmed before excising the coronary arteries. NB

NB Division of the Aorta

It can be helpful to divide the aorta slightly above the midpoint so as to procure more ascending aorta (neopulmonary root) and thereby reduce tension on the Lecompte. By design, this maneuver also places the aortic root more posteriorly (Fig. 25.4). NB

The pulmonary artery confluence is brought anterior to the distal ascending aorta (Fig. 25.5). The most proximal portion of the transected distal aorta is then grasped with a forceps or straight vascular clamp. The initial cross-clamp

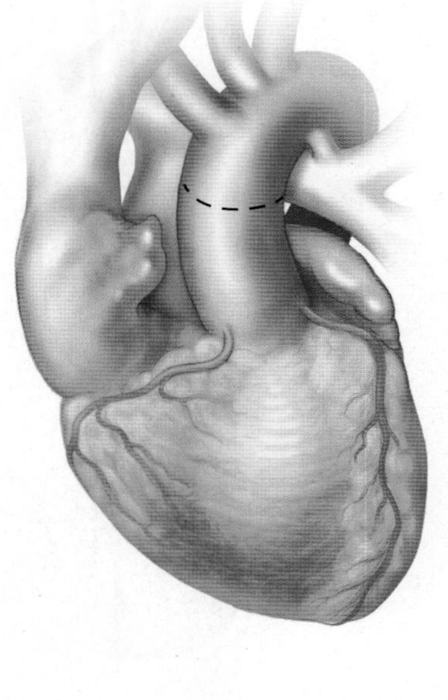

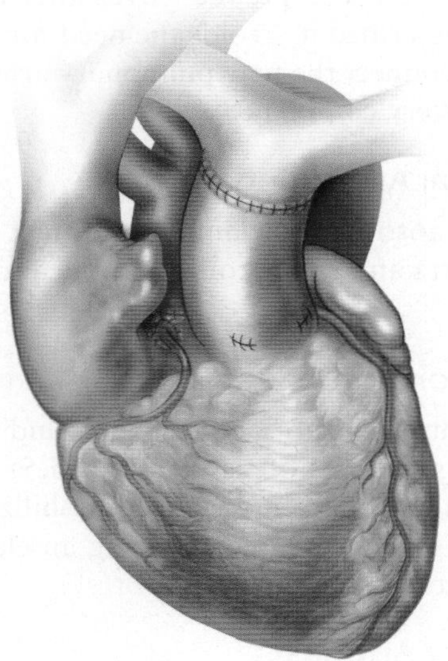

FIG. 25.4 By dividing the ascending aorta at or just beyond its midpoint, and the pulmonary artery closer just above the commissures, the neoaorta will be foreshortened (and somewhat posteriorly directed) and the neopulmonary root slightly longer to reduce the chance of stenosis from stretching after Lecompte.

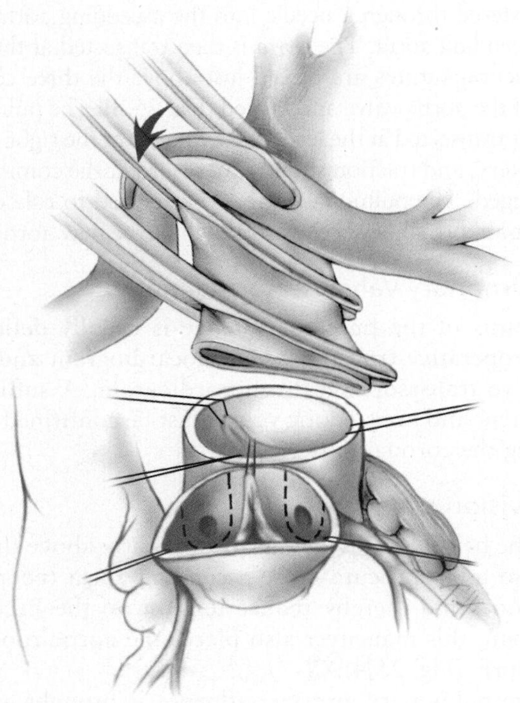

FIG. 25.5 The Lecompte maneuver: Pulmonary artery confluence is brought in front of the aorta and a second aortic clamp is applied. Arrow shows distal aortic clamp reapplied below the pulmonary artery confluence. Dotted lines indicate excision for the coronary tongues.

is then reapplied proximal to the pulmonary artery confluence as high as possible on the ascending aorta. This technique, referred to as the Lecompte maneuver after the surgeon who originally described it, avoids the need for an interposition conduit to connect the new pulmonary artery base to the pulmonary artery confluence.

⊘ Distorting the Distal Ascending Aorta

When repositioning the aortic cross-clamp, care must be taken not to twist the aorta and create torsion at the aortic suture line. ⊘

⊘ Excision of the Coronary Ostia

The coronary ostia and at least 2 to 3 mm of surrounding aortic wall are excised as tongues of tissue (Fig. 25.5) or as buttons. The proximal coronary arteries are mobilized from the epicardium for several millimeters using an electrocautery on low current. ⊘

⊘ Kinking of Coronary Arteries

Adequate dissection of the coronary arteries must be carried out to allow successful translocation of each coronary ostium to the corresponding sinus of the pulmonary artery. Insufficient mobilization may lead to tension on the coronary anastomosis or kinking of the coronary artery. ⊘

NB Mobilization of the Right Coronary Artery

Conal branches may rarely need to be ligated and divided to allow adequate mobilization of the right coronary artery. NB

NB Juxtacommissural Ostia

When one or both coronary ostia arise immediately adjacent to the commissure, the adjacent commissure must be excised along with the coronary ostia. This may lead to mild neopulmonary valve insufficiency. NB

NB Intramural Coronary Artery

A generous cuff of aortic wall must be included in the tongue of tissue containing the coronary ostium to avoid injury to the intramural portion of the coronary artery. NB

Coronary Artery Reimplantation

The reimplantation sites for the coronary ostia are determined by holding the mobilized coronary arteries up against the anterior facing sinuses of the pulmonary root, ensuring that no distortion of the proximal course of the coronary arteries is created. The coronary arteries can be reimplanted into the pulmonary root as tongues of tissue by making a U-shaped incision in the appropriate location (Fig. 25.6). Alternatively, the coronary flaps are reattached

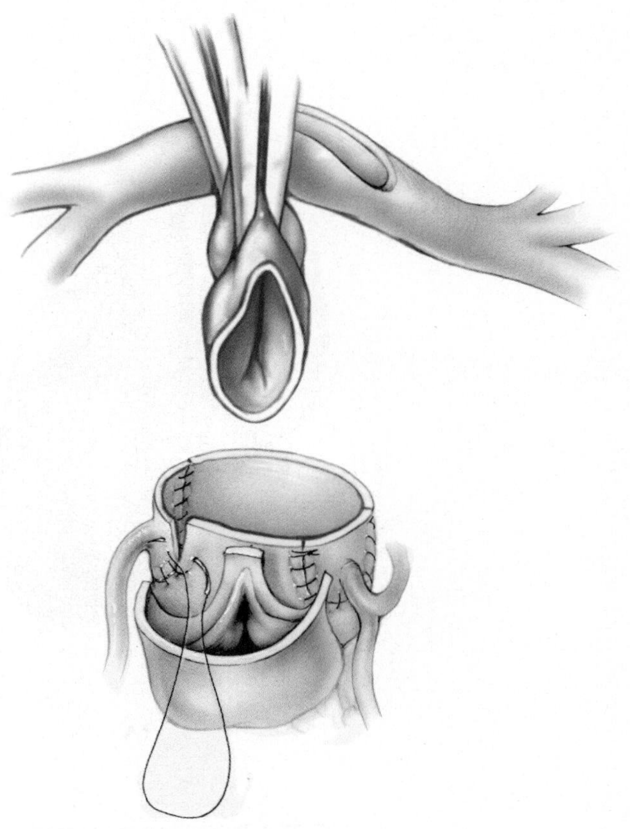

FIG. 25.6 Reattachment of the coronary tongues to the pulmonary root.

as buttons of tissue, trimming the distal end of the flap before completing the suture line. In this case, a small slit is made at the appropriate location for coronary reimplantation in the pulmonary root. This site may be enlarged free hand, or with a small aortic punch. The coronary artery is sutured to the opening in the pulmonary root using 7-0 or 8-0 Prolene suture (Fig. 25.7). After each coronary anastomosis, cold blood cardioplegic solution is infused directly into each coronary ostium with a 2-mm olive-tipped cannula, allowing assessment of any kinking or distortion of the coronary artery. If any problems are detected, they should be rectified now by either freeing up any restrictive adventitial or epicardial bands or redoing the anastomosis.

⊘ Coronary Implantation

Many surgeons favor creating the incisions for coronary implantation with the aortic root filled. To achieve this, the Lecompte maneuver is performed, and the neoaorta is anastomosed with marking sutures placed on the outside exactly at the site of the three commissures. The cross-clamp can either be removed, or a cardioplegia catheter placed and the root filled to demonstrate the orientation and extent of the root prior to choosing sites for coronary implantation. The incision into the root is done with the root fully distended to reduce the chance of injury to the neoaortic valve (Fig. 25.8). ⊘

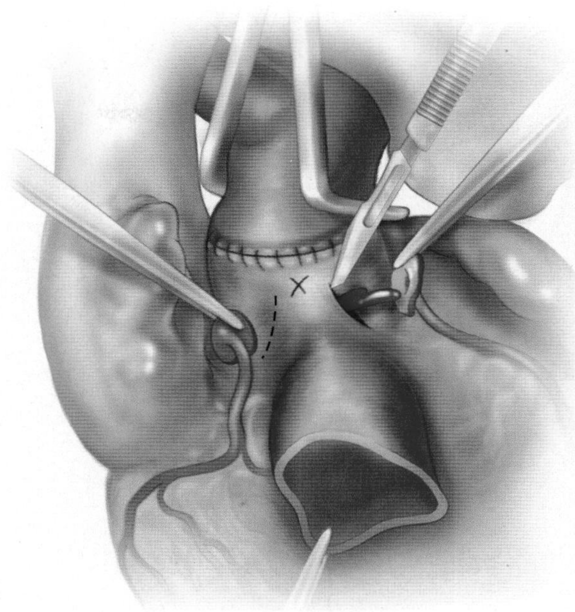

FIG. 25.8 "Closed" technique for coronary reimplantation. Note the angulation of the incisions slightly toward the midline. The "X" marks the location of the top of the commissure, and is marked on the outside of the neoaorta with a marking suture.

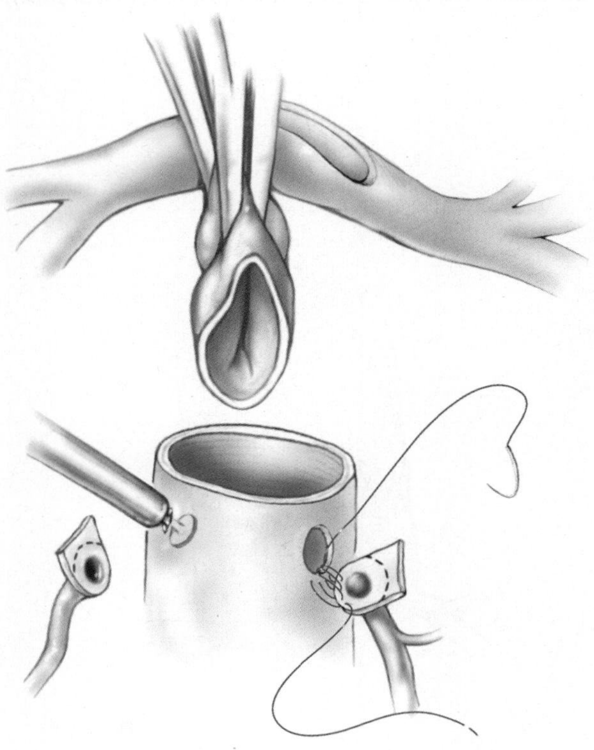

FIG. 25.7 Reattachment of the coronary ostia as buttons to the pulmonary root.

⊘ Torsion of the Coronary Artery

Some surgeons prefer to excise the coronary ostia as buttons, instead of tongues of tissue from the aortic root. When this technique is used, extreme care must be taken to prevent rotation and distortion of the coronary artery button during reimplantation. ⊘

NB Circumflex Coronary Artery Arising from the Right Coronary Artery

If the circumflex coronary artery arises from the right coronary artery, a trapdoor may be created in the neoaorta to prevent kinking of the takeoff of the circumflex branch (Fig. 25.9). Alternatively, the right coronary artery ostium may be implanted higher on the neoaorta. When the circumflex arises from the right coronary artery, the pulmonary artery should be transected as far distally as possible to allow a high reimplantation of the right coronary button. Occasionally, the anastomosis must be performed on the ascending aorta distal to the suture line joining the neoaortic root to the distal aorta (Fig. 25.10). NB

NB Intramural Coronary Artery

A shallow, U-shaped incision is made in the proximal neoaorta adjacent to the location of the previously prepared aortic tongue of tissue containing the involved coronary ostium

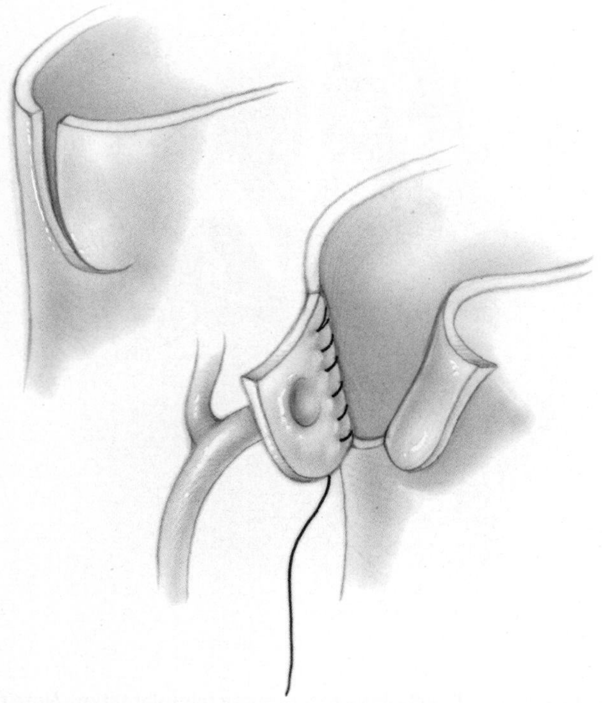

FIG. 25.9 Trapdoor technique when the circumflex coronary artery arises from the right coronary artery.

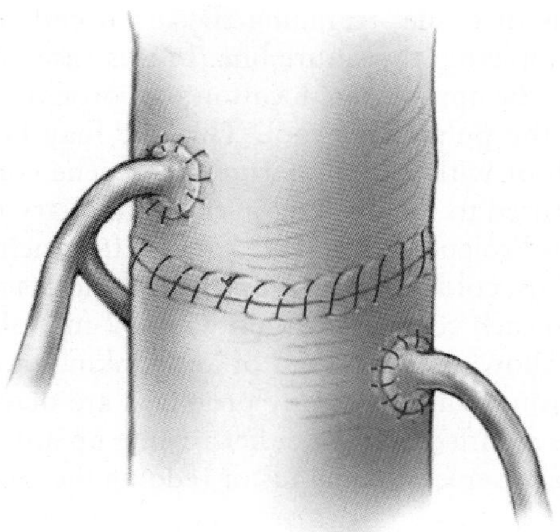

FIG. 25.10 Placing an anastomosis of the right coronary artery above the anastomosis of the neoaortic root to the ascending aorta.

or ostia. The upper edge of the aortic tongue is sutured to the lower portion of this U-shaped opening in the neoaortic root with a 7-0 Prolene suture (Fig. 25.11A). The suture line is secured at both ends. The neoaortic root is anastomosed to the ascending aorta posteriorly, securing the suture line on both sides where it meets the coronary artery anastomosis. A piece of autologous pericardium is cut in the appropriate shape, and sewn into place to create a convex roof over the remaining opening (Fig. 25.11B). This technique allows the coronary artery to maintain its original orientation, and

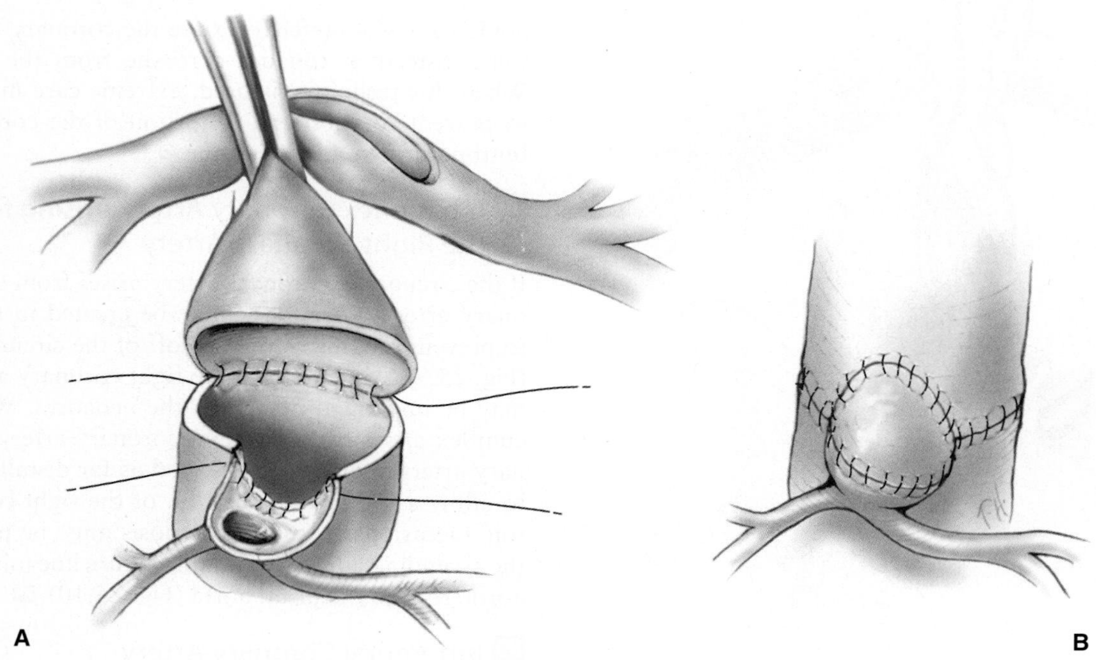

FIG. 25.11 **A:** Anastomosing a single intramural coronary artery to the neoaorta maintaining the native orientation of the coronary ostium. **B:** Using a pericardial hood to complete the anastomosis.

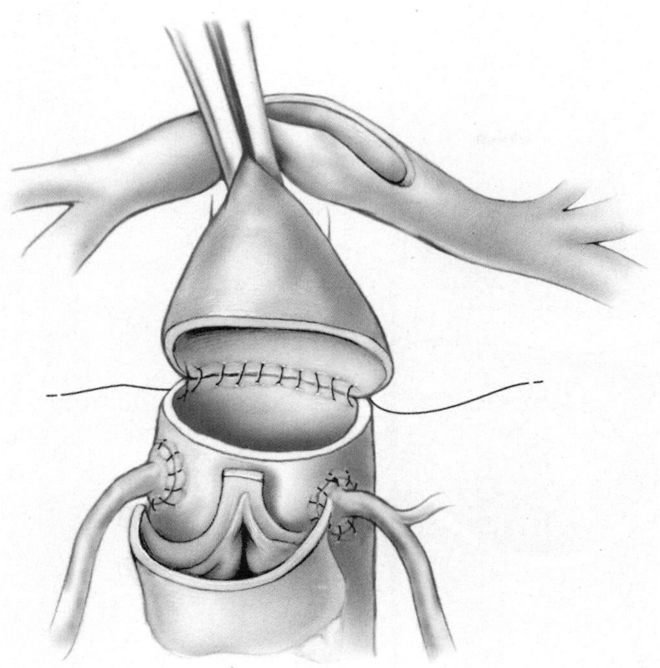

FIG. 25.12 Anastomosis of the neoaortic root to the distal aorta.

minimizes the risk of twisting or tension on the proximal course of the coronary artery. NB

⊘ Injury to the Neoaortic Leaflets

Care must be taken when making the opening in the neoaortic root first with the knife blade and then with the punch to protect the valve leaflets from injury. The assistant may gently retract the leaflet with the back of a fine forceps. ⊘

Reconstructing the Aorta

The distal ascending aorta is anastomosed to the neoaortic root with running 6-0 or 7-0 Prolene suture (Fig. 25.12).

NB Size Difference between the Neoaortic Root and Ascending Aorta

If a discrepancy between the diameter of the distal ascending aorta and neoaortic root exists, the excess tissue can usually be gathered in the posterior suture line. Gathering tissue anteriorly can distort the coronary artery anastomoses. This is especially true if the coronary arteries have been reimplanted as flaps. NB

NB Hemostasis of the Posterior Suture Line

Care must be taken to ensure hemostasis of the aortic suture line, especially posteriorly, because this is relatively inaccessible after the repair is completed. NB

NB Side-by-Side Great Vessels

When the aorta and pulmonary artery are side by side, the Lecompte maneuver may not be performed. The distal ascending aorta is mobilized laterally and anastomosed to the neoaortic base. NB

Intracardiac Repair

The atrial septal defect or balloon atrial septostomy and a ventricular septal defect, if present, are closed through a right atriotomy incision (see Chapters 19 and 21). Alternatively, a ventricular septal defect can be closed through one of the semilunar valves. If this is done through the posterior (pulmonary) valve, great care must be taken to avoid the conduction system. After closing the right atrium, the aortic cross-clamp may be removed or left in place until the pulmonary artery reconstruction is finished. If it is left in place, another dose of cardioplegia is given through a butterfly needle in the neoaortic root, allowing the surgeon to check the lie and filling of the coronary arteries as well as the suture lines for bleeding.

Reconstructing the Pulmonary Artery

If the aorta is to remain clamped, the clamp must now be moved to the ascending aorta above the pulmonary artery confluence. The defect created in the neopulmonary base is filled either with two separate patches, or with a rectangular patch of glutaraldehyde-treated pericardium ("pantaloon"). The patch should be approximately twice as long as the remaining neopulmonary sinus. A slit-like or V-shaped incision is made halfway along the long edge of this rectangular patch. This fits into the posterior commissure of the neopulmonary base. The patch is sewn into place with a running 6-0 or 7-0 Prolene suture. The resultant neopulmonary root is then anastomosed to the pulmonary artery confluence with a 6-0 Prolene suture (Fig. 25.13).

⊘ Supravalvular Pulmonary Stenosis

A well-recognized late complication of arterial switch procedures is supravalvular pulmonary stenosis. This can be minimized by leaving a generous cuff of pericardium when reconstructing the neopulmonary root. ⊘

NB Side-by-Side Great Vessels

When the Lecompte maneuver is not performed, the pulmonary artery confluence is oversewn with a 6-0 Prolene suture. A longitudinal opening is made on the underside of the right pulmonary artery. The reconstructed neopulmonary artery base is anastomosed to this opening in the right pulmonary artery with a 6-0 Prolene suture. NB

Completing the Operation

The aortic cross-clamp is removed, and deairing carried out through the cardioplegic needle hole, which is subsequently closed with a 7-0 Prolene horizontal mattress suture. When rewarming is completed, the patient is weaned off cardiopulmonary bypass, taking care not to overfill the heart.

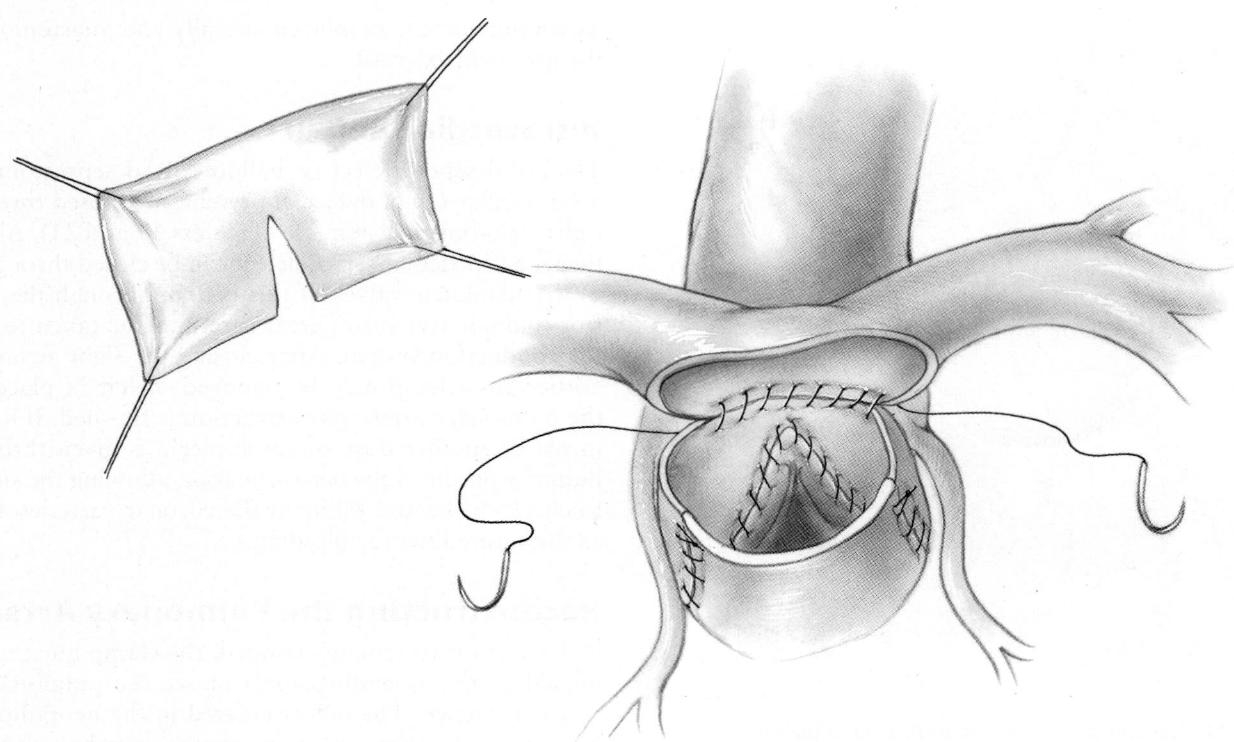

FIG. 25.13 Reconstruction of the neopulmonary root with pericardium and its attachment to the pulmonary artery confluence.

NB Examining Coronary Perfusion

After the aortic cross-clamp is removed, the heart is examined for perfusion in all coronary distributions. Abnormalities of perfusion must be corrected. Further mobilization of the coronary artery in question may be required, or a coronary anastomosis may need to be repositioned. If it is determined that the coronary anatomy is not suitable for further revision, or that the patient will not tolerate an additional period of cross-clamping, a bypass procedure should be performed. Most often, this consists of mobilizing the left or right internal thoracic artery from the chest wall as an *in situ* conduit. It is anastomosed to the involved coronary artery. Occasionally, the left subclavian artery may be ligated distally, transected, and the distal end anastomosed to the proximal left anterior descending or circumflex coronary artery. NB

⊘ Dysrhythmias

Rhythm disturbances during rewarming or soon after cardiopulmonary bypass is discontinued are most often secondary to coronary perfusion problems in the absence of preoperative tachyarrhythmias. The cause must be determined and corrected promptly. ⊘

⊘ Stretching of the Coronary Arteries

Overdistention of the heart in the immediate postbypass period may stretch the transposed coronary arteries. This can lead to decreased coronary flow. Therefore, volume should be administered carefully to these patients for the first 24 to 48 hours postoperatively to avoid this potentially fatal complication. ⊘

⊘ Suture Line Bleeding

Bleeding can be a problem because of the extensive suture lines. Hemostasis should be checked after removing the aortic cross-clamp. Bleeding sites should be carefully sutured with adventitial horizontal mattress 7-0 Prolene sutures. If bleeding from the aorta is noted after discontinuation of cardiopulmonary bypass, reinstitution of bypass may be required. Takedown of the pulmonary artery anastomosis to allow access to the aortic suture line may be necessary. ⊘

⊘ Coronary Artery Spasm

The transposed coronary arteries are susceptible to spasm in the postbypass and early postoperative periods. Intravenous nitroglycerin infusion is indicated in these patients. Intravenous calcium solution should be given very cautiously to prevent coronary artery spasm. ⊘

CONGENITALLY CORRECTED TRANSPOSITION OF THE GREAT ARTERIES

Congenitally corrected transposition of the great arteries is a congenital heart defect in which both atrioventricular discordance and ventriculoarterial discordance are present. Physiologically, this combination allows for a normal circulation if other defects are not present. Most of these patients also have ventricular septal defects, pulmonary valve abnormalities, and/or Ebsteinoid changes of the tricuspid valve. The traditional surgical approach ("functional repair") has been to repair the associated lesions only. This leaves the patient with a morphologic right ventricle and tricuspid valve as the systemic ventricle and atrioventricular valve. More recently, some centers have advocated an anatomic repair, the "double switch" procedure, in certain subgroups of these patients. Patients with two adequate ventricles and a normal pulmonic valve undergo an arterial switch procedure combined with a Senning or Mustard atrial switch. If the pulmonic valve is not suitable for an arterial switch, a Senning and Rastelli procedure may be an option if there is an appropriate ventricular septal defect for baffling the morphologic left ventricle to the aortic valve. Theoretically, a double switch procedure should improve the long-term outcome of these patients, who often develop progressive tricuspid regurgitation and right ventricular failure, by making the morphologic left ventricle the systemic ventricle and placing the abnormal tricuspid valve in the lower pressure pulmonary circulation. However, proper patient selection is critical, and many patients require a multistaged pulmonary banding procedure to train the left ventricle.

When performing the double switch operation, either the arterial switch or the atrial switch can be performed first. Some modifications to both procedures may be required because of previous pulmonary artery banding and anatomic considerations.

NB Closure of Ventricular Septal Defect

The ventricular septal defect is closed through the mitral valve. Sutures are placed on the morphologic right ventricular side of the septum to avoid the conduction system. NB

NB Previous Pulmonary Banding

Dissection between the aorta and pulmonary artery should be carried out carefully in the presence of a previously placed pulmonary band. The proximal pulmonary root (neoaorta) may be dilated. This may require V-shaped excisions of tissue from the sinuses before coronary transfer to ensure a competent valve. In addition, the area of the band must be excised or enlarged to prevent supravalvar stenosis and distortion of the sinotubular junction. NB

THE SENNING PROCEDURE

Cannulation

The distal ascending aorta is cannulated and direct superior and inferior vena caval cannulation is achieved with right-angled cannulas. The site of the superior vena cava cannula should be as high as possible above the cavoatrial junction (Fig. 25.14). Individual caval cannulation must be done carefully to minimize interference with venous return and avoid hypotension and serious dysrhythmias. Partial cardiopulmonary bypass may be initiated after one cannula is inserted to facilitate placement of the second cannula. Under moderate hypothermia, the aorta is cross-clamped and cardioplegia is delivered into the aortic root.

Atrial Incision

Access to the inside of the right atrium is gained through a longitudinal incision made 3 to 4 mm anterior and parallel to the sulcus terminalis (Fig. 25.15).

NB Incision Length

The incision should be well away from the sinoatrial node, and its superior extension should be limited to 0.5 cm from the superior margin of the right atrium. If additional length is required, the incision can be extended onto the right atrial appendage (Fig. 25.15). NB

NB Direction of the Incision

Only after the surgeon has inspected the inside of the right atrium should the incision be extended inferiorly so that it can be directed toward the lateral insertion of the valve of the inferior vena cava (Eustachian valve) (Fig. 25.15). NB

The Atrial Septum

The fossa ovalis is usually torn if a balloon septostomy has been performed earlier. The trapezoid septal flap is developed starting in the most anterior part of the foramen ovale and is incised superiorly for a distance of approximately 7 mm. The direction of the incision is then changed posteriorly toward the superior margin of the right superior pulmonary vein and extends to the base of the interatrial septum. Similarly, an incision from the lower part of the fossa ovalis is continued downward toward the inferior margin of the right inferior pulmonary vein (Fig. 25.16). The raw margins of the septum are then endothelialized with interrupted sutures of 6-0 or 7-0 Prolene taking superficial bites and approximating the endothelium (Fig. 25.16, inset). This atrial septal flap is now connected only at its base, which corresponds outside the atria to the interatrial groove.

⊘ Injury to the Sinoatrial Node Artery

The artery to the sinoatrial node traverses the anterosuperior quadrant of the medial wall of the right atrium. Development of the atrial septal flap should spare the vascular supply of the sinoatrial node by not deviating the superior extension of the incision anteriorly. ⊘

⊘ Perforation of the Medial Wall of the Right Atrium

Similarly, the direction of the superior incision in the septum is significant. If this incision is deviated anteriorly toward the muscular aortic mound, it may lead into the

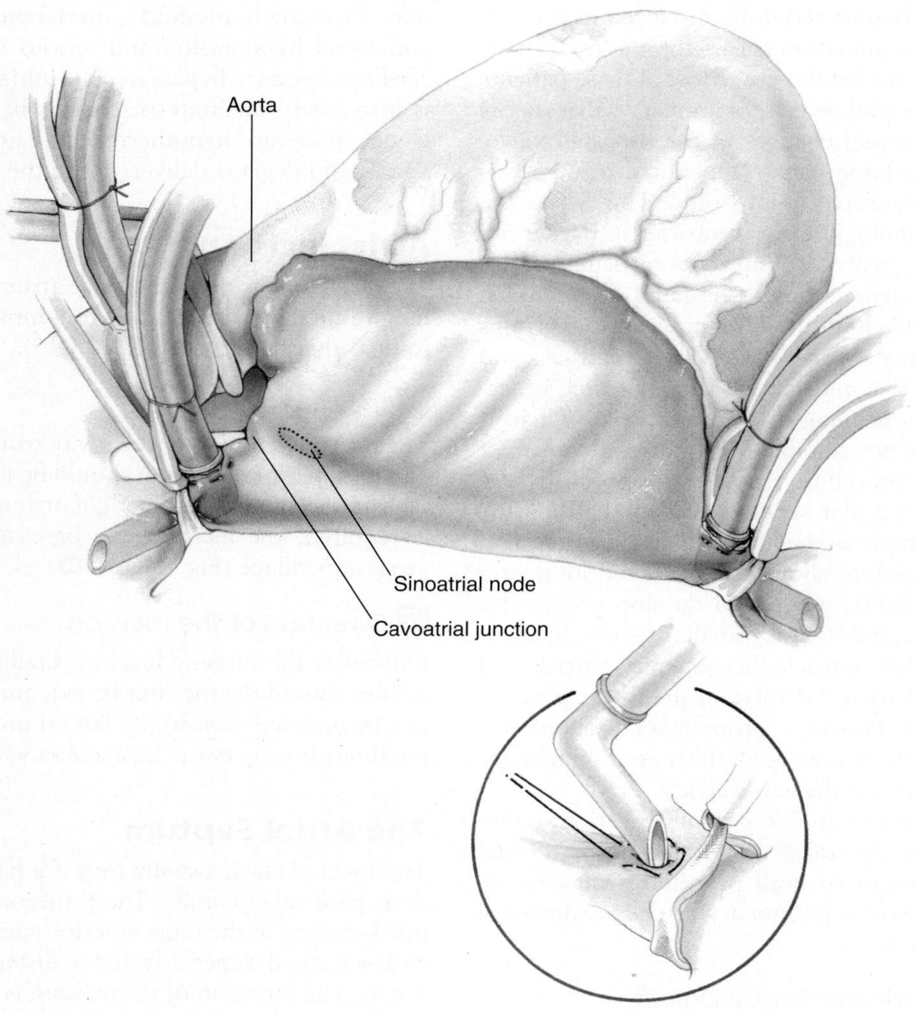

FIG. 25.14 Technique for caval cannulations. Inset: Direct cannulation using a right-angled cannula.

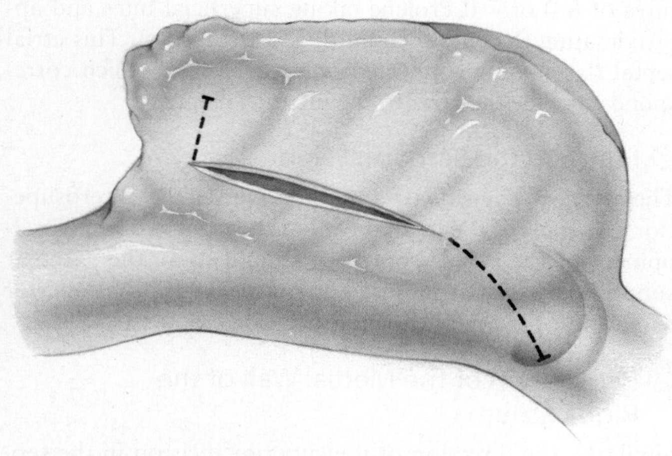

FIG. 25.15 Atriotomy.

pericardium outside the heart. If this happens, it must be immediately detected and the defect reapproximated with multiple fine Prolene sutures. ⊘

⊘ Preferential Conduction Tracts

There are three main preferential conduction tracts or muscle bands joining the sinoatrial node to the atrioventricular node (Fig. 25.17). These probably correspond to the crista terminalis and limbic muscle bundles. The anterior conduction tract passes anterior to both the fossa ovalis and coronary sinus. The middle tract also lies anterior to the fossa ovalis but may pass through or just posterior to the coronary sinus. The posterior preferential tract crosses the posterior wall of the right atrium between the venae cavae and then curves forward toward the coronary sinus. During the development of the flap, the middle tract will be sacrificed in

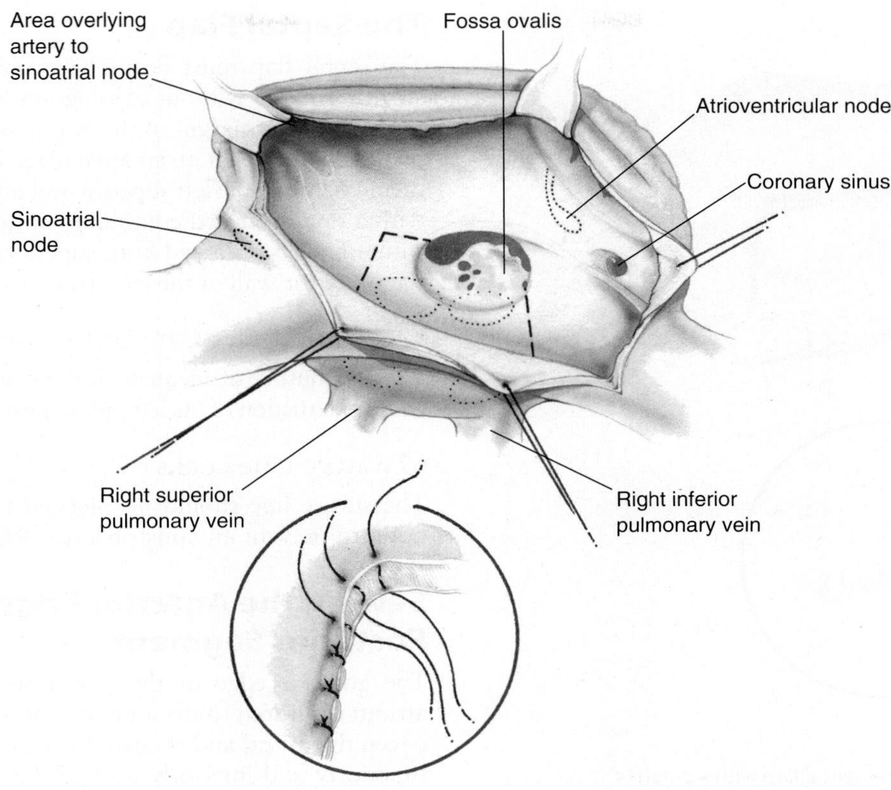

FIG. 25.16 Preparation of the atrial septal flap. Inset: Endothelial approximation.

most cases. Great care should be taken to prevent injury to the other conduction pathways. ⊘

The defect in the flap from the fossa ovalis is filled by attaching an appropriately sized patch of Gore-Tex or glutaraldehyde-treated autologous pericardium. The size of the atrial septal flap thereby developed is remarkably constant and has a base of approximately 3 cm, a height of 2 cm, and an anterior side of 1.5 to 2 cm in infants 6 to 12 months of age.

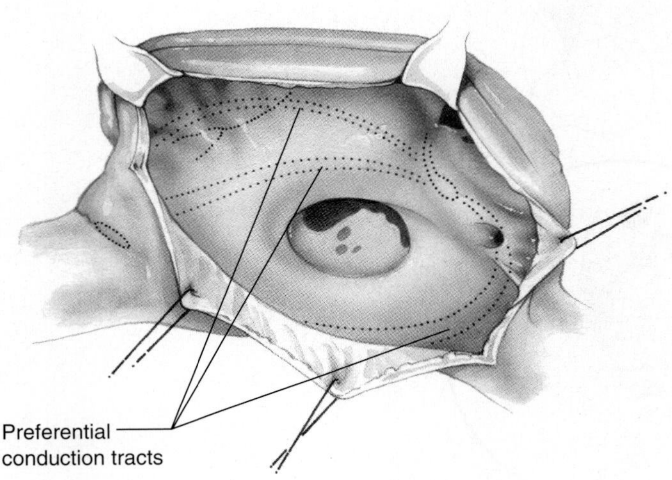

FIG. 25.17 The three main preferential conduction tissue pathways joining the sinoatrial node to the atrioventricular node.

NB Inadequate Flap Size

The flap often must be enlarged by attaching a patch of appropriately sized Gore-Tex or glutaraldehyde-treated autologous pericardium with a continuous suture of 6-0 Prolene (Fig. 25.18). NB

⊘ Tearing the Fossa Ovalis

A segment of the fossa ovalis is usually torn open by an earlier balloon septostomy. It is also thin and sometimes full of perforating holes. This segment should be excised because it may tear at the suture line and produce a defect in the newly constructed atrial septum. ⊘

The interatrial groove is dissected to free as much of the posterior atrial wall as possible. Traction on the septal flap brings the left atrium and pulmonary veins into view. A longitudinal incision is made parallel with and posterior to the groove into the left atrium (Fig. 25.18).

⊘ Small Left Atrial Opening

A transverse incision may be made down into the right superior pulmonary vein or between the right superior and inferior pulmonary veins to ensure a larger left atrial opening. ⊘

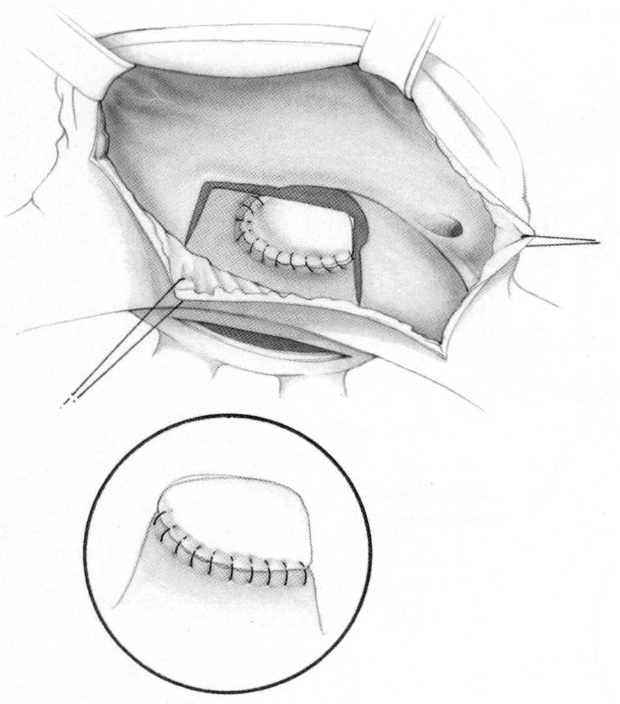

FIG. 25.18 Enlarging the septal flap with a patch of autologous pericardium or Gore-Tex.

The Septal Flap

The septal flap must be mobile enough so that it can be slightly rotated without causing any tension. The midpoint of the anterior margin of the flap is sutured to the left atrial wall behind the left atrial appendage beginning just in front of and between the left superior and inferior pulmonary veins with a double-armed continuous suture of 6-0 Prolene. The suture line is continued both superiorly and inferiorly along the posterior wall of the left atrium to the base of the flap.

⊘ Obstruction of the Left Pulmonary Veins

The flap must be of adequate size or it will be under tension and cause obstruction of the left pulmonary veins at their orifices. ⊘

⊘ Suture Line Leaks

The suture line should be checked for leaks with a nerve hook to prevent any postoperative shunting. ⊘

Sewing the Anterior Edge of the Posterior Segment

The anterior edge of the posterior segment of the right atrium is sutured to the anterior part of the septal defect between the mitral and tricuspid valves. Suturing is continued superiorly and inferiorly around the lateral margins of the orifices of the superior and inferior venae cavae (Fig. 25.19).

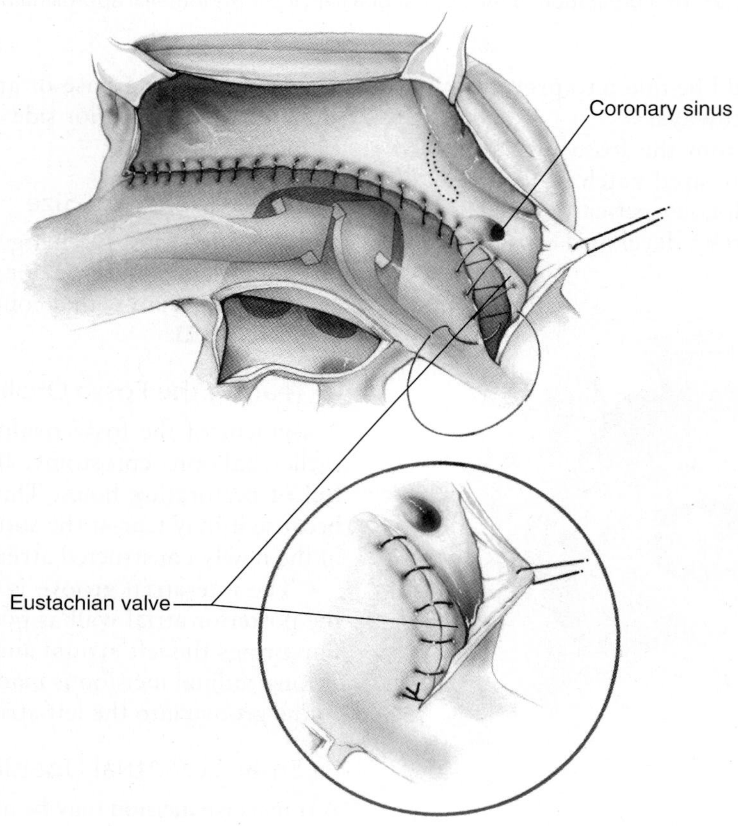

FIG. 25.19 Direction of the suture line to prevent injury to the atrioventricular node. Inset: Close-up of the suture line below the coronary sinus.

⊘ Injury to the Atrioventricular Node

The suture line, when continued down toward the inferior vena cava, should pass behind the coronary sinus to avoid any injury to the atrioventricular node. ⊘

⊘ Obstruction of the Inferior Vena Cava

The medial aspect of the Eustachian valve of the inferior vena cava, when well developed, is an important landmark because it signifies the medial limit of the orifice of the inferior vena cava. The approximation of the atrial wall flap to the medial margin of the Eustachian valve ensures an adequate inflow channel for the inferior vena cava. ⊘

⊘ Underdeveloped or Absent Eustachian Valve

If the Eustachian valve is absent or underdeveloped, a venous cannula of appropriate size may be introduced through the left atrial appendage and the newly constructed atrial septal defect into the inferior vena cava. The atrial wall flap is then sutured in place using the cannula as a stent (Fig. 25.20). ⊘

⊘ Caval Obstruction

If suturing impinges on the orifices of the superior or inferior vena cava, the resultant constriction may cause obstruction to the venous return. This can be particularly troublesome with the superior vena cava (Fig. 25.21). ⊘

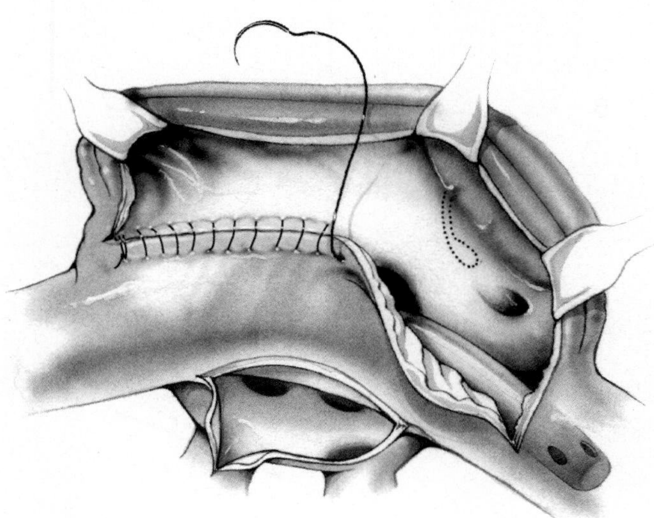

FIG. 25.20 Introduction of a venous cannula into the inferior vena cava when the Eustachian valve is absent or underdeveloped to ensure adequate flow.

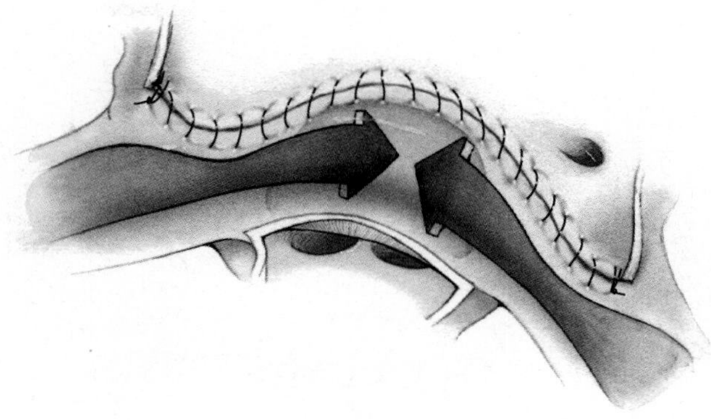

FIG. 25.21 Obstruction to venous return due to constriction at the orifices of the venae cavae.

Sewing the Posterior Edge of the Anterior Segment

The posterior edge of the anterior segment of the right atrial wall is now sewn to the left atrial opening and the right atrial wall around the caval channel (Fig. 25.22).

⊘ Injury to the Sinoatrial Node

To prevent injury to the sinoatrial node, suturing is done with interrupted sutures 0.5 to 1 cm above the superior cavoatrial junction. Alternatively, superficial bites with a 6-0 or 7-0 Prolene running suture are taken in this area. ⊘

⊘ Caval Constriction

The caval snares are loosened so that both cavae become filled, fully distended, and stretched before suturing is continued. This prevents any caval constriction. ⊘

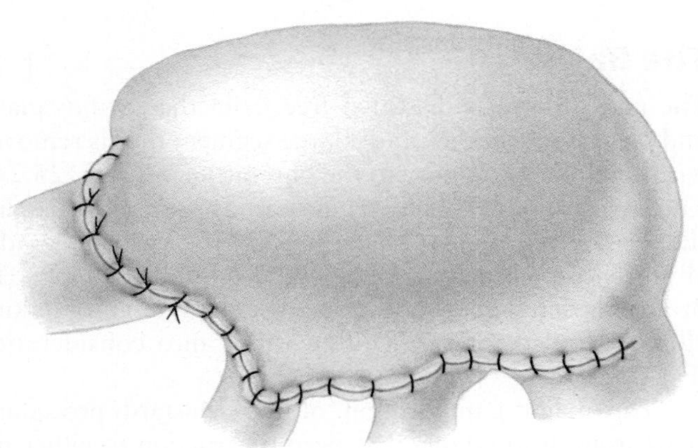

FIG. 25.22 Closure of the right atrium.

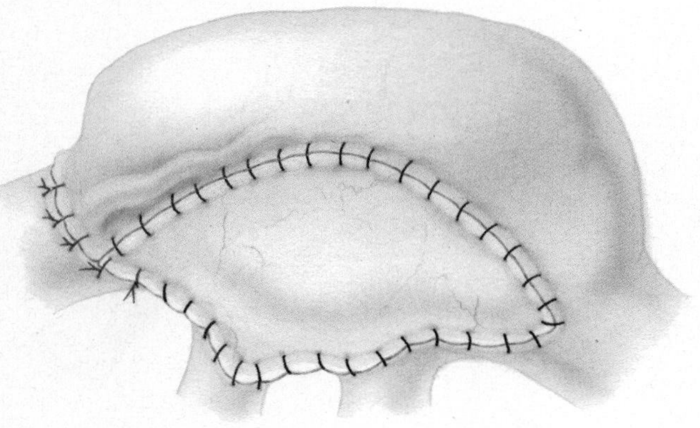

FIG. 25.23 Use of a patch of pericardium or Gore-Tex to enlarge the right atrial wall.

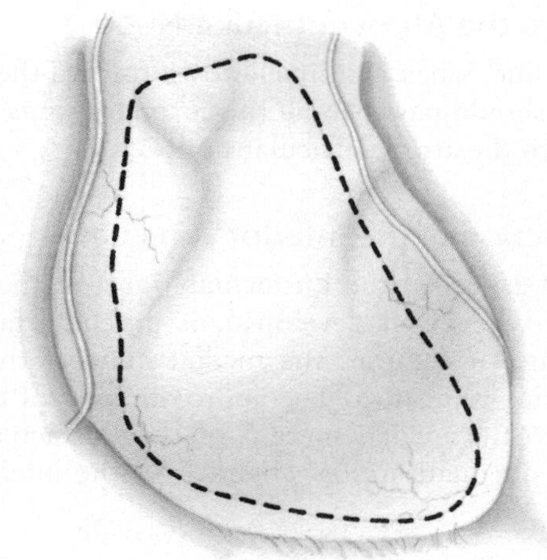

FIG. 25.24 Segment of pericardium for use as a baffle in the Mustard procedure.

⊘ Inadequate Right Atrial Wall

Occasionally, the anterior part of the right atrial wall may not be adequate to provide a satisfactory roof over the new systemic venous chamber, and allow for a generous pulmonary venous chamber. This problem can be overcome by adding a patch of pericardium or Gore-Tex to enlarge the right atrial wall (Fig. 25.23). This is particularly useful when the atrial appendages are juxtaposed. In these cases, there is always too little atrial wall, and enlargement with a patch becomes mandatory. In some patients undergoing a double switch procedure, the free wall of the morphologic right atrium is narrow, and extra tissue is required to enlarge the pulmonary venous atrium. A segment of *in situ* pericardium along the right side of the heart can be used instead of a separate patch, taking shallow bites over the phrenic nerve. ⊘

THE MUSTARD PROCEDURE

The incision, cannulation, and myocardial protection are carried out as for the Senning procedure.

The Baffle

The pericardium is dissected free from the thymus gland and pleural reflections, and a large segment of it is removed with care to avoid injury to the phrenic nerves (Fig. 25.24). The pericardium is then cut into an appropriate size and shape. The rectangular shape used in the past has gradually been replaced by a wedge or a dumbbell shape. The Brom trouser-shaped baffle has the advantage of taking all the detailed intraatrial dimensions into consideration (Fig. 25.25).

The major complication of the Mustard procedure, apart from dysrhythmia, has been obstruction to either the systemic or the pulmonary venous system, which can be

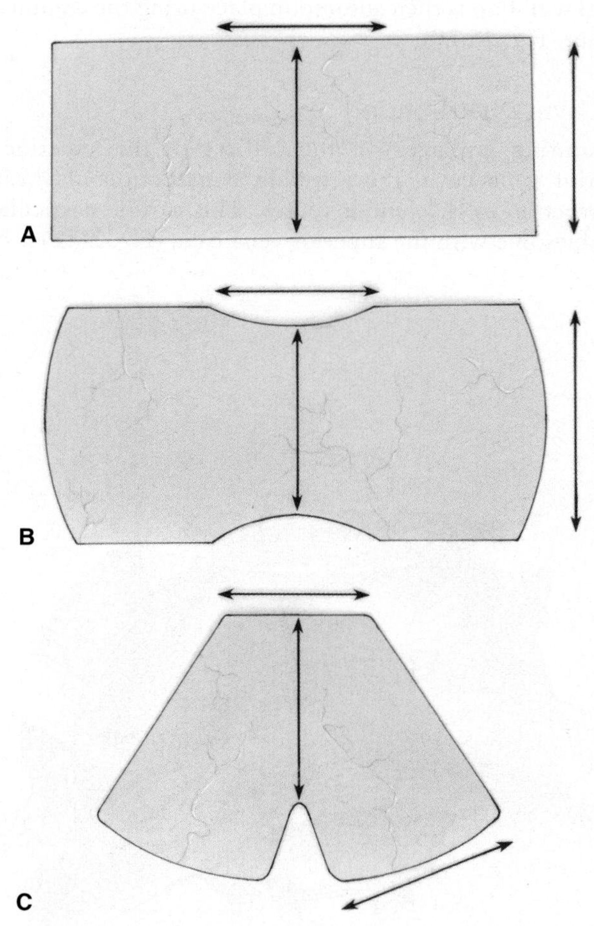

FIG. 25.25 Appropriate sizes and shapes of pericardium for a baffle. **A:** Traditional rectangle shape. **B:** Dumbbell shape. **C:** Trouser shape. See legend to Fig. 25 .24 for explanation of dimensions.

attributed to baffle malfunction. Therefore, a clear and accurate understanding of the functional anatomy of the Mustard procedure is essential to prevent subsequent complications. The atrial septum must be excised as completely as possible (taking care not to injure the sinoatrial node artery and the preferential conduction pathways; see hazards in Senning Procedure section). The baffle then becomes the new interatrial septum and functions as part of the inflow tract for drainage from the caval veins through the mitral valve.

NB The Posterior Margin of the Baffle

The posterior margin of the baffle should be 0.5 cm longer than the combined diameters of both left pulmonary veins (they can each be measured with calibrated Hegar dilators). In small infants younger than 6 months or weighing less than 5 kg, the pulmonary veins measure approximately 7 mm in diameter. Therefore, the posterior margin of the baffle in the small infant is 2 to 2.5 cm (Fig. 25.26). NB

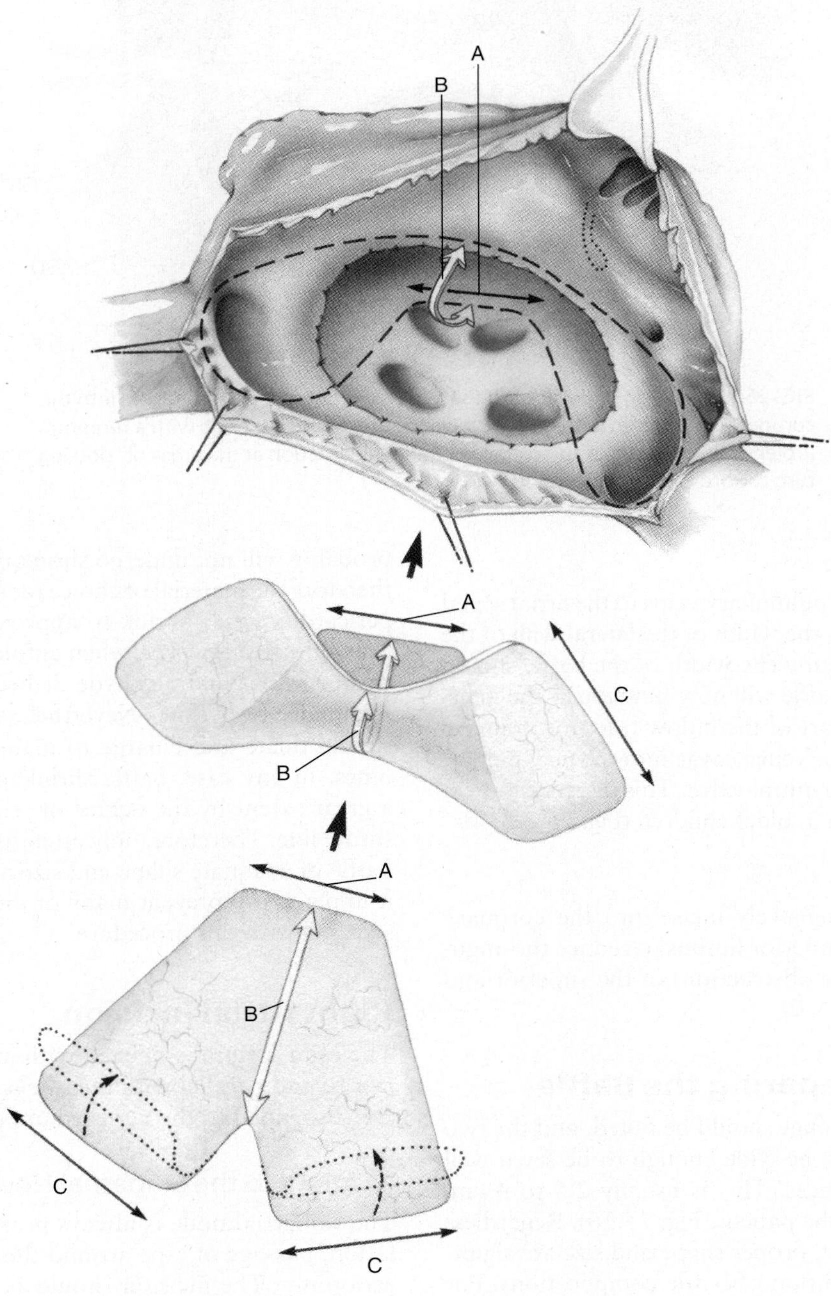

FIG. 25.26 Size of the baffle corresponding to the age of the patient. The dorsal margin **(A)** in small infants is 2 to 2.5 cm. the width of the baffle **(B)** is approximately 3 cm in infants and 3 to 5 cm in older children. Caval openings **(C)** are 2.5 to 4 cm.

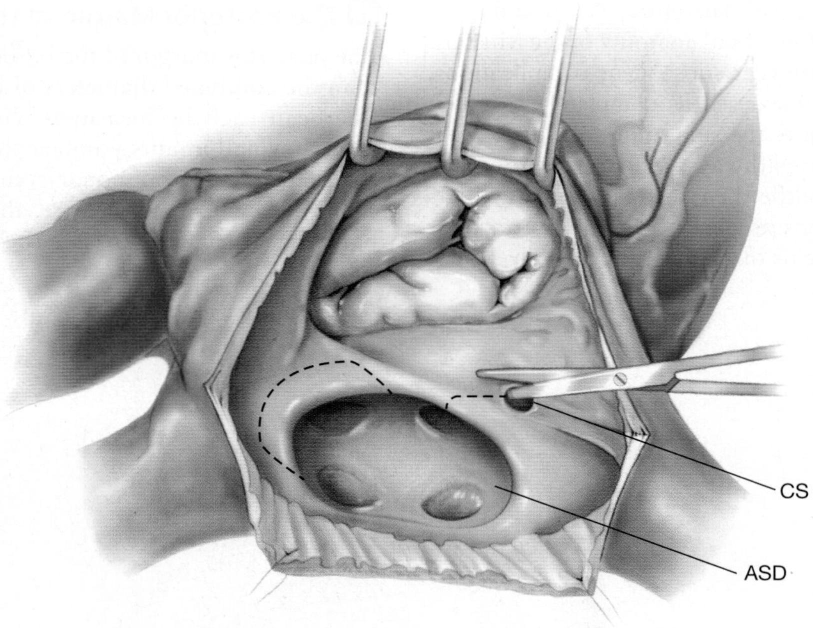

FIG. 25.27 Excision of portions of the superior limbus as well as cutting into the coronary sinus (often with re-endothelialization of the cut edge with a running Prolene suture) reduces the chance of baffle obstruction at the areas of "dog leg" turn toward the tricuspid valve.

NB Width of the Baffle

The distance from the left pulmonary veins to the atrial septal remnant at its midpoint is the width of the lateral wall of the new systemic venous atrium. The width of the baffle should be the same because the baffle will now function as the interatrial septum and form part of the inflow tract for drainage of the superior and inferior venae cavae into the new pulmonary ventricle through the mitral valve. This distance is 3 cm in infants and 3.5 to 5 cm in older children (Fig. 25.26). NB

NB Coronary Sinus

It is often helpful to extensively incise into the coronary sinus as well as into the superior limbus to reduce the angulation (and thereby baffle obstruction) of the superior and inferior limbs (Fig. 25.27). NB

Technique for Preparing the Baffle

The size of the caval openings should be noted, and the two limbs of the baffle should be wide enough to be sewn well away from the caval orifices. This is usually 2.5 to 4 cm, depending on the size of the patient (Fig. 25.26). Regardless of the baffle material used, proper shape and size are significant factors in the prevention of baffle complications. For this reason, Brom designed metallic patterns for different age groups. This pattern is placed on the sheet of pericardium, and the baffle is prepared by cutting around the pattern with a knife. Gore-Tex is easier to handle than pericardium and probably will not undergo shrinkage or deformation, and is therefore the material of choice for some surgeons. Untreated pericardium may shrink to approximately two-thirds of its original size. However, when autologous pericardium is pretreated with glutaraldehyde, it becomes fixed and changes minimally over time. Nevertheless, the normal atrial wall should dilate and enlarge to maintain adequate atrial volumes. In any case, baffle shrinkage is generally limited to a great extent by the degree of tension created by a secure suture line. Therefore, only attention to detail in preparing a baffle of adequate shape and size and meticulously suturing it in place will prevent many of the complications often associated with this procedure.

Right Atrial Incision

The right atrium is opened with an oblique incision, anterior to and parallel with the sulcus terminalis, and its edges are suspended to the pericardium or skin towels.

⊘ Injury to the Sinoatrial Node

The sinoatrial node is always prone to injury from cannulation, passage of tape around the superior vena cava, and atriotomy. The incision should be well away from the sinoatrial node, and its superior extension should be limited to 0.5 cm from the superior margin of the right atrium. If additional length is required, the incision can be extended anteriorly onto the right atrial appendage (Fig. 25.15). ⊘

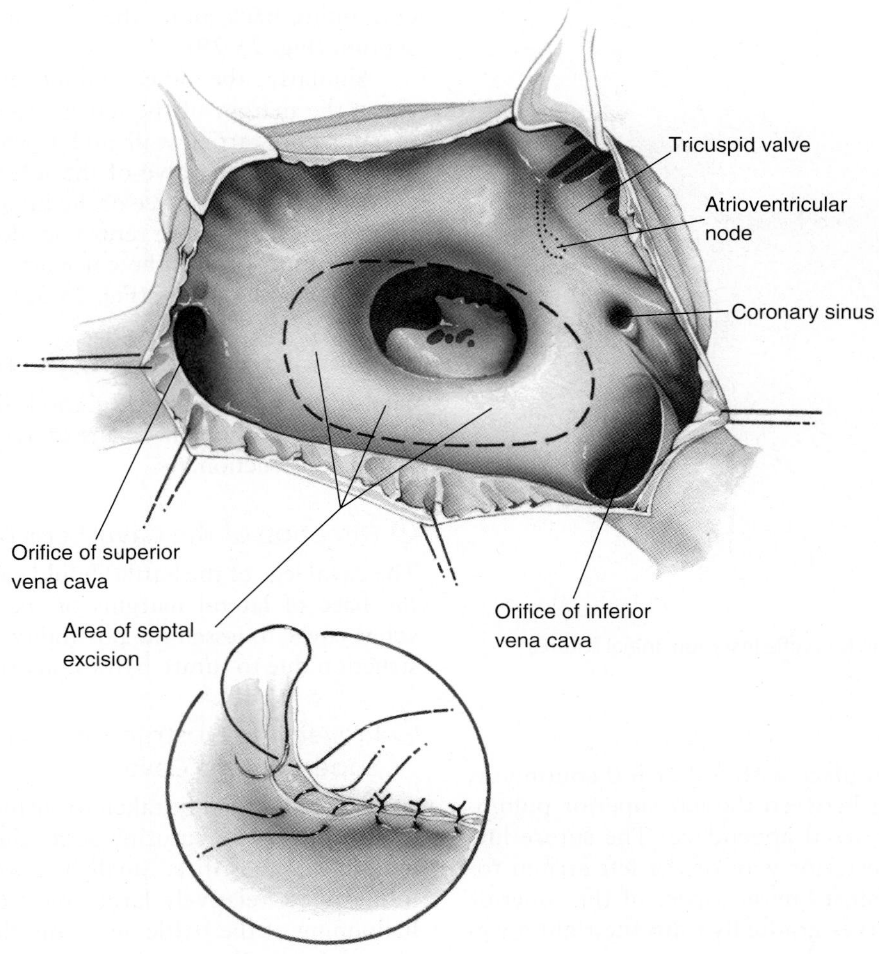

FIG. 25.28 Excision of the atrial septum. Inset: Endothelialization of the cut edges of the septum.

Excision of the Atrial Septum

The atrial septum, including the fossa ovalis (which may have already been torn by a previous balloon septostomy), is now partially excised. The line of incision begins in the foramen ovale and is extended superiorly toward the center of the superior vena cava orifice for a short distance (approximately 7 mm). It is then continued posteriorly toward the base of the interatrial septum and is finally curved inferiorly (parallel with the septum) (Fig. 25.28). An incision is made from the anterior margin of the fossa ovalis inferiorly, avoiding the coronary sinus, and is extended toward the ostium of the inferior vena cava. The septal remnant is now removed, and the raw edges of the septum are endothelialized using interrupted sutures of 6-0 Prolene (Fig. 25.28, inset). This technique ensures safe removal of as large a segment of atrial septum as possible.

⊘ Excision of the Septum

The artery to the sinoatrial node traverses the anterosuperior quadrant of the atrial wall. Excision of the septum should spare the vascular supply of the sinoatrial node. This can be achieved by starting the excision through the foramen ovale superiorly and then continuing it posteriorly toward the interatrial groove (Fig. 25.28). ⊘

NB Preferential Conduction Tracts

There are three main preferential conduction tracts joining the sinoatrial node to the atrioventricular node (Fig. 25.17). These probably correspond with the crista terminalis and limbic muscle bundles. The anterior tract passes anterior to both the fossa ovalis and coronary sinus. The middle tract also lies anterior to the fossa ovalis but may pass through or just posterior to the coronary sinus. The posterior preferential tract crosses in the posterior wall of the right atrium between the cavae and then curves forward toward the coronary sinus. Although the middle tract and the posterior tract are more likely to be sacrificed during excision of the atrial septum, every precaution should be made not to injure or traumatize the anterior conduction tract. NB

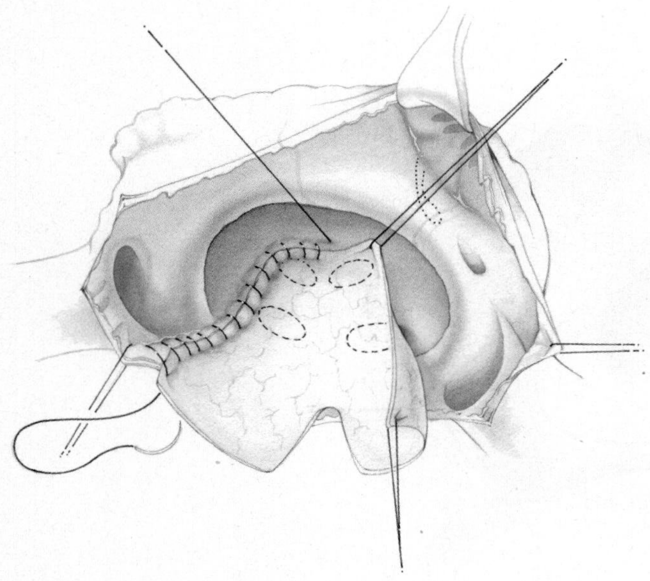

FIG. 25.29 Technique for baffle insertion: Initial sutures.

Baffle Insertion

The baffle is sutured in place with 5-0 or 6-0 continuous Prolene suture starting between the left superior pulmonary vein and the left atrial appendage. The suture line continues along the posterior wall of the left atrium toward the base of the most lateral aspect of the superior vena cava and then curves gradually onto the right atrial wall around the orifice of the superior vena cava before continuing back along the edge of the already cut atrial septum (Fig. 25.29).

Similarly, the other end of the suture is continued along the margin of the left inferior pulmonary vein and the posterior atrial wall and toward the lateral margin of the Eustachian valve of the inferior vena cava. It then curves around the orifice of the inferior vena cava onto the right atrial wall before returning along the cut edge of the atrial septum behind the coronary sinus to be tied to the other end of the suture (Fig. 25.30).

⊘ Pulmonary Venous Obstruction

The suture line should be a good distance away from orifices of the pulmonary veins to avoid causing pulmonary venous obstruction. ⊘

⊘ Direction of the Caval Legs of the Baffle

The caval legs of the baffle should extend obliquely toward the base of lateral margins of the superior and inferior venae cavae to lessen the possibility of pulmonary vein obstruction due to future baffle constriction (Fig. 25.31). ⊘

⊘ Preventing Obstruction to the Superior Vena Cava

Special care should be taken to ensure a wide superior vena caval opening by suturing some distance away from the margin of the orifice. Small bites of the right atrial wall followed by relatively larger bites on the baffle result in ballooning of the baffle, lessening the possibility of future obstruction to the superior vena cava (Fig. 25.32A). ⊘

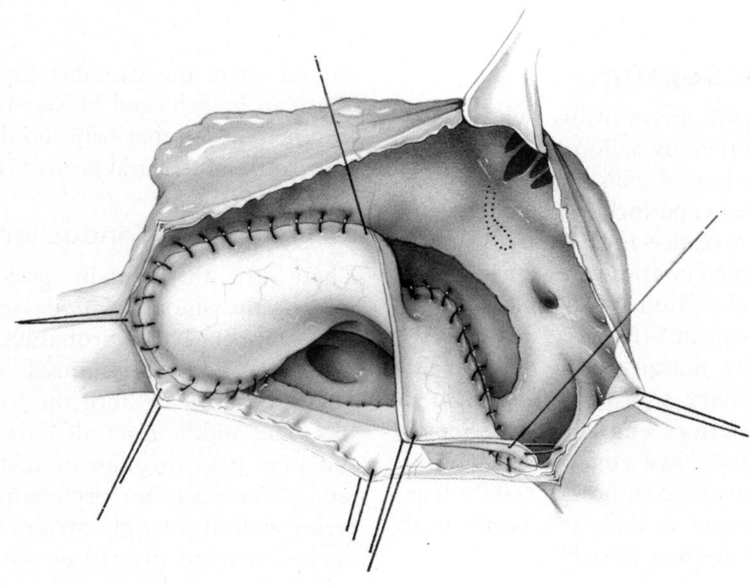

FIG. 25.30 Technique for baffle insertion: Completing the sutures.

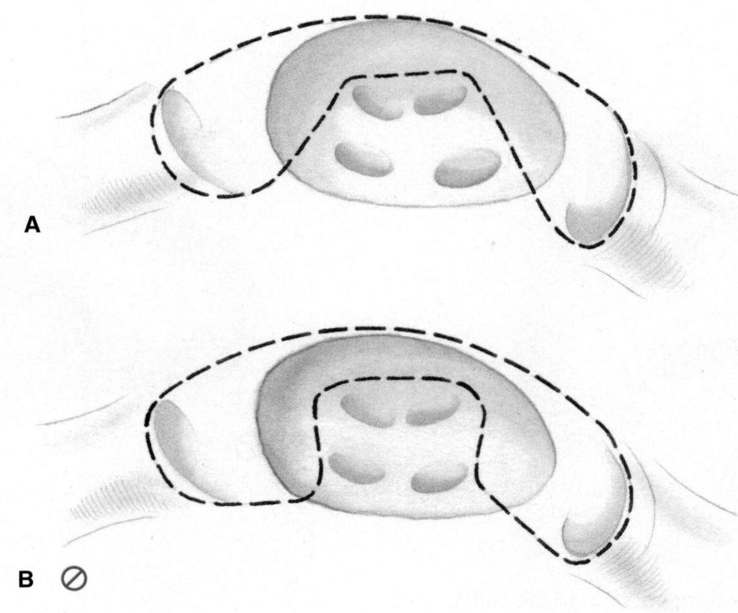

FIG. 25.31 Direction of the caval legs of the baffle. A: Correct. B: Incorrect.

⊘ Preventing Obstruction to the Inferior Vena Cava

The same precautions should be taken to prevent obstruction to the inferior vena cava. The suture line of the baffle is continued along the border of the Eustachian valve so as not to impinge on the inferior vena caval orifice (Fig. 25.32B). ⊘

NB Relationship of the Coronary Sinus to the Baffle

Because of the close proximity of the conduction tracts and atrioventricular node to the coronary sinus, the baffle suture line is continued behind the coronary sinus. This allows its drainage to mix with the pulmonary venous return (Fig. 25.33). NB

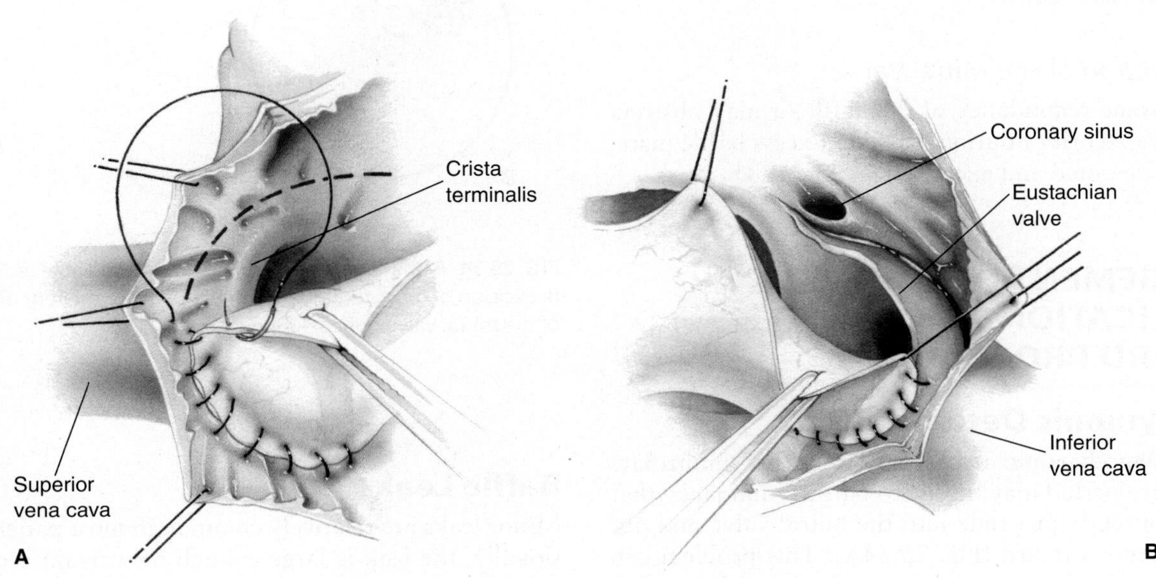

FIG. 25.32 Technique to prevent future obstruction at the orifice of the superior vena cava (A) and inferior vena cava (B).

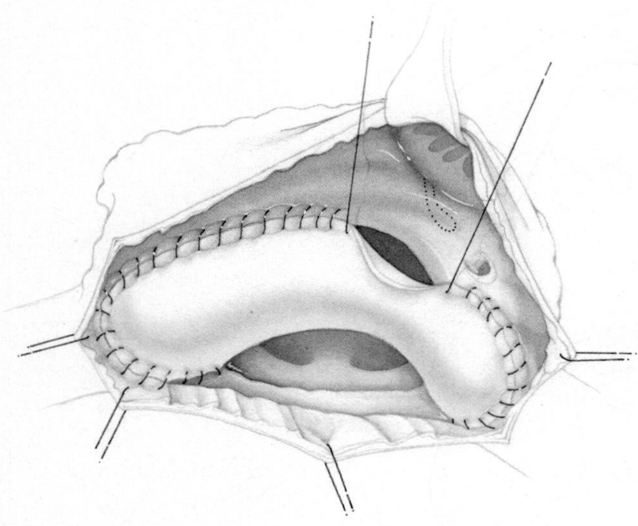

FIG. 25.33 Relationship of the coronary sinus to the baffle.

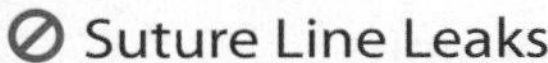

⊘ Suture Line Leaks

With the aid of a fine nerve hook, the surgeon must check the suture line for possible leaks that may be corrected with additional sutures at this time to prevent postoperative shunting. This can also be accomplished by releasing the caval tapes, and briefly occluding the venous cannulas. The baffle will balloon out and reveal any possible leaks, and also provide an opportunity to assess the size and configuration of the caval baffle. ⊘

⊘ Obstruction of the Mitral Valve

If there is some redundancy of the baffle, it may obstruct the mitral valve orifice during diastole. Excess baffle material should be noted and excised (Fig. 25.34). ⊘

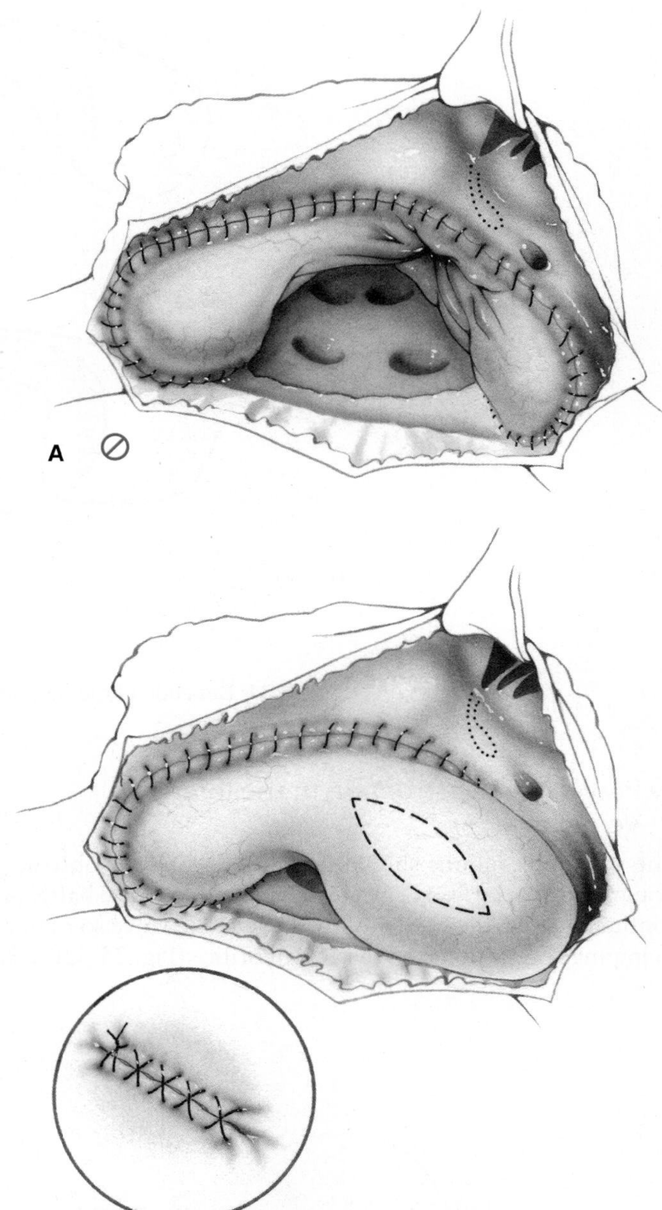

FIG. 25.34 **A:** Mitral valve obstruction from the baffle redundancy. **B:** Excision of gross redundancy of the baffle to prevent obstruction of the mitral valve orifice during diastole.

MANAGEMENT OF LATE COMPLICATIONS OF THE MUSTARD PROCEDURE

Hemodynamic Deterioration

Episodic hemodynamic deterioration in the immediate postoperative period may be due to baffle redundancy that may intermittently protrude into the mitral valve and obstruct the venous return (Fig. 25.34A). This problem can easily be diagnosed by two-dimensional echocardiography. The patient must undergo another operation as soon as possible, the redundant area must be excised, and the defect sutured together (Fig. 25.34B).

Baffle Leaks

Minor leaks are relatively common in most patients. Occasionally, the leak is large enough to warrant reoperation. At the time of surgery, primary closure may be possible, but more commonly a patch of Gore-Tex or pericardium is used to make up for the shrunken pericardium and to reduce tension on the suture line (Fig. 25.35).

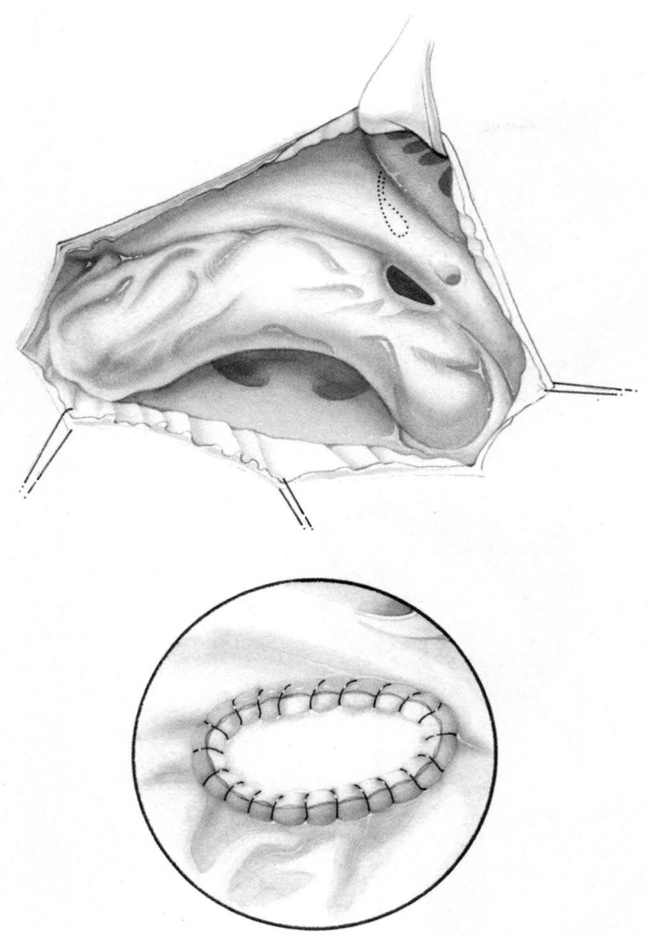

FIG. 25.35 Patching a baffle leak.

Obstruction to the Superior Vena Cava

Obstruction to the superior vena cava may have important sequelae related to elevated central venous pressure in the upper body. Obstruction is usually due to inadequate width and length of the superior limb of the baffle or due to suturing too close to the ostium of the superior vena cava. Unless the gradient across the caval ostium is minimal, these patients should undergo surgical correction of the obstruction. At the time of reoperation, the baffle looks thickened, shrunken, and wrinkled. It is incised longitudinally, and the superior vena cava inflow is enlarged by suturing an appropriately sized Gore-Tex patch in place. The right atrium is also enlarged with the same patch material (Fig. 25.36).

Obstruction to the Inferior Vena Cava

Obstruction to the inferior vena cava is seen less commonly, but when it occurs, it can be approached in the same manner as obstruction to the superior vena cava.

NB Stenosis of the systemic venous baffle involving the superior or inferior vena caval portion can be successfully managed with balloon dilation in the cardiac catheterization laboratory in most instances. NB

Obstruction to the Pulmonary Veins

Fibrosis and cicatrization around the lumen of the right pulmonary veins may cause obstruction to the pulmonary venous return. These patients should undergo surgical correction. The technique entails extension of a transverse right atriotomy that crosses the interatrial groove between the superior and inferior pulmonary veins for a short distance. The defect can be repaired by an appropriately sized patch; alternatively, the parietal pericardium can be sewn to the edges of the atriotomy to a point well above the right pulmonary veins. This substantially enlarges the pulmonary inflow tract. The remaining right atriotomy can be closed either directly or with a separate patch of pericardium or Gore-Tex. Alternatively, if the pulmonary venous obstruction has led to pulmonary hypertension, the left ventricle may be prepared for an arterial switch procedure. If the pulmonary artery pressure is at least two-thirds systemic, a combined arterial switch procedure and removal of the interatrial baffle and atrial reseptation can be performed in one stage.

HEMI-MUSTARD/RASTELLI

Because approximately 75% of patients with congenitally corrected transposition of the great vessels have an associated ventricular defect and pulmonary stenosis, a version of the "double switch" often performed is an atrial switch (Senning or Mustard) with a Rastelli-type reconstruction (VSD closure and RV-PA conduit). More recently, some have promoted the so-called hemi-Mustard/Rastelli, in which a bidirectional Glenn procedure is performed with only the lower limb of the Mustard, and Rastelli. The purported advantages are avoidance of suture in the sinus node area, technical simplicity of the Mustard patch (especially for patients with dextrocardia), and the speculated increased durability of the RV-PA conduit. The Glenn will be "pulsatile" because of the RV-PA conduit in proximity to the cavopulmonary connection, but this is rarely a problem. Because of the lifetime risk of complete heart block with L-TGA, and the later difficulty in placing transvenous pacing leads, it can be beneficial to place "prophylactic" epicardial pacing electrodes, leaving their capped leads in a subcutaneous pocket.

NB Unlike with usual technique in performing a bidirectional Glenn, it can be helpful to leave the azygous vein intact because the Glenn pressures may be elevated in the presence of the RV-PA connection. The azygous vein in this system functions as a "pop off" for the cerebral circulation. NB

The bidirectional Glenn is performed at any point during the operation. The inferior limb of the hemi-Mustard

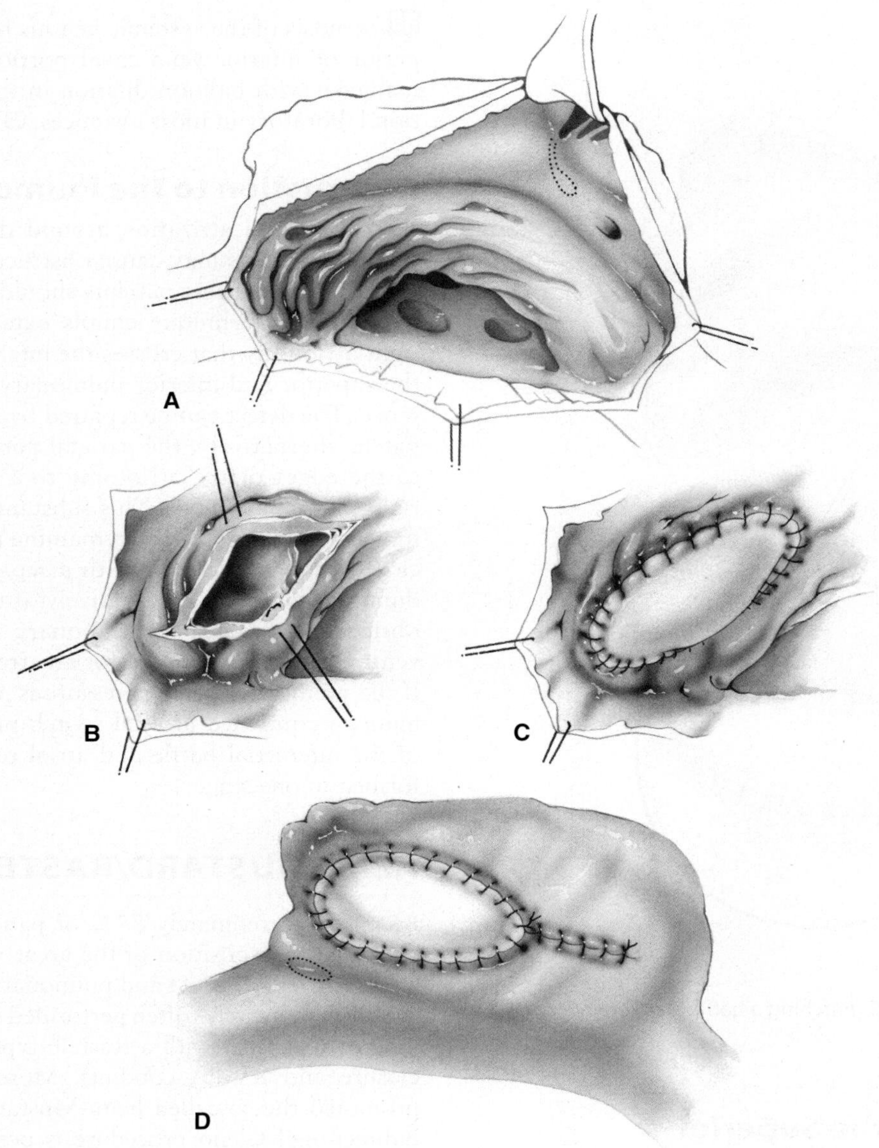

FIG. 25.36 A–D: Stepwise technique for a patch enlargement of an obstructive baffle.

connection is prepared much as with the Mustard, with particular attention paid to "laying open" the coronary sinus and reflecting the inferior edge of the atrial septum posteriorly so as to reduce any "dog leg" turn to IVC flow as it courses leftward.

The Hemi-Mustard patch is simple to create and essentially a disc, whose diameter is roughly the distance from the superior most aspect of the tricuspid valve to the entrance of the IVC (or Eustachian valve). It is helpful to create this patch out of a material that has less flexibility (e.g., thick-walled PTFE rather than autologous pericardium) to most effectively direct the IVC blood leftward without billowing into the pulmonary venous atrium (Fig. 25.37).

The patch is sewn into place beginning at the cranial aspect of the left-sided tricuspid valve. The suture line follows up along the tricuspid valve annulus until it reaches the atrial septum, and then is run inferiorly toward the IVC (or Eustachian valve). The left atrial appendage marks the border along which the suture line extends anteriorly in its first quarter. The opposite suture line runs along the inferior aspect of the inferior pulmonary veins and up to the other side of the IVC (Fig. 25.38).

A schematic of the completed operation demonstrates the flow of blood from the IVC leftward toward the tricuspid valve and ultimately out the RV-PA conduit. Note that often this conduit crosses the midline at a 45-degree

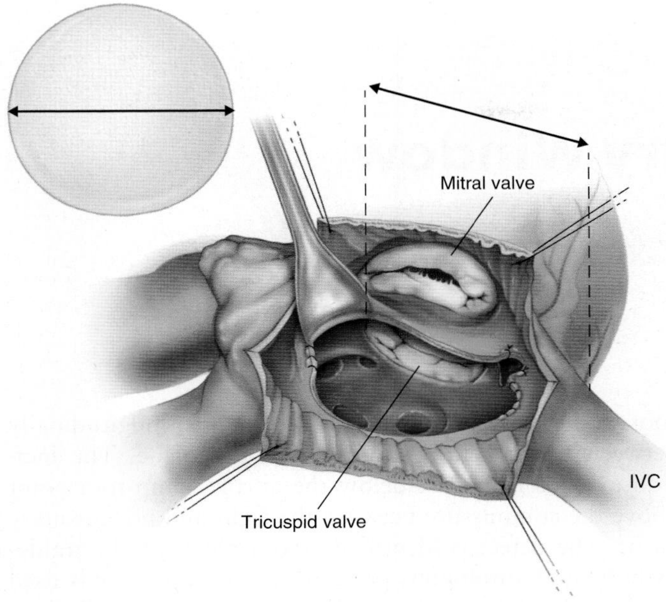

FIG. 25.37 Creation of the hemi-Mustard baffle from PTFE.

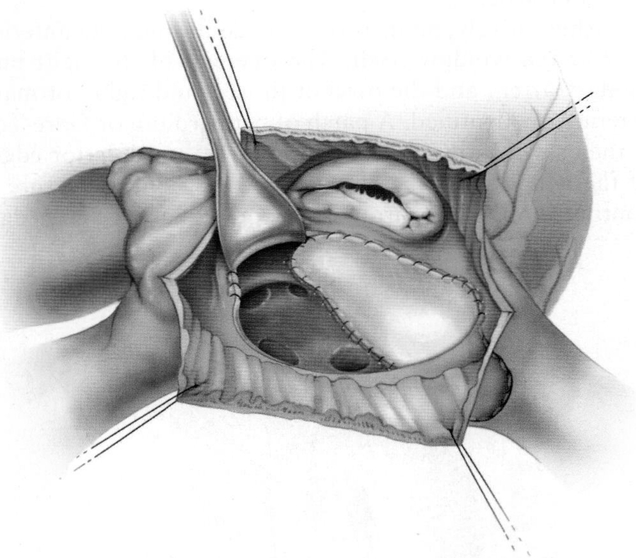

FIG. 25.38 Insertion of the hemi-Mustard baffle.

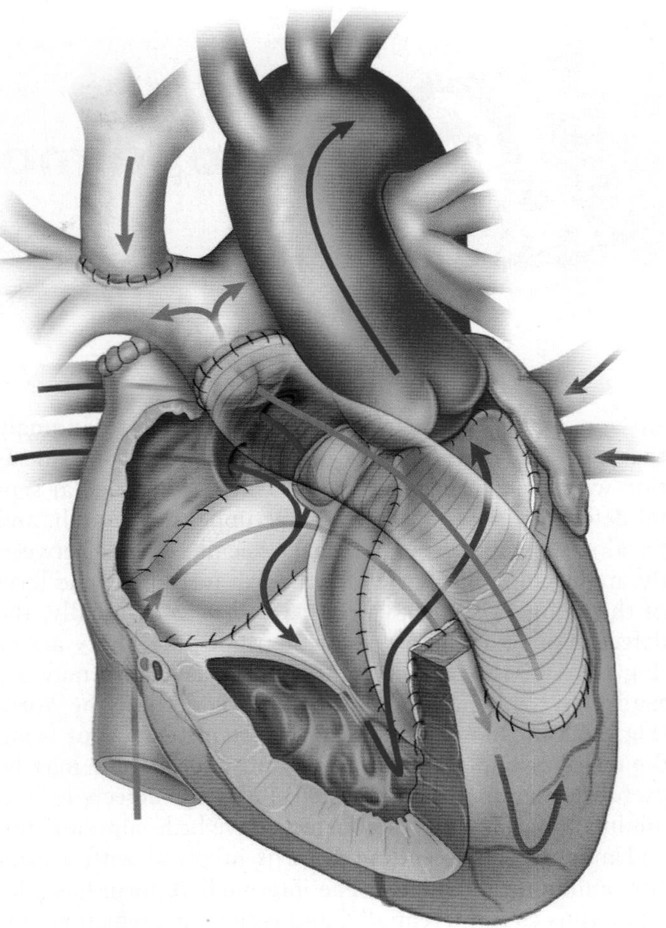

FIG. 25.39 A schematic of the completed hemi-Mustard/Rastelli operation

angle to meet the main PA (because of the L-TGA relation); this can also be made to the left of the aorta to eliminate the need to have the conduit sit immediately retrosternal. The bidirectional Glenn is also demonstrated. Often the conduit may be smaller than would be calculated by body surface area, since the flow will be diminished in the presence of the Glenn (Fig. 25.39).

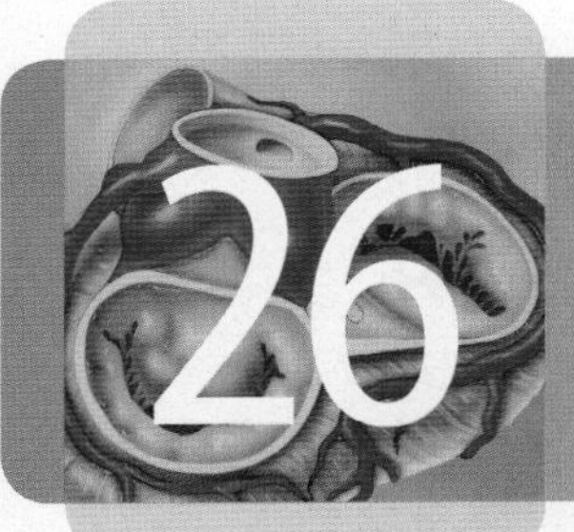

26 Aortopulmonary Window

An aortopulmonary window is a relatively rare anomaly that can occur either as an isolated defect or in association with other congenital lesions, such as ventricular septal defect, atrial septal defect, interrupted aortic arch, and tetralogy of Fallot. The defect classically occurs between the main pulmonary artery and aorta just above the level of the sinuses of Valsalva (Fig. 26.1A). Occasionally, the defect may be at the origin of the right pulmonary artery (Fig. 26.1B). Rarely, the right pulmonary artery may actually have a separate anomalous origin from the aorta (Fig. 26.1C). Many classification systems exist, but using the terms proximal, distal, total, and intermediate may be useful in planning the approach. Proximal defects have a minimal inferior rim, distal defects have little superior rim, and most of the ascending aorta is involved with a total aortopulmonary window. The intermediate form has adequate rims circumferentially, and is the type, which potentially could be closed by a transcatheter device.

Although simple ligation or division between clamps has been successfully performed in the past, closure of the defect under direct vision with the aid of cardiopulmonary bypass is now the method of choice. This prevents serious hemorrhagic complications that can occur because of the fragility of the great vessel walls, distortion of the aorta and coronary ostia, and allows precise closure of the various forms of the defect. The diagnosis is made with echocardiography, and closure of the aortopulmonary window is indicated without delay to prevent the development of pulmonary vascular disease.

TECHNIQUE

Through a standard median sternotomy, the aorta is cannulated distally on the aortic arch and a single venous cannula is placed in the right atrium. Snares are placed around the right and left pulmonary arteries, and the ductus arteriosus is occluded with a metal clip. With the onset of cardiopulmonary bypass, the pulmonary artery snares are snugged down. A vent is placed in the right superior pulmonary vein, and cooling to 28°C–34°C is carried out. The ascending aorta is clamped at the takeoff of the innominate artery. Cardioplegic solution is administered into the aortic root, and the ascending aorta is then incised longitudinally between two traction sutures of fine Prolene. The incision extends from just below the aortic clamp to a point above the commissure between the right and noncoronary cusps. The defect is identified, and a patch of glutaraldehyde-treated autologous pericardium or Gore-Tex is used to close the defect with a 5-0 or 6-0 continuous Prolene suture (Fig. 26.2). The suture line is completed anteriorly, and both needles are passed outside the vessel and tied. The aortotomy is then closed with a continuous suture of 5-0 or 6-0 Prolene.

Alternatively, an incision is made through the anterior part of the window itself. The opening of the right pulmonary artery and the ostia of the left and right coronary arteries are identified. A patch of pericardium or Gore-Tex is then sewn to the posterior, superior, and inferior edges of the window. At the edges of the incision, the suture is continued, passing through the pulmonary artery edge,

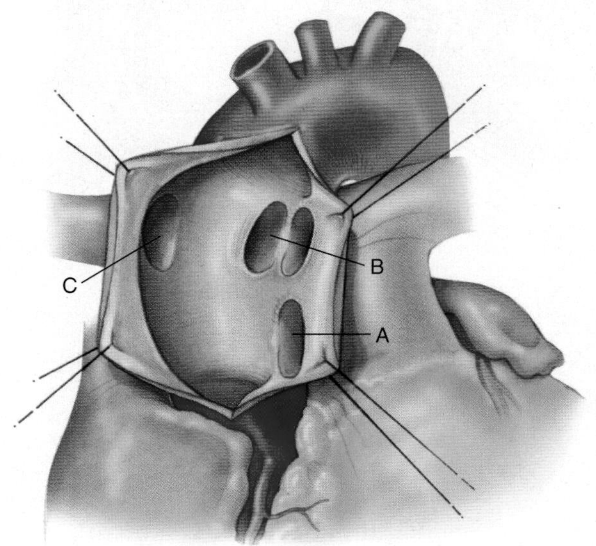

FIG. 26.1 Types of aortopulmonary window. **A:** Defect just above the level of the sinuses of Valsalva. **B:** Defect at the origin of right pulmonary artery. **C:** Anomalous origin of the right pulmonary artery from the aorta.

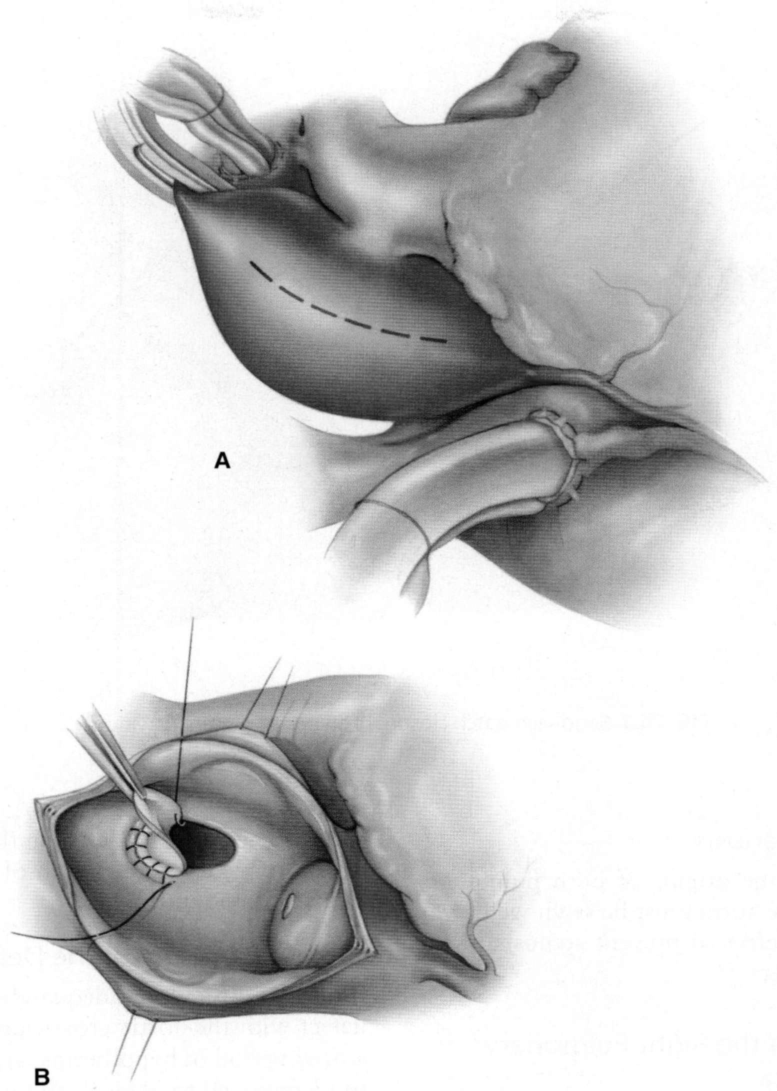

FIG. 26.2 Technique for closure of an aortopulmonary window. **A:** Incision on the aorta. **B:** Patch closure of the defect.

the patch, and then the aortic wall until the entire opening is closed. In this manner, the patch is sandwiched between the aorta and pulmonary artery to close the window (Fig. 26.3).

The aortic clamp is removed, and deairing completed. The patient is rewarmed, and weaned from cardiopulmonary bypass.

⊘ Aortic Cannulation

Aortic cannulation must be done high on the ascending aorta, or preferably on the aortic arch, so that cross-clamping will still allow good visualization of the defect. ⊘

⊘ Occluding the Pulmonary Arteries

Both right and left pulmonary arteries must be occluded with snares with the initiation of cardiopulmonary bypass to prevent flooding of the pulmonary circulation. The snares must be kept in place while cardioplegia is delivered into the aortic root. ⊘

⊘ Injury to the Left Coronary Ostium

The lower margin of a proximal defect may be in close proximity to the left coronary artery ostium; therefore, closure of the defect must be performed in such a manner as to avoid injury to the coronary ostium. ⊘

⊘ Anomalous Origin of the Coronary Arteries

Occasionally, the right coronary artery, and rarely the left coronary artery, may arise from the pulmonary trunk close to the edge of the defect. In these cases, the patch must be modified to baffle the coronary opening into the aorta. ⊘

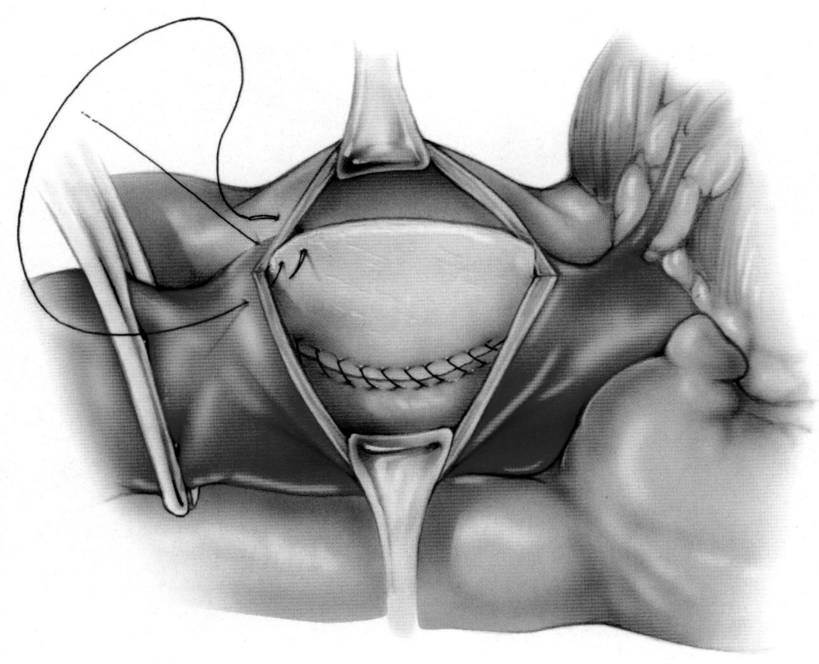

FIG. 26.3 Sandwich patch closure of an aortopulmonary window.

⊘ Pulmonary Artery Stenosis

When the defect involves the origins of both pulmonary arteries, the patch inside the aorta must be sewn well away from the margins of the defect to prevent stenosis of the right or left pulmonary artery. ⊘

NB Anomalous Origin of the Right Pulmonary Artery from the Aorta

If the right pulmonary artery has an anomalous origin from the aorta, it is detached from the aorta and anastomosed to the main pulmonary artery with a continuous 6-0 Prolene suture. The resulting defect in the aorta is then closed with an appropriately sized patch of Gore-Tex or piece of pulmonary homograft. NB

⊘ Poor Exposure of the Defect

It may be difficult to adequately expose and repair a distal defect with the aortic cross-clamp in place. In these cases, a brief period of hypothermic arrest allows the cross-clamp to be removed to identify and patch the defect precisely. It also is sometimes helpful to approach the repair with *both* aortotomy and distal main pulmonary arteriotomy to fully delineate the exact anatomy. ⊘

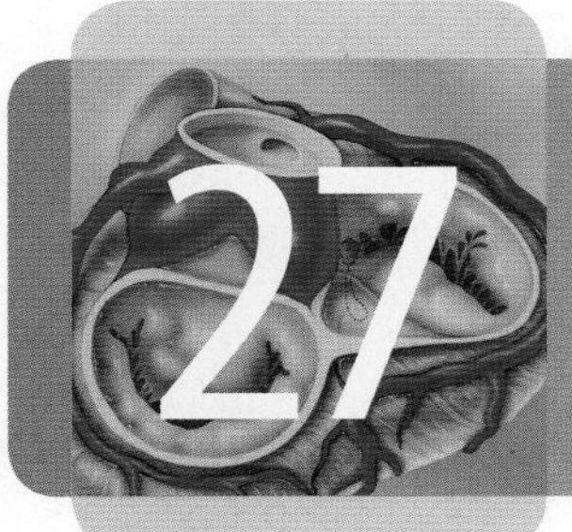

27 Truncus Arteriosus

Persistent truncus arteriosus is characterized by the emergence of a single common arterial trunk from the heart overriding the interventricular septum. The main pulmonary artery or the right and left pulmonary arteries originate from the side or posterior aspect of the truncal artery at varying distances above the truncal valve. Most commonly, the truncal valve is trileaflet or quadrileaflet and overrides a high ventricular septal defect. Nearly one-half of the valves have two or four leaflets; all truncal valves exhibit varying degrees of dysplasia and may be regurgitant, stenotic, or both. Often, the main pulmonary artery originates from the left side of the truncus arteriosus and divides into left and right branches that traverse in the usual manner to their respective lungs. This form has been classified as type I by Collett and Edwards. In type II, the right and left pulmonary arteries originate adjacent to each other from the side or back of the truncal artery. In type III, each pulmonary artery originates from different parts of the truncal artery (Fig. 27.1). Type IV, when the lungs are supplied by two pulmonary arteries originating from the descending thoracic aorta, is now considered not a true truncus arteriosus but a form of pulmonary atresia with ventricular septal defect. Associated anomalies include interrupted aortic arch as well as coronary artery abnormalities.

Most centers now perform primary repair of truncus arteriosus at the time of presentation to prevent the development of irreversible pulmonary vascular disease. Pulmonary artery banding is no longer recommended because it carries a high mortality. In symptomatic neonates who respond to medical management of their heart failure, surgery may be delayed for a few weeks. However, continued symptoms should prompt urgent surgical intervention. Patients presenting at older than 12 months of age should have preoperative cardiac catheterization to assess pulmonary vascular resistance and suitability for repair.

INCISION

A median sternotomy is the approach of choice.

TECHNIQUE

The ascending aorta is cannulated as distally as possible, and bicaval cannulation is achieved. The anatomy is well evaluated, and the right and left pulmonary arteries are dissected circumferentially. Tapes are passed around the pulmonary arteries so that they can be occluded just before the initiation of cardiopulmonary bypass.

NB Aortic Cannula Position

The aortic cannula should be placed at the level of the innominate artery to ensure adequate exposure of the pulmonary arteries after the cross-clamp is applied. NB

⊘ Flooding of the Lungs

It is essential to dissect both pulmonary arteries so that they can be encircled and occluded as soon as cardiopulmonary bypass is initiated. This prevents runoff of arterial flow from the pump into the lungs, which leads to inadequate systemic and coronary perfusion and flooding of the pulmonary circulation. ⊘

When cardiopulmonary bypass is initiated, the pulmonary artery snares are tightened, and systemic cooling is begun.

⊘ Truncal Valve Insufficiency

If significant truncal valve insufficiency is present, the heart may distend as soon as cardiopulmonary bypass is begun. A vent should be immediately placed through the right superior pulmonary vein into the left ventricle (see Chapter 4). If regurgitation is severe, a large amount of the aortic line return may be retrieved by the left ventricular vent, leading to inadequate systemic perfusion. In this case, the truncal artery must be clamped immediately and opened so that cardioplegic solution can be administered directly into the coronary arteries. ⊘

The truncus is cross-clamped, and cardioplegic solution is administered into the truncal root. The main pulmonary artery is detached from the truncal artery, and the defect is closed, usually with a patch, with a continuous 6-0 Prolene suture (Fig. 27.2A, B). In type II or III defects, the pulmonary arteries are detached in continuity, leaving a rim of aortic tissue attached to their origins. The resulting defect in the truncal artery is closed.

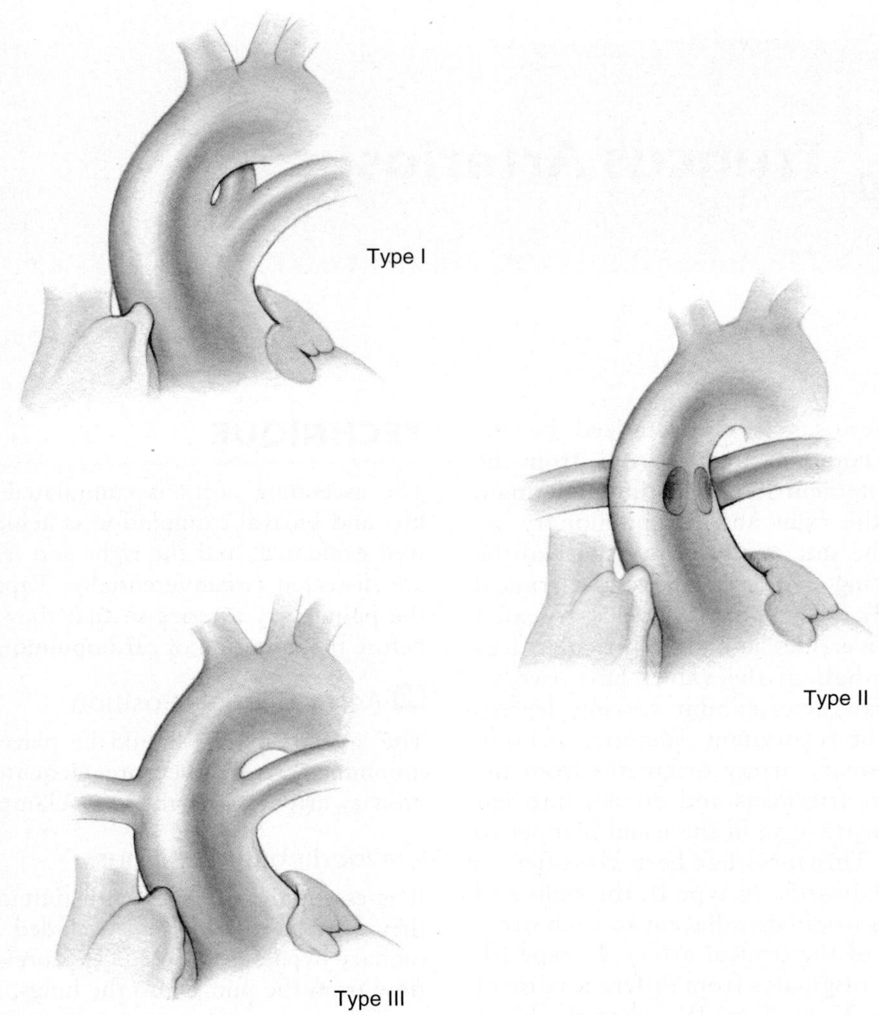

FIG. 27.1 Forms of truncus arteriosus.

NB Adequate Tissue Surrounding the Pulmonary Arteries

The main or right and left pulmonary arteries should be excised in continuity with adequate surrounding tissue. Often, this can be best accomplished by transecting the truncal artery just above the pulmonary arteries, excising the orifices of the pulmonary arteries, and then performing an end-to-end anastomosis of the ascending aorta to the truncal root. This technique necessitates adequate mobilization of the distal ascending aorta, aortic arch, and arch vessels to prevent undue tension on the aortic suture line. NB

⊘ Injury to the Coronary Ostium

The left coronary artery may be located high on the posterior wall of the truncal root. Care must be taken when closing the aortic defect not to injure the left coronary artery. ⊘

⊘ Inadequate Cardioplegic Protection

The snares on the pulmonary arteries must be kept in place until after the cardioplegic solution has been delivered. Otherwise, the cardioplegia will run off into the pulmonary circulation and inadequate amounts will reach the coronary bed. When significant truncal valve insufficiency is present, cardioplegic solution should be delivered directly into the coronary ostia. ⊘

A high, longitudinal right ventriculotomy is made, and the ventricular septal defect is identified. Usually, the septal defect is a subarterial infundibular type with a thick lower rim (Fig. 27.3). Occasionally, it may be a large perimembranous type extending to the annulas of the tricuspid valve.

⊘ Abnormal Coronary Artery Branches

The ventriculotomy should be positioned to avoid any major coronary arteries on the anterior surface of the right

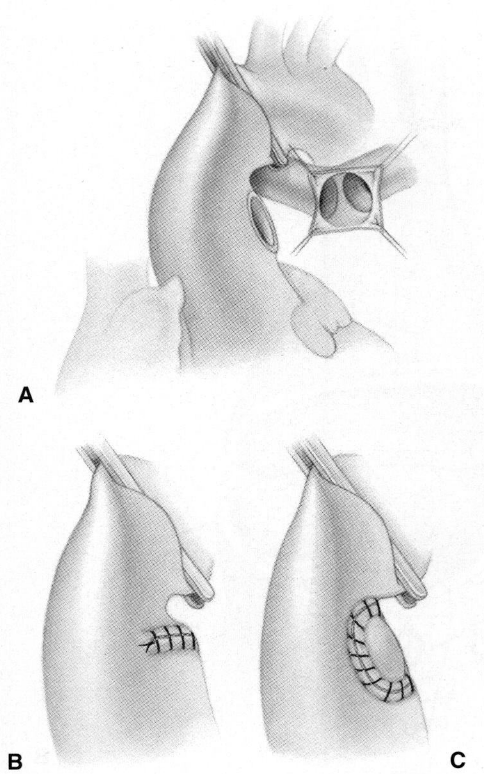

FIG. 27.2 **A:** Detachment of the pulmonary artery from the truncal artery. **B:** Patch closure of the defect.

ventricle. The left anterior descending coronary artery is particularly at risk when it takes origin from the right coronary artery. ⊘

⊘ Too High Right Ventriculotomy

Care must be taken when extending the ventriculotomy superiorly to avoid cutting or injuring the truncal valve and annulus. ⊘

NB Truncal Valve Repair

If truncal regurgitation is mild to moderate, most surgeons recommend a conservative approach. The sinotubular junction can be narrowed if it appears that this will improve the coaptation of dysplastic valve leaflets. The aorta is transected just above the sinotubular ridge. After excising the pulmonary arteries, a wedge of tissue is removed anteriorly from the distal aorta so that, when closed, the new diameter of the distal aorta will be the new sinotubular diameter. The aortic root is symmetrically gathered during the suturing process, bringing the proximal and distal aortic segments together. Some surgeons close the defect created by excising the pulmonary arteries from the truncus longitudinally when mild to moderate valvular insufficiency is present. This plicates the sinotubular junction and may increase the coaptation of the valve leaflets. NB

In cases of moderate to severe truncal insuffiency, a reparative procedure should be undertaken. In these cases, the truncus should be divided just above the pulmonary arteries, and cardioplegia administered directly into the coronary ostia. After excising the pulmonary arteries as a confluence, the valve is carefully inspected. If the valve is trileaflet, subcommissural sutures at one or more commissures may increase the central coaptation of the leaflets. Most commonly, the significantly insufficient valves are quadricuspid. These valves may be converted to a tricuspid valve by approximating the margins of two

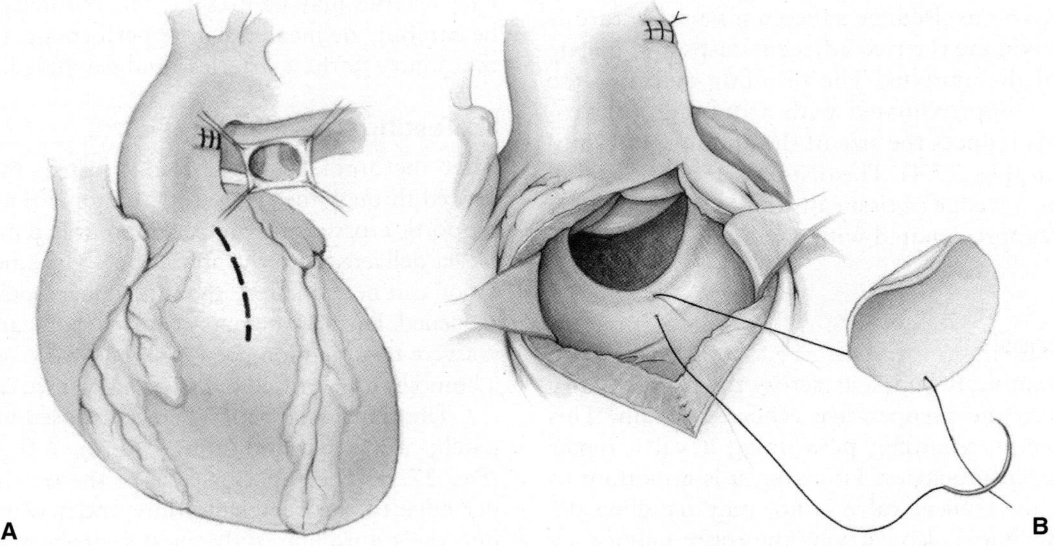

FIG. 27.3 Technique for closure of the associated ventricular septal defect. **A:** Right ventriculotomy. Note traction sutures on the detached pulmonary confluence. **B:** Patch closure of the ventricular septal defect. Note proximity of truncal valve to ventriculotomy and ventricular septal defect.

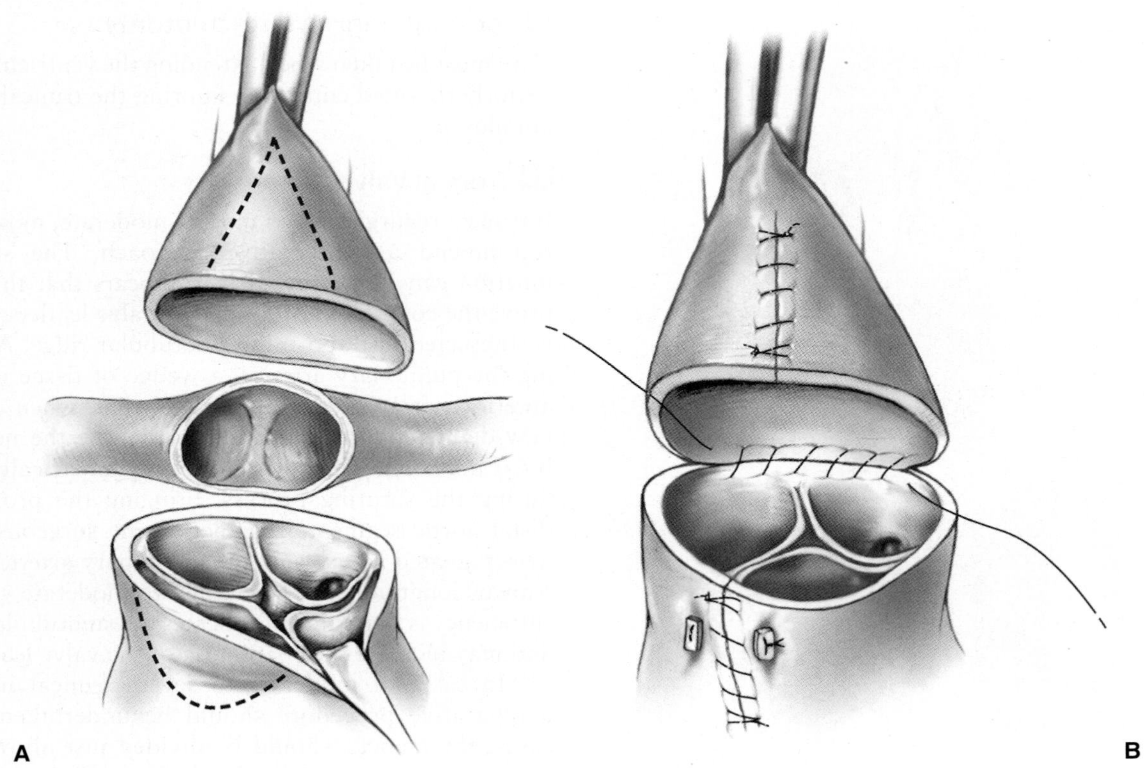

FIG. 27.4 Truncal valvuloplasty. **A:** Excision of one leaflet and the attached aortic wall. **B:** Reconstruction of a new truncal root, tailoring the distal ascending aorta. Anastomosis of the reconstructed root and ascending aorta.

cusps, and reinforcing the repair with subcommissural sutures to increase leaflet coaptation. Alternatively, the smallest cusp of the four-leaflet valve and the attached aortic wall may be excised. A subcommissural suture is placed to approximate the two adjacent cusps and plicate this segment of the annulus. The resulting defect in the truncal root is reapproximated with a running 6-0 Prolene suture. This reduces the size of the annulus and sinotubular junction (Fig. 27.4). The distal aorta is reduced in size by resecting a wedge of tissue of similar width and the two ends are reapproximated with a running 6-0 Prolene suture.

NB Aortic Stenosis

Frequently, a significant gradient across the truncal valve is appreciated on the preoperative echocardiogram. This may raise concerns regarding performing a valve repair for truncal valve insufficiency. However, it is important to remember that the truncal valve is not only handling the regurgitant flow, but is also carrying the entire pulmonary blood flow. Therefore, the measured gradient across the valve is artificially increased by the large volume crossing the valve, which will be markedly reduced by separating the pulmonary circulation and correcting the regurgitation. NB

NB Anomalous Coronary Artery

Abnormally located coronary ostia and intramural coronary arteries may be present. The coronary anatomy must be carefully delineated before performing a valve repair so that injury to these arteries can be avoided. NB

NB Testing the Valve Repair

After the aorta has been reconstructed, the valve can be viewed through the right ventriculotomy (Fig. 27.3B). Either the aortic cross-clamp can be temporarily removed, or cardioplegia delivered into the aortic root. The amount of regurgitation can be estimated, and if it is unacceptable, the aorta is reopened. Further attempts at valve repair can be made. Only if severe regurgitation persists should valve replacement with a homograft be carried out (see Chapter 5). NB

The ventricular septal defect is closed with a Gore-Tex patch, using a continuous 5-0 or 6-0 Prolene suture (Fig. 27.5). The superior edge of the patch meets the upper edge of the ventriculotomy and will be incorporated into the suture line of the right ventricular–pulmonary artery conduit. The aortic cross-clamp is removed and deairing maneuvers performed. The construction of the right ventricle to pulmonary connection is carried out during rewarming.

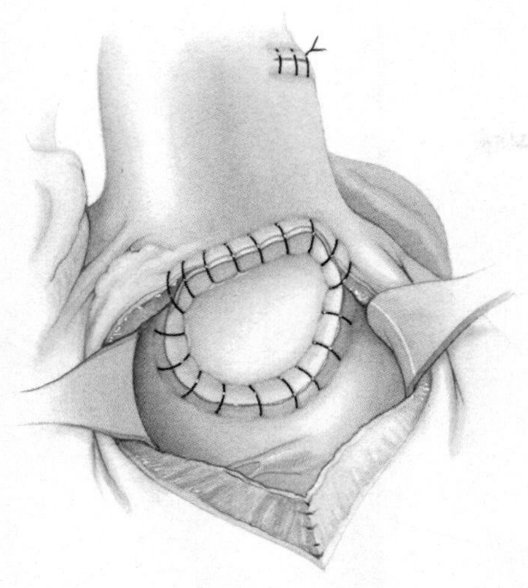

FIG. 27.5 Superior edge of the ventricular septal defect patch meets the upper edge of the ventriculotomy.

⊘ Left Ventricular Distention

If residual aortic regurgitation is present, left ventricular distention may occur when the cross-clamp is removed. This may respond to manual decompression until the heart is warm enough to eject. ⊘

NB Patent Foramen Ovale

In a patient younger than 2 to 3 months, a patent foramen ovale is normally left open to provide decompression of the right-sided circulation during the early postoperative period. NB

Ideally, a pulmonary or aortic homograft is used to reconstruct the right ventricular outflow tract. More recently, bovine jugular vein conduits have been used, and porcine pulmonary or aortic roots are available in smaller sizes. The distal pulmonary artery is appropriately tailored. Four traction sutures are used on its adventitia to maintain the correct orientation (Fig. 27.3A).

⊘ Nonvalved Right Ventricular to Pulmonary Artery Connections

Some surgeons advocate direct connections using autologous tissue and a pericardial or Gore-Tex patch for reconstruction of the right ventricular outflow tract. Although this approach provides the potential for growth and may reduce the need for reoperation on the right ventricular outflow tract, it leaves the infant with pulmonary insufficiency that may be poorly tolerated (Fig. 27.6). ⊘

⊘ Too Small a Pulmonary Artery Lumen

The lumen of the pulmonary artery can be enlarged by extending the opening onto both its branches. A piece of the homograft wall can be used to patch and enlarge these openings. ⊘

The homograft or conduit is cut to the appropriate length and anastomosed to the pulmonary artery with 5-0 or 6-0 Prolene suture. The posterior layer of the anastomosis is completed first (Fig. 27.7).

⊘ Homograft Length

The homograft should be trimmed at a level just above the commissures of the valve. If the homograft is left too long, it will produce kinking of the pulmonary artery bifurcation. ⊘

⊘ Anastomotic Leaks from the Posterior Wall

An anastomotic leak from the posterior wall is practically impossible to control once the surgery has been completed. For this reason, small bites close to each other should be taken. ⊘

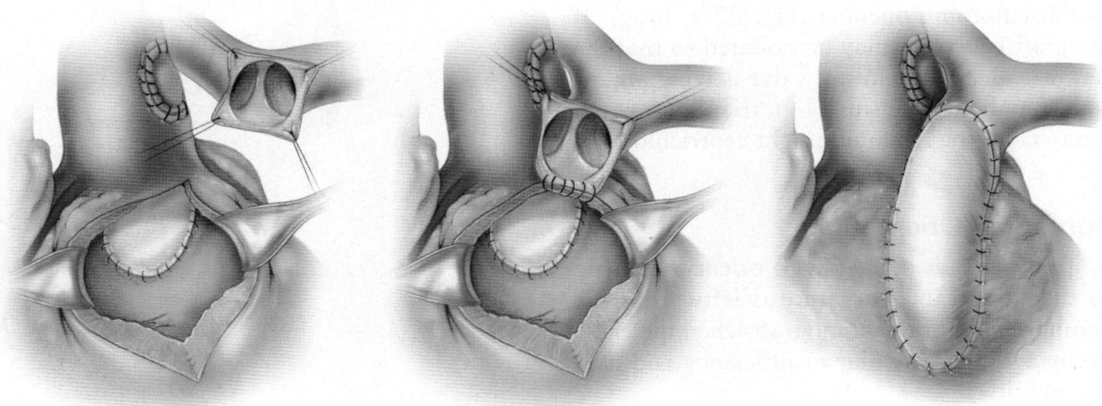

FIG. 27.6 With the "direct connection" or "Brazilian" technique, the branch pulmonary arteries are anastomosed directly to the cranial edge of the right ventriculotomy. A prosthetic patch (or autologous pericardial patch) is used to reconstruct the remainder of the defect.

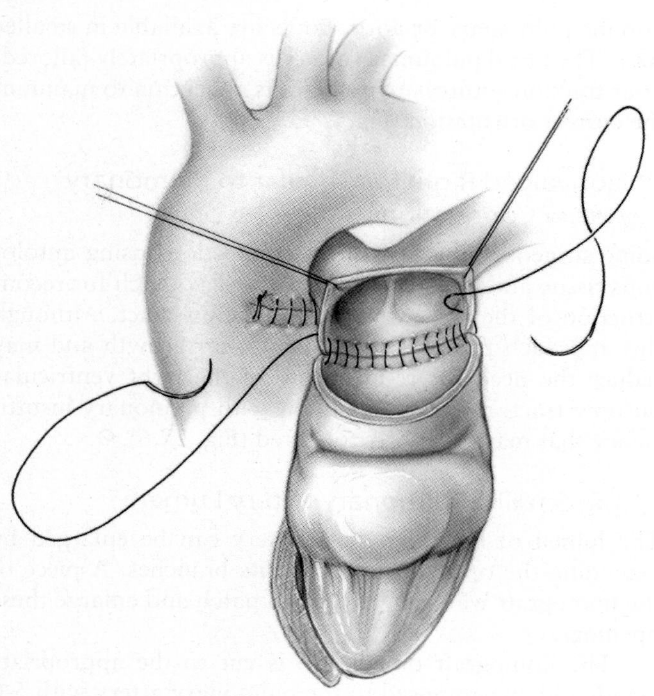

FIG. 27.7 Technique for placement of the conduit (homograft) from the right ventricle to the pulmonary artery. Posterior aspect of a distal anastomosis.

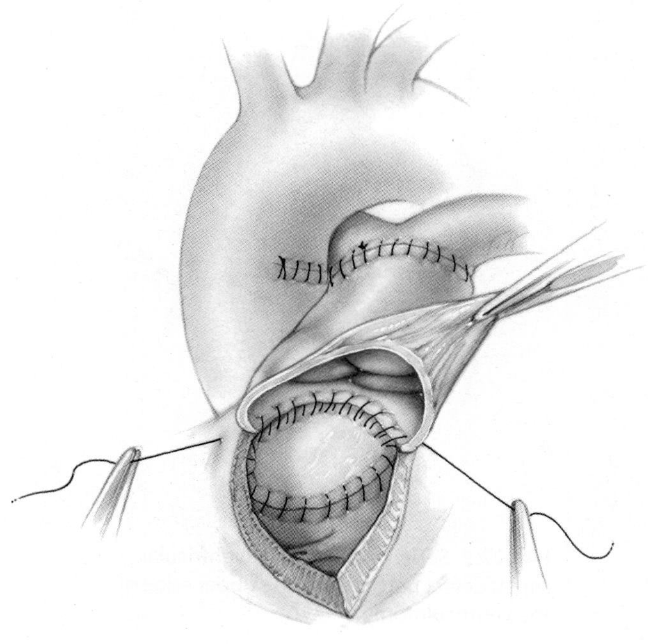

FIG. 27.8 Technique for placement of a homograft from the right ventricle to the pulmonary artery.

The anterior distal anastomosis is completed and the suture secured. The proximal end of the homograft is anastomosed to the right ventriculotomy beginning posteriorly, using a 5-0 Prolene running suture (Fig. 27.8). After approximately 40% of the circumference of the homograft has been attached in this manner, the remainder of the opening is closed with a triangular patch of glutaraldehyde-treated autologous pericardium using a running 5-0 or 6-0 Prolene suture. The patch is attached along the anterior circumference of the homograft and the remainder of the right ventriculotomy opening (Fig. 27.9, inset). If an aortic homograft is used, it may be oriented so that the attached anterior leaflet of the mitral valve is lying anteriorly. This tissue may be used instead of a triangular patch of pericardium to close the remaining right ventriculotomy (Fig. 27.9).

NB Aortic Homograft Orientation

Alternatively, it may be advantageous to orient the aortic homograft so that its greater curvature is leftward. This may prevent compression of the homograft when the chest is closed, thereby avoiding valvular insufficiency and narrowing of the conduit. NB

⊘ Twisting of the Conduit

Care must be taken when performing the proximal anastomosis to maintain the correct orientation of the homograft to avoid distortion of the pulmonary artery confluence. ⊘

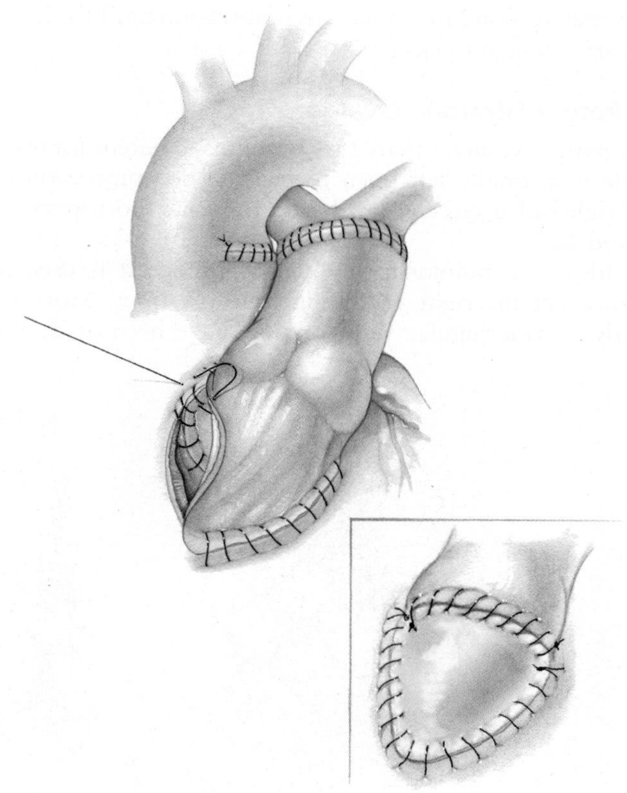

FIG. 27.9 Completion of placement of the aortic homograft conduit from the right ventricle to the pulmonary artery. Inset: Augmentation of a proximal anastomosis with pericardium when using a pulmonary homograft.

When the procedure is completed and the patient is warmed, the process of air removal is completed and the patient is weaned off cardiopulmonary bypass.

TRUNCUS ARTERIOSUS WITH INTERRUPTED AORTIC ARCH

These patients are candidates for primary simultaneous repair of both lesions. Adherence to the technique of extensive mobilization of the descending aorta and arch vessels is especially important in these patients (see Chapter 29). A direct anastomosis of the descending aorta to the arch can usually be accomplished superiorly, and the inferior opening patched with a piece of homograft wall. In addition, complete division of the truncus proximal to the pulmonary arteries results in a rightward shift of the new aorta after removal of the pulmonary arteries and reanastomosis of the two ends. These maneuvers should minimize the risk of left bronchial compression. Some surgeons have found it useful to perform a Lecompte maneuver, translocating the pulmonary bifurcation anterior to the truncal artery, to avoid narrowing the aortopulmonary window and compressing the right pulmonary artery.

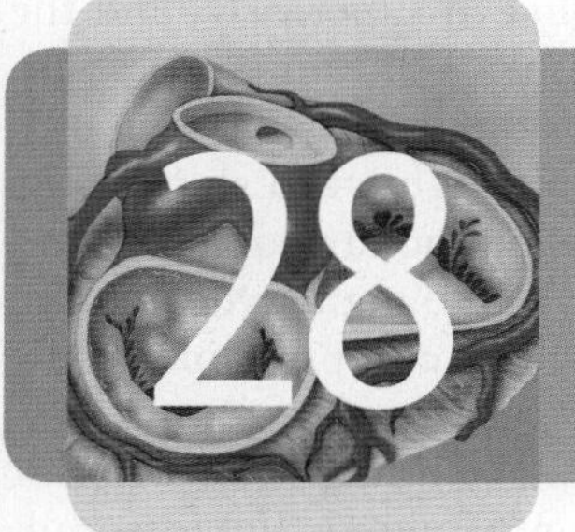

28 Ebstein Anomaly

Ebstein anomaly is a rare disease. The pathologic anatomy consists of displacement of part or all of the tricuspid valve orifice into the right ventricle. Attachments of all valve leaflets are abnormal, especially the septal and posterior leaflets, which are dysplastic and displaced downward. This gives rise to the extension of the right atrium into the right ventricle, resulting in an "atrialized" portion of the right ventricle above the valve. The anterior leaflet is large and usually has an abnormal insertion, sometimes producing obstruction in the right ventricular cavity. The atrioventricular node and conduction bundle lie within the triangle of Koch as in the normal heart, but because of the downward displacement of the valve below the true atrioventricular junction, the atrialized ventricle separates the penetrating bundle from the valve proper. An atrial septal defect or a patent foramen ovale is usually present (Fig. 28.1).

PRESENTATION

There is a wide range of anatomic variations of Ebstein anomaly. The least severe form has a true right ventricle with adequate volume. These patients have very mild cyanosis and may be asymptomatic even as adults. The most severe form consists of nearly complete atrialization of the right ventricle. These patients present as neonates with massive cardiomegaly, severe heart failure, cyanosis, and acidosis.

SURGERY FOR THE NEONATE

Neonates who demonstrate a need for mechanical ventilation and dependence on prostaglandin E_1 to maintain ductal patency have a universally poor outcome with medical management. The surgical approach is designed to create a reliable source of pulmonary flow, reduce the massive cardiomegaly, and prevent severe tricuspid insufficiency. If there is a tripartite ventricle with an open right ventricular outflow tract and adequate valve tissue, a reparative procedure may be attempted. Most severely symptomatic neonates have unfavorable anatomy and marked dilation of the right side of the heart with impingement on the left ventricle and lungs. A right ventricular exclusion procedure decompresses the right side and can palliate these critically ill patients. This procedure creates a single ventricle physiology allowing for a future Fontan operation (see Chapter 31).

Technique

A median sternotomy is used, and standard aortic and bicaval cannulation is performed. The ductus arteriosus is ligated with the institution of cardiopulmonary bypass. Cooling to 28°C to 32°C is carried out. The aorta is cross-clamped, and cold blood cardioplegic solution is administered into the aortic root. Tapes around the cavae are snared snugly and cardiopulmonary bypass is continued with low perfusion flow. The right atrium is opened through an oblique incision. A piece of autologous pericardium treated with glutaraldehyde or GORTEX is sewn at the anatomic level of the tricuspid valve annulus, deviating into the true right atrium in the area of the conduction system. A fenestration is created in the patch with a 4-mm coronary punch and the atrial septum is excised (Fig. 28.2).

⊘ Injury to the Conduction System

In the past, the patch was sewn to the right atrial wall above the coronary sinus to avoid the conduction tissue. However, this resulted in increased blood flow into the excluded right ventricle and an elevated coronary venous pressure. By suturing inside the coronary sinus, injury to the conduction system can be avoided and the coronary sinus remains in the right atrium. ⊘

NB Right Ventricular Outflow Tract Obstruction

Before the introduction of patch fenestration, patients with pulmonic stenosis or atresia required the placement of a small pulmonary homograft between the right ventricle and pulmonary artery to decompress the right ventricle. The fenestration allows adequate decompression of the right ventricle without the use of a homograft and reduces the likelihood of thrombus formation if an RV-PA conduit has not been used. This simplifies and shortens the procedure, and avoids the need for reintervention on the right ventricular outflow tract. NB

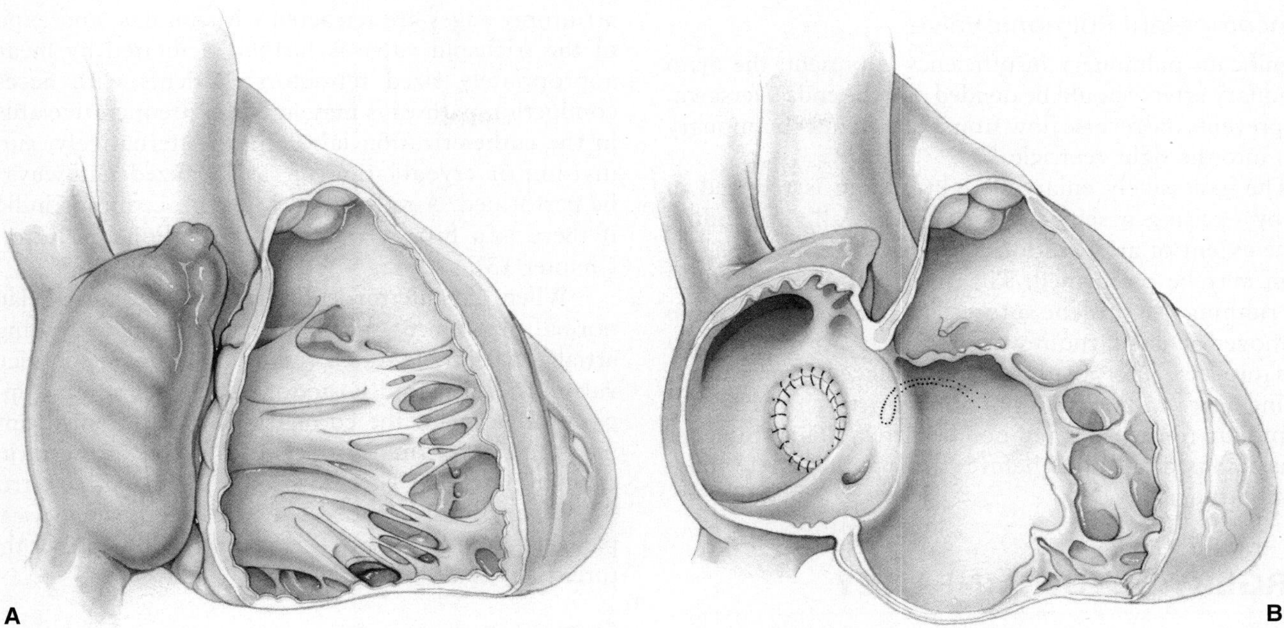

FIG. 28.1 Surgical view of Ebstein anomaly. **A:** Right anterior oblique view of the heart with the anterior wall of the right ventricle cut away. The abnormally large anterior leaflet with its multiple anomalous attachments, as shown in this heart, sometimes impedes blood flow into the distal ventricle and pulmonary outflow tract. **B:** Same view as in **(A),** but with the anterolateral wall of the right atrium and the anterior tricuspid leaflet removed to show the dilated area of the atrialized ventricle and the displaced remnants of the septal and posterior tricuspid leaflets. The atrial septal defect has been closed with a patch.

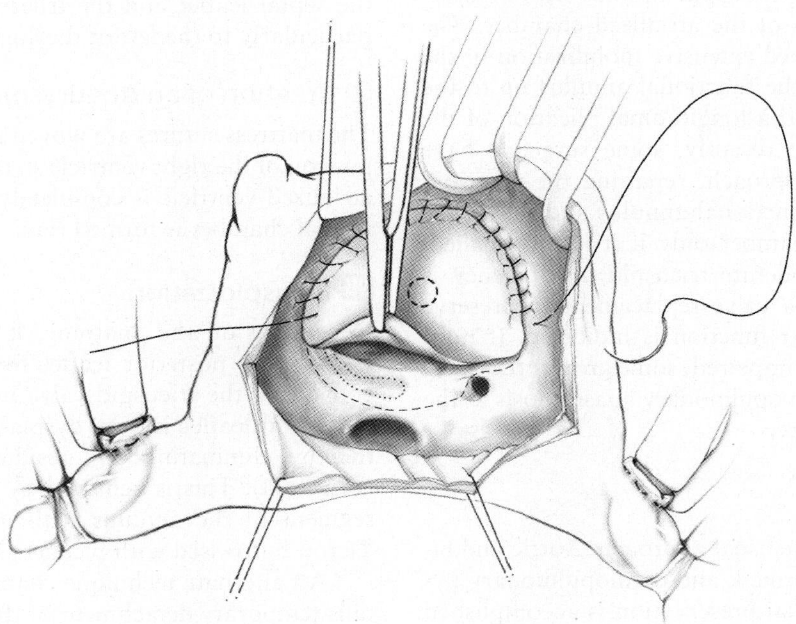

FIG. 28.2 The pericardial patch is sewn around the right ventricular orifice deviating into the true right atrium (*dashed line*). A 4-mm fenestration is created.

NB Incompetent Pulmonic Valve

If significant pulmonary insufficiency is present, the main pulmonary artery should be divided and the ends oversewn. This prevents the reverse flow from the systemic–pulmonary shunt into the right ventricle. NB

The excessively enlarged right atrium is reduced in size by excising a segment of its free wall. Depending on the extent of atrialization of the right ventricle, a plication may be performed. The atriotomy is then closed with running 6-0 Prolene sutures. The aortic cross-clamp is removed. During the rewarming phase, a 3.5- to 4.0-mm Gore-Tex interposition graft is placed from the ascending aorta to the main pulmonary artery or from the innominate to the right pulmonary artery. This shunt remains clamped until just before cardiopulmonary bypass is discontinued.

SURGERY BEYOND INFANCY

Most patients do not become symptomatic until adolescence or adulthood. Symptoms include progressive heart failure secondary to tricuspid insufficiency and right ventricular dysfunction, and cyanosis due to right-to-left shunting through a patent foramen ovale or atrial septal defect. Many of these patients can have biventricular repairs with surgery designed to restore normal tricuspid valve function and improve right ventricular contractility. Traditionally, one of two approaches has been utilized. The first is plication of the tricuspid annulus with or without a transverse plication of the atrialized chamber. The other approach has involved extensive mobilization of the anterior leaflet, bringing the functional annulus up to the true tricuspid annulus, and a longitudinal plication of the atrialized chamber. More recently, some surgeons have advocated a simplified approach, repairing the tricuspid valve at the level of the functional annulus and selectively plicating the atrialized chamber only if it is thin walled. If more than mild to moderate tricuspid insufficiency is present following repair, a valve replacement to preserve long-term right ventricular function is indicated. If right ventricular contractility is impaired, some groups routinely perform a bidirectional cavopulmonary anastomosis at the conclusion of the procedure.

Technique

A median sternotomy is the usual approach. Aortic and bicaval cannulation is performed, and cardiopulmonary bypass is initiated. Myocardial preservation is accomplished with cold blood potassium cardioplegic solution administered into the aortic root after aortic cross-clamping. This may be complemented by the retrograde technique (see Chapter 3).

A longitudinal atriotomy is made 1 cm posterior to and parallel with the atrioventricular groove. The atriotomy edges are retracted with sutures, and exposure of the tricuspid valve is further facilitated by means of appropriately sized retractors. Patients with accessory conduction pathways may undergo preoperative ablation in the catheterization laboratory. Alternatively, surgical division or cryoablation of the localized pathways may be performed. A right-sided Maze procedure is indicated if there is a history of atrial fibrillation or flutter (see Chapter 13).

When the anterior leaflet is large and has a relatively normal attachment, an annular plication, excluding the atrialized ventricle, often results in a competent tricuspid valve. The displaced posterior and septal annuli (up to a point adjacent to the coronary sinus) are pulled upward into the right atrium proper to the level of the atrioventricular junction. This is accomplished with interrupted 3-0 Ticron sutures buttressed with Dacron or pericardial pledgets on both the atrial and ventricular sides of the sutures (Fig. 28.3).

⊘ Right Coronary Artery Injury

The ventricular plication sutures must be placed carefully after identifying the right coronary artery and its branches to avoid direct injury to, or distortion of, the coronary arteries, which can result in myocardial infarction. ⊘

⊘ Injury to Conduction Tissue

Because of the proximity of the atrioventricular node to the bundle of His, placement of sutures that extend between the septal leaflet and the true right atrium is hazardous, particularly to the left of the coronary sinus. ⊘

⊘ Creation of an Aneurysmal Cavity

The mattress sutures are woven in and out of the atrialized portion of the right ventricle so that when they are tied, the atrialized ventricle is completely obliterated and no aneurysmal chamber is formed (Fig. 28.3). ⊘

NB Bicuspidization

Depending on the anatomy, it is sometimes possible to exclude the posterior leaflet by a modified annuloplasty converting the tricuspid valve into a bicuspid valve (or if the septal leaflet is very dysplastic, a monocuspid valve), thereby eliminating any residual tricuspid insufficiency (Fig. 28.4). This is achieved by constricting the posterior segment of the annulus with interrupted sutures of 3-0 Ticron buttressed with pledgets. NB

An alternate technique championed by Carpentier entails temporary detachment of the anterior leaflet from the anteroseptal commissure to the junction with the posterior leaflet, if present (Fig. 28.5A). Extensive mobilization is achieved by dividing the fibrous band connections of the leaflets to the muscular wall of the right ventricle. The interchordal spaces on the leaflets may require conservative fenestration.

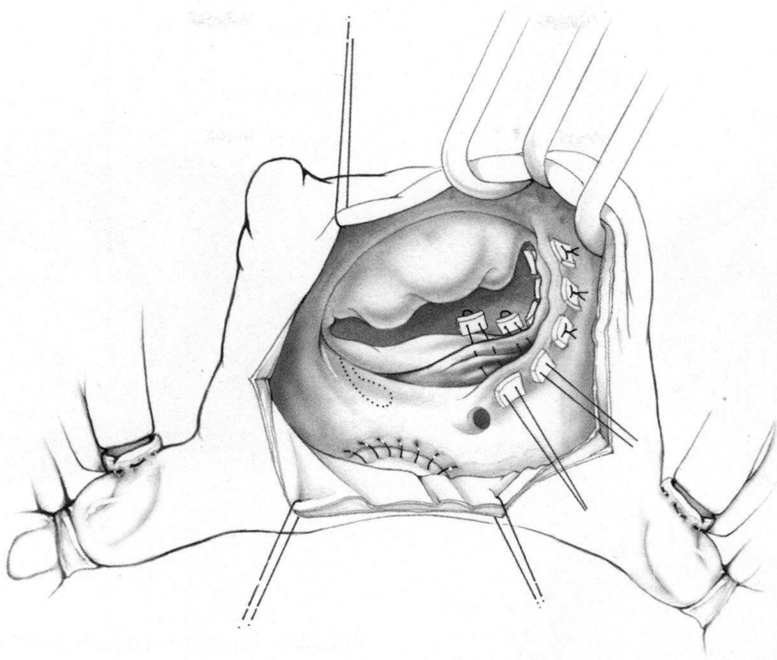

FIG. 28.3 Repair of the tricuspid valve and obliteration of atrialized ventricle with pledgeted sutures.

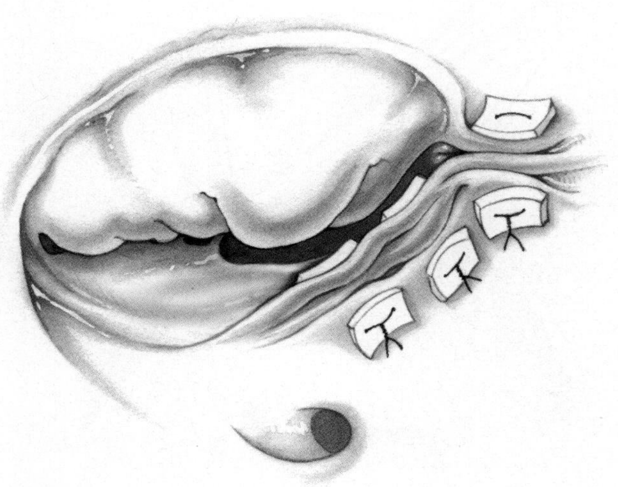

FIG. 28.4 Converting the tricuspid valve to a bicuspid valve.

The atrialized segment of the right ventricle can now be clearly visualized. It is plicated with multiple interrupted sutures of 3-0 Ticron, and the posterior annulus is similarly reduced in size to achieve a relatively normal right ventricular geometry. The redundant atrial wall behind the coronary sinus may also need to be plicated with continuous suture of 4-0 Prolene. The anterior leaflet is then reattached to the fibrous annulus using continuous 5-0 Prolene suture. This repair is often reinforced with an annuloplasty ring after clockwise rotation of the valve that uses the redundant anterior leaflet to augment the deficiency along the septal leaflet (Fig. 28.5B).

⊘ Excess Traction on the Leaflets

If the anterior papillary muscle is malpositioned, it must be cut at its base and reimplanted at a higher level in the septum or the ventricular wall with pledgeted 3-0 Prolene sutures. ⊘

⊘ Injury to the Conduction System

The right atrial plication must be accomplished to the right side of the coronary sinus to avoid the conduction system. ⊘

NB Bidirectional Cavopulmonary Anastomosis

If right ventricular function is impaired, a bidirectional cavopulmonary anastomosis can decrease the right ventricular preload and may improve patient survival. This procedure does eliminate catheter access from the upper extremities in these patients who may need future ablation procedures or pacemakers. Because some of these patients have associated left ventricular dysfunction, it is important to document low left atrial and pulmonary pressures before performing a bidirectional cavopulmonary shunt (see Chapter 31). NB

NB Atrial Septal Defect Closure

The patent foramen ovale or atrial septal defect should be closed by primary suture or patching with pericardium or Gore-Tex (see Chapter 19). If right ventricular function is

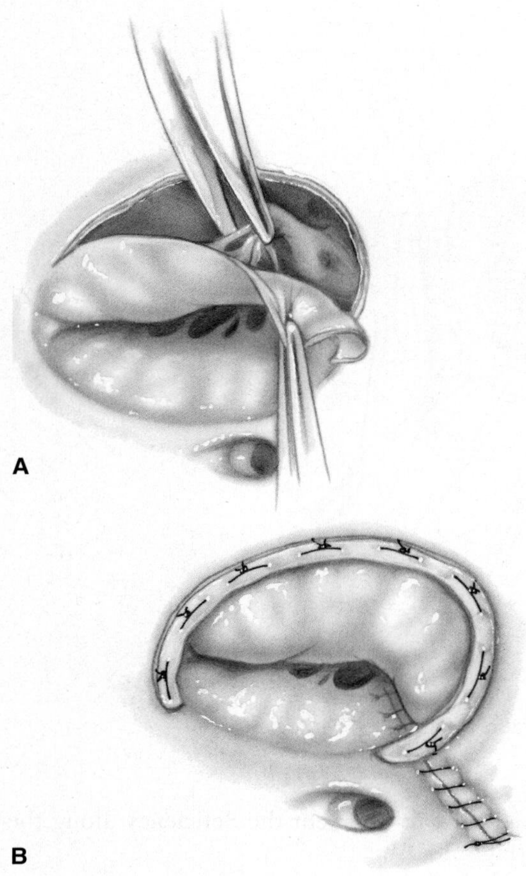

FIG. 28.5 **A:** The anterior leaflet is detached from the annulus to expose and divide the fibrous bands. **B:** The atrialized ventricle and redundant atrial tissue are plicated. The anterior leaflet is reconstructed and the annulus is reinforced.

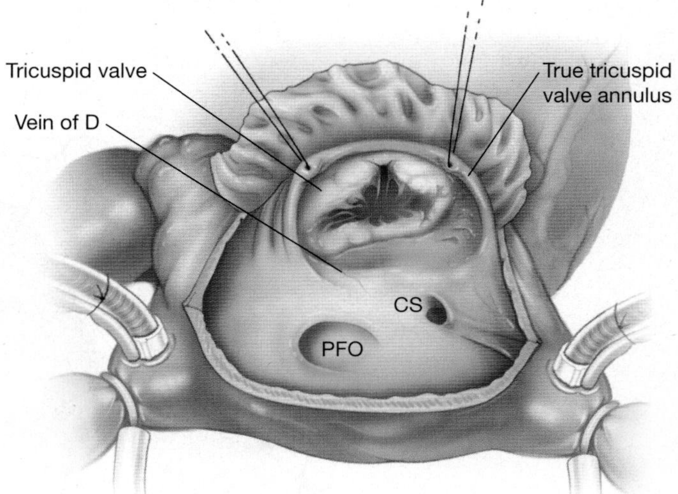

FIG. 28.6 Exposure in preparation for valve repair. Note the location of the "true" tricuspid annulus to which the repaired valve will be secured, as well as the vein of D, which often denotes the region of the conduction system.

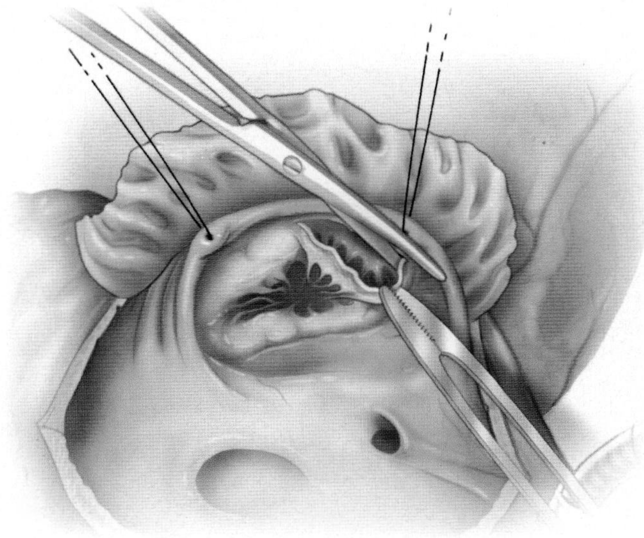

FIG. 28.7 Initial incision in the anterior leaflet extended clockwise while dividing underlying fibrous attachments.

marginal, an adjustable atrial septal defect, encircled with a pledgeted suture threaded through a snare, can be left and closed later under local anesthesia when right ventricular contractility improves (see Chapter 31). NB

An alternative to the Carpentier repair is the so-called Cone procedure. After standard bicaval cannulation and cardioplegic arrest, the anatomy is inspected (Fig. 28.6) with the addition of stay sutures placed through the "true" annulus. Notable in this is the small vein of D, which marks the membranous septum and AV node. The anterior leaflet is then taken down, in particular, capitalizing on the true area of delamination between the anterior leaflet and the right ventricle (Fig. 28.7). All fibrous and muscular attachments of the leading edge of the leaflet are extensively taken down, with attention paid not to divide true chordal support to the leading edge. The dissection is then extended clockwise to include the septal leaflet all the way to the anteroseptal commissure; the septal leaflet often is quite diminutive (nearly absent) and may have multiple fenestrations that require closure (Fig. 28.8). With the anterior, inferior, and septal leaflets all fully mobilized, the cut edge of the inferior leaflet is rotated clockwise to the proximal edge of the septal leaflet (as in the Carpentier repair), and the two are approximated with interrupted 6-0 prolene sutures completing the "cone" (Fig. 28.9). In doing so, there are now 360 degrees of leaflet tissue that can comprise the new tricuspid

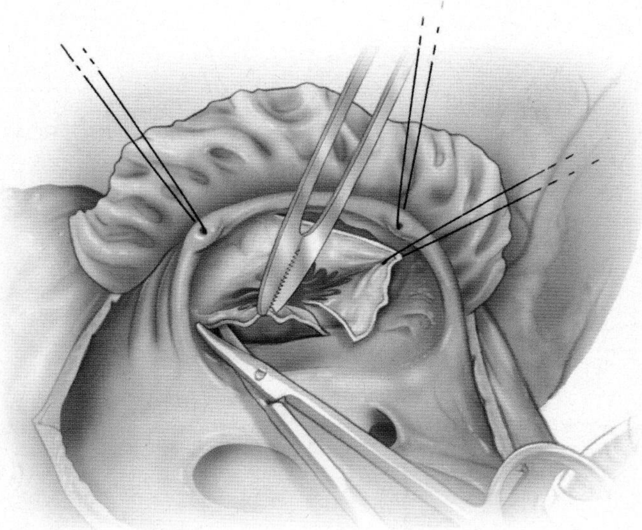

FIG. 28.8 Extension of the incision to include the septal leaflet, no matter how diminutive.

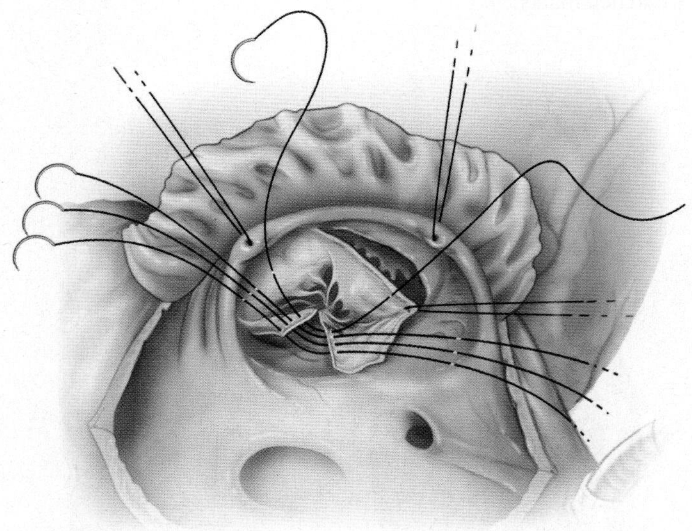

FIG. 28.9 Approximation of septal and anterior leaflet edges to begin creating the cone.

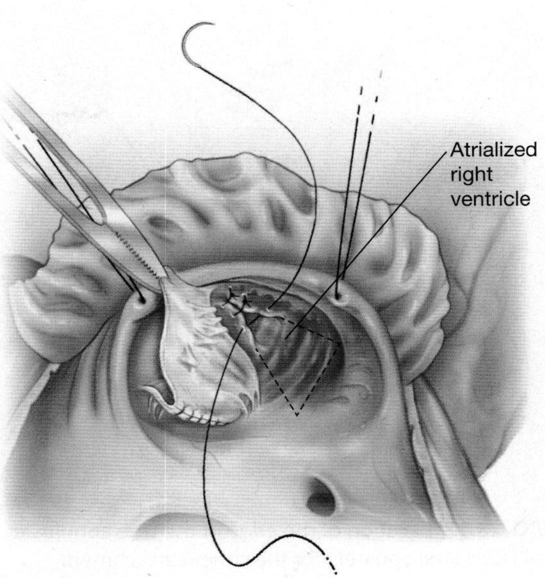

FIG. 28.10 The triangular area of atrialized right ventricle to be excluded. Attention needs to be paid to the depth of these sutures so as not to compromise the right coronary artery.

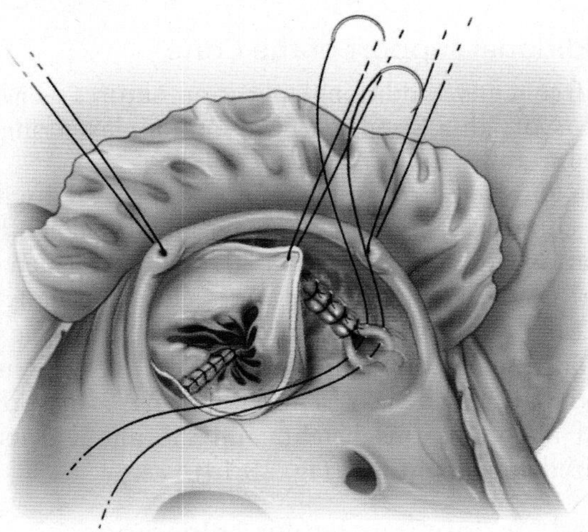

FIG. 28.11 Completion of the exclusion, with interrupted sutures that eliminate any "blind pouch" at the top of the excluded segment.

orifice, in particular creating leaflet along the area of the prior diminutive septal leaflet. With the cone retracted, the area of atrialized right ventricle is closed vertically, with attention paid to the preservation of the right coronary artery (which lies just outside this area). The epicardium will appear "puckered" inward (Fig. 28.10). As with the Carpentier repair, vertical plication (unlike horizontal plication) will preserve the height of the true tricuspid annulus, and not artificially displace it further downward.

NB Closure of the atrialized ventricle

The suture line is advanced toward the AV groove, but limited so as not to distort the course of the right coronary artery (shown in Fig. 28.11). NB

Interrupted sutures are placed carefully to eliminate the blind pouch of the excluded atrialized segment. The newly constructed "cone" (tricuspid valve) is then reattached at the level of the true annulus; here several interrupted sutures are recommended as reinforcement should a

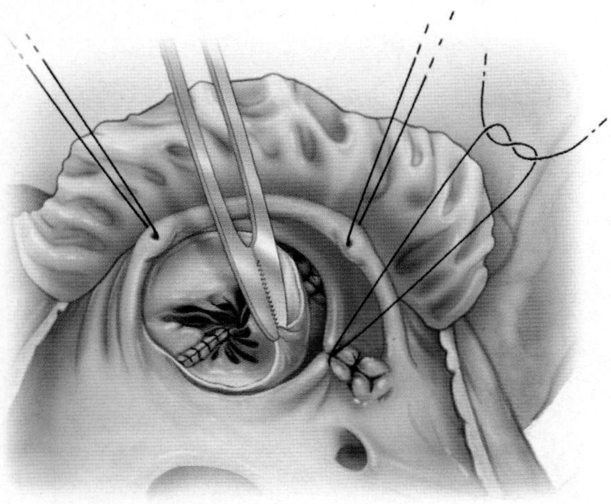

FIG. 28.12 Plication of the edge of the true annulus to be sized appropriately for the cone reattachment.

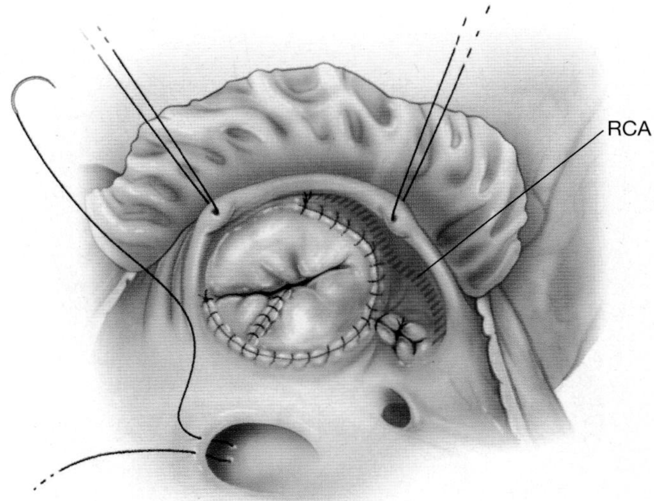

FIG. 28.13 Reattachment of the cone to the true annulus, which may require interrupted sutures and even annuloplasty reduction. The course of the right coronary artery is noted in hatched marks.

running technique be employed. Often the annulus must be plicated to meet the smaller circumference of the "cone." Again, although the sutures need to be deep enough to be durable, attention to the adjacent right coronary artery is of utmost importance (Fig. 28.12).

NB Additional support of the Cone

Not infrequently, additional plication sutures—or if the patient is of adult size, an entire annuloplasty ring—are required to fully support the cone. NB

The completed reconstruction is static tested with saline to confirm competency. Any residual leak or leaflet fenestrations are addressed, as is the patent formen ovale (shown) (Fig. 28.13). The atrium is closed, usually after some form of reduction atrioplasty. In the schematic form, the reconstructed cone is now at the level of the true annulus, the atrialized right ventricle having been vertically plicated maintains this height, and the annulus itself is downsized and supported (Fig. 28.14).

NB Need for right ventricular unloading

To note, if the right ventricle appears inadequate to support full cardiac output, a Glenn cavopulmonary connection can be created to offload some of this volume. NB

Tricuspid Valve Replacement

When the abnormality produces obstruction within the right ventricle, the tricuspid valve is excised and replaced with an appropriate prosthesis. If more than mild to moderate tricuspid insufficiency is present following valve repair, replacement is indicated. The septal and posterior leaflet tissues are resected, but the anterior leaflet tissue is often incorporated in the suture technique of anchoring the prosthesis. Because of the ambiguous location of the conduction system owing to displacement of the tricuspid valve, the true atrial wall above the coronary sinus is used to construct a new annulus to which the prosthesis is sutured with multiple, interrupted, and everting mattress sutures of 2-0 Tevdek buttressed with pledgets (see Chapter 8).

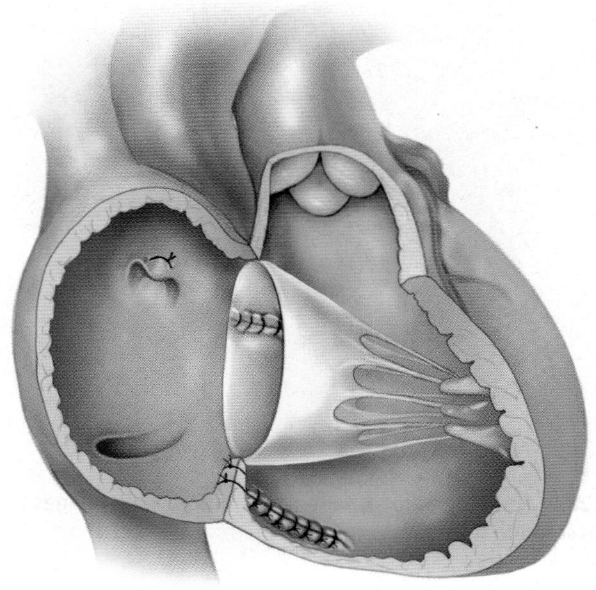

FIG. 28.14 Schematic of the completed cone, now reattached at the true annulus with vertical plication of the atrialized ventricle.

⊘ Injury to Conduction Tissue

Incorporating the true atrial wall, rather than the septal annulus, in the suturing process prevents damage to the conduction system. Alternatively, a patch of glutaraldehyde-treated autologous or bovine pericardium may be sewn to the right atrial wall, beginning at the anteroseptal commissure, continuing above the level of the atrioventricular node and inside the coronary sinus, back to the posterior annulus. The valve sewing ring is then attached to this patch to avoid placing sutures in the septal annulus. ⊘

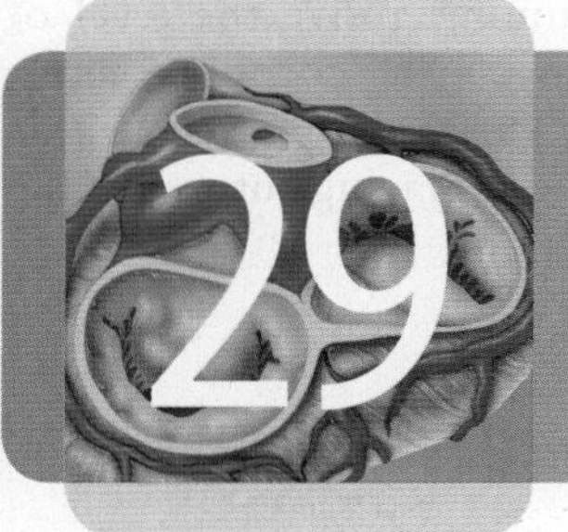

29 Interrupted and Hypoplastic Aortic Arch

INTERRUPTED AORTIC ARCH

Interruption of the aortic arch is a rare condition that requires a patent ductus arteriosus for survival. A ventricular septal defect is often present and may be associated with left ventricular outflow obstruction due to malalignment of the conal septum. Other associated anomalies may include a bicuspid aortic valve, truncus arteriosus, and aortopulmonary window. The aortic arch may be interrupted at one of three sites. The interruption may be just distal to the left subclavian artery (type A), between the left carotid and left subclavian arteries (type B), or between the innominate and left carotid artery (type C) (Fig. 29.1). Type B is the most common form of interrupted aortic arch, and type C is very rare.

HYPOPLASTIC AORTIC ARCH

Hypoplasia of the aortic arch may occur with or without a discrete coarctation. Hypoplasia of the proximal arch between the innominate and left carotid arteries is defined as a diameter less than 60% of that of the ascending aorta. The distal arch between the left carotid and left subclavian arteries is considered hypoplastic if the diameter is less than 50% that of the ascending aorta. A hypoplastic aortic arch may be associated with a ventricular septal defect and other congenital heart lesions.

Patients with an interrupted or hypoplastic aortic arch usually present as neonates when the ductus arteriosus closes and flow to the descending aorta ceases or is severely restricted. Low cardiac output with metabolic acidosis is soon evident. Infusion of prostaglandin E_1 is immediately started to reopen the ductus arteriosus to perfuse the distal aorta. When the patient's general condition has improved and the low output state has been corrected, semiurgent surgical intervention is contemplated. One-stage complete repair of the aortic arch and associated cardiac defects is the preferred technique.

Incision

A median sternotomy is performed. Most of the thymus gland (if present) is removed to allow adequate mobilization of the branches of the aortic arch.

Cannulation

Traditionally, deep hypothermic arrest has been used for surgery involving the aortic arch. More recently, low-flow antegrade cerebral perfusion has been advocated during reconstruction of the arch to avoid or minimize circulatory arrest and cerebral ischemia.

A purse-string suture is placed on the far right side of the distal ascending aorta near the origin of the innominate artery. In patients with an interrupted aortic arch, a second purse-string suture is placed on the proximal main pulmonary artery. The right and left pulmonary arteries are dissected and encircled with Silastic tourniquets. Dual arterial cannulation with flexible 8 to 10-French aortic cannulas is achieved using a Y-connector on the arterial line for interrupted aortic arch. Single aortic cannulation is used with a hypoplastic aortic arch. The right atrial cannula is then placed through a purse-string suture on the right atrial appendage. If intracardiac defects need to be addressed, bicaval cannulation is performed. A vent is placed through the right superior pulmonary vein (see Chapter 4). As cardiopulmonary bypass is initiated, the snares on the right and left pulmonary arteries are tightened to prevent flooding of the pulmonary bed.

Technique: General

While cooling is being carried out, the innominate artery, left common carotid artery, and left subclavian artery are mobilized, and snares are placed around them. The ductus arteriosus is also dissected, and the descending aorta is mobilized distally beyond the level of the left bronchus. Also during this period, the intracardiac lesions can be repaired after cross-clamping the aorta and administering cardiopegia into the aortic root. Following the intracardiac procedure, the aortic cannula is advanced into the innominate artery, and the snare around the innominate artery is tightened. The pump flow is reduced to 10 to 20 mL per kilogram per minute, and adjusted to maintain a right radial pressure of 30 to 40 mm Hg. The left carotid and left subclavian tourniquets are snugged down, and a curved vascular clamp is applied to the distal descending aorta.

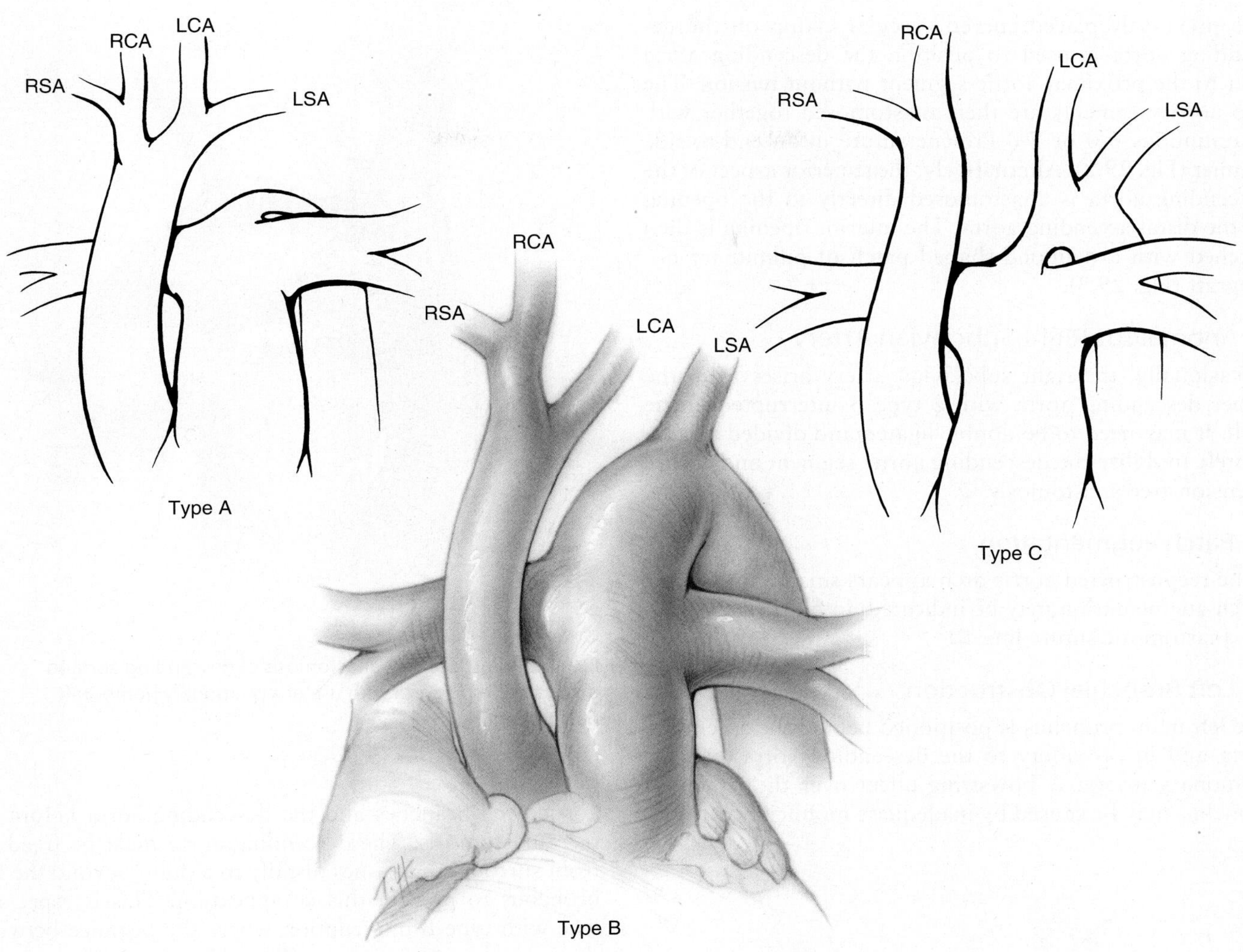

FIG. 29.1 Interrupted arch, types A, B, and C. RSA, right subclavian artery; RCA, right carotid artery; LCA, left carotid artery; LSA, left subclavian artery.

NB Anomalous Right Subclavian Artery

If an anomalous origin of the right subclavian artery from the descending aorta is present, the pressure in the right temporal artery can be monitored during low-flow cerebral perfusion or more commonly bilateral near infrared spectroscopy (NIRS) can aid in assessing bilateral cerebral hemispheric flow. NB

NB Alternate Cannulation Techniques

Whether or not the cardiac lesion requires a systemic–pulmonary shunt, the surgeon may elect to sew a 3- or 3.5-mm Gore-Tex tube end-to-side to the innominate artery, and secure an olive-tipped or small arterial cannula inside the graft. Low-flow cerebral perfusion is then performed after clamping the takeoff of the innominate artery. Alternatively, a brief period of hypothermic arrest is used to open the arch. The arterial cannula is then placed into the innominate artery under direct vision. The tourniquet around the innominate artery is then snugged down, and low-flow cerebral perfusion is begun. The arch repair can now proceed. NB

NB Before snaring the head vessels and beginning low-flow cerebral perfusion, ice is placed around the patient's head. NB

Technique: Interrupted Aortic Arch

The ductus arteriosus is divided and its pulmonary artery end is oversewn with 6-0 or 7-0 Prolene suture. All the ductal tissue on the aortic end must be aggressively resected. An incision is made along the left posterolateral aspect of the distal ascending aorta. The opening may be enlarged to approximate the lumen of the descending aorta by extending the incision onto the left carotid (with type B interruption) or left subclavian artery (with type A interruption).

The previously placed curved vascular clamp on the descending aorta is used to position the descending aorta next to the proximal aortic segment without tension. The two aortic segments are then anastomosed together with a continuous 6-0 or 7-0 Prolene suture in an end-to-side manner (Fig. 29.2). Alternatively, the superior aspect of the descending aorta is anastomosed directly to the opening on the distal ascending aorta. The inferior opening is then patched with a diamond-shaped patch of pulmonary homograft (Fig. 29.3).

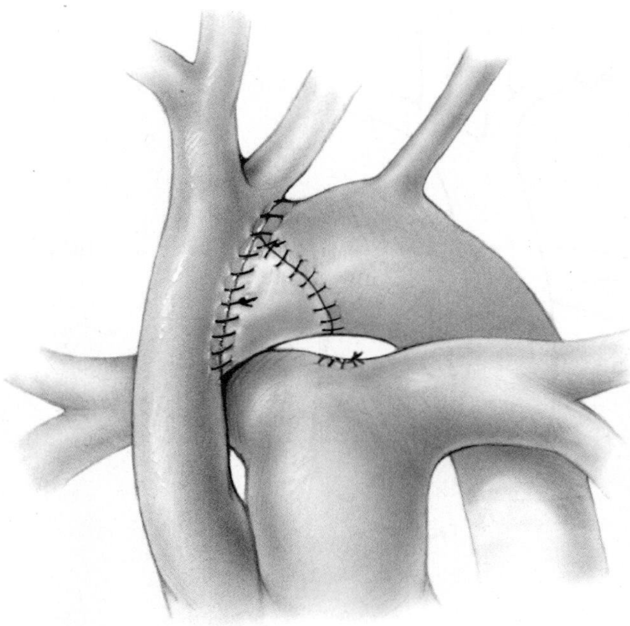

FIG. 29.3 Partial direct anastomosis of descending aorta to distal ascending aorta with use of a pulmonary homograft patch inferiorly.

⊘ Anomalous Right Subclavian Artery

Occasionally, the right subclavian artery arises from the upper descending aorta with a type B interrupted aortic arch. It may need to be double ligated and divided to adequately mobilize the descending aortic segment and ensure a tension-free anastomosis. ⊘

NB Patch augmentation

If the reconstructed aortic arch appears small, a full onlay patch augmentation may be indicated, in particular across the anastomotic suture line. NB

NB Left Bronchial Obstruction

The left main bronchus is positioned behind the ascending aorta and in proximity to the descending aorta and left pulmonary artery. A bowstring effect over the left main bronchus may be caused by inadequate mobilization of the aortic arch branches and the descending aorta before direct anastomosis. The descending aorta must be freed up from surrounding tissues distally to a point beyond the left bronchus to prevent this complication. This is especially true with type B interruption where the distance between the two segments is greater. NB

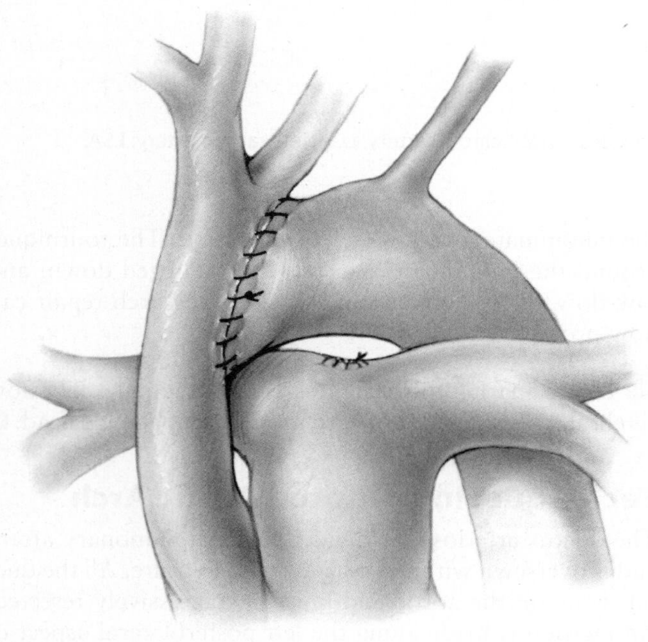

FIG. 29.2 Complete primary repair of type B interrupted arch. The ductal tissue has been removed and the fully mobilized descending aorta is anastomosed to the posterolateral aspect of the distal ascending aorta.

NB Rarely, despite adequate mobilization of the arch vessels and descending aorta, a direct anastomosis or partial direct anastomosis with patch augmentation is not possible. If this occurs with a type B interruption, the left subclavian artery may be doubly ligated and divided to increase the mobility of the descending aortic segment (Fig. 29.4). Alternatively, the left subclavian artery may be used to create a tube extension consisting of subclavian artery wall laterally and a pulmonary homograft patch medially. The subclavian artery is dissected distally to its first branches, ligated at this level, and transected. For type A interruption, the subclavian artery is opened longitudinally along its lateral aspect from the distal end of the arch. It is reflected inferiorly and sutured to the lateral aspect of the descending aorta with a running 7-0 Prolene suture. For type B interruption, the incision along the length of the subclavian artery extends on its medial aspect from the end of the descending aorta. In this case, it is swung superiorly and anastomosed to the superior aspect of the distal arch. In both types of interruption, the remaining opening on the underside of the arch and medial aspect of the descending aorta is patched with a piece of pulmonary homograft. NB

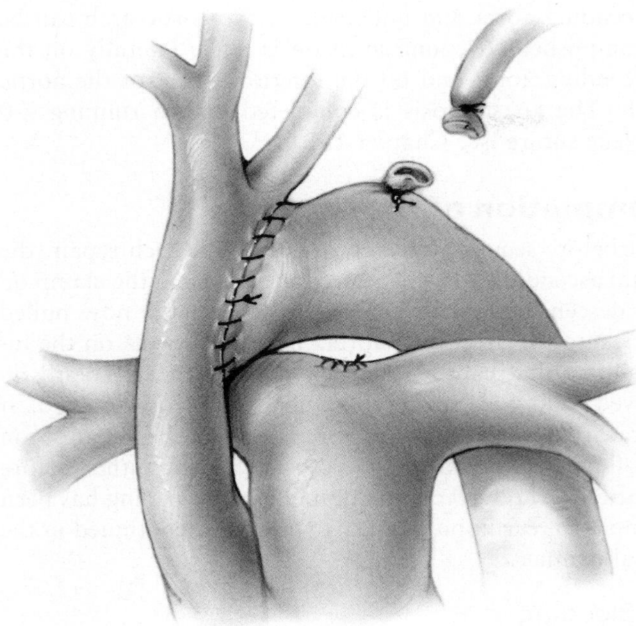

FIG. 29.4 If excess tension is noted on the anastomosis, division of the left subclavian artery allows for further mobilization of the descending aortic segment.

NB Aberrant Subclavian Arteries

In the event of an aberrant right subclavian artery, full mobilization of the descending aorta can involve sacrifice of both subclavian arteries so as to reduce the likelihood of left bronchial obstruction or excess tension on the anastomosis. This considerably complicates postoperative monitoring of anastomotic gradients. NB

Technique: Hypoplastic Aortic Arch

The ductus arteriosus is divided, and the pulmonary end oversewn with fine Prolene suture. All the ductal tissue must be excised. The resultant opening on the underside of the aortic arch is now extended distally onto the descending aorta. Reverse Potts scissors or a Beaver blade is used to incise the underside of the arch from the ductal opening back to the ascending aorta (Fig. 29.5). A rectangular patch of pulmonary homograft is sewn into the opening beginning at the descending aortic end with a 7-0 Prolene suture (Fig. 29.6). The posterior suture line is accomplished before completing the anterior portion of the anastomosis.

⊘ Residual Ductal Tissue

Leaving ductal tissue behind in the aortic arch may lead to bleeding from the suture line or even dehiscence of the patch from this area due to friability. Residual ductal tissue may also lead to late constriction and stenosis of the aortic arch. ⊘

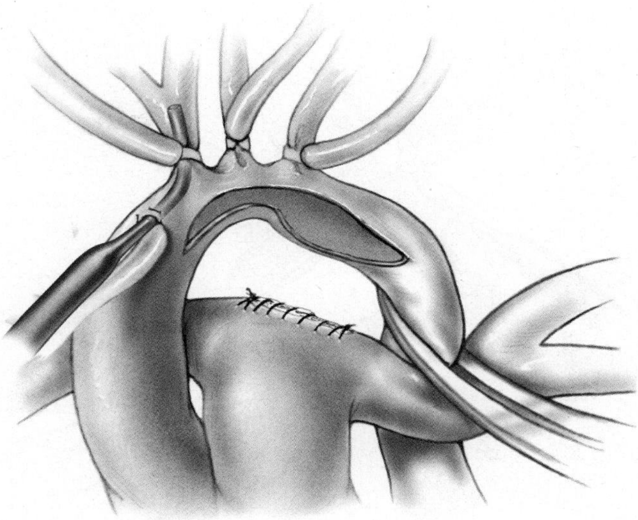

FIG. 29.5 Hypoplastic aortic arch: division and resection of ductal tissue and opening on the inferior aspect of the arch. Aortic cannula has been advanced into innominate artery for low-flow cerebral perfusion.

NB Recurrent Arch Obstruction

One of the most important causes of recurrent aortic arch narrowing following the surgical repair of hypoplastic aortic arch is the incomplete resection of ductal tissue. For this reason, many surgeons circumferentially excise the portion of the aorta attached to the ductus. The resultant distal end of the arch and proximal end of the descending aorta are anastomosed together in an end-to-end fashion on their posterolateral aspects with a running 7-0 Prolene suture (Fig. 29.7). Both ends of the stitch are secured.

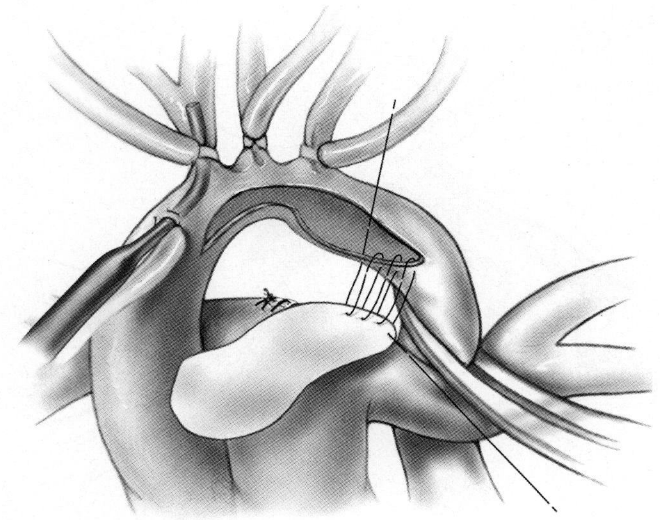

FIG. 29.6 Pulmonary homograft patch enlargement of the aortic arch.

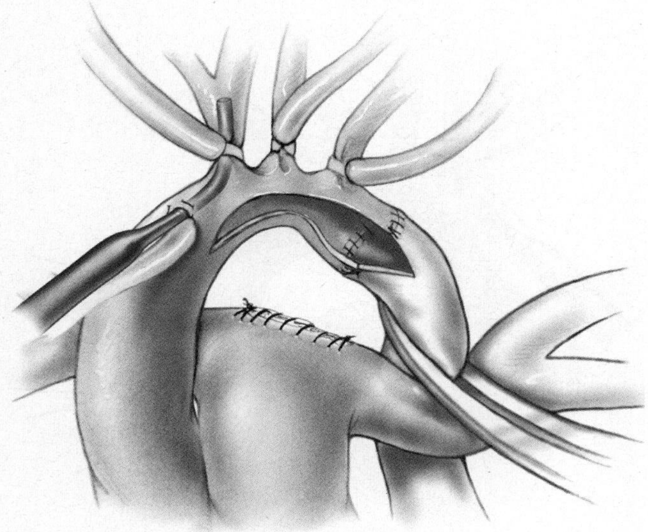

FIG. 29.7 The periductal aorta is excised circumferentially. The posterolateral aspect of the descending aorta and distal arch are reapproximated.

A longitudinal incision is made on the anteromedial wall of the descending aorta, thereby splitting any residual ductal tissue. A patch of pulmonary homograft is then used to reconstruct the remaining opening in the arch and descending aorta with a continuous 7-0 Prolene suture (Fig. 29.8). NB

NB Discrete Coarctation

If a discrete coarcted segment of aorta is present, it is resected. With adequate mobilization of the descending aorta, an extended end-to-end anastomosis between the descending aorta and underside of the aortic arch can be accomplished. A counterincision is made laterally on the descending aorta and on the inferior aspect of the aortic arch. The anastomosis is completed with a running 7-0 Prolene suture (see Chapter 15). NB

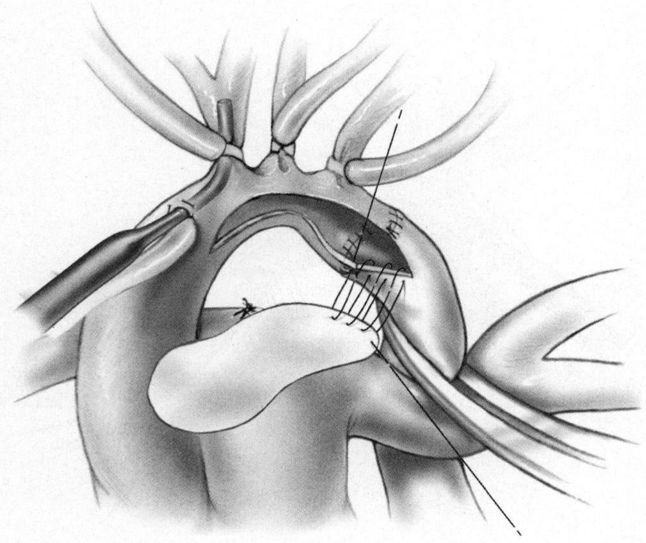

FIG. 29.8 The remaining opening in the arch and proximal descending aorta is closed with a patch of pulmonary homograft.

Completion of the Operation

Just before securing the suture line of the arch repair, the distal ascending aorta is deaired by removing the clamp on the descending aorta. The arterial cannula is now pulled back into the ascending aorta. The tourniquets on the innominate, left carotid, and left subclavian artery are removed, and full cardiopulmonary bypass is resumed. If intracardiac defects are present, they can be repaired on full-flow bypass with aortic cross-clamping either before or after the arch reconstruction. After rewarming has been completed, cardiopulmonary bypass is discontinued in the usual manner.

⊘ Bleeding

If there is excessive tension on the arch anastomosis, bleeding is fairly common. Tissue friability also contributes to the risk of bleeding, and often retention of ductal tissue in the suture line is the cause. Needle hole bleeding may respond to the topical application of fibrin glue. Continued bleeding may respond to superficial adventitial figure-of-eight sutures surrounding the tear site. More major tearing requires reinstitution of cardiopulmonary bypass, systemic cooling, and low-flow cerebral perfusion to redo the arch reconstruction. This may require further mobilization of the descending aorta and/or resection of retained ductal tissue. ⊘

⊘ Injury to Recurrent Laryngeal and Phrenic Nerves

Both the recurrent laryngeal and the phrenic nerves are at risk during repair of an interrupted or hypoplastic aortic arch. Careful attention should be given to identifying and protecting these nerves. ⊘

NB Postoperative Compression of the Left Bronchus

Despite extensive mobilization of the descending aorta, a few patients show signs of left bronchial compression following arch repair. Traditionally, this complication has been dealt with by fixing the ascending aorta to the back of the sternum. Results with this procedure are inconsistent, and aortopexy may be contraindicated if further cardiac procedures are anticipated, as in single ventricle patients. Lengthening of the ascending aorta or aortic arch with a tube graft may be required. This is usually accomplished with a Gore-Tex or Hemashield conduit. NB

NB Left ventricular outflow tract obstruction

In some cases of interrupted aortic arch/VSD, considerable concern is raised about a small left ventricular outflow

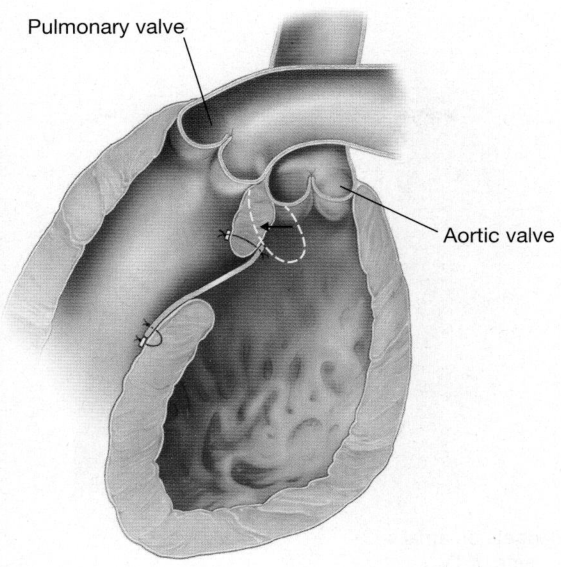

FIG. 29.9 VSD Closure tethering the posteriorly deviated septum rightward.

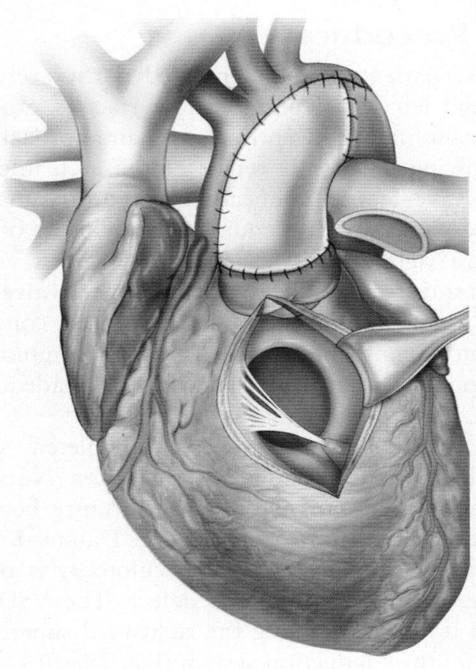

FIG. 29.10 Vertical right ventriculotomy exposing the perimembranous defect, and demonstrating the "safe area" should the VSD require enlargement.

tract obstruction, which can be challenging to measure in the setting of a posteriorly deviated septum. In these cases, the obstructing septum can sometimes be resected, or more often is used to secure the ventricular septal defect patch in a manner that "pulls" the septum out of the subvalvar region (Fig. 29.9). Other patients with prohibitively small left ventricular outflow tracts may require a Yasui-type reconstruction. NB

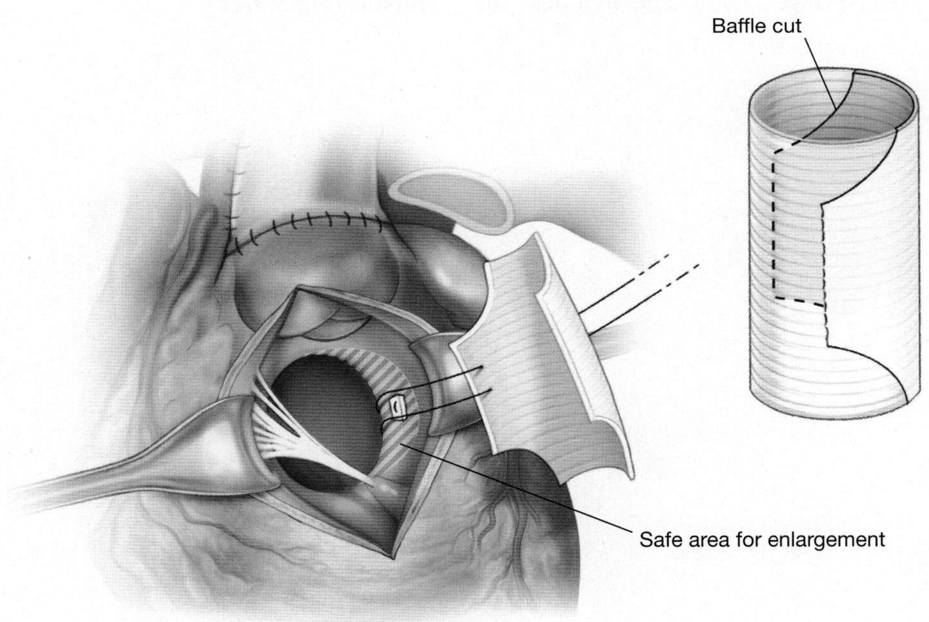

FIG. 29.11 Use of a bisected Dacron graft to create the baffle.

Yasui Procedure

For those patients with interrupted aortic arch/VSD for whom the left ventricular outflow tract is prohibitively small, an alternative biventricular repair approach involves the following tenets: (1) repair of the arch interruption, Damus–Kaye–Stansel connection of the proximal pulmonary artery and small ascending aorta, closure of the VSD through a right ventriculotomy allowing left ventricular blood to traverse the VSD to the pulmonary valve, and creation of a right ventricle to pulmonary artery conduit. This operation has also been used for the uncommon patient with hypoplastic left heart syndrome, two adequate-sized ventricles, and a ventricular septal defect.

The aortic arch repair is completed with the Damus-Kaye-Stansel similar to that of a Norwood reconstruction so as to make a gentle taper between the smaller descending aorta and the large Damus–Kaye–Stansel neo-aortic root. A right ventriculotomy is performed exposing the perimembranous defect. The VSD may be enlarged if necessary along the rightward superior aspect away from the conduction system (Fig. 29.10).

NB The right ventriculotomy in this operation, like that in a Ross procedure, must acknowledge that the pulmonary valve extends quite inferiorly and may need to be lower on the right ventricular free wall. NB

A PTFE patch or bisected Dacron graft (as with a Rastelli procedure) can be used to baffle flow through the VSD to the pulmonary valve. The superior tip of the baffle will be secured to the most superior/anterior portion of the ventriculotomy, and the inferior tip of the baffle near the muscle of Lancisi (Fig. 29.11). The area near the tricuspid valve may be approached best through the tricuspid valve.

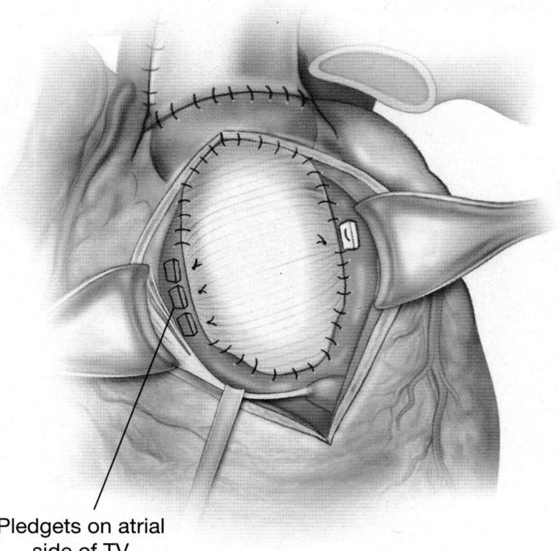

FIG. 29.12 Completed intracardiac baffle with sutures from the septal leaflet of the tricuspid valve shown (these usually are interrupted). The right ventriculotomy is then used for the proximal site of the right ventricle to pulmonary artery connection.

Using the right ventriculotomy, a homograft connection is created between the right ventricle and transected main pulmonary artery, thus creating a two-ventricle repair. (Fig. 29.12)

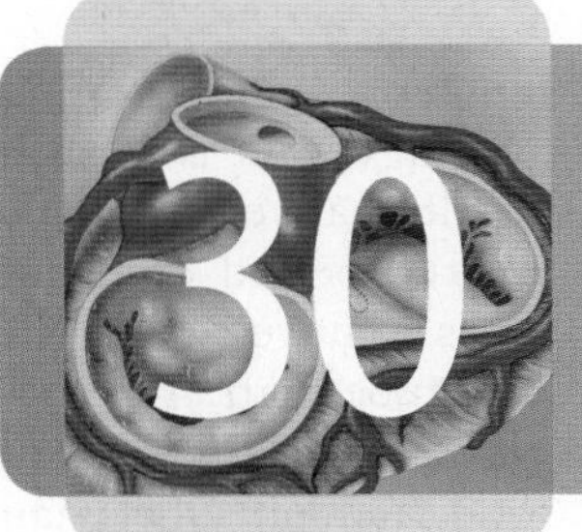

30 The Norwood Principle

Hypoplastic left heart syndrome is the most common form of congenital heart disease in which there is only one fully developed ventricle and is the fourth most common congenital heart defect presenting in the first year of life. The anatomic features include aortic valve atresia or severe stenosis, with marked hypoplasia or absence of the left ventricle. The ascending aorta is small, usually only 2 to 3 mm in diameter, and the mitral valve is hypoplastic or atretic. A patent ductus arteriosus is the only route for adequate systemic perfusion.

Other single-ventricle complexes may present with evident or potential left ventricular outflow tract obstruction. These include tricuspid atresia with transposition of the great arteries and single ventricles with left ventricular outflow chambers. Narrowing of the bulboventricular foramen may cause subaortic obstruction. Pulmonary artery banding in this subgroup of patients may predispose to the development of subaortic obstruction.

The Norwood principle can be applied to all patients with single-ventricle morphology and real or potential obstruction to systemic flow. It involves the creation or preservation of optimal hemodynamics and anatomy in preparation for a successful Fontan procedure.

There are three important basic concepts in the initial palliation phase:

1. The aorta must be associated directly with the single ventricle in such a way as to provide unobstructed flow from the single ventricle to the systemic circulation and to allow potential for growth.
2. Pulmonary blood flow must be regulated to avoid the development of pulmonary vascular disease, and minimize the volume load on the single ventricle to preserve long-term ventricular function. This must be achieved without distorting the pulmonary arteries.
3. When there is stenosis or atresia of the left-sided atrioventricular valve, a large interatrial communication must be created to avoid the development of pulmonary venous obstruction and hypertension.

STAGE I PALLIATIVE RECONSTRUCTION FOR HYPOPLASTIC LEFT HEART SYNDROME

Diagnosis may be made prenatally with a fetal echocardiogram, which then allows for prospective management of the neonate from the time of delivery. Preoperative management includes continuous infusion of prostaglandin E_1 to maintain patency of the ductus arteriosus. A balanced pulmonary and systemic circulation is critical to the survival of these patients. A particularly restrictive interatrial communication limits pulmonary overcirculation, and a balloon atrial septostomy or blade septectomy may result in hemodynamic deterioration and should be avoided. In contrast, a truly restrictive atrial component may increase pulmonary vascular resistance and significantly increase perioperative mortality. In this scenario, a careful balloon septostomy may relieve this obstruction without incurring pulmonary overcirculation. In addition, hyperventilation and increased inspired oxygen concentrations may decrease pulmonary vascular resistance, leading to increased pulmonary blood flow at the expense of decreased systemic perfusion. Hypoventilation with room air is most often indicated in these patients.

Traditionally, this operation has been performed with the use of deep hypothermic arrest for the aortic reconstruction. More recently, techniques using selective cerebral perfusion to avoid or minimize circulatory arrest have been adopted in most institutions.

Incision

A median sternotomy is performed, and the thymus is excised. If a Sano-type right ventricle–to–pulmonary artery conduit is to be used, the "top hat" can be created prior to sternotomy with a tube graft (usually 5 to 6 mm) and a piece of Gore-Tex patch with an appropriate-sized defect created with a skin punch (Fig. 30.1).

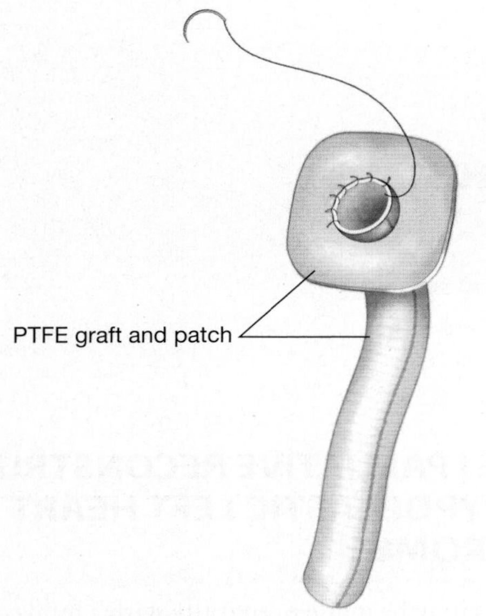

FIG. 30.1 Creation of the Sano insertion site using PTFE graft and "skirt."

Cannulation

Regardless of the type of shunt ultimately planned for pulmonary blood flow, a 3.0- or 3.5-mm Gore-Tex tube graft is anastomosed to the innominate artery with a continuous 7-0 Prolene suture. A purse-string suture is placed on the right atrial appendage. The right and left pulmonary arteries are encircled with Silastic tapes. The arterial cannula is deaired and introduced several millimeters into the Gore-Tex chimney, and the purse-string suture is tightened. A single venous cannula is placed in the right atrial appendage and cardiopulmonary bypass is begun. The tapes around the pulmonary arteries are placed on traction to prevent pulmonary blood flow and ensure satisfactory systemic perfusion. During the cooling period, the ascending aorta is dissected away from the main pulmonary artery and the branch vessels of the aortic arch are mobilized. The innominate, left carotid, and left subclavian arteries are looped with Silastic tapes on tourniquets. The distal aortic arch and descending aorta are mobilized down to the level of the left bronchus with blunt dissection.

NB Before cannulation, ice is placed around the patient's head. NB

NB For patients with significant transverse aortic arch hypoplasia, a second ductal cannula may improve lower body perfusion and cooling. NB

NB Patients with severe aortic atresia (ascending aorta <2 mm) require careful handling of the aorta during dissection so as not to distort the great vessel and cause coronary ischemia. NB

Procedure

After cooling for at least 15–20 minutes to a temperature of 18°C, the second limb of the arterial circuit is flushed and secured to the Gore-Tex tube. Alternatively, a single arterial line is used, and during a brief period of hypothermic arrest, the arterial cannula is removed from the pulmonary artery and placed into the tube graft. The previously placed tourniquets are used to occlude the proximal innominate artery, the left carotid, and left subclavian artery (Fig. 30.2). The cannula in the pulmonary artery is removed. A curved clamp is placed on the distal descending aorta. The pump flow is reduced to 10 to 20 mL per kilogram per minute. The ductus arteriosus is transected, and the pulmonary end is ligated or oversewn with a running 6-0 Prolene suture. The main pulmonary artery is transected at the level of the takeoff of the right pulmonary artery (Fig. 30.2). The defect in the distal pulmonary artery is then closed with either a patch of Gore-Tex if an aortopulmonary shunt is to be used, or with the Sano "top hat" created previously (Fig. 30.3).

NB Myocardial Preservation

With the descending thoracic aorta and arch vessels occluded, cold blood cardioplegic solution is infused into the side port of the arterial cannula. This perfuses the coronary circulation by retrograde flow through the ductus, arch, and ascending aorta. NB

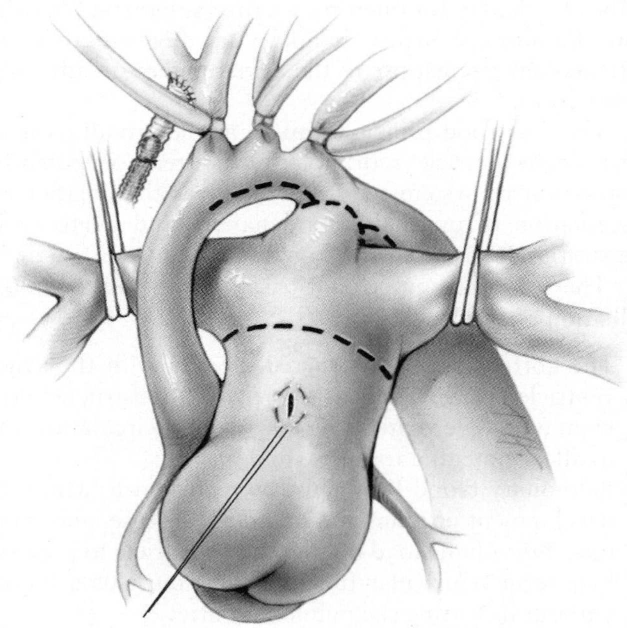

FIG. 30.2 Occlusion of pulmonary arteries during cooling. Gore-Tex tube anastomosed to innominate artery for cerebral perfusion. Tourniquets are tightened around innominate, left carotid, and left subclavian arteries during low-flow cerebral perfusion. The purse-string marks the location of the ductal cannula if used.

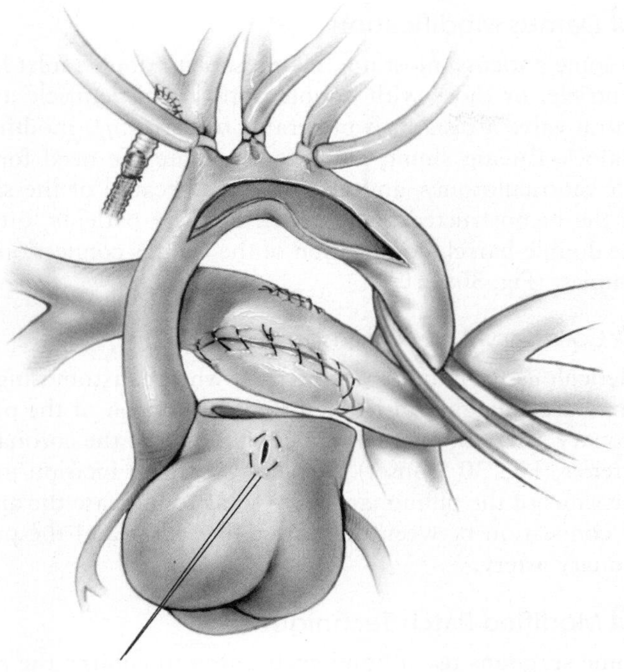

FIG. 30.3 Transection of main pulmonary artery and patch closure of confluence. Oversewing of pulmonary end of ductus and opening of proximal descending aorta and arch.

A brief period of circulatory arrest or continued low-flow cerebral perfusion providing venous return with a pump sucker is used to excise the septum primum. This can be accomplished through the right atrial cannulation site by temporarily removing the venous cannula. Alternatively, a small right atriotomy is made and closed with a 6-0 Prolene suture after creating an adequate interatrial communication.

AORTIC ARCH RECONSTRUCTION

Patch Reconstruction Technique

The aortic opening of the ductus arteriosus is extended distally for 10 to 15 mm on the medial aspect of the descending aorta. The opening is carried proximally along the lesser curvature of the aortic arch and down the left side of the ascending aorta. This incision should stop at the level of the transected proximal pulmonary artery.

⊘ Retained Ductal Tissue

All the ductal tissue in the aortic arch and descending aorta must be excised, including resection of the coarctation ridge, if present. Sewing to ductal tissue may result in bleeding from the suture line or even dehiscence of a portion of the anastomosis. In addition, residual ductal tissue may lead to late stenosis of the reconstructed arch. In most patients, this may require the excision of a circumferential portion of the periductal aorta. The descending aortic segment is then anastomosed to the posterolateral aspect of the distal arch opening with a running Prolene suture. Both suture ends are secured before proceeding with the patch. ⊘

An oval patch of pulmonary homograft is tailored to reconstruct the proximal descending aorta, aortic arch, and ascending aorta. The anastomosis of the pulmonary homograft to the aorta is started at the most distal extent of the incision on the descending aorta with a 7-0 Prolene double-armed suture. The posterior suture line is continued onto the ascending aorta, stopping 5 mm above the proximal extent of the incision. The anterior suture line is accomplished with the other needle, again ending the suture line 5 mm short of the proximal ascending aortic opening.

NB Patch Material

A patch cut from an adult-sized pulmonary homograft has a natural curved shape, which mimics the curve of the underside of the aortic arch. It is easy to handle, and has good hemostatic properties. However, there are availability and cost issues, as well as concerns regarding viral transmission and the generation of cytotoxic antibodies, which may limit transplant options. Some surgeons have advocated the use of bovine pericardium or other substitutes, using two pieces cut in a curved shape and sewn together along their concave aspect to create an appropriately shaped aortic arch patch. NB

NB Suturing along Arch

Alternating traction on the left carotid tourniquet and the innominate artery tourniquet improves the exposure for performing the posterior and anterior suture line on the underside of the aortic arch. NB

The main pulmonary artery is anastomosed to the ascending aorta, taking care not to distort the aortic root. This is accomplished with multiple interrupted 7-0 Prolene sutures to avoid "purse-stringing" of the opening into the aortic root. This interrupted suture line is carried up to meet the suture lines connecting the ascending aorta to the pulmonary homograft patch. The interrupted sutures are tied, and the continuous suture lines secured (Fig. 30.4). The pulmonary homograft patch and base of the pulmonary artery are pulled upward, and the patch trimmed to create an appropriate hood. The pulmonary base is sewn to the patch with a running 7-0 Prolene suture (Fig. 30.5).

⊘ Compression of Pulmonary Artery by Neoaorta

The homograft patch must not be too large or left too long because it may compress the central pulmonary artery. This is especially problematic if the original ascending aorta is larger than 3 to 4 mm in diameter. Pulmonary homograft tissue is fairly distensible, and this must be taken into consideration when fashioning the patch. ⊘

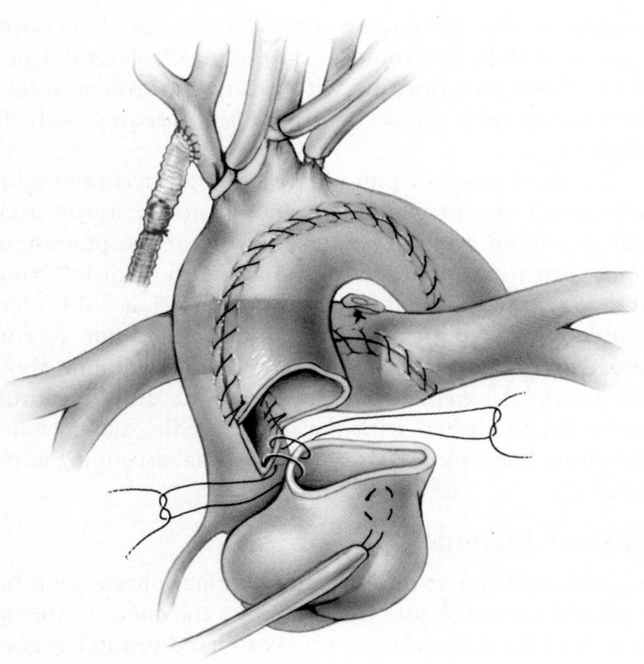

FIG. 30.4 Reconstructing aorta with triangular patch of pulmonary homograft. Anastomosing proximal pulmonary artery to aortic root with interrupted sutures.

NB Damus Modification

In some patients, most notably those with double inlet left ventricle, or those with double outlet right ventricle and mitral valve atresia, it is preferable to perform a modified Blalock-Taussig shunt, so as to eliminate the need for a left ventriculotomy, and also for ease because of the size of the reconstructed great vessel. In these patients, often the double-barrel modification of the Damus connection is simplest (Fig. 30.6). NB

⊘ Coronary Artery Compromise

Meticulous technique must be used when anastomosing a small ascending aorta to the proximal portion of the pulmonary artery to avoid obstructing flow into the coronary arteries (Fig. 30.5, inset). Some advocate an incision into the sinus of the pulmonary valve so as to increase the area of connection between the diminutive aorta and the pulmonary artery. ⊘

NB Modified Patch Technique

Some surgeons use a homograft patch to enlarge the entire opening beginning in the descending aorta, across the aortic arch, and down the ascending aorta to just above the sinotubular junction. Most of the patch is sewn in place with a running 7-0 Prolene suture, but the

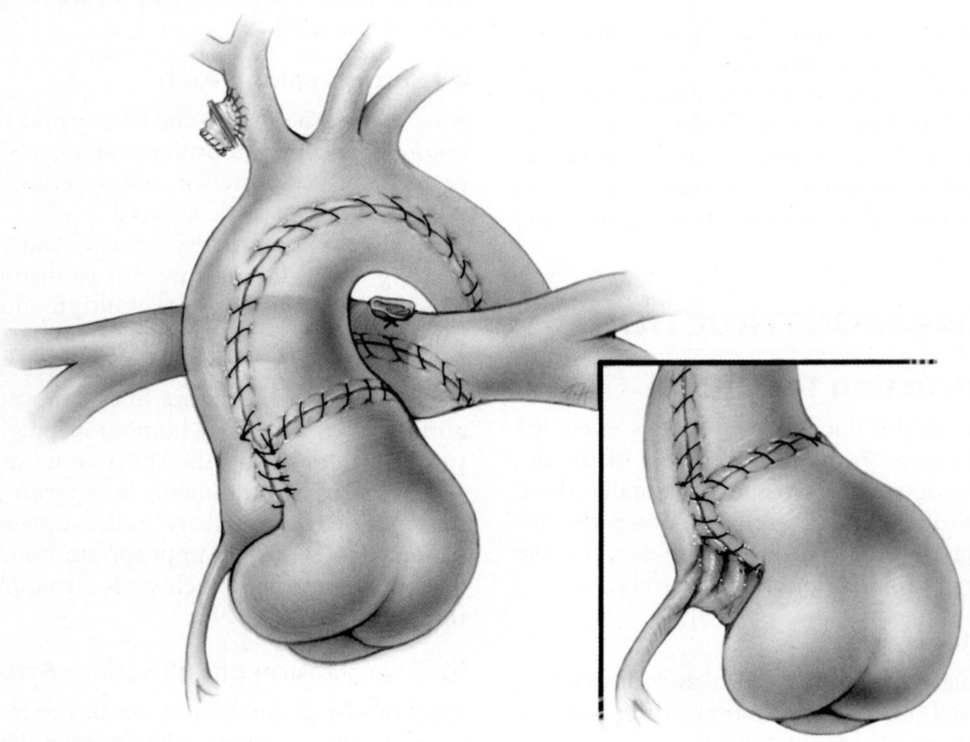

FIG. 30.5 Completed aortic reconstruction with metal clip on innominate graft site. **Inset:** Distortion of proximal aorta by inaccurate alignment of proximal pulmonary artery to aortic opening or purse-stringing of anastomosis.

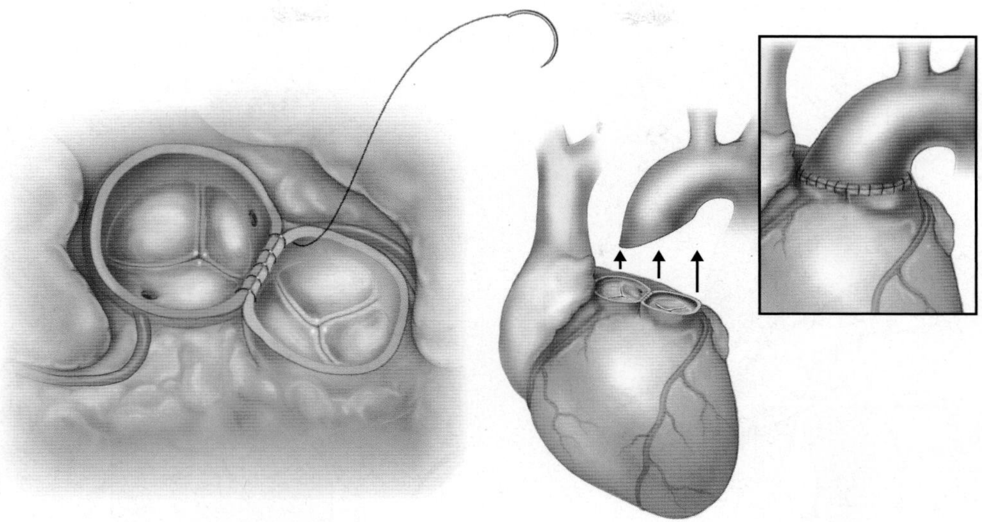

FIG. 30.6 Double-barrel modification of the Damus–Kaye–Stansel reconstruction with two large-sized semilunar valves.

proximal ascending aortic suture line is accomplished with interrupted sutures. An incision is made in the patch under the aortic arch, and the pulmonary base is anastomosed to this opening. A disadvantage of this technique is the lack of growth potential of the homograft patch, which is circumferentially attached to the pulmonary base. NB

Direct Anastomotic Arch Reconstruction

The ductus arteriosus and periductal aorta are excised (Fig. 30.7). The opening is carried proximally along the inferior aspect of the aortic arch to the level of the innominate artery (Fig. 30.8). The descending aorta is anastomosed to the aortic arch posterolaterally (Fig. 30.9).

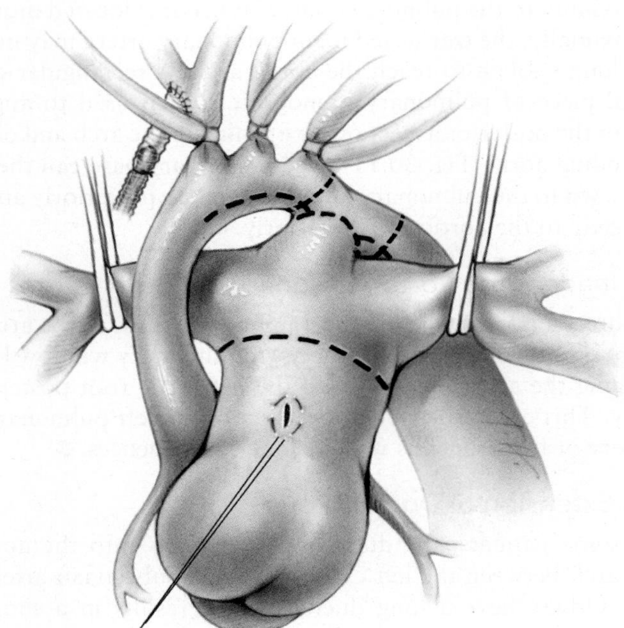

FIG. 30.7 Occlusion of the pulmonary arteries during cooling. The innominate, left carotid, and left subclavian arteries are snared down during low-flow cerebral perfusion. Dotted lines represent proposed incisions excising all ductal tissue.

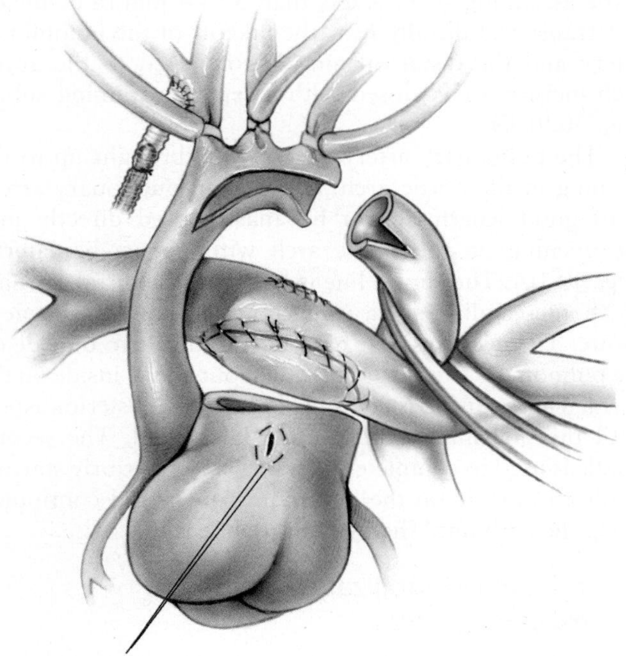

FIG. 30.8 Transection of the main pulmonary artery and a patch closure of the confluence. Oversewing of the pulmonary arterial end of the ductus arteriosus. Resection of periductal aortic segment and opening of the arch.

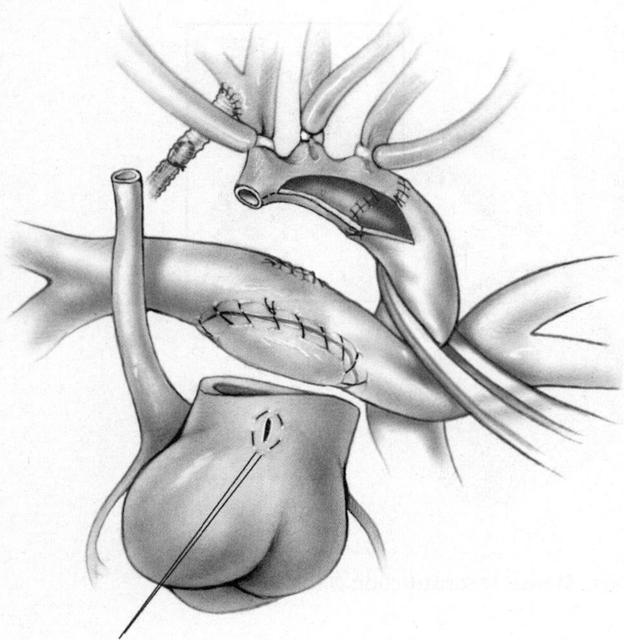

FIG. 30.9 Transecting the small ascending aorta. The distal opening may be connected to the incision on the inferior aspect of the aortic arch (dotted line).

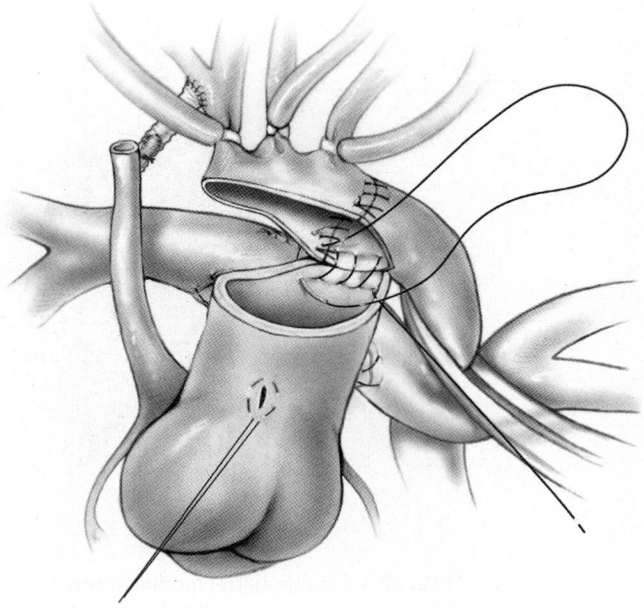

FIG. 30.10 All autologous tissue Norwood anastomosis joining the pulmonary artery base to the proximal descending aorta and underside of the arch. Note incision on medial aspect of descending aorta to divide any residual ductal tissue.

NB Small Ascending Aorta

If the ascending aorta is less than 3 to 4 mm in diameter, it is transected distally near the takeoff of the innominate artery and the distal opening is connected to the aortic arch incision or is closed with a separate running suture (Fig. 30.9). NB

The pulmonary artery base is now brought up to the opening in the aortic arch. If the main pulmonary artery is of good length, it can be anastomosed directly into the opening on the aortic arch with no patch material (Fig. 30.10). The suture line is begun at the distal opening on the descending aorta using double-armed 7-0 Prolene suture. The needle is first passed from inside to outside on the pulmonary artery base and then outside to inside on the aorta. This suturing is continued along the posterior aspect until the proximal arch opening is reached. The second needle is used to complete the suture line anteriorly starting inside to outside on the descending aorta and continuing along the arch until the first suture line is met.

⊘ Inadequate Mobilization of the Descending Aorta

The descending aorta must be aggressively mobilized at least 1 cm beyond the ductal insertion to allow a tension-free anastomosis. The curved clamp placed on the descending aorta helps to hold it in place and provides improved exposure for the distal extent of the anastomosis (Fig. 30.10). ⊘

⊘ Inadequate Length of the Main Pulmonary Artery

The takeoff of the right pulmonary artery is variable in its proximity to the pulmonary valve. When it is located more proximally, the transected main pulmonary artery may not be long enough to reach the aortic arch. A rectangular or oval piece of pulmonary homograft is then used to augment the posterior aspect of the opening in the arch and descending aorta (Fig. 30.11). The pulmonary base can then be sewn to the pulmonary homograft patch posteriorly and directly to the aortic arch anteriorly. ⊘

⊘ Inadequate Aortopulmonary Window

A direct anastomosis of a short pulmonary base to the arch may result in narrowing of the aortopulmonary window by pulling the arch inferiorly and the neoaortic root posteriorly. This can result in compression of the left pulmonary artery or left bronchus with serious consequences. ⊘

NB Extension of Ductal Tissue

In some patients, the ductal tissue extends into the aortic arch between the left carotid and left subclavian arteries. Others have a long ductus, which results in a short descending aorta after the ductal tissue is excised. A direct anastomosis in these circumstances is contraindicated. NB

NB Incision on Descending Aorta

Some surgeons advocate making a 5- to 10-mm opening on the medial aspect of the transected descending aorta

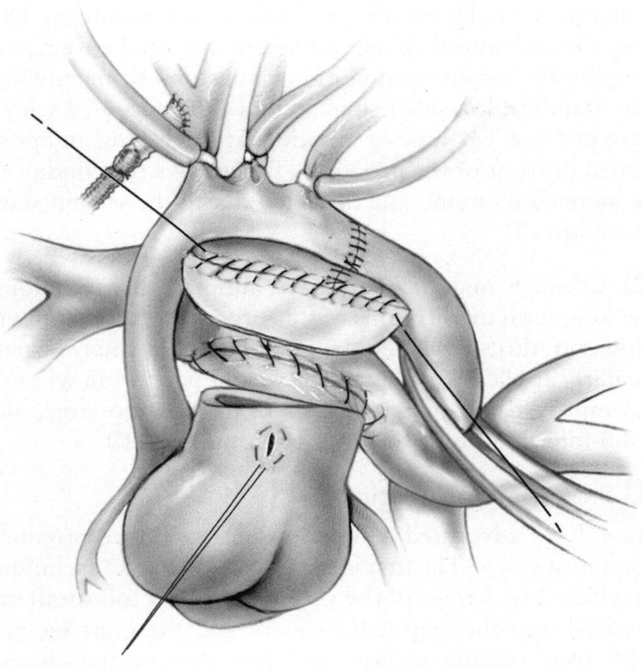

FIG. 30.11 Augmenting the posterior aspect of the aortic arch opening with a patch of pulmonary homograft.

(Fig. 30.10). This divides any potential residual ductal tissue. The pulmonary base is then anastomosed to the opening in the descending aorta and aortic arch. NB

If the ascending aorta has been transected, it is now trimmed to a length of 10 to 15 mm and the open end is beveled (Fig. 30.12). A 2.8-mm aortic punch is used to create a circular opening of the appropriate size on the posterolateral aspect of the main pulmonary artery. The anastomosis is performed in an end-to-side manner using a 7-0 or 8-0 Prolene suture.

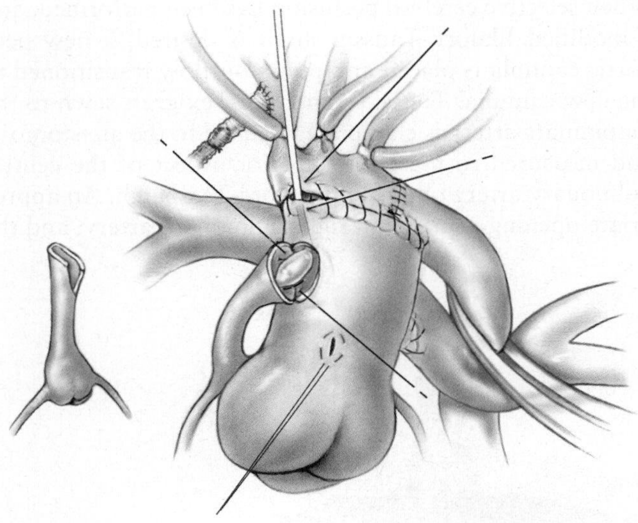

FIG. 30.12 Anastomosing the diminutive ascending aorta to the posterolateral aspect of the main pulmonary artery (neoaortic root). Note the probe introduced through the open arch anastomosis to prevent purse-stringing of the ascending aortic suture line.

⊘ Too Long an Ascending Aorta

If the diminutive aorta is left too long, it may kink, thereby causing coronary ischemia. ⊘

⊘ Purse-Stringing the Anastomosis

When the ascending aorta is 2 mm or less in diameter, the suture line of the main pulmonary artery to aortic arch may be left untied. When the ascending aortic anastomosis is complete, a 1.5- or 2-mm coronary probe is passed through the arch anastomosis into the ascending aorta, and the suture is tied over the probe to avoid purse-stringing the anastomosis (Fig. 30.12). ⊘

PULMONARY BLOOD FLOW

Traditionally, a small systemic-to-pulmonary shunt with a Gore-Tex tube from the innominate artery to the proximal right pulmonary artery has been used to supply controlled pulmonary blood flow in these patients. More recently, many centers have adopted a right ventricle–to–pulmonary artery graft to provide pulmonary blood flow. The potential advantages of this shunt include a higher diastolic blood pressure in these patients, leading to improved coronary perfusion, and a decreased risk of shunt thrombosis perioperatively. Some questions remain regarding the optimal shunt size and material, the effect on pulmonary artery growth, and the impact of the right ventriculotomy on ventricular function. After transecting the main pulmonary artery just below the bifurcation, an appropriate site for the right ventriculotomy is marked on the right ventricular outflow tract. This is carefully positioned 1.5 to 2.0 cm below the pulmonic valve. The confluence patch with the attached Gore-Tex tube is anastomosed to the opening at the pulmonary artery bifurcation.

Right Ventricle-Pulmonary Artery Shunt

During rewarming, a right ventriculotomy is made at the previously marked site. The proximal end of the tube graft is cut obliquely at the appropriate length and anastomosed to the ventriculotomy (Fig. 30.13).

⊘ Injury to Pulmonic Valve

The right ventriculotomy must be carefully positioned below the pulmonary valve leaflets as this is the patient's neoaortic valve. Marking the position with the pulmonary root open is the best way to avoid injuring this valve. ⊘

⊘ Size of Ventriculotomy

Dynamic narrowing of the inflow to these shunts has been observed. Ingrowth of tissue from the ventricular endocardium

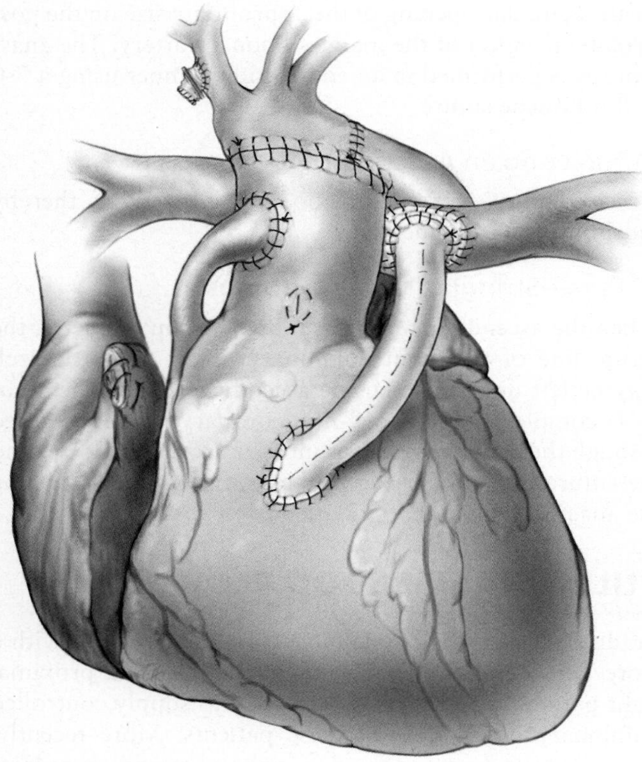

FIG. 30.13 Right ventricle-pulmonary artery shunt. Distal end attached to patch on pulmonary artery confluence. Proximal anastomosis to right ventriculotomy.

has also been reported. An adequate core of muscle must be removed along with a slice of underlying endocardium. However, it must be kept in mind that this is the patient's systemic ventricle. The ventriculotomy should be no larger than required for unobstructed shunt inflow. Some use a coronary arotic punch to remove the right ventricular muscle underlying the incision. If the "dunk" technique (See below) is utilized, a skin punch of appropriate size is used (Fig. 30.14). ⊘

NB To facilitate the second-stage procedure, some surgeons place the conduit from the right ventricle to the right pulmonary artery on the right side of the neoaorta. This may make removal of the prosthetic material easier, and simplify the reconstruction of any anastomotic narrowing. The standard left-sided shunt can also be encircled with a strip of Gore-Tex tape or Silastic that is left long and positioned in front of the neoaorta. This allows the conduit to be more easily found and dissected free at the second-stage procedure. NB

NB Although many centers have adopted this technique, the long-term implications of this procedure are unknown. However, this source of pulmonary blood flow may be particularly applicable in low-birth-weight patients in whom a 3.5-mm systemic–pulmonary shunt may be too large, and a 3.0-mm shunt may be prone to thrombosis. NB

NB Proximal Connection

Some have advocated several options to reduce proximal conduit stenosis. The first is the so-called "dunk" technique in which 2 to 3 rings of the ringed Gore-Tex tube graft are inserted into the ventricular cavity and the graft secured with four tacking sutures and two purse-string sutures (Fig. 30.15). Others have advocated for creating a hood on the proximal graft of homograft so as to reduce the angulation required in a direct connection (Fig. 30.16). NB

NB Gore-Tex Graft on Innominate Artery

If a right ventricle-pulmonary artery shunt is constructed, the tube graft sewn to the innominate artery is occluded with a large metal clip near the anastomosis, cut short, and the end oversewn (Fig. 30.13). NB

Systemic–Pulmonary Shunt

When selective cerebral perfusion has been performed, and a modified Blalock-Taussig shunt is desired, a new neoaortic cannula is placed and pump outflow transitioned to the new cannula. The 3.5-mm Gore-Tex graft sewn to the innominate artery is clamped just distal to the anastomosis and measured to meet the superior aspect of the central pulmonary artery opposite the Gore-Tex patch. An appropriate opening is made on right pulmonary artery, and the

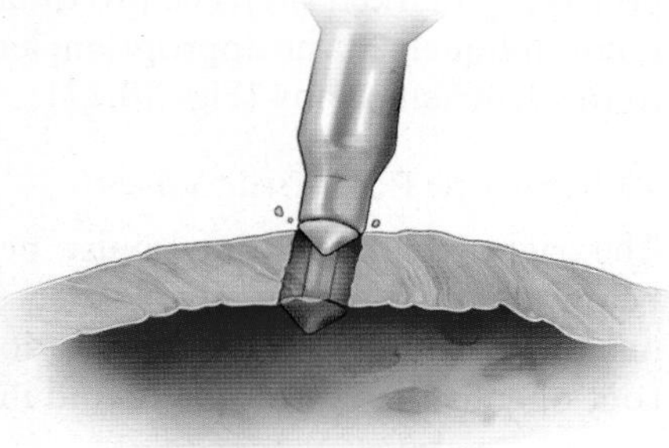

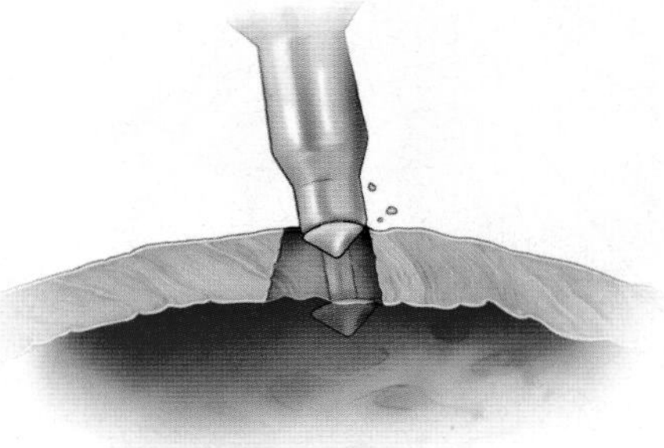

FIG. 30.14 Use of a punch to enlarge the proximal ventriculotomy by undermining the muscle.

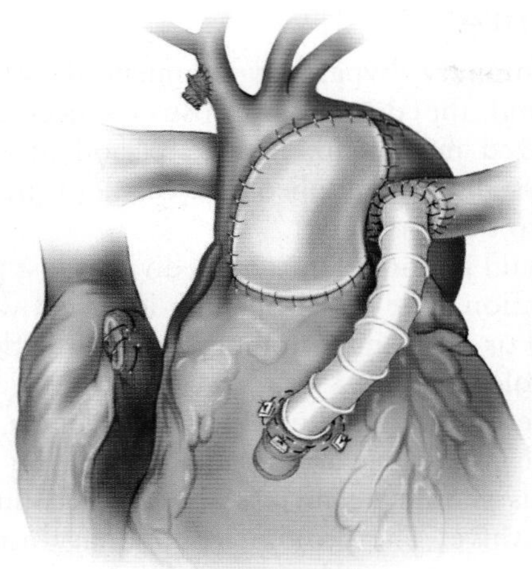

FIG. 30.15 "Dunk" technique for the proximal Sano (with graft shown inside the ventricle, and concentric purse-string sutures).

tube graft is anastomosed in an end-to-side manner with a running 7-0 Prolene suture (Fig. 30.17). The shunt is then clamped with a bulldog vascular clamp for the remainder of the rewarming period.

NB Shunt Placement on Pulmonary Artery

The distal end of the shunt should be placed as centrally as possible, close to the oversewn ductus on the proximal pulmonary artery. This theoretically should allow more uniform growth of both pulmonary arteries. In addition, it may

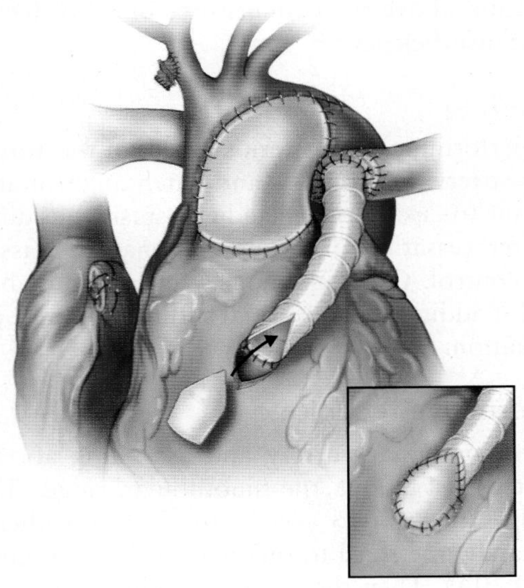

FIG. 30.16 Modification of the proximal Sano to reduce angulation using a prosthetic hood of pentagon-shaped material.

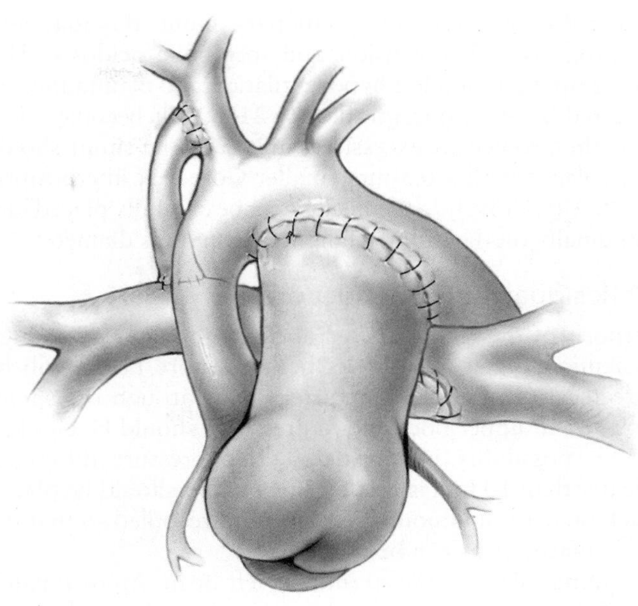

FIG. 30.17 Completed aortic reconstruction when the ascending aorta is not diminutive. Gore-Tex tube graft from the innominate to proximal right pulmonary artery.

allow the bidirectional Glenn procedure to be performed without cardiopulmonary bypass (see Chapter 31). NB

After rewarming is completed, the shunt is opened and the patient is weaned off cardiopulmonary bypass. Pulmonary vascular resistance is often high for the first 15 to 30 minutes after weaning off bypass. It may be necessary to hyperventilate the patient aggressively during this time with 100% FIO_2. Nitric oxide may be useful in these patients. The oxygen saturation may be as low as 50% to 60% during this period. If adequate ventricular function appears to be maintained, these low saturations should be tolerated.

⊘ Persistent Low Oxygen Saturation

If very low oxygen saturations persist, the cause must be determined. One cause of low systemic oxygen saturation is low cardiac output with very low mixed venous saturations. Direct visualization of the heart or, preferably, transesophageal assessment of ventricular function is useful. If decreased function is noted, an increase in inotropic support may improve the situation. If the myocardial contractility remains poor, extracorporeal membrane oxygenator support may be indicated. ⊘

If a systemic–pulmonary shunt has been used, and shunt flow is thought to be inadequate, the patient should be placed back on cardiopulmonary bypass and the shunt revised. It may be appropriate to up size the shunt from 3.0 to 3.5 mm, or 3.5 to 4.0 mm.

⊘ Persistent High Oxygen Saturations

High oxygen saturations greater than 85% usually indicate excessive pulmonary blood flow. If the source of pulmonary blood flow is a systemic–pulmonary shunt, this may lead to progressive hypotension and metabolic acidosis. This may respond to modest hypoventilation and maintaining an inspired oxygen concentration of 21%. If it becomes clear that the problem is excessive shunt size, the shunt should be replaced with a 0.5-mm smaller Gore-Tex interposition graft. Alternatively, a metal clip may be carefully placed longitudinally on the shunt tubing to decrease its diameter. ⊘

⊘ Residual Arch Obstruction

Stenosis of the reconstructed aortic arch may lead to high systemic oxygen saturations because more blood will be directed to the innominate artery and through the shunt. Lower and upper body blood pressures should be checked if this possibility is considered. If a pressure difference greater than 10 mm is present, the patient should be placed back on cardiopulmonary bypass, and recooled so that the arch anastomosis can be revised. ⊘

In many cases, the sternum is left open. An oval patch of Silastic is sutured to the skin edges over the mediastinal chest tube. Povidone iodine (Betadine) ointment is applied to the suture line, and the entire chest is covered with a Betadine-impregnated Vi-Drape.

⊘ Dysrhythmias

After weaning off cardiopulmonary bypass, dysrhythmias often indicate inadequate coronary perfusion. If discoloration of the ventricle is observed or inadequate coronary arterial filling is noted, cardiopulmonary bypass should be recommenced. The anastomosis between the ascending aorta and proximal main pulmonary artery may need to be revised. ⊘

DAMUS–KAYE–STANSEL PROCEDURE

Patients with a single ventricle and mild or potential obstruction to systemic blood flow probably are best served by application of the Norwood principle. Banding the pulmonary artery in such patients may encourage the development of a subaortic obstruction and should be avoided. In these cases, two outlets for systemic perfusion are created by anastomosing the pulmonary artery to the ascending aorta, often referred to as the Damus–Kaye–Stansel procedure. Controlled pulmonary blood flow is then established by interposing a Gore-Tex graft from the innominate artery to the right pulmonary artery.

Incision

A median sternotomy is performed. The thymus is excised, and a patch of autologous pericardium is harvested and prepared in 0.6% glutaraldehyde solution.

Cannulation

The distal ascending aorta and right atrium are cannulated, and the ductus arteriosus is dissected free from surrounding structures.

Procedure

Cardiopulmonary bypass is commenced with systemic cooling, and the ductus arteriosus is occluded with a medium-sized metal clip. After a period of cooling, the aortic cross-clamp is applied and cardioplegic solution is infused into the aortic root.

The main pulmonary artery is divided just proximal to the bifurcation. The distal opening is closed with an oval pericardial or pulmonary homograft patch with a continuous 6-0 Prolene suture.

A generous longitudinal incision is made on the left side of the ascending aorta, adjacent to the pulmonary artery. This should begin just above the commissures of the aortic valve. The proximal pulmonary artery is then opened longitudinally adjacent to the incision in the aorta (Fig. 30.18).

The proximal portion of the anastomosis is started at the inferior extent of the incisions on the aorta and pulmonary artery with a running 6-0 or 7-0 Prolene suture. To prevent distortion of the pulmonary root, the distal aspect of the anastomosis is completed by using a hemicone-shaped patch of pericardium or pulmonary homograft to augment the pulmonary artery to aorta confluence with a continuous 6-0 or 7-0 Prolene suture (Fig. 30.19).

⊘ Tension on the Valvular Apparatus

Care must be taken not to distort either the pulmonary or aortic valves when performing this anastomosis. Any tension on the valve annulus may result in valvular insufficiency. ⊘

⊘ Injury to the Valve

When opening the ascending aorta, it is important to keep the incision above the commissures of the valve to avoid valvular insufficiency. ⊘

⊘ Bleeding

While performing the posterior aspect of the aorta to pulmonary artery anastomosis and patch augmentation, it is important to ensure complete hemostasis. Bleeding in this area after cessation of cardiopulmonary bypass is difficult to control. Cardiopulmonary bypass must be recommenced if additional adventitial sutures are to be placed in this situation. ⊘

NB Alternative Technique

Both the pulmonary artery and ascending aorta can be transected just above the sinotubular ridge. The adjacent edges of the two vessels are sewn together for approximately one-third to one-half of their circumferences (Fig. 30.20A). Then the distal ascending aorta is anastomosed to the posterior aspect of the double-barrel root with a 5-0 or 6-0 Prolene suture. The anterior opening is then closed with an oval piece of pulmonary homograft (Fig. 30.20B). NB

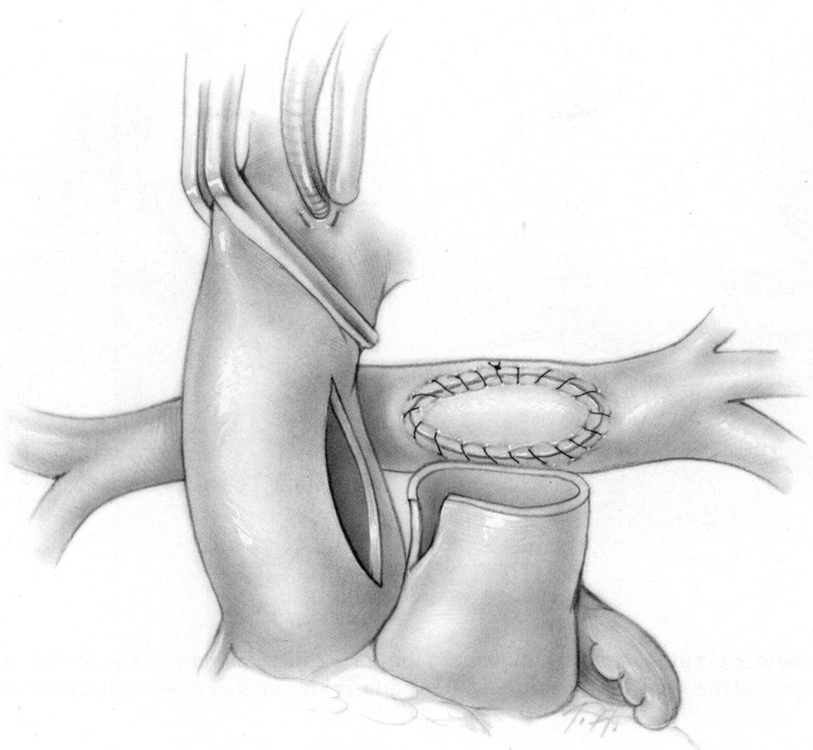

FIG. 30.18 Damus–Kaye–Stansel procedure. The distal pulmonary artery opening is closed with a patch. The medial aspect of the aorta is opened and a corresponding opening is made in the proximal pulmonary artery.

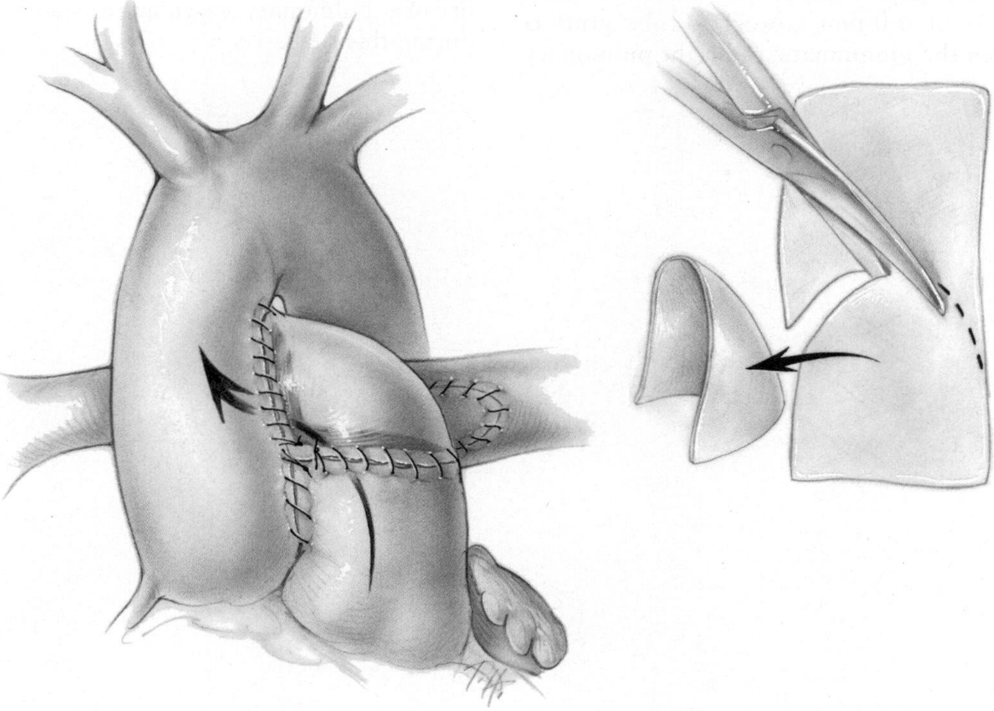

FIG. 30.19 The completed Damus–Kaye–Stansel anastomosis. Inset: Fashioning the hemicone-shaped patch to complete the pulmonary artery–aortic anastomosis.

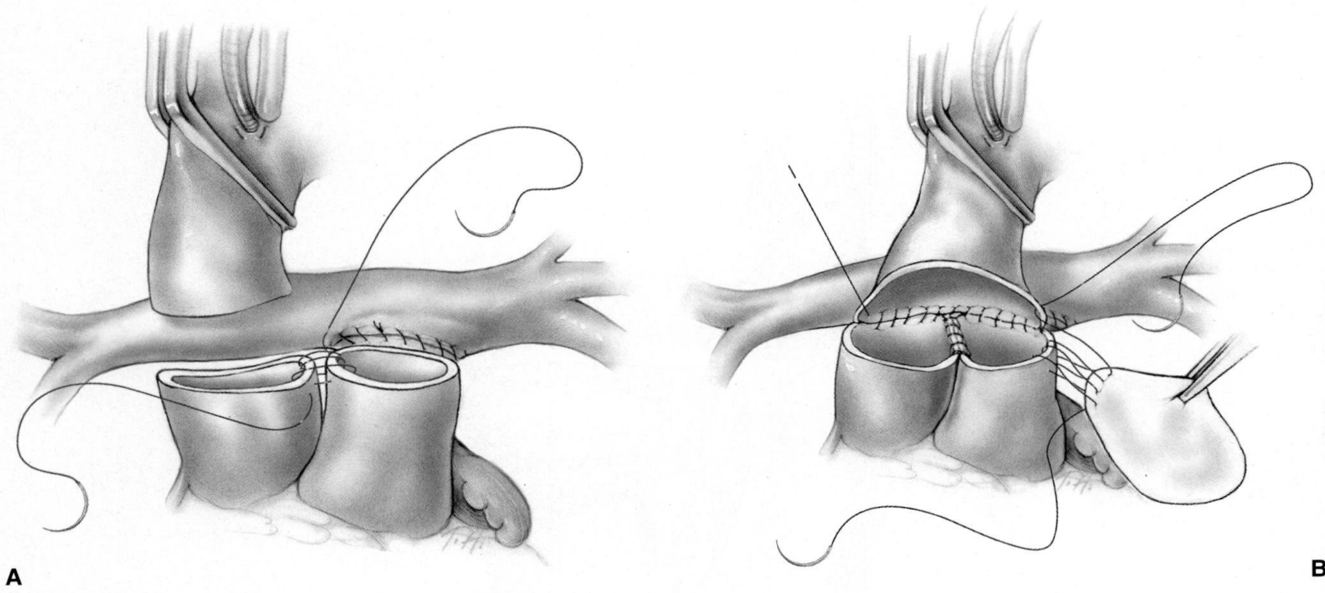

FIG. 30.20 Creating a double-barrel outflow tract by transecting the aorta and pulmonary artery. **A:** The two roots are anastomosed together along adjacent sides and then attached to the ascending aorta. **B:** The anterior opening is closed with a patch of a pulmonary homograft.

Completion of the Operation

This is also the preferred method if any augmentation is required of the transverse aortic arch. After removal of the aortic cross-clamp, a modified Blalock–Taussig shunt using a 3.5- or 4.0-mm Gore-Tex tube graft is performed between the innominate and right pulmonary arteries during systemic rewarming. The shunt should be clamped until cardiopulmonary bypass is discontinued, at which point the shunt is opened. Vigorous hyperventilation may be required in the early postbypass period because pulmonary vascular resistance is often elevated during this time.

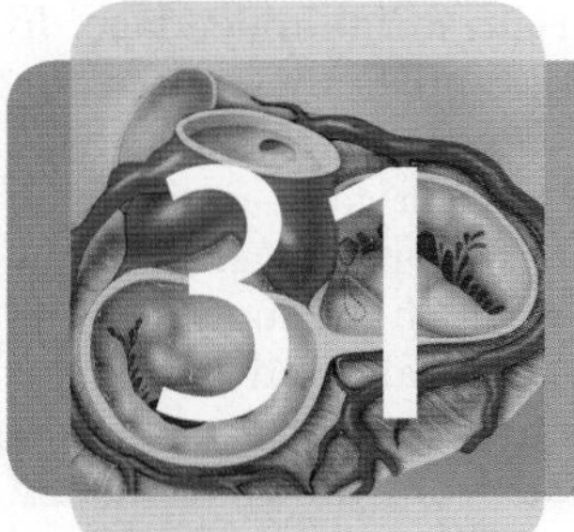

31 The Fontan Principle

The Fontan principle is applied to patients with single-ventricle congenital heart disease. The ultimate goal is to achieve a circulation in which the systemic venous return is delivered directly to the pulmonary arteries, and the single ventricle is used for systemic blood flow. The original Fontan operation utilized an atriopulmonary connection for patients with tricuspid atresia. Since then, the procedure and its indications have evolved, allowing for a Fontan circulation in many single-ventricle patients.

PATHOPHYSIOLOGY OF A SINGLE VENTRICLE

The patient with a single ventricle may present in a variety of ways depending on the presence or absence of obstruction to pulmonary or systemic flow. Severe obstruction to pulmonary flow results in cyanosis. Obstruction to systemic flow may lead to inadequate systemic perfusion and a low cardiac output state. The flow of blood through a patent ductus arteriosus bypasses the obstruction in either the pulmonary or systemic circulation, maintaining a clinically stable state. However, when the ductus starts to close, clinical deterioration becomes evident. In a small group of patients, there is no or minimal obstruction to systemic or pulmonary blood flow. Initially, these patients may demonstrate well-balanced pulmonary and systemic circulations. However, as the pulmonary vascular resistance diminishes over the first several weeks of life, pulmonary blood flow increases and congestive heart failure develops. If pulmonary venous obstruction is present, the patient may be cyanotic owing to increased pulmonary vascular resistance.

Management of the neonate with a single ventricle is directed at achieving adequate systemic oxygenation while preventing the development of pulmonary vascular disease. Surgical intervention may be required to achieve unimpeded outflow from the single ventricle into the systemic circulation. Adequate mixing of systemic and pulmonary venous blood must be ensured. These hemodynamic parameters allow the patient to become a candidate for a subsequent Fontan procedure.

Surgical Management

Infants younger than 3 months with inadequate pulmonary blood flow require a systemic–pulmonary artery shunt (see Chapter 18). Infants with excessive pulmonary blood flow with no obstruction to systemic outflow require early intervention aimed at reducing the volume load on the systemic ventricle and reducing pulmonary blood flow to prevent pulmonary vascular disease. In the past, pulmonary artery banding has been used to accomplish these goals (see Chapter 16). However, pulmonary artery banding may not limit pulmonary blood flow sufficiently or may result in distortion of the right or both pulmonary arteries. Therefore, many surgeons believe that division and oversewing of the proximal main pulmonary artery with construction of a systemic–pulmonary shunt is the best palliation in these cases. Patients who have both excessive pulmonary blood flow and obstruction to systemic outflow are best treated with a combined Damus–Kaye–Stansel procedure and a shunt (see Chapter 30).

Management after the Neonatal Period

The goal in these patients is to minimize both the pressure and volume load on the single ventricle as soon as possible. All patients should undergo routine cardiac catheterization at 4 to 6 months of age. If signs or symptoms of ventricular dysfunction, atrioventricular valve problems, or increased pulmonary vascular resistance are noted, the study should be performed earlier. These patients are prone to develop aortopulmonary collateral vessels. Therefore, during cardiac catheterization, a search for collateral vessels should be made, and, if present, they should be occluded with coils.

Any aortic arch or subaortic obstruction that has not been dealt with previously must be corrected before proceeding with any other surgical interventions. Subaortic obstruction may require a Damus–Kay–Stansel procedure (see Chapter 30) or enlargement of the bulboventricular foramen. Aortic arch obstruction or discrete coarctation may respond to balloon angioplasty or may require surgical intervention (see Chapters 15 and 29). Any situation that requires the single ventricle to pump blood to both the systemic and pulmonary circulations puts a so-called volume load on that ventricle. All single-ventricle complexes initially have an extra volume load on the ventricle. This is true whether the pulmonary blood flow is provided through a systemic–pulmonary artery shunt, or through controlled forward flow from the single ventricle, as is seen with pulmonic stenosis or following a pulmonary artery banding procedure. A superior cavopulmonary connection removes some of the volume load from the ventricle because all pulmonary blood flow is directly from the superior vena cava. The ventricle provides forward flow into the systemic circulation only. This procedure can be performed successfully once the elevated pulmonary vascular resistance has fallen, usually after 3 months of age. Early removal of the volume load on the ventricle will potentially improve its long-term function.

By performing the Fontan connection in two stages, the operative risk for the completion Fontan operation has been reduced. When the volume load is acutely removed from the ventricle, the afterload of the single ventricle has been shown to increase. This afterload increasing effect is smaller when only the superior vena cava is connected to the pulmonary artery as compared to the Fontan procedure in which all systemic venous return is diverted into the pulmonary artery. The staged approach lessens the impact of afterload mismatch at each stage. The decrease in diastolic ventricular volume is also less with the superior cavopulmonary connection. By staging the Fontan, the sometimes fatal combination of ventricular hypertrophy and a sudden decrease in diastolic volume can be avoided.

BIDIRECTIONAL GLENN PROCEDURE

The classic cavopulmonary, or Glenn, shunt achieved by anastomosing the transected superior vena cava to the transected right pulmonary artery is rarely performed today. The bidirectional superior cavopulmonary anastomosis, or bidirectional Glenn, allows superior vena caval return to enter both the right and left pulmonary arteries. Because only 40% to 50% of the systemic venous return is presented to the pulmonary arterial bed, patients who would not be candidates for a full Fontan procedure may be able to undergo a bidirectional Glenn shunt. This procedure is often used as part of a staged approach for the patient with a single ventricle. The bidirectional Glenn may also be used in patients with small or dysfunctional right ventricles to create a so-called one and one-half ventricle repair. This may allow some patients who are not candidates for a two-ventricle repair to have the right ventricle manage part of the systemic venous return.

Cannulation

A standard median sternotomy is performed. A bidirectional Glenn may be performed without cardiopulmonary bypass, using a shunt between the most proximal aspect of the superior vena cava and the right atrial appendage. In this case, two right-angled venous cannulas are selected, approximating the size of the superior vena cava. Purse-string sutures are placed at the superior vena cava–innominate vein junction and in the right atrial appendage. Systemic heparin is then administered, after which the superior vena caval cannula is placed. The cannula is allowed to fill with blood and clamped. A second cannula is then placed in the right atrial appendage. The blood from the right atrium is allowed to fill this cannula, which is then connected to the first cannula, making sure no air is trapped in the connector. The shunt is opened to allow flow from the superior vena cava into the right atrium. Any previously placed systemic to pulmonary artery shunts are dissected circumferentially. The azygos vein is doubly ligated with fine silk ties and divided between the ligatures to allow full mobilization of the superior vena cava and prevent later venous runoff after the Glenn. A tape around the superior vena caval cannula is now snared, and an angled vascular clamp is placed just above the right atrium–superior vena cava junction. The superior vena cava is then transected (Fig. 31.1). The right atrium–superior vena cava junction is oversewn with a running 6-0 Prolene suture, and the vascular clamp is removed.

⊘ Torsion of the Superior Vena Cava

A marking suture should be placed on the superior vena cava to maintain the orientation of the vessel during the anastomosis. ⊘

The superior aspect of the right pulmonary artery is either grasped with a curved clamp or the branch pulmonary

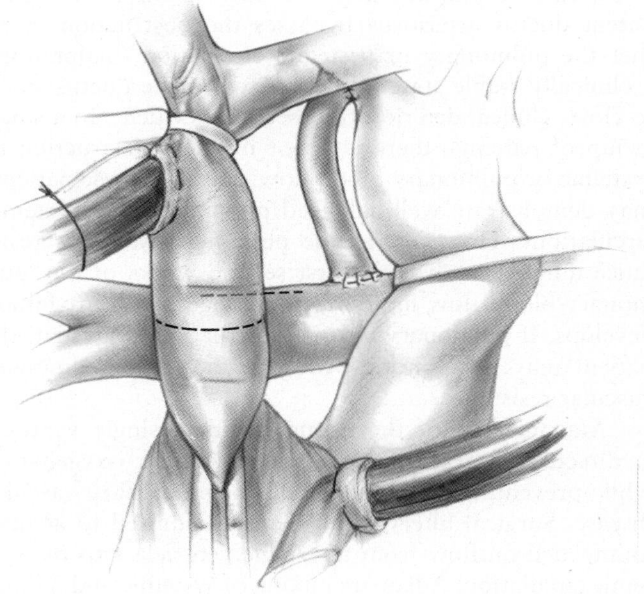

FIG. 31.1 Bidirectional Glenn shunt: Transection of the superior vena cava and a longitudinal opening on the superior aspect of the right pulmonary artery.

arteries are controlled with silastic tapes, and an opening on the superior aspect of the right pulmonary artery is made with a knife blade and Potts scissors. The anastomosis of the superior vena cava to the right pulmonary artery is then accomplished with a running 6-0 or 7-0 Prolene suture beginning at the most medial aspect of the pulmonary arteriotomy, completing the posterior row with one needle, and then the anterior aspect with the second needle (Fig. 31.2).

NB If the bidirectional Glenn is to be performed off pump, the source of pulmonary blood flow must be maintained during the construction of the anastomosis. If the pulmonary flow is from the ventricle through a native valve, pulmonary band, or ventricular–pulmonary shunt, placement of the clamp on the right pulmonary artery should be well tolerated. However, if a systemic–pulmonary shunt to the right pulmonary artery is present, the clamp on the right pulmonary artery must be placed carefully. Unless the previous shunt is centrally located on the right pulmonary artery, it may not be possible to perform the bidirectional Glenn without cardiopulmonary bypass. NB

⊘ Tension on the Superior Vena Cava–Pulmonary Artery Anastomosis

Tension on the anastomosis between the superior vena cava and right pulmonary artery must be avoided by leaving the superior vena cava as long as possible and placing the opening on the right pulmonary artery as close to the transected superior vena cava as feasible. This avoids any tension on the anastomosis that may lead to intraoperative bleeding from the suture line, dehiscence of the suture line, or long-term fibrosis and narrowing of the anastomosis. ⊘

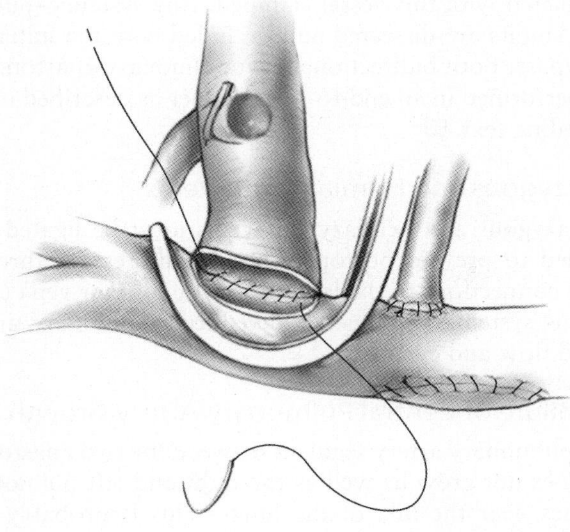

FIG. 31.2 Bidirectional Glenn shunt: Completing the posterior suture line.

⊘ Purse-Stringing the Anastomosis

It may be prudent to use interrupted sutures on the anterior aspect of the anastomosis to prevent a purse-string effect and narrowing of the anastomosis. This is especially important if the superior vena cava is small in diameter, as is seen when bilateral superior venae cavae are present. Some surgeons advocate the use of intermittent lock sutures along the anterior suture line to mitigate this problem. ⊘

Completing the Shunt

The clamp on the pulmonary artery is removed, and the anastomosis is inspected for bleeding and patency. The shunt tubing is clamped, the superior vena caval cannula is taken out, and the purse-string suture is secured. Any previously placed systemic–pulmonary or ventricular–pulmonary shunt is occluded with metal clips. If forward flow from the ventricle is present, the pulmonary artery may be tightly banded or transected and oversewn. The right atrial cannula is removed, and protamine is administered.

⊘ Injury to the Sinoatrial Node

The sinoatrial node is located on the lateral aspect of the junction between the atrium and superior vena cava and is prone to injury. The surgeon should place the clamp well away from this area, and suturing should be carried out with this potential complication in mind. ⊘

⊘ Ligation of Pulmonary Artery

Ligation of the pulmonary artery creates a space between the pulmonic valve and the ligature where stasis occurs and thrombus frequently develops. The main pulmonary artery either should be transected just above the valve, the pulmonic valve oversewn, and both ends closed with a running 5-0 or 6-0 Prolene suture or the leaflets excised in their entirety under direct vision. ⊘

NB Additional Pulmonary Blood Flow

Some surgeons believe that an additional source of pulmonary blood flow is important is these patients. This can be achieved by leaving a systemic–pulmonary or ventricular–pulmonary shunt in place, with or without narrowing the conduit. If forward flow from the ventricle is present, the pulmonary artery can be tightly banded. The beneficial effects of these procedures are an increase in the oxygen saturation levels and potentially better pulmonary artery growth. The downside is increasing the volume load on the ventricle. If additional pulmonary flow is maintained, the pulmonary artery pressure must be monitored. NB

NB Development of Pulmonary Arteriovenous Malformations

The incidence of pulmonary arteriovenous malformations increases with time following a bidirectional Glenn procedure. This is felt to be due to the exclusion of hepatic venous blood from the pulmonary arterial circulation. This can lead to progressive cyanosis if patients are left with the bidirectional Glenn circulation for a prolonged period of time. Because the bidirectional Glenn is most often performed as part of a staged Fontan procedure, pulmonary arteriovenous malformations are usually not an issue. Bidirectional Glenn should not be the final procedure for patients who are not candidates for a full Fontan procedure because of the significant risk of developing these pulmonary arteriovenous malformations. The restoration of hepatic venous flow to the pulmonary arterial bed leads to the regression of these malformations. Prevention of these pulmonary arteriovenous malformations is one argument made by surgeons who prefer to maintain an additional source of pulmonary blood flow when performing the bidirectional Glenn procedure. NB

⊘ High Pulmonary Artery Pressure

A pulmonary artery pressure greater than 20 mm Hg will not be tolerated and this circumstance may necessitate interrupting additional sources of flow into the pulmonary artery. ⊘

If superior vena caval pressures remain high, direct needle measurements of the pressure in the pulmonary artery and superior vena cava should be made to rule out an anastomotic problem. If pulmonary artery pressures remain at 20 or above despite maneuvers to reduce pulmonary vascular resistance, the bidirectional Glenn must be taken down, the superior vena cava reanastomosed to the right atrium, and a systemic to pulmonary artery shunt performed.

⊘ Leaving Shunt Tubing Intact

If the previously placed systemic–pulmonary or ventricular–pulmonary shunt is simply occluded with a metal clip and not divided, the pulmonary artery may become distorted. It is preferable to clip the shunt tubing proximally and distally and divide it. ⊘

⊘ Narrowing of the Superior Vena Cava at the Cannulation Site

Simply tying down the purse-string suture at the superior vena caval cannulation site may result in significant distortion and obstruction to flow into the distal superior vena cava and pulmonary artery. If this occurs, the superior vena cava should be grasped with a shallow curved clamp, the purse-string suture removed, and the opening meticulously repaired with a running or interrupted 7-0 Prolene sutures. ⊘

BIDIRECTIONAL GLENN ON CARDIOPULMONARY BYPASS

In some patients, it is necessary or preferable to perform the bidirectional Glenn shunt on cardiopulmonary bypass. This is particularly true when patients require reconstruction of the pulmonary arteries, or in patients with bilateral superior venae cavae who require bilateral bidirectional Glenn shunts. In these cases, cannulation of the ascending aorta, very proximal superior vena cava, and right atrium is performed. Cardiopulmonary bypass is commenced, and previously placed systemic–pulmonary or ventricular–pulmonary shunts are closed. The previously described procedure for anastomosis of the superior vena cava to the right pulmonary artery can then be performed with the heart decompressed.

⊘ Distally Placed Shunt

If a previous systemic–pulmonary shunt has been positioned close to the takeoff of the right upper lobe branch of the pulmonary artery, the bidirectional Glenn must be carried out on cardiopulmonary bypass. The shunt is clipped proximally and divided. The pulmonary artery end of the shunt is removed, and the resultant opening in the pulmonary artery is enlarged and anastomosed to the superior vena cava. ⊘

NB Bilateral Superior Venae Cavae

Most patients with bilateral superior venae cavae require bilateral bidirectional Glenn shunts. Rarely, there is a sizable bridging vein, which may allow the smaller of the two superior venae cavae to be ligated, and a unilateral bidirectional Glenn shunt performed with the larger vena cava. The operation is most often performed on cardiopulmonary bypass with a beating heart. Both superior venae cavae may be cannulated as superiorly as possible. Alternatively, the left superior vena cava may be test occluded while monitoring the pressure above the site of occlusion. If the pressure is above 20 mm Hg, the left superior vena cava is cannulated for cardiopulmonary bypass. If the pressure is less than 20 mm Hg, the anastomosis of the left superior vena cava to the left pulmonary artery may be completed with this vessel clamped. Any systemic–pulmonary shunts are dissected and occluded with the initiation of bypass. Both bidirectional cavopulmonary anastomoses are performed in an end-to-side manner as described in the preceding text. NB

⊘ Azygous and Hemiazygous Veins

The azygous and hemiazygous veins must be ligated and divided to prevent postoperative decompression through these connections to the lower pressure inferior vena caval venous system. This results in reduced pulmonary artery blood flow and cyanosis. ⊘

⊘ Failure of Central Pulmonary Artery Growth

The pulmonary artery segment between the two anastomoses does not grow as well as the right and left pulmonary arteries near the hila of the lungs. This is probably due to selective flow into the lungs, and may result in relative stasis in the central pulmonary artery and even thrombus formation. Each vena cava should be anastomosed to the pulmonary artery as medially as possible to minimize this segment. ⊘

⊘ Thrombosis of Cavopulmonary Circulation

The risk of thrombus developing in the cavopulmonary circuit is increased in patients with bilateral superior venae cavae. This may be related to the smaller size of the vessels with lower flow and a higher risk of anastomotic problems. Meticulous attention to detail in performing these suture lines is critical, and interrupted sutures for the entire anastomosis may be indicated. Some surgeons prefer to wait until the patient is 6 to 9 months of age to perform a bilateral bidirectional Glenn procedure when the vessels are somewhat bigger. In addition, central lines involving the superior venae cavae should be avoided or removed as early as possible following surgery. ⊘

NB Interrupted Inferior Vena Cava with Azygous Continuation

A bidirectional Glenn shunt in patients with heterotaxy syndrome and interrupted inferior vena cava with azygous continuation to the superior vena cava incorporates approximately 85% of the systemic venous return into the pulmonary circulation. Only the coronary sinus and hepatic venous flow are excluded. In these cases, the azygous vein obviously must not be ligated, as it carries most of the subdiaphragmatic systemic venous return. This procedure was initially viewed as definitive therapy for these patients. However, over time, many of these patients develop pulmonary arteriovenous malformations and progressive cyanosis. These patients should undergo a simultaneous or staged procedure to divert the hepatic veins to the pulmonary artery through a lateral tunnel or extracardiac conduit (see subsequent text). Some surgeons advocate a direct connection of the hepatic veins to the azygous vein. NB

NB Anomalous Pulmonary Venous Connection

Intracardiac types of anomalous pulmonary venous drainage do not require intervention. Other types may be dealt with by anastomosing the pulmonary venous confluence to the left or common atrium and ligating the connecting vein. In certain supracardiac types with anomalous drainage into the right or left superior vena cava close to the atrium, the involved vena cava may be divided above the pulmonary vein entrance site. The proximal end is anastomosed to the pulmonary artery, and the distal portion is carefully oversewn to allow the anomalous veins to enter the atrium. NB

HEMI-FONTAN PROCEDURE

The bidirectional Glenn has the advantage of being relatively simple to carry out and can be accomplished without cardiopulmonary bypass or on cardiopulmonary bypass with a beating heart. It prepares the patient for an extracardiac conduit from the inferior vena cava to the pulmonary artery as the completion Fontan procedure. However, patients who require extensive augmentation of the pulmonary arteries may be better served by a so-called hemi-Fontan procedure. Some surgeons use this operation routinely as the second-stage procedure in patients with hypoplastic left heart syndrome. The hemi-Fontan procedure prepares the patient for a lateral tunnel intraatrial baffling of the inferior vena caval flow to the pulmonary artery as the completion Fontan operation.

Technique

A median sternotomy approach is used. The procedure may be carried out under hypothermic arrest or with continuous cardiopulmonary bypass and moderate hypothermia. The ascending aorta is cannulated in the usual manner. A single right-angled cannula is placed in the right atrial appendage if hypothermic arrest is used. Alternatively, a right-angled cannula is placed at the superior vena caval–innominate vein junction and a second right-angled cannula is placed at the junction of the right atrium and inferior vena cava.

Cardiopulmonary bypass is initiated, and any previously placed shunt is mobilized and closed with a metal clip. If hypothermic arrest is to be used, cooling is carried out for at least 10 to 15 minutes to a rectal temperature of 18°C or lower. A single dose of cold blood cardioplegia is injected into the ascending aorta after the aorta is cross-clamped. The volume is emptied into the pump circuit, and the venous cannula is removed. If continuous bypass is used, cooling to 28°C is performed and intermittent cardioplegia is given every 15 to 20 minutes during the cross-clamp interval. Tapes are snugged down around both vena caval cannulas.

A longitudinal opening is made on the anterior surface of the right pulmonary artery and extended behind the aorta to the pulmonary artery confluence and rightward to a point directly behind the superior vena cava (Fig. 31.3).

NB Previous Shunt Site

Often a Gore-Tex tube graft has been anastomosed to the right pulmonary artery or pulmonary artery confluence. The tube graft should be mobilized, secured with two metal clips as far from the pulmonary artery as possible, and transected. The remaining Gore-Tex tube attached to the pulmonary artery should be removed and the resultant opening in the pulmonary artery incorporated into the longitudinal incision. NB

⊘ Small Pulmonary Artery Confluence

If the proximal right or left pulmonary artery is small or stenotic, the longitudinal incision should be extended to the hilum of the left lung. ⊘

An opening is made in the superior aspect of the right atrium and carried superiorly onto the medial aspect of the superior vena cava. The incision ends posteriorly on the superior vena cava 3 to 4 mm above the longitudinal incision in the pulmonary artery. A 6-0 Prolene suture is used to

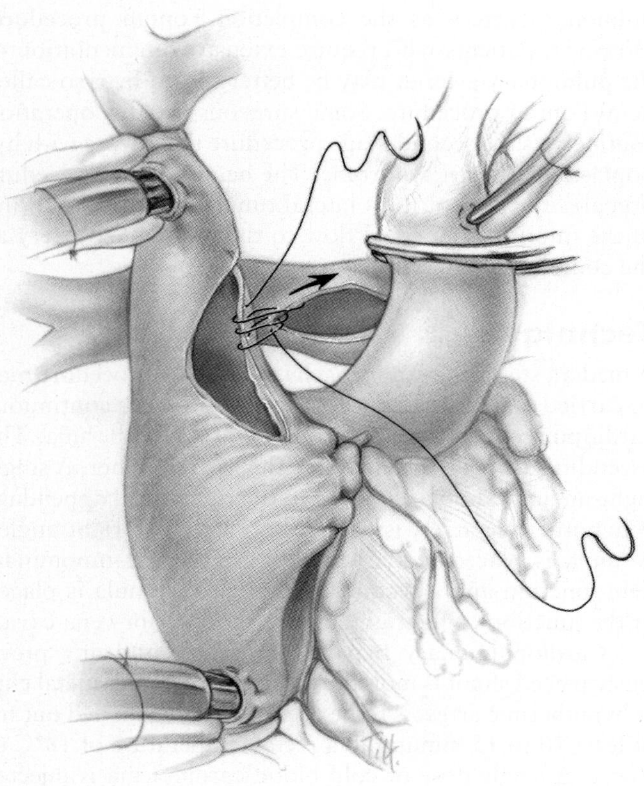

FIG. 31.3 Hemi-Fontan procedure: Opening of the right atrial–superior vena caval junction and right pulmonary artery.

anastomose the rightward extent of the pulmonary artery opening to the posterior edge of the superior vena cava (Fig. 31.3). A large triangular patch of autologous pericardium or pulmonary homograft is used to augment the anterior opening of the pulmonary artery and superior vena cava. The suture line is begun at the leftward extent of the pulmonary artery opening and continued until the suture line meets the initial pulmonary artery–superior vena caval suture (Fig. 31.4). These sutures are tied securely together. The inferior aspect of the triangular patch is then sewn to the endocardium of the right atrium, extending from the right atrial opening posteriorly and up along the lateral aspect to meet the right atrial incision. A separate "dam" of Gore-Tex is used as (Fig. 31.5) a patch to close the superior vena caval–right atrial junction (Fig. 31.6). When the completion Fontan procedure is undertaken, this pericardial or homograft patch is excised through the right atrial opening to reestablish flow through this junction.

⊘ Blood Supply to Sinoatrial Node

It is important to start the right atrial incision in the most superior part of the atrium. The incision must be continued on the medial aspect of the superior vena cava to avoid injuring the blood supply to the sinoatrial node. ⊘

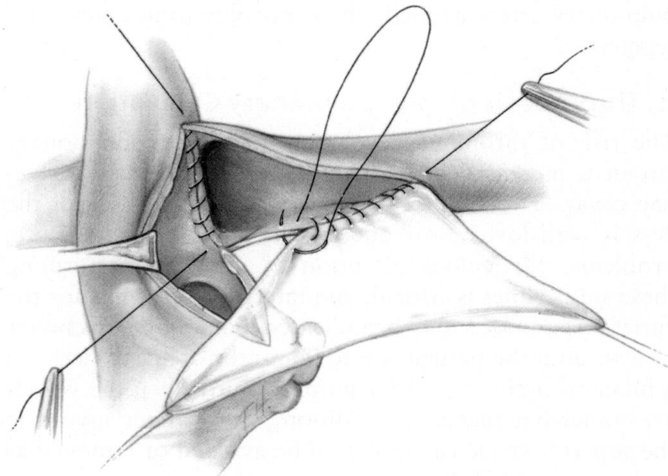

FIG. 31.4 Hemi-Fontan procedure: Patching the pulmonary artery and superior vena cava with pericardium or piece of pulmonary homograft.

⊘ Ligating the Pulmonary Artery

The hemi-Fontan procedure is most often used for patients after stage I palliation for hypoplastic left heart syndrome. If there is forward flow through the pulmonary valve, the main pulmonary artery should be transected at the valve level, not ligated. Ligating the pulmonary artery creates a dead space above the pulmonic valve where thrombus may form. The proximal end is oversewn with interrupted pledgeted 4-0 Prolene sutures incorporating valve tissue

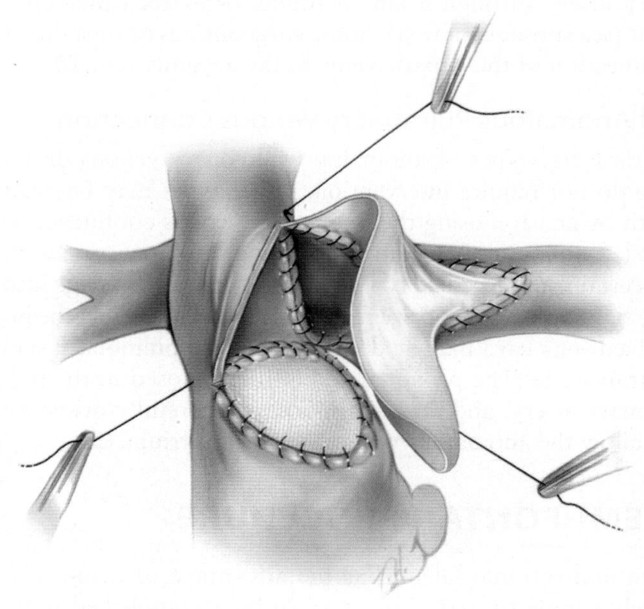

FIG. 31.5 Hemi-Fontan procedure: Folding patch to close the right atrial–superior vena caval junction.

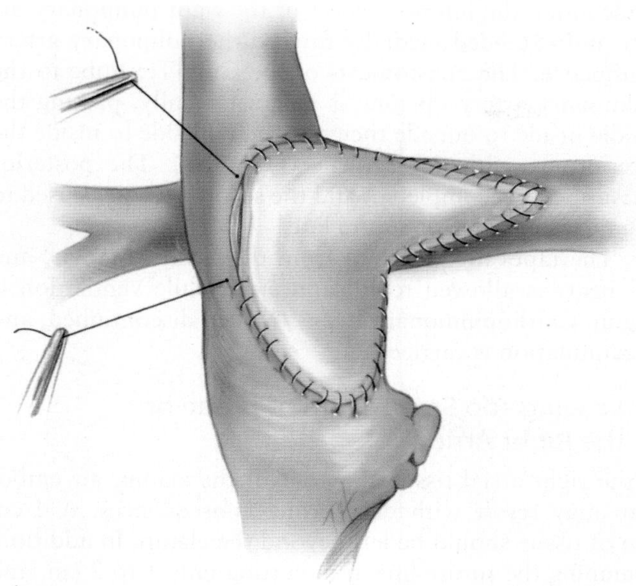

FIG. 31.6 Hemi-Fontan procedure: Completing the anterior patch of the right pulmonary artery–superior vena caval anastomosis.

reinforced by a running 5-0 Prolene suture. The resultant opening in the distal main pulmonary artery is then extended onto the right pulmonary artery. ⊘

NB Atrioventricular Valve Regurgitation

The presence of more than moderate atrioventricular valve regurgitation has been demonstrated to negatively affect the function of the single ventricle, and to elevate the pulmonary artery pressure. Both these sequelae may prevent the patient from becoming a candidate for the completion Fontan operation. It is important to perform a valve repair before or at the time of the second-stage procedure, whether a bidirectional Glenn or hemi-Fontan is undertaken. NB

COMPLETION FONTAN PROCEDURE

The full Fontan operation can be accomplished when the child is at least 2 years of age. Today, the Fontan procedure is usually performed as part of a staged approach in patients with a single ventricle following a bidirectional Glenn shunt or hemi-Fontan procedure.

The original Fontan procedure involved an atriopulmonary connection. The benefit of atrial contraction is greatly limited by the low resistance to backflow in the systemic veins. Today, a total cavopulmonary connection is performed to create the Fontan circulation. This consists of directing superior vena caval flow directly into the pulmonary artery and channeling inferior vena caval return through a straight conduit or baffle to the pulmonary artery. This connection is believed to provide improved flow patterns with presumed hemodynamic advantages, less stasis with decreased risk of thrombus formation, and fewer arrhythmias secondary to atrial distention.

TOTAL CAVOPULMONARY CONNECTION

Incision

This is usually a reoperative procedure because the Fontan connection is usually staged. A standard median sternotomy provides excellent exposure.

Cannulation

Cannulation of the ascending aorta is carried out in the usual manner. The superior vena cava should be cannulated near its junction with the innominate vein. The inferior vena caval cannula must be placed very low on the inferior vena cava itself or at the right atrial–inferior vena caval junction.

Technique for the Extracardiac Fontan Procedure

Patients who have undergone a previous bidirectional Glenn shunt are ideally suited to have an extracardiac Fontan procedure. This can be performed on cardiopulmonary bypass without aortic cross-clamping. The potential advantages of this technique are improved flow dynamics through the conduit tubing into the pulmonary artery and decreased arrhythmias secondary to limited atrial suture lines and atrial distention. In addition, certain anatomic considerations such as the location of pulmonary veins that might complicate an intraatrial baffle procedure, or the position of the inferior vena cava may make the extracardiac conduit the best option. The disadvantage of this technique is the lack of growth potential. Therefore, this operation is generally performed in somewhat older and larger children to allow an adult-sized conduit to be implanted.

On cardiopulmonary bypass with the heart decompressed and beating, the lateral aspect of the right atrium and inferior aspect of the right pulmonary artery are completely dissected. With the inferior caval tape tightened, a Satinsky clamp is placed 2 to 3 cm above the junction of the right atrium with the inferior vena cava (Fig. 31.7). The right atrium is divided approximately 1 cm from the edges of the clamp, and the edges are oversewn with a double running 4-0 Prolene suture.

An 18- or 20-mm Gore-Tex tube graft is cut straight transversely and anastomosed to the transected inferior vena caval cuff using a 6-0 or 5-0 Prolene suture. The graft is then measured to the appropriate length to lie posterolateral to the right atrium and meet the inferior edge of the right pulmonary artery (Fig. 31.8). The graft is trimmed, leaving the tube slightly longer medially. With the superior vena caval snare tightened, a longitudinal incision is

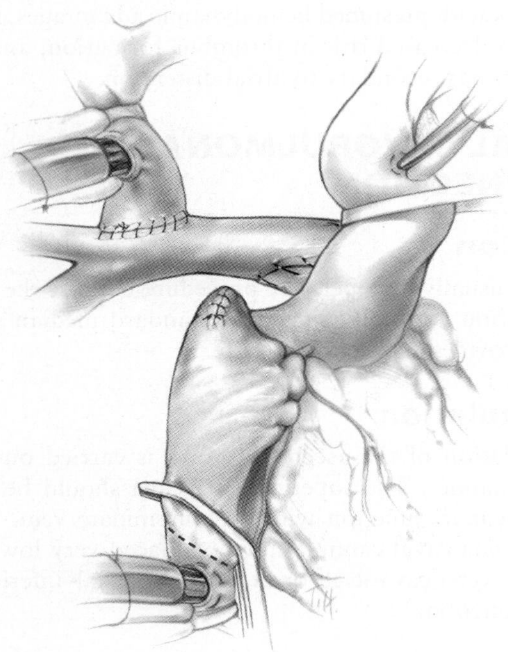

FIG. 31.7 Extracardiac Fontan procedure: A clamp placed on the wall of the right atrium 2 to 3 cm above the inferior vena cava.

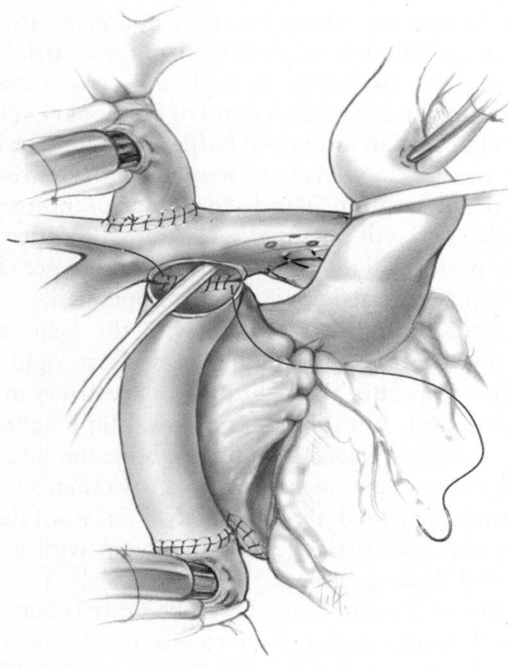

FIG. 31.8 Extracardiac Fontan procedure: The inferior vena caval anastomosis is completed. Sewing Gore-Tex conduit to the inferior aspect of the pulmonary artery. Note the vent in the pulmonary artery.

made along the inferior aspect of the right pulmonary artery and extended medially toward the pulmonary artery confluence. The anastomosis of the Gore-Tex tube to the pulmonary artery opening is begun medially, passing the needle inside to outside the graft then outside to inside the arteriotomy with 6-0 Prolene (Fig. 31.8). The posterior anastomosis is completed, and the second needle is used to complete the anterior suture line.

The tapes are removed from the caval cannulas, and the heart is allowed to fill and eject while ventilation is begun. Cardiopulmonary bypass is then discontinued, and decannulation is carried out.

⊘ Leaving Too Small a Rim of Tissue on the Right Atrium

If the right atrial tissue slips out of the clamp, air embolism may result with devastating consequences. A 1-cm rim of tissue should be left beyond the clamp. In addition, beginning the suture line after cutting only 1 to 2 cm, and continuing to cut and sew after each centimeter along the incision ensures that if the clamp should slip off, the right atrial opening will be controlled. ⊘

⊘ Injury to the Coronary Sinus

Before and after placing the clamp on the right atrium, the heart should be inspected to ensure that the coronary sinus or right coronary artery is not included. ⊘

⊘ Forward Flow into the Pulmonary Artery

If forward flow from the single ventricle into the pulmonary artery is present, the main pulmonary artery needs to be ligated or divided. To prevent the possible development of thrombus above the pulmonary valve and below the level of ligation due to stasis, the preferred approach is to divide the pulmonary artery just above the valve and oversew the proximal end, incorporating valve tissue in the suture line or to excise all the leaflets under direct vision. This requires a short period of aortic cross-clamping. The distal end can then be oversewn, patched, or used as the most medial aspect of the extracardiac conduit anastomosis. ⊘

⊘ Pulmonary Artery Stenosis

Any areas of pulmonary arterial narrowing must be addressed, usually with a longitudinal opening across the stenotic area and placement of a pulmonary homograft patch. Narrowing of the proximal right pulmonary artery can often be managed by placing the Gore-Tex tube graft across this area. ⊘

NB Maintaining Laminar Flow into the Pulmonary Arteries

Many studies have suggested that the least disturbance to forward flow from the superior vena cava and inferior vena cava into the pulmonary arteries is achieved when the

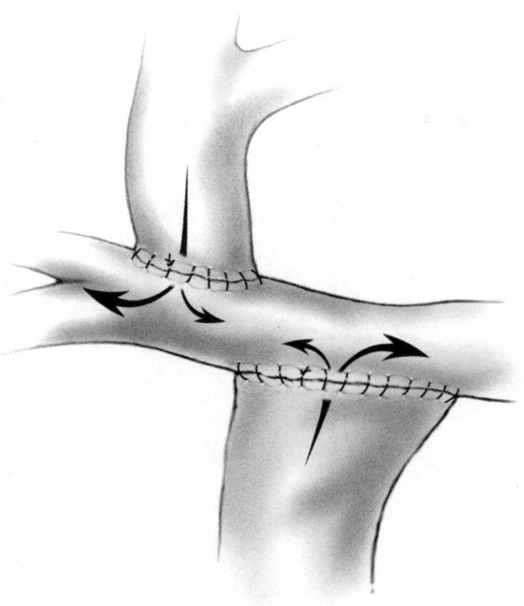

FIG. 31.9 Offset of superior and inferior vena caval flows.

two flows are offset (Fig. 31.9). Therefore, every attempt should be made to place the Gore-Tex conduit as medially as possible to offset its opening to the left of the superior vena caval anastomosis. Alternatively, if the bidirectional Glenn shunt has been placed centrally on the very proximal right pulmonary artery, the extracardiac conduit will be placed distally on the inferior aspect of the right pulmonary artery near its lower lobe branch. NB

⊘ Excessive Backflow from the Pulmonary Arteries

A significant amount of collateral flow may be noted when the opening in the pulmonary artery is made. Placing a vent sucker into the pulmonary artery will control this flow while the anastomosis is performed (Fig. 31.8). ⊘

NB Size of Conduit

The extracardiac conduit has two potential growth limitations. One is the diameter and the other is the length of the tube. There is concern that oversizing the diameter more than one and a half times the size of the patient's inferior vena cava may result in stasis and increased risk of thrombosis. By the age of 2 to 4 years and a body weight of 12 to 15 kg, the diameter of the inferior vena cava at the right atrium and the distance from the inferior vena cava to the right pulmonary artery are both 60% to 80% of adult size. Therefore, the extracardiac Fontan can be performed when the patient reaches this age and weight limit without significant oversizing and hopefully avoiding the need for reoperation. NB

NB Interrupted Inferior Vena Cava

Patients with interrupted inferior vena cava with azygous continuation have relatively small diameter hepatic veins entering the right atrium. The completion extracardiac Fontan procedure in these patients therefore requires a smaller diameter conduit to avoid stasis and thrombosis. The long-term use of anticoagulation may be indicated in these patients. Alternatively, some surgeons advocate disconnecting the hepatic veins with a cuff of right atrial tissue. The cuff is fashioned into a vascular pedicle, which is anastomosed directly to the azygous vein during a brief period of hypothermic arrest. NB

NB Bilateral Superior Venae Cavae

Patients with previous bilateral bidirectional Glenn procedures often have a somewhat hypoplastic central pulmonary artery segment. For optimal flow characteristics in this situation, the conduit from the inferior vena cava should be positioned between the two superior vena caval anastomoses. If the local anatomy permits this arrangement, the conduit itself may be used to enlarge the central pulmonary artery segment. If it appears that this will compress the pulmonary veins, the conduit can be placed on the right pulmonary artery and a separate patch used to enlarge the narrowed segment. NB

Technique for a Lateral Tunnel Fontan Procedure

Patients who have previously undergone a hemi-Fontan procedure are good candidates for the lateral tunnel Fontan procedure. In these patients, the anastomosis of the top of the right atrium to the pulmonary artery has already been completed. A portion of a tube graft is used to create a baffle from the inferior vena cave to the right atrial-pulmonary artery anastomosis. This type of Fontan operation has growth potential of the pathway from the inferior vena cava to the pulmonary artery, which allows it to be used in smaller patients.

Bicaval cannulation and cardiopulmonary bypass with moderate hypothermia are used. The aortic cross-clamp is applied, and cold blood cardioplegic solution is infused into the aortic root. A longitudinal right atriotomy is made starting at a point 0.5 to 1 cm anterior to and parallel with the sulcus terminalis after tightening the tape around the inferior vena caval cannula. Residual atrial septal tissue is excised to ensure unobstructed drainage of pulmonary venous return through the atrioventricular valve.

A piece of Gore-Tex tube graft, 10 to 12 mm in diameter, is cut to a length corresponding with the distance between the inferior vena caval–right atrial junction and the right superior vena caval–right atrial junction. The graft is cut in half lengthwise and its width adjusted as appropriate to the size of the patient to create an intraatrial baffle from the inferior vena cava to the superior vena cava. The baffle is placed inside the atrium, and the posterior suture line is begun inferiorly using a running 5-0 Prolene suture (Fig. 31.10). The baffle is sutured in front of the opening of the right-sided pulmonary veins. The suture line is carried around the opening of the inferior vena cava into the right atrium, up to the right atriotomy where the suture is brought outside the right atrium. The remainder of the posterior suture line of the baffle is completed. If a previous hemi-Fontan procedure has been performed, the patch ("dam") closing off the right atriopulmonary artery anastomosis is excised completely. The tape on the superior vena caval cannula must be tightened. Superiorly, the suture line is continued onto the crista terminalis, around the opening of the superior vena cava into the right atrium until the suture line meets the right atriotomy. The suture is brought outside the right atrium. The baffle often needs to be trimmed in this area because the lateral distance between the inferior and superior venae cavae is shorter than the medial distance between the two structures. The baffle is completed by closing the right atriotomy, including the baffle in the suture line (Fig. 31.11). Just before this suture line is completed, a 16G catheter can be placed through the suture line into the pulmonary venous side of the baffle to monitor pulmonary venous pressures in the postoperative period.

NB Anastomosis of Right Atrium to Pulmonary Artery

The lateral tunnel Fontan is most often performed following a hemi-Fontan procedure. These patients have a

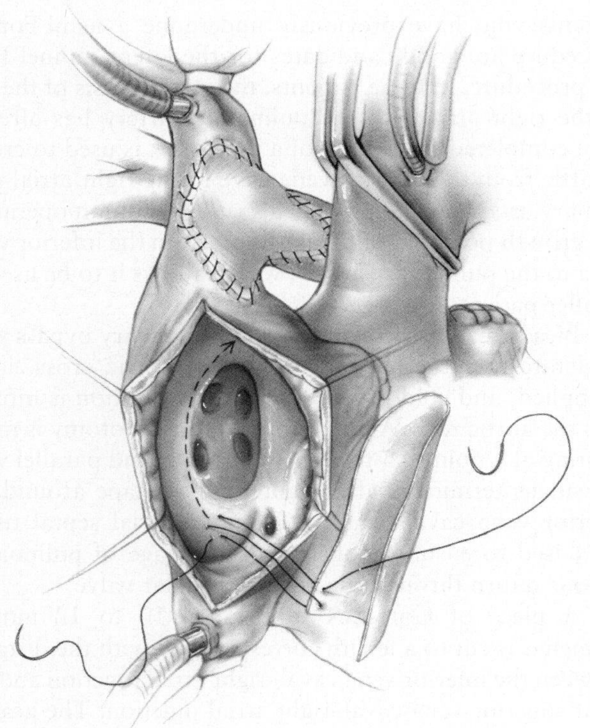

FIG. 31.10 Fontan procedure: Intraatrial baffle.

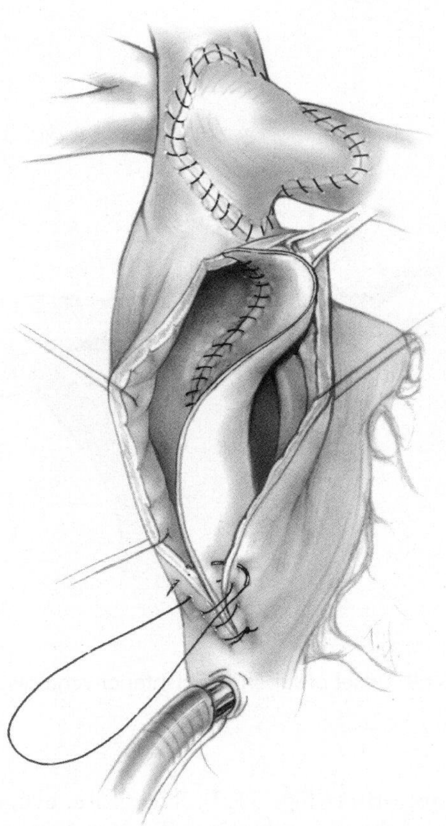

FIG. 31.11 Fontan procedure: Completion of an intraatrial baffle.

previously constructed anastomosis of the superior vena cava, pulmonary artery, and superior aspect of the right atrium. The folded patch, which was used to close off the right atrium from this confluence must be completely excised to allow for unobstructed flow from the inferior vena cava through the baffle into the pulmonary artery. Alternatively, if the patient previously had a bidirectional Glenn procedure, an extra step is required to join the right atrium to the pulmonary artery. The superior aspect of the right atrium is opened, usually at the site where the stump of the superior vena cava was previously oversewn. An incision is made on the inferior aspect of the right pulmonary artery corresponding to the right atrial opening. The anastomosis is completed with a running suture of 6-0 or 5-0 Prolene. NB

Completing the Operation

Deairing maneuvers are carried out, and the aortic cross-clamp is removed. Ventilations are begun, and flow is allowed into the pulmonary arteries by removing the tapes from the caval cannulas. If a monitoring catheter has not been previously placed into the superior vena cava or inferior vena cava preoperatively, a second catheter should be placed into the baffle through the right atriotomy and secured with a pledgeted 5-0 Prolene suture for monitoring pulmonary arterial pressures. After systemic rewarming is completed, cardiopulmonary bypass is discontinued.

NB Pulmonary Artery Pressure

Pulmonary artery pressures are monitored, and if the pressure is persistently 20 mm Hg or higher, efforts to identify correctable problems must be made. Individual pressure measurements with a 25G needle should be made in the superior vena cava, inferior vena cava, right atrial side of the baffle, and the pulmonary artery directly to rule out any anastomotic narrowing and pressure gradient. If pulmonary venous pressures are noted to be elevated, efforts to improve ventricular function and decrease ventricular end-diastolic pressure should be made. Transesophageal echocardiography may identify significant atrioventricular valve regurgitation. If this is present, repair or even replacement of the atrioventricular valve may be necessary. NB

NB In older children or young adults who do not require growth potential, a 16- or 18-mm Gore-Tex tube graft can be placed from the opening of the inferior vena cava to the opening of the superior vena cava, rather than using a baffle. NB

NB Patients who have hepatic veins entering the base of the right atrium separately from the inferior vena cava require a more complicated intraatrial baffle to ensure that all systemic venous return is directed to the pulmonary artery. NB

NB Recently, some patients who have undergone a previous hemi-Fontan procedure have had completion of the Fontan procedure performed in the cardiac catheterization laboratory. This is accomplished by placing a covered stent within the atrium extending from the opening of the inferior vena cava to the superior vena caval–right atrial junction. The patch closing off the right atrial–pulmonary artery anastomosis is perforated with a catheter and balloon dilated to accommodate the stent. NB

High-Risk Candidates for the Fontan Procedure

Staging the Fontan by performing a bidirectional Glenn or hemi-Fontan procedure first may allow some patients who otherwise would not qualify for a full Fontan procedure to show improvement in ventricular function or decrease in pulmonary vascular resistance after removal of the volume load. Patients who have somewhat elevated pulmonary vascular resistance or mild to moderate ventricular dysfunction may be candidates for a Fontan procedure with the creation of a small fenestration between the extracardiac conduit and the right atrium or in the intraatrial baffle (Fig. 31.12). A simple punch is placed in the lateral tunnel patch prior to insertion. The price to be paid for improved systemic perfusion and lower systemic venous pressure is a decrease in systemic arterial oxygen saturation.

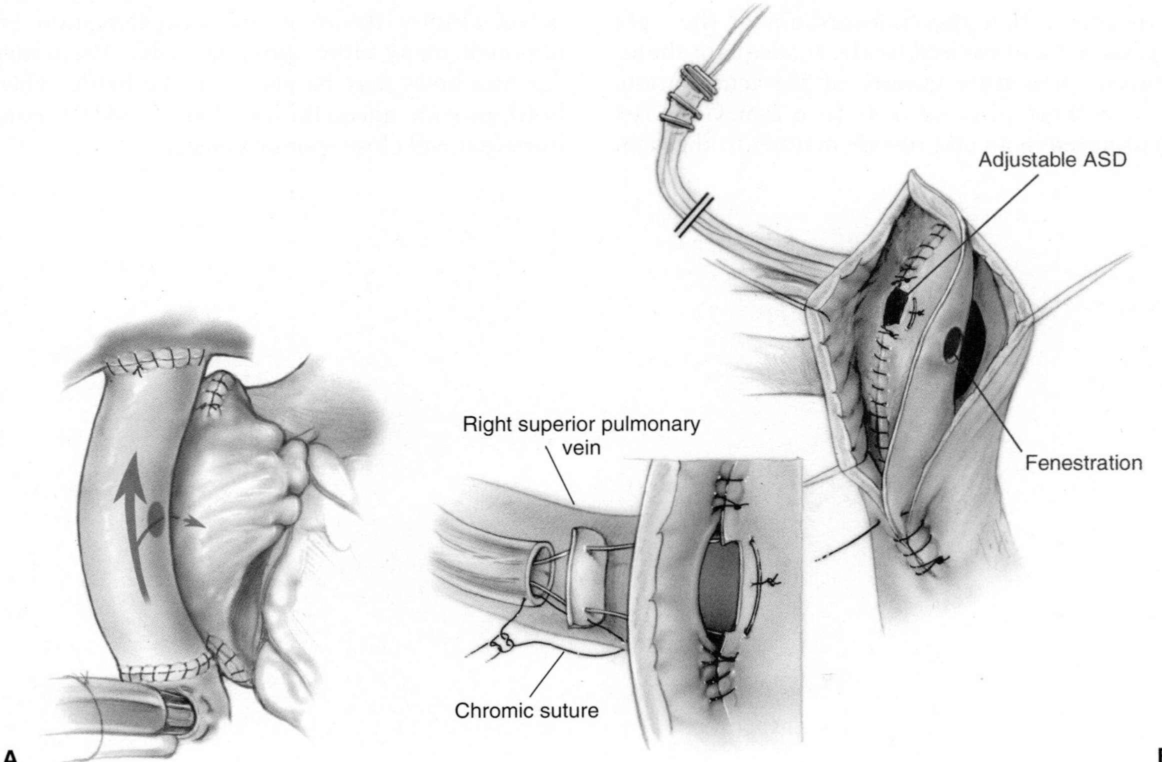

FIG. 31.12 **A:** Extracardiac Fontan procedure with fenestration. **B:** Fenestration in extracardiac conduit.

In addition, there is a risk of paradoxic embolus, and the possible need for a catheter intervention to close the fenestration. Some centers routinely fenestrate all their Fontan patients, believing that this reduces the duration of postoperative pleural effusions and operative risk.

Technique

For patients with an extracardiac conduit, the fenestration can be created while on cardiopulmonary bypass in borderline Fontan procedure candidates, or after separation from cardiopulmonary bypass if the pulmonary artery pressures remain above 20 mm Hg. The extracardiac conduit and right atrium are marked at a location where they are adjacent to one another. Side-biting clamps are placed on the conduit and wall of the right atrium. A 4-mm aortic punch is used to create an opening in both structures, which are joined in a side-to-side manner with a 6-0 Prolene suture (Fig. 31.12A). With care taken to sew only the free edge of the atriotomy to the area *around* the fenestration in the Gore-Tex tube (and not the fenestration itself), the likelihood of fenestration obstruction by atrial tissue is minimized (Fig. 31.13) Deairing is carried out through the anastomosis as the clamps are removed. This defect can be later closed with an atrial septal defect closure device in the cardiac catheterization laboratory if necessary.

NB When a side-to-side anastomosis is performed, it is important to ensure that the endocardium of the right atrium is visualized and excised to allow adequate shunting and prevent premature closure of the fenestration. Alternatively, a short piece of a 4- to 6-mm Gore-Tex tube is anastomosed in an end-to-side manner to the right atrial wall and the side of the conduit with side-biting clamps in place. NB

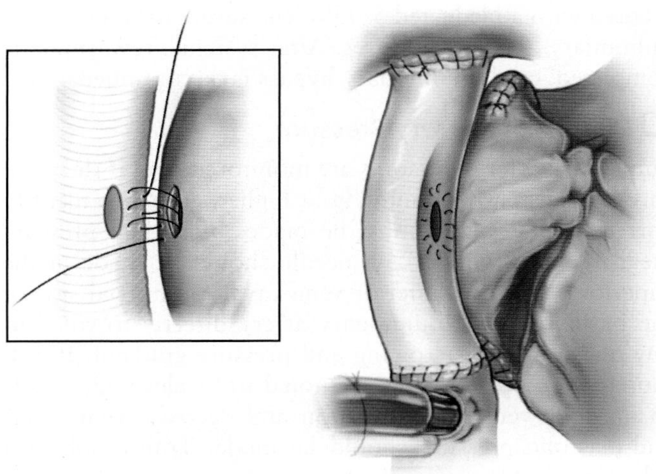

FIG. 31.13 Suture technique for creating a fenestration in an extracardiac conduit.

For patients undergoing a lateral tunnel Fontan procedure, either a fenestration must be created in the intraatrial baffle during the period of aortic cross-clamping, usually prior to insertion of the patch itself. The fenestration is created using a 4-mm aortic punch in the middle of the Gore-Tex baffle. This can be closed with an atrial septal defect closure device in the catheterization laboratory, although many close spontaneously. Alternatively, three 2.5 mm holes may be placed in the baffle. These smaller holes provide adequate initial right-sided decompression, but often will close spontaneously.

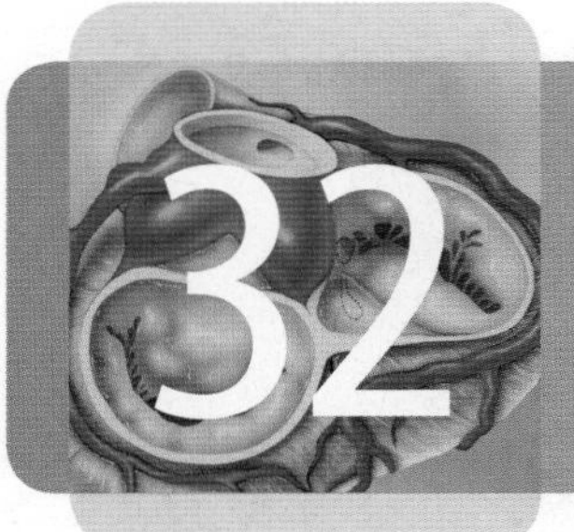

32 Coronary Artery Anomalies

Anomalies of the coronary arteries are rare and include left coronary artery origin from the pulmonary artery, coronary artery fistula, and aberrant origin of the left or right coronary artery with subsequent coursing between the great vessels.

ANOMALOUS LEFT CORONARY ARTERY FROM THE PULMONARY ARTERY

Origin of the left coronary artery from the pulmonary artery is the most common congenital coronary artery anomaly and occurs in 1 of every 300,000 live births. This anomaly is compatible with *in utero* life because of the presence of relatively high pulmonary artery pressure and oxygen saturation. However, over the first 1 to 3 months of life as the pulmonary vascular resistance decreases, the flow into the left coronary artery decreases, resulting in inadequate coronary perfusion. This may lead to progressive dilatation of the left ventricle, myocardial infarction, and secondary mitral regurgitation. Lack of adequate perfusion stimulates the development of collateral circulation from the right coronary artery to the left system. Significant left-to-right shunting secondary to run off from these collateral vessels into the pulmonary artery may occur. The clinical course of the patient depends on the relative dominance of the right and left coronary arteries and the rapidity and extent of collateral development.

Surgical Anatomy

The ostium of the anomalous left main coronary artery may be located anywhere in the main pulmonary artery or the proximal right or left pulmonary artery. Most commonly, it is found leftward in the posterior sinus of the pulmonary root (the sinus facing the aortic sinus, which normally gives rise to the left main coronary artery).

Incision

An anomalous left coronary artery from the pulmonary artery is best approached through a median sternotomy with standard cardiopulmonary bypass.

Technique

Before commencing cardiopulmonary bypass, the right and left pulmonary arteries are dissected and encircled with snares. High cannulation of the ascending aorta is performed and a single venous cannula is used. Immediately after starting cardiopulmonary bypass, the snares around the pulmonary arteries are tightened. A vent is placed into the left ventricle through the right superior pulmonary vein (see Chapter 4). Cooling to 28°C is carried out, and antegrade cardioplegic solution is delivered into the aortic root after the cross-clamp is applied.

A transverse incision is made on the pulmonary artery just above the sinotubular ridge. Snares around the right and left pulmonary arteries are removed. The ostium of the anomalous coronary artery is identified. It is often possible to administer cardioplegic solution directly into this vessel with an appropriately sized olive-tipped catheter for optimal myocardial protection. The main pulmonary artery is now transected, and the ostium of the anomalous left coronary artery is excised with a generous margin of tissue as a button or a U-shaped flap from within the pulmonary sinus (Fig. 32.1).

The anterior edge of the pulmonary artery root is pulled downward with a traction suture. This maneuver will improve visualization of the anomalous left coronary artery. It is mobilized and dissected free from the surrounding tissues with a low-current electrocautery. The coronary artery, now well mobilized, is brought up toward the left posterior aspect of the ascending aorta (Fig. 32.2). A small vertical or transverse incision is made on the aorta to identify the precise location of the aortic leaflets and commissures. Under direct vision, a slit is made on the posterior aspect of the aortic wall, taking meticulous care not to injure the aortic valve components. The opening is then enlarged appropriately to accommodate the left coronary using a 4-mm coronary aortic punch. The left coronary button or flap is then anastomosed to the aortic opening with 6-0 or 7-0 Prolene suture. The aortotomy is closed with continuous 6-0 Prolene suture. The defect in the pulmonary root is patched with a piece of autologous pericardium using a running 6-0 or 7-0 Prolene suture. The pulmonary root is then reattached to the pulmonary artery confluence with a continuous suture of 5-0 Prolene (Fig. 32.3).

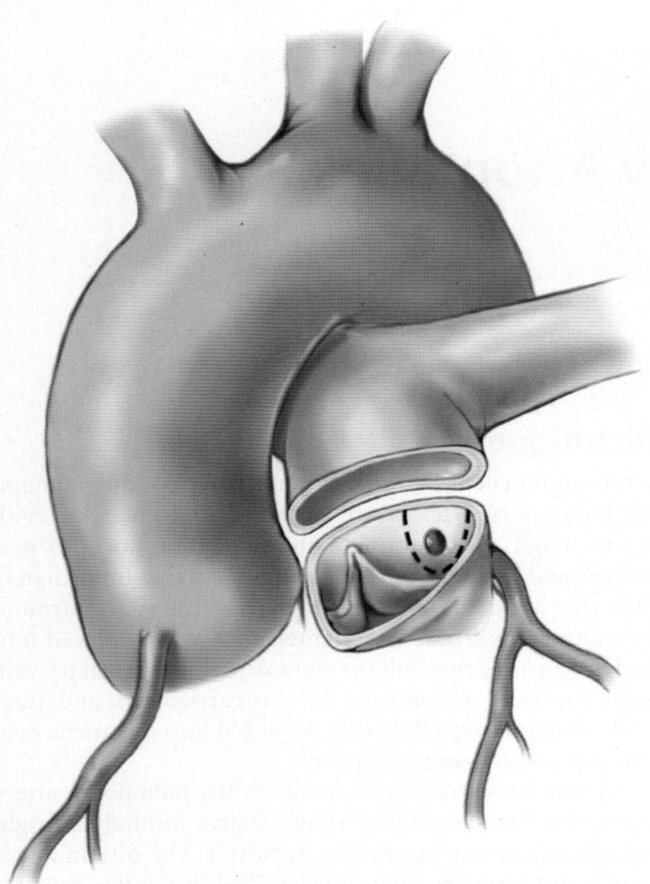

FIG. 32.1 Transected pulmonary artery. Dotted line demonstrates excision of the left main coronary artery.

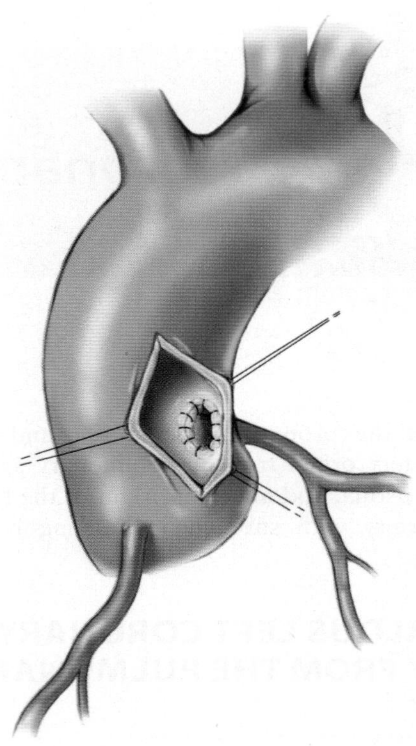

FIG. 32.2 Mobilizing the left main coronary artery for reimplantation into the posterolateral aspect of the aorta.

⊘ Coronary Artery Steal

It is essential to occlude the right and left pulmonary arteries with the initiation of cardiopulmonary bypass. Otherwise, the right coronary artery flow may runoff into the decompressed pulmonary artery through the coronary artery collaterals. This right coronary artery steal may cause global myocardial ischemia. ⊘

⊘ Left Ventricular Distention

Most of these patients have dilated, compromised left ventricles and do not tolerate left ventricular distention. Snaring the pulmonary arteries helps to prevent a large volume of blood return through the pulmonary veins into the left atrium. Venting through the right superior pulmonary vein provides excellent decompression of the left ventricle (see Chapter 4). ⊘

⊘ Inadequate Length of the Anomalous Left Coronary Artery

It is usually possible to mobilize an adequate length of the left coronary artery to reach the aorta. When this does not appear to be feasible, an extension technique should be contemplated. ⊘

NB Extension of the Left Anomalous Coronary Artery

Before excising the left coronary button or flap from the pulmonary artery, a judgment should be made regarding the ability to mobilize the left coronary for a tension-free direct anastomosis to the aorta. If the distance between the *in situ* left coronary artery and aorta is too large, the artery should be lengthened with an attached tongue of pulmonary artery wall (Fig. 32.4). The upper (superior) and lower (inferior) segments of the extension are sewn together with 6-0 or 7-0 Prolene suture to create a tube the same size or a little larger than the coronary artery. The end of this tube is anastomosed to the left side of the aorta. The defect in the pulmonary artery is patched with autologous pericardium. NB

NB Correct Lie of the Left Coronary Artery

It is useful to unclamp the aorta before reconstructing the pulmonary artery. This allows the surgeon to check the pressurized transferred coronary artery for distortion. If twisting of the artery is noted, the aortic anastomosis needs to be redone. Sometimes division of adventitial bands will compensate for minor degrees of torsion. NB

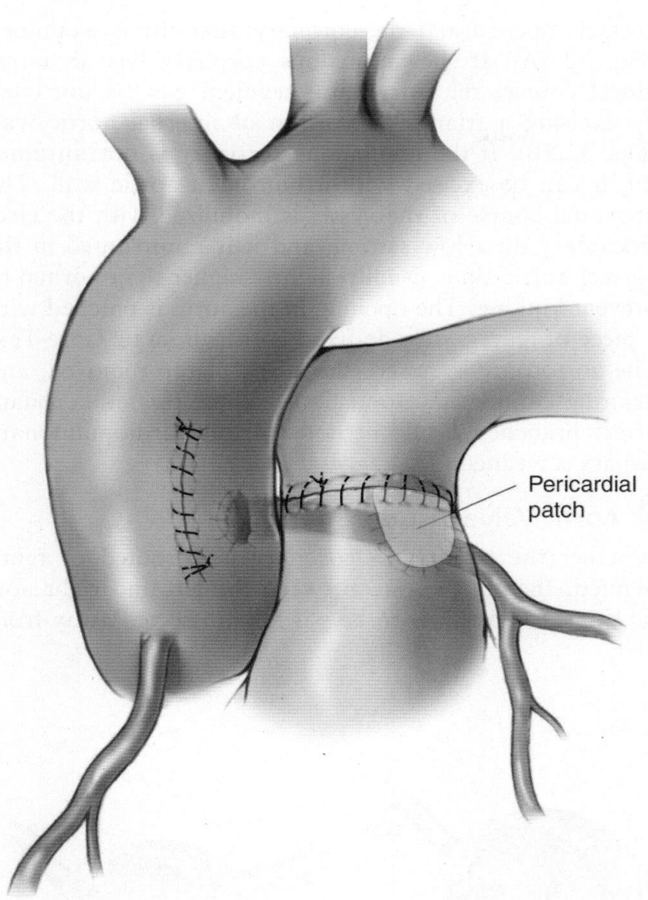

FIG. 32.3 Completed repair with autologous pericardial patch reconstruction of an excised pulmonary sinus and reanastomosis of the main pulmonary artery.

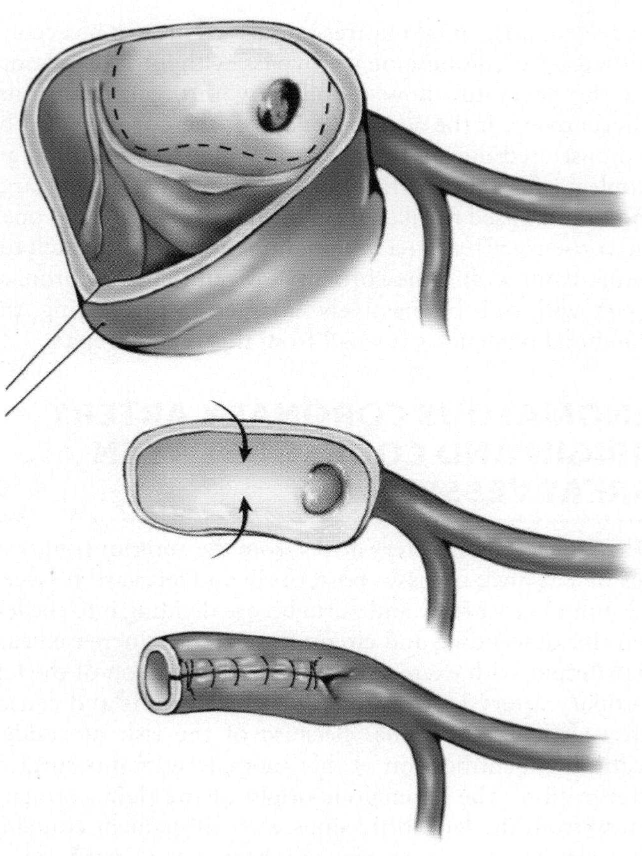

FIG. 32.4 Lengthening left main coronary artery with attached tongue of pulmonary artery wall to create a tube extension.

⊘ Tension on the Pulmonary Anastomosis

Extensive mobilization of the main, right, and left pulmonary arteries and division of the ligamentum or ductus arteriosus allows a tension-free anastomosis. ⊘

NB Because many of these patients have very compromised left ventricular function, left ventricular support with a left ventricular assist device or extracorporeal membrane oxygenator may be required for a few days postoperatively. NB

CORONARY FISTULAE

It is very rare for coronary artery fistulae to be seen early in life. Many fistulae are small and cause no symptoms and no measurable left-to-right shunting. Patients who are symptomatic with angina from coronary steal or congestive heart failure owing to a significant left-to-right shunting should undergo surgery for an isolated coronary artery fistula. Not infrequently, patients undergoing coronary artery bypass surgery may be noted to have an incidental coronary artery fistula that can be closed at the time of the coronary artery bypass procedure. Many are treatable by interventional techniques in the cardiac catheterization laboratory.

Technique

A median sternotomy is used. The fistula may be directly oversewn without cardiopulmonary bypass. To avoid myocardial ischemia or infarction, the fistula can be ligated just at its entrance into the cardiac chamber while monitoring the electrocardiogram; however, often this can be inexact. Digital pressure to occlude the fistula before oversewing it may also be useful.

When the fistula drains into the right atrium or pulmonary artery, cardiopulmonary bypass is used to close the distal (and often the proximal) opening under direct vision. Often the fistula has multiple openings into the recipient chamber. When the fistula empties into the right atrium, bicaval cannulation is used. When the fistula opens into the pulmonary artery, a single atriocaval cannula is usually adequate. Through a standard oblique right atriotomy or a vertical pulmonary arteriotomy, the orifices of the fistula are identified. They are then oversewn with multiple pledgeted, horizontal mattress sutures. This can be accomplished on cardiopulmonary bypass without cross-clamping the aorta to allow blood flow through the fistula. Alternatively, if the aorta is clamped, the openings can be demonstrated during the antegrade administration of cardioplegia into the aortic root. For those extremely large and broad-based fistulae, it can be most efficacious to open the coronary artery in a longitudinal fashion and patch the fistula from within the coronary. Given that the coronary artery will itself be massively enlarged in this setting, the likelihood of stenosis is small from this type of repair.

ANOMALOUS CORONARY ARTERY ORIGIN AND COURSE BETWEEN GREAT VESSELS

When the left main artery arises from the anterior (right) sinus of Valsalva, it passes posteriorly and leftward between the pulmonary artery and aorta before dividing into the left anterior descending and circumflex arteries. Increased cardiac output with exercise results in compression of the left coronary artery between the two great vessels and causes left ventricular ischemia. Because of the risk of sudden death, the identification of this anomaly warrants surgical intervention. The anomalous origin of the right coronary artery from the left aortic sinus with subsequent coursing between the great vessels has also been recognized as a risk for myocardial ischemia and sudden death. It should be noted that patients with this anomaly may have normal exercise stress tests and cardiac perfusion scans. In asymptomatic patients, surgery is usually delayed until age 10 because the risk of sudden death is low before adolescence. Echocardiography can usually define the proximal course of the coronary arteries, and therefore make the diagnosis. It is recommended that all patients undergo coronary angiography or magnetic resonance imaging before surgical intervention.

Several surgical approaches have been used in these patients, including the use of one or both internal thoracic arteries to bypass the left anterior descending artery and a branch of the circumflex coronary artery in the case of anomalous origin of the left main. Concern has been raised that competitive flow through the normally unobstructed native left main coronary could lead to a so-called string sign with minimal flow reserve through the internal thoracic vessel(s). Others have suggested translocating the main pulmonary artery toward the left pulmonary hilum to create additional space between the great vessels, thereby reducing the risk of dynamic coronary obstruction with exercise. However, the best option is to restore the normal coronary anatomy if possible.

Technique

On cardiopulmonary bypass, the aorta is cross-clamped and cardioplegia is administered into the aortic root. The aorta is opened and the coronary anatomy is examined (Fig. 32.5A). If the anomalous coronary has an intramural course, the intramural segment can be unroofed by excising a triangular portion of internal aortic wall (Fig. 32.5B). If the anomalous coronary is not intramural, it can be excised with a button of aortic wall. The proximal course of the vessel is mobilized with the electrocautery on a low setting, and it is reimplanted in the correct aortic sinus usually slightly higher than normal to prevent kinking. The opening in the aorta is patched with a piece of glutaraldehyde-fixed pericardium or Gore-Tex. The aortotomy is closed, the aortic clamp removed, and deairing completed. Good filling of the treated coronary artery branches should be noted before cardiopulmonary bypass is weaned.

⊘ Aortic Valve Insufficiency

Whether the anomalous coronary is unroofed or reimplanted, the commissure between the left and right aortic sinuses may needs to be partially dissected away from

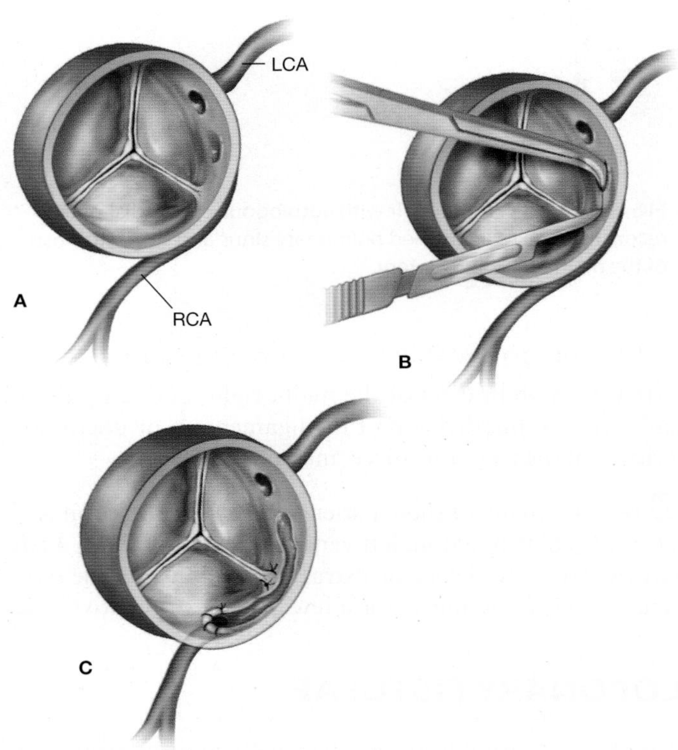

FIG. 32.5 **A:** Anomalous origin of the right coronary artery from the left sinus. **B:** With a right angle clamp as a guide, the intramural section is 'unroofed'. **C:** When the unroofing is complete, if the commissure requires resuspension this can be completed. Note also the 'tacking back' of the cut edge of the right coronary at its exit point from the aorta.

the aortic wall. It must be subsequently resuspended to the aortic wall or patch to prevent aortic valve dysfunction (Fig. 32.5C). ⊘

NB Cardioplegia

During the procedure, additional doses of cardioplegic solution are delivered directly into the coronary ostia with an olive-tipped cannula. NB

NB Difficult Anatomy

If inspection of the anomalous coronary anatomy suggests a technically difficult transfer or disruption of the intercoronary commissure by an unroofing procedure, the aorta should be closed and coronary bypass graft considered (the left or both internal thoracic arteries to the left system or the right internal thoracic artery to the right coronary). NB

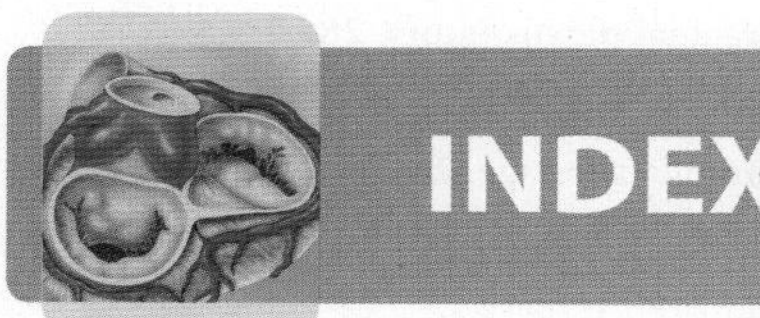

INDEX

Note: Page numbers in **bold** refer to pitfalls/errors and those followed by '*f*' indicate figures.

N

O

P

U

V

W

Y

Z